AF778024

Percutaneous Revascularization Techniques

Edited by

Manuel Maynar-Moliner, M.D.
Professor of Radiology
Director of Vascular Interventional Radiology
Hospital Nuestra Señora del Pino
Las Palmas
Islas Canarias, Spain

Wilfrido R. Castañeda-Zúñiga, M.D.
Professor of Radiology
Department of Radiology
The University of Minnesota Hospital
and Clinic
Minneapolis, MN

Francis Joffre, M.D.
Professor of Radiology
Service Central de Radiologie
Chu Rangueil
Toulouse Cedex, France

Christoph L. Zollikofer, M.D.
Chairman, Department of Radiology
Radiologisches Institut
Kantonsspital Winterthur
Winterthur, Switzerland

1993
Thieme Medical Publishers, Inc., New York
Georg Thieme Verlag, Stuttgart • New York

Thieme Medical Publishers, Inc.
381 Park Avenue South
New York, New York 10016

Percutaneous Revascularization Techniques
Manuel Maynar-Moliner, M.D.
Francis Joffre, M.D.
Christoph L. Zollikofer, M.D.
Wilfrido R. Castañeda-Zúñiga, M.D.

Library of Congress Cataloging-in-Publication Data

Percutaneous revascularization techniques / edited by Manuel Maynar
-Moliner . . . [et al.].
p. cm.
Includes bibliographical references and index.
ISBN 0-86577-441-2. — ISBN 3-13-783301-9
1. Arterial occlusions—Interventional radiology. 2. Peripheral
vascular diseases—Interventional radiology. I. Maynar-Moliner,
Manuel.
[DNLM: 1. Angioplasty, Transluminal. 2. Vascular Diseases—
surgery. 3. Vascular Surgery—methods. WG 170 P4285]
RD598.67.P47 1993
617.4′13059—dc20
DNLM/DLC
for Library of Congress 92-49670
CIP

Copyright © 1993 by Thieme Medical Publishers, Inc. This book, including all parts thereof, is legally protected by copyright. Any use, exploitation or commercialization outside the narrow limits set by copyright legislation, without the publisher's consent, is illegal and liable to prosecution. This applies in particular to photostat reproduction, copying, mimeographing or duplication of any kind, translating, preparation of microfilms, and electronic data processing and storage.

Important note: Medicine is an ever-changing science. Research and clinical experience are continually broadening our knowledge, in particular our knowledge of proper treatment and drug therapy. Insofar as this book mentions any dosage or application, readers may rest assured that the authors, editors, and publishers have made every effort to ensure that such references are strictly in accordance with the state of knowledge at the time of production of the book. Nevertheless, every user is requested to carefully examine the manufacturers' leaflets accompanying each drug to check on his own responsibility whether the dosage schedules recommended therein or the contraindications stated by the manufacturers differ from the statements made in the present book. Such examination is particularly important with drugs that are either rarely used or have been newly released on the market.

Some of the product names, patents, and registered designs referred to in this book are in fact registered trademarks or proprietary names even though specific reference to this fact is not always made in the text. Therefore, the appearance of a name without designation as proprietary is not to be construed as a representation by the publisher that it is in the public domain.

Printed in the United States of America.

5 4 3 2 1

TMP ISBN 0-86577-441-2
GTV ISBN 3-13-783301-9

CONTENTS

CONTRIBUTORS

George S. Abela, M.Sc., M.D.
Director of Interventional Research
Department of Cardiology
Co-Director, Institute for the Prevention of Cardiovascular Disease
New England Deaconess Hospital
Boston, MA

Kurt Amplatz, M.D.
Professor of Radiology
Department of Radiology
The University of Minnesota Hospital and Clinic
Minneapolis, MN

Francesco Antonucci, M.D.
Staff Radiologist
Radiologisches Institut
Kantonsspital Winterthur
Winterthur, Switzerland

Gerald R. Barbeau, M.D.
Division of Cardiology
Hopital Laval
Quebec, Canada

Klemens H. Barth, M.D.
Professor of Radiology
Director, Vascular/Interventional Radiology
Georgetown University Hospital
Washington, D.C.

Richard Baxter, M.D.
Cardiovascular/Interventional Radiology
Voluntary Clinical Faculty
Stanford University Medical Center
Stanford, CA

Wolfgang Beinborn, M.D.
Staff Radiologist
Department of Radiology
University Hospital Bonn
Bonn, Germany

Michael Berns, Ph.D.
Professor of Surgery
Beckman Laser Institute
University of California Irvine
Irvine, CA

Joseph J. Bookstein, M.D.
Professor of Radiology
Department of Radiology
University of California at San Diego Medical Center
San Diego, CA

Diane K. Burnside, A.A.S.
American Medical Systems
Pfizer Hospital Products Group
Minnetonka, MN

John E. Carlson, M.D., Ph.D.
Medical Fellow Specialist
Department of Radiology
The University of Minnesota Hospital and Clinic
Minneapolis, MN

C. Humberto Carrasco, M.D.
Professor of Radiology
Department of Radiology
The University of Texas M.D. Anderson Cancer Center
Houston, TX

Moises Casal, M.D.
Radiologia Vascular Intervencionista
Hospital Xeral de Vigo
Vigo, Spain

Flavio Castañeda, M.D.
Department of Angiography
St. Francis Medical Center
Peoria, IL

Wilfrido R. Castañeda-Zúñiga, M.D.
Professor of Radiology
Department of Radiology
The University of Minnesota Hospital and Clinic
Minneapolis, MN

Chusilp Charnsangavej, M.D.
Professor and Deputy Department Chair of Radiology
Department of Diagnostic Radiology
The University of Texas M.D. Anderson Cancer Center
Houston, TX

Rami Chemali, M.D.
Service Central de Radiologia
Hopital de Toulouse
Toulouse Cedex, France

Miguel Correia, M.D.
Professor
Faculdade de Ciências Mèdicas
Departamento de Anatomia
Campo de Santana 130
Lisboa Codex, Portugal

Andrew H. Cragg, M.D.
Department of Radiology
Riverside Medical Center
Minneapolis, MN

Mariano DeBlas, M.D.
Jefe del Servicio de Radiologia
Gipuzkaoko Ospitalea
Hospital de Guipúzcoa
Donostia San Sebastian, Spain

Luis Aires de Sousa, M.D.
Professor and Chairman
Universidade Nova de Lisboa
Lisboa, Portugal

Larry-Stuart Deutsch, M.D., C.M., F.R.C.P.
Associate Clinical Professor of Radiology and Cardiology
Department of Radiological Sciences
University of California Irvine Medical Center
Orange, CA

Riccardo Di Segni, M.D.
Aiuto Radiologo
Reparto Centrale di Radiologia e Diagnostica per Immagini
Ospedale S. Giovanni
Roma, Italy

Janette D. Durham, M.D.
Department of Radiology
University of Colorado Health Sciences Center
Denver, CO

Christopher E. Engeler, M.D.
Assistant Professor of Radiology
Department of Radiology
The University of Minnesota Hospital and Clinic
Minneapolis, MN

Deborah Fein-Miller, M.D.
Staff Radiologist
Department of Radiologic Science and Diagnostic Imaging
Shadyside Hospital
Pittsburgh, PA

José Manuel Felices, M.D.
Radiologia Vascular Intervencionista
Hospital Provincial de Murcia
Murcia, Spain

Charitha C. Fernando, B.H.B., MB.ChB, D.R.A.C.R.
Consultant Radiologist
Radiology Department
Wairau Hospital
Blenheim, New Zealand

Nikolaus L. Freudenberg, M.D.
Professor of Pathology
Pathologisches Institut der Universität
Freiburg/Br, Germany

Vladimir G. Germashev, M.D.
Research Collaborator
National Research Center for Surgery
USSR Academy of Medical Science
Moscow, Russia

Phillippe P. Giacomino, M.D.
Research Fellow from the Division of Radiology
University of Toulouse
France

Robert S. Ginsberg, M.D.
Director, Unit for Cardiovascular Intervention
University Hospital
Denver, CO

Elias Gorriz, M.D.
Radiologia Vascular Intervencionista
Hospital Nuestra Senora dēl Pino
Islas Canarias, Spain

Edward J. Grogan, C.C.E.
Director, Biomedical Engineering and Safety
The Alexandria Hospital
Alexandria, VA

Warren Grundfest, M.D.
Assistant Director of Surgery
Director of Laser Surgery and Surgical Research
Cedars-Sinai Medical Center
Los Angeles, CA

Walter Henry, M.D.
Vice Chancellor—Dean CCM
College of Medicine
University of California Irvine
Irvine, CA

Robert W. Holden, M.D.
Professor and Chairman
Department of Radiology
Indiana University Hospital
Indianapolis, IN

David Hunter, M.D.
Professor of Radiology
Department of Radiology
The University of Minnesota Hospital and Clinic
Minneapolis, MN

Noni Jenkins, R.N.
Nurse Coordinator, Interventional Cardiology
Division of Cardiovascular Medicine
Stanford University Medical Center
Stanford, CA

Francis Joffre, M.D.
Professor of Radiology
Service Central de Radiologie
Chu Rangueil
Toulouse Cedex, France

Martin Kaltenbach, M.D.
Professor
Klinikum-Zentrum
Abteilung Cardiologie
Frankfurt, Germany

Kenneth R. Kensey, M.D.
Kensey Nash Corporation
Marsh Creek Corporation Center
Exton, PA

Günther Erich Klein, M.D.
Assistant Professor of Radiology
University Hospital Graz
Department of Radiology
Graz, Austria

Jürgen Kollath, M.D.
Professor of Radiology
Center of Radiology
University Hospital Frankfurt
Frankfurt/Main, Germany

David A. Kumpe, M.D.
Professor of Radiology
Department of Radiology
University Hospital
Denver, CO

Catherine A. Kusnick, M.D.
Staff Physician
Department of Radiology
San Ramon Regional Medical Center;
Assistant Clinical Faculty Staff
Stanford University Medical Center
Stanford, CA

Johannes Lammer, M.D.
Professor of Radiology
Department of Radiology
Angiography and Interventional Radiology
Hospital AKH-University Hospital of Vienna
Angiography and Interventional Radiology
Vienna, Austria

Helmut Landgraf, M.D.
Professor
Center of Internal Medicine
Department of Angiology
University Hospital Frankfurt
Frankfurt/Main, Germany

David Lawrence, M.D.
Associate Professor
Department of Radiology
University of Texas M.D. Anderson Cancer Center
Houston, TX

Robert G. Levitt, M.D.
Staff Radiologist
Barnes County West Hospital
Creve Coeur, MO

Dieter Liermann, M.D.
Staff Radiologist
Z. Rad. am Klinikum der J.W. Goethe-Universitat
Frankfurt am Main, Germany

Frank Litvak, M.D.
Assistant Professor of Medicine
Co-Director, Cardiac Catheterization Laboratory
Ceders-Sinai Medical Center
Los Angeles, CA

Dierk Maass, M.D.
Professor of Medicine
Zürich, Switzerland

John T. Mail, M.D.
Assistant Professor of Radiology
Department of Radiology
Indiana University Hospital
Indianapolis, IN

Alan H. Matsumoto, M.D.
Department of Radiology
University of Virginia Health Sciences Center
Charlottesville, VA

Manuel Maynar-Moliner, M.D.
Professor of Radiology
Director of Vascular Interventional Radiology
Hospital Nuestra Señora del Pino
Las Palmas, Islas Canarias, Spain

Michael McRae, M.D.
Pathologist
Long Beach V.A. Medical Center
Long Beach, CA

John T. Mehigan, M.D.
Clinical Associate Professor
Stanford University Medical Center
Stanford, CA

Donald L. Miller, M.D.
Director, Vascular/Interventional Radiology
Diagnostic Radiology Department
National Institutes of Health
Bethesda, MD

Cres P. Miranda, M.D.
Clinical Instructor
University of California Irvine Medical Center
Orange, CA

Harold A. Mitty, M.D.
Professor of Radiology
The Mount Sinai School of Medicine of the City University of New York
New York, NY

Masahito Moriuchi, M.D.
Assistant Professor of Medicine
Division of Cardiology
Second Department of Internal Medicine
Nihon University, School of Medicine
Tokyo, Japan

Amir Motarjeme, M.D.
Illinois Institute of Vascular Diseases
Downers Grove, IL

Leonard A. Nordstrom, M.D.
Department of Cardiology
Park Nicollet Medical Center
St. Louis Park, MN

Christa Paasch, R.N.
Medical Nurse
Center of Radiology
University Hospital Frankfurt
Frankfurt/Main, Germany

Julio C. Palmaz, M.D.
Professor of Radiology
Department of Radiology
University of Texas Health Science Center
San Antonio, TX

Ernst Pilger, M.D.
Professor of Medicine
Department of Medicine, Division of Angiology
University Hospital of Graz
Graz, Austria

José A. Esperança Pina, M.D.
Professor and Chairman
Faculdade de Ciências Mèdicas
Departamento de Anatomia
Campo de Santana 130
Lisboa Codex, Portugal

João Martins Pisco, M.D.
Chairman and Professor
Hospital de Santa Marta
Lisboa, Portugal

Eugenio Ponomar-Sulepov, M.D., Ph.D.
Servico de Radiodiagnostico
Hospital "Carmen y Severo Ochoa"
Asturias, Spain

Ingeborg Prignitz, M.D.
Staff Radiologist
Department of Radiology
Aggertalklinik Engelskirchen
Engelskirchen, Germany

Juan M. Pulido-Duque, M.D.
Radiologia Vascular Intervencionista
Hosptital Nuestra Señora del Pino
Las Palmas, Islas Canarias, Spain

Joseff K. H. Rabkin, M.D.
Professor
Chief Roentgenologist of the USSR Ministry of Health
Head of Roentgeno-Radiology Department
National Research Center of Surgery
USSR Academy of Medical Science
Moscow, Russia

Thomas M. Rassmussen
Clinical Program Manager for Bradycardia Projects
Intermedics, Inc.
Angleton, TX

Falah H. Redha, D.V.M.
Research Section
Department of Surgery
University Hospital of Zurich
Zürich, Switzerland

Ricardo Reyes, M.D.
Radiologia Vascular Intervencionista
Hospital Nuestra Señora del Pino
Las Palmas, Islas Canarias, Spain

William R. Richli, M.D.
Associate Professor of Radiology
Department of Diagnostic Radiology
The University of Texas M.D. Anderson Cancer Center
Houston, TX

Franz-Josef Roth, M.D.
Professor
Department of Radiology
Aggertalklinik Engelskirchen
Engelskirchen, Germany

Hervé Rousseau, M.D.
Professor of Radiology
Service Central de Radiologie
Chu Rangueil
Toulouse Cedex, France

Erich Salomonowitz, M.D.
Professor of Radiology
St. Poelten Hospital
St. Poelten, Austria

Timothy A. Sanborn, M.D.
Director, Cardiac Catheterization Laboratory
Professor of Medicine
New York Hospital-Cornell Medical Center
New York, NY

Michael Savin, M.D.
Radiology Resident
Department of Radiology
University of Washington Hospital
Seattle, WA

Beate Schneider, M.D.
Department of Radiology
Diakonissen-Krankenhaus Karlsruhe-Rüppurr
Akademisches Röntgendiagnostik und Nuklearmedizin
Karlsruhe, Germany

Werner Schoop, M.D.
Professor
Department of Radiology
Aggertalklinik Engelskirchen
Engelskirchen, Germany

Donald E. Schwarten, M.D.
Director of Cardiovascular Laboratory
St. Vincent's Hospital and Health Science Center
Indianapolis, IN

James S. Seeger, M.D.
Chief of Vascular Surgery
Department of Surgery
University of Florida
Gainesville, FL

Jacob Segalowitz, M.D.
Department of Surgery
Cedars-Sinai Hospital
Los Angeles, CA

Tony P. Smith, M.D.
Department of Radiology
Neurovascular Medical Group, Inc.
University of California Medical Center
San Francisco, CA

Reingard Sörensen, M.D.
Priv.-Doz. Doctor of Medicine
Entwicklunge und Forschungszentrum für Mikrotherapie (EFMT), Bochum
Freie Universität Berlin
Klinikum Steglitz
Abt. Röntgendiagnostik
Berlin, Germany

Erhard Starck, M.D.
Rotes Kreuz Krankenhaus Frankfurt
Frankfurt, Germany

D. Eugene Strandness, Jr., M.D.
Professor of Surgery
University of Washington
Seattle, WA

Ernst-Peter Strecker, M.D.
Professor and Chairman
Department of Radiology
Diakonissen-Krankenhaus Karlsruhe-Rüppurr
Akademisches Lehrkrankenhaus der Universität Freiburg
Abt. Röntgendiagnostik und Nuklearmedizin
Karlsruhe, Germany

G. Stuckmann, M.D.
Department of Radiology
Kantonsspital Winterthur
Winterthur, Switzerland

S. Murthy Tadavarthy, M.D.
Associate Clinical Professor
Co-Director, Cardiovascular and Interventional Radiology
Department of Radiology
Abbott-Northwestern Hospital
Minneapolis, MN

George P. Teitelbaum, M.D.
Assistant Professor of Radiology
Division of Interventional Neuroradiology
Department of Radiology
UCSF Medical Center
San Francisco, CA

Patricia E. Thorpe, M.D.
Assistant Professor of Radiology
Chief, Vascular and Interventional Radiology
Department of Radiology
Creighton University Medical Center
Omaha, NE

Jonathan M. Tobis, M.D.
Professor of Medicine and Radiology
Acting Chief, Division of Cardiology
University of California Irvine Medical Center
Orange, CA

Panagiotis Tsikuras, M.D.
Department of Gynecology and Obstetrics
University Clinics Göttingen
Göttingen, Germany

Karim Valji, M.D.
Assistant Professor of Radiology
Department of Radiology
University of California Medical Center
San Diego, CA

Christian Vallbracht, P.D., M.D.
University Lecturer (Associate Professor)
Center of Internal Medicine
Department of Cardiology
University Hospital Frankfurt
Frankfurt/Main, Germany

Martin J.C. van Gemert, Ph.D.
Professor and Head, Laser Center
Academic Medical Center
Amsterdam, The Netherlands

Renu Virmani, M.D.
Chairman
Armed Forces Institute of Pathology
Washington, D.C.

Thomas Vollrath, M.D.
Director of Medicine
Institut für Röntgendiagnostik
Stadtspital Waid
Zürich, Switzerland

Sidney Wallace, M.D.
Professor and Chair of Radiology
Department of Diagnostic Radiology
The University of Texas M.D. Anderson Cancer Center
Houston, TX

Hans Joachim Wagner, M.D., O.A.
Staff Radiologist
Städtische Kliniken Kassel
Institut für Röntgendiagnostik
Kassel, Germany

Ashley J. Welch, Ph.D.
Marion E. Forsman Centennial Professor of Electrical and Computer Engineering
The University of Texas at Austin
Department of Electrical and Computer Engineering
Austin, TX

Soraya Wenig, M.D.
Staff Radiologist
Krankenhaus Zehlendorf
Röntgen Diagnostik
Bereich Heckeshorn
Berlin, Germany

Michael Westphal, M.D.
Chief, Department of Radiology
Krankenhaus Neukolln
Berlin, Germany

Lewis Wexler, M.D.
Professor of Radiology and Medicine (Cardiology)
Department of Radiology
Stanford University Hospital
Stanford, CA

Mark H. Wholey, M.D.
Professor of Radiology
The Pittsburgh Vascular Institute
Department of Radiological Sciences and Diagnostic Imaging
Shadyside Hospital
Pittsburgh, PA

Hellmut R.D. Wolf, M.D.
Staff Radiologist
Department of Internal Medicine
Akademisches Lehrkrankenhaus der Universität Freiburg
Abt. Röntgendiagnostik und Nuklearmedizin
Freiburg, Germany

Alan Wright, M.D.
Director, Interventional Radiology
Good Samaritan Hospital;
Voluntary Clinical Faculty
Stanford University Medical Center
Stanford, CA

Kenneth C. Wright, M.D.
Department of Diagnostic Radiology
University of Texas M.D. Anderson Cancer Center
Houston, TX

Joseph W. Yedlicka, Jr., M.D.
Assistant Professor
Northwestern University
Evanston, Illinois

Christoph L. Zollikofer, M.D.
Chairman, Department of Radiology
Radiologisches Institut
Kantonsspital Winterthur
Winterthur, Switzerland

PREFACE

In the 1980s the field of vascular and interventional radiology has seen the development and growth of multiple new diagnostic and interventional procedures. Their impact on the longterm outcome in patients with severe occlusive vascular disease is still unknown.

Unfortunately, this explosion in technology has not been adequately controlled with scientific rigor. Therefore, comparison of the results reported in the multiple series found in the literature with the results of the more traditional percutaneous transluminal balloon dilatation of vascular occlusive disease is impossible at this time. This is unfortunate because overutilization of techniques has been seen without clearly defined improvement in the final outcome of the procedures, and clearly, with an increase in the health cost expenditures.

We hope that randomized prospective clinical trials that compare all of these technologies with the longterm results of transluminal balloon dilatation will be undertaken in the future, in order to learn the real place of each of these technologies in the management of patients with vascular occlusive disease.

In this book, we have included world authorities on the different developments in vascular interventional radiology, and attempted to organize them in a comprehensive fashion in order to facilitate the reader's familiarization with new developments.

We hope we have included most of the new developments, but are sure some of them have been left out. Furthermore, by the time of publication, some of the information provided might already be outdated. However, we hope that the information presented will be of help to the reader in understanding the advances in the field of vascular and interventional radiology.

Manuel Maynar-Moliner, M.D.
Francis Joffre, M.D.
Christoph Zollikofer, M.D.
Wilfrido R. Castañeda-Zúñiga, M.D., M.Sc.

ACKNOWLEDGMENTS

We thank all of those who preceded us in the field of vascular interventional radiology, starting with Sven Seldinger, who pioneered the technique of percutaneous vascular access; also, Charles Dotter, who looked into the future and described most of the current techniques used in interventional radiology; Kurt Amplatz, whose genius and inventions have advanced the field of interventional radiology in giant steps; Josef Rösch, whose dream of a new specialty of interventional therapy might one day become a reality; Eberhard Zeitler, who kept the dream of transluminal angioplasty alive for so many years before one of his disciples, Andreas Grüntzig, developed the balloon technology that made angioplasty a reality in the early 1970s.

I am afraid the list is never-ending, as it crosses specialties and goes outside of the medical profession into the engineering and industrial laboratories where the new devices are developed. To all of these people, our thanks for their efforts in building up interventional radiology.

The field of vascular interventional radiology has seen an explosion of technology in the 1980s and early 1990s so the need for a large number of contributors can be explained easily. We are indebted to our contributors for their outstanding participation in this textbook that we hope will become a classic in the field of vascular interventional radiology.

We thank all of our coworkers and support staff. Without their help, our efforts to put this work together would have been very difficult. We would especially like to acknowledge the patience and dedication of Ms. Carla J. Nelson, who typed numerous revisions of the chapters of this book.

Finally, we would like to thank the editors and staff of Thieme Medical Publishers for their help in providing uniform editing of manuscripts from individuals from so many parts of the world.

On a more personal level, we give our love and thanks to our families, whose help and encouragement over the years kept us going forward during the many times our bodies wanted to give up, even though our souls wanted to keep looking forward.

Manuel Maynar-Moliner, M.D.
Francis Joffre, M.D.
Christoph Zollikofer, M.D.
Wilfrido R. Castañeda-Zúñiga, M.D., M.Sc.

1 A Surgeon's Appraisal of the Future of Percutaneous Revascularization Techniques

D.E. Strandness, Jr., M.D.

The introduction of percutaneous transluminal angioplasty by Dotter and Judkins in 1964[1] heralded a new era in the treatment of vascular diseases. The method was met by a great deal of skepticism and even scorn by some surgeons. However, experience has shown it to be an acceptable method of treatment, particularly for stenoses in the aortoiliac area where the long-term results appear to be nearly equal to those obtained by surgical means. The method became more widely applied following the introduction of the balloon catheter by Grüntzig and Hopff in 1974.[2]

The procedure appears to work by the production of a longitudinal tear in the artery wall adjacent to the plaque that narrows the vessel. The plaque is not removed but the artery is enlarged due to this disruption of the wall that extends into the adventitia. This type of injury to the wall would appear to be destined to lead to failure due to thrombosis. Surprisingly for large arteries such as the iliac, the results appear to defy logic, since the long-term outcome can be very good.[3] For medium-sized arteries (femoral, popliteal, tibial), the results with angioplasty are not as durable, although the immediate results can be quite satisfactory.

Although there was continued interest in expanding the role of balloon angioplasty, the field became relatively stable with the indications for the procedure quite well defined. However, the scene began to change as new methods designed to treat the atherosclerotic plaque began to appear. The major impetus for the new look was the development of laser technology[4] and atherectomy catheters.[5] These new methods held promise because of their potential for crossing total occlusions and perhaps even for removing the lesion itself. The intended target site was the coronary artery, where the restenosis rate with balloon angioplasty remains in the 20 to 30% range. If the newer methods could result in a lower restenosis rate, this would represent a major advance for the field. Not surprisingly, the coronary arteries could not be used as the initial testing ground for both lasers and the mechanical atherectomy devices. The potential risks were too great. Since the atherosclerosis involving the superficial femoral artery was identical to that found in the coronary arteries, why not start there? A complication at this site would not generally be life threatening and could be dealt with immediately by the vascular surgeon. Thus, it was primarily the cardiologists who began to utilize some of these new methods in the arteries of the lower limb. The introduction of these new percutaneous methods has changed the direction of the field and the indications for treatment.

Traditionally, any intervention, be it surgery or angioplasty, has been limited primarily to patients with lifestyle-limiting claudication and those with threatened limb loss due to far advanced ischemia. Although some might disagree, both surgeons and radiologists consider the patients with iliac artery stenosis and with short stenoses (<7 cm) of the superficial femoral and popliteal arteries (<3 cm) to be candidates for balloon angioplasty. Although patients with total arterial occlusions can also be dilated if a guide wire will traverse the lesion, the complication rate is higher and the long-term results are not as good as those seen with stenotic lesions alone.

With the new methods, the superficial femoral artery was the initial target. It was discovered that the hot-tipped laser could create a channel through some total arterial occlusions and could be followed by balloon angioplasty. Early reports were encouraging, but the studies were not well controlled and the follow-up period was short. The early successes were enthusiastically accepted, leading to a nationwide proliferation of "Laser Centers" and advertisements by both physicians and hospitals to attract patients.

Unfortunately, this was done without a review or consideration of past experience in the field. Why was past experience important? In the early days of vascular surgery, endarterectomy of the superficial femoral artery was a common procedure. It completely removed the plaque down to the outer portion of the media, leaving a glistening surface of smooth muscle exposed to flowing blood. This was the type of endpoint that the advocates of the newer percutaneous methods are hoping to achieve. The immediate results with endarterectomy were usually excellent but often followed by reocclusion and failure. At the time, the failures were thought to be due to either thrombosis or recurrence of the atherosclerosis. However, as we now know, this was not the entire answer.[6]

ATHEROSCLEROSIS

Before dealing with the present and future of percutaneous methods, it is important to review our knowledge about the disease we are intending to treat. Atherosclerosis produces problems by the development of high-grade stenoses (>50% diameter reduction) that can progress to total occlusion. In order to improve the patient, it is necessary to increase pressure and flow to the limb by either removing or bypassing the areas of disease. The surgeon most often bypasses areas of disease because it is the most efficient way of restoring flow and preserving existing collaterals. For percutaneous methods, if a guide wire can cross the areas of disease, it should be possible to treat the narrowed segment by either dilation or removal of the lesion. The bypass approach is the most versatile, since it can successfully treat even multiple levels of occlusion. The percutaneous approaches have generally been limited to treating only a single segment.

Those patients with one arterial segment narrowed or occluded present with intermittent claudication. Limb viability is not a concern. The most commonly involved areas are the aortoiliac segment and the femoropopliteal region. The most common surgery for such problems is bypass grafting or endarterectomy for the aortoiliac area and bypass grafting for lesions distal to the inguinal ligament. The long-term results are particularly good for the aortoiliac region, where 90% patency rates at 5 years are common. For femoropopliteal disease, long-term patency rates of 70 to 80% can be achieved, particularly if saphenous vein grafts are used. The results are not as good when prosthetic grafts are employed. With balloon angioplasty, a successful dilation of an iliac artery stenosis is as good as a surgical procedure. In the femoropopliteal area, most dilations were performed for short stenotic segments (<7cm). The longer lesions and the total occlusions were generally left to the surgeon.

The problems associated with either operation or the percutaneous methods become more difficult when multiple levels of the arterial system are occluded. From a practical standpoint, multisegment disease commonly occurs with the following combinations: (1) aortoiliac and superficial femoral involvement; and (2) femoropopliteal and tibioperoneal occlusions. From a theoretical standpoint, when the most proximal arterial segment is removed or bypassed in patients with multiple segmental lesions, the key factor to success will be the exit collaterals. For example, correction of an iliac artery lesion in the presence of a superficial femoral artery occlusion will increase flow to the profunda femoris artery, the most important exit collateral in the leg. This can increase flow to the extent that intermittent claudication is improved and rest pain is relieved. For superficial femoral and tibioperoneal disease and with correction of the proximal disease alone, the outcome is less certain because the exit collaterals are more variable and uncertain in terms of their capacity to carry the new volume of blood.

To evaluate the potential of the newer transcutaneous methods, their roles must be discussed with regard to the patterns of disease commonly seen.

SINGLE-SEGMENT DISEASE

For the iliac arteries with stenotic lesions, it is unlikely that the newer methods will offer any advantages over the use of balloon angioplasty. Since the immediate and long-term good results (up to 5 years) of both surgery and angioplasty approach 90%, it would take a very large series of cases to prove the superiority of any new method for this region. For total occlusions, the new methods may be superior if they are not associated with a high rate of peripheral embolization and better long-term results. This is an area that will need exploration and comparison with current approaches.

For femoropopliteal stenosis or occlusion, the long-term results of angioplasty by any method for long areas of stenosis and occlusions have not begun to approach those achieved with direct arterial surgery.[7] Why? The reason is clear—restenosis frequently occurs, which is responsible for failure of the method and recurrence of the symptoms. If the new percutaneous methods are to be better than balloon angioplasty, they will have to result in a lower incidence of restenosis. Isolated stenoses or occlusions of the tibial and peroneal arteries are an uncommon cause of ischemia unless found in conjunction with proximal disease.

MULTISEGMENT DISEASE

Therapy with multiple levels of occlusion requires more thought, since it may not be feasible to correct all areas of involvement. When considering therapy for such lesions, it is common practice to focus attention on the status of the "runoff" arteries. What are these vessels and why are they important? Simply defined, they are all arteries distal to the intended site of intervention. The success of any procedure often depends on these arteries. A few examples will be given to illustrate what this means:

1. *Aortoiliac and femoropopliteal disease*. For iliac artery reconstruction, the profunda femoris and its reconstitution with the tibioperoneal arteries constitutes the runoff. If successful, the patient is left with the superficial femoral occlusion that is commonly associated with moderately severe intermittent claudication.

2. *Femoropopliteal and tibioperoneal involvement*. These patients commonly appear with limb-threatening ischemia. Treatment of the proximal lesion will apply a new pressure head to the below-knee arteries, which are further classified as one, two, and three vessel runoff. If all three of the below-knee arteries are occluded, the popliteal artery—if open—is commonly referred to as a blind segment. Long-term results are best if there are one or more patent arteries to the level of the foot.

3. *Tibioperoneal disease*. In this setting, the plantar arch and its continuity appear to play a role in determining long-term results. It is unlikely that any percutaneous method will be able to open completely all arteries that are involved. Disease confined to these arteries alone is not common and when seen is almost exclusively found in type II diabetics. These lesions can be treated by distal bypass grafts if there are patent arteries at the level of the ankle and foot. If percutaneous methods are to work here, they will have to be successful in removing long segments involved with disease. Although this may be feasible, it appears that the rate of restenosis will be prohibitively high.

METHODS

An important question relates to the type of percutaneous procedure used and whether this makes any difference in the immediate and long-term results. The hot-tipped laser simply provides the avenue for passage of the dilating balloon. Thus, its only advantage is that it may be able to cross more totally occluded segments than is possible with currently available guide wires.

What of selective ablation of the plaque without damage to the underlying media and adventitia? Some of the newer pulsed ultraviolet or selective wavelength lasers are attempting to move in this direction. It is hoped that the end result would be similar to total removal of the lesion, as is accomplished with endarterectomy. In theory, the restenosis rate should be the same with both approaches. This will remain the limiting factor for its application to the longer stenoses and total occlusions, which are the major problem for all of the percutaneous methods.

The mechanical devices work by removing the plaque down to the level of the underlying media. These appear to work best for stenotic lesions that are not heavily calcified—the very lesion that is best suited for balloon angioplasty. Their only advantage would be a lower rate of restenosis, which remains to be shown. It is clear that these methods may have problems with the long occlusions where passage of the device may be difficult.

There have been preliminary efforts to assist in the use of the newer methods by the incorporation of angioscopy and intraluminal ultrasound.[8] These will be of value only if they can assist in the complete removal of the lesion with the hoped-for reduction in the development of restenosis within the treated segment.

PREDICTORS OF OUTCOME

Given all of the considerations previously mentioned, the major limiting factor in the success of all of the percutaneous methods will be the problem of restenosis that commonly occurs. It is now known that the lesion responsible for the restenosis is myointimal hyperplasia.

It is clear that the outcome of any therapy will depend on many variables. Johnston[9] used the Cox proportional hazard model to evaluate 39 variables that might affect and in turn be predictive of outcome with transluminal angioplasty. There were only four that proved to be significant ($p < 0.01$) predictors of long-term success:

1. Indication. Those with claudication had a better long-term outcome than those with limb-threatening ischemia.
2. The site of intervention. The common iliac was better than any other site.
3. Severity of lesions. Stenoses fared better than occlusions.
4. Runoff. The better the runoff, the better the outcome.

These can serve as guidelines that will apply not only to current percutaneous methods, but to the newer ones as well.

MYOINTIMAL HYPERPLASIA

Those areas of the arterial circulation most frequently treated by any interventional method include the coronary arteries, the carotid bulb, and the peripheral arteries. Immediate success in restoring flow regardless of the approach used will exceed 90%. However, with the passage of time (up to 2 years), failure in up to 30% may occur, not because of recurrent atherosclerosis but because of myointimal hyperplasia. These white, smooth, firm lesions are similar to those that occur with the balloon injury model in animals. Although the cause is undetermined, it appears to be the arterial wall response to injury.[10] It is observed with all forms of intervention, be it in bypass grafts, at endarterectomy sites, or where balloon angioplasty has been performed. Efforts to control its occurrence by the use of antiplatelet agents have been unsuccessful.[6]

Will the new methods, such as laser technology and the atherectomy devices, be any better? If they require the use of a balloon to complete the treatment, the failure rate particularly for the small and medium-sized arteries will remain high. If the plaque is entirely removed, the restenosis rate will likely be the same as that which follows endarterectomy. The only hope for a lower restenosis rate will be the control of the proliferative response by pharmacologic means or perhaps by rapid resurfacing with normal endothelium.

From a clinical standpoint, the prevalence of the myointimal hyperplasia and its rate of development for nearly all segments of the arterial circulation is well known. The process can develop within weeks and is usually complete by the end of 2 years. The clinical importance of the restenosis depends on the site where it occurs. A recurrent stenosis in the carotid bulb may not be serious, since the recurrent lesion is smooth and is rarely the site from which emboli can arise. On the other hand, in the coronary and peripheral arteries, a high-grade recurrent stenosis will again limit flow and lead to the development of the symptoms for which the treatment was given.

There is no question that research into the use of the newer percutaneous methods should proceed. Given all of the problems and unanswered questions, the use of the newer methods should be confined to centers where meaningful basic and clinical research can be carried out. It is no longer acceptable to continue to exploit these methods for economic gain when the promise of success for many of the applications remains so uncertain.

REFERENCES

1. Dotter CT, Judkins MP. Transluminal treatment of arteriosclerotic obstruction: description of a new technic and a preliminary report of its application. Circulation 1964;30:654–70.
2. Grüntzig A, Hopff H. Perkutane rekanalisation Chronischer arterieller verschlusse mit einem neuen dilationskather: Modification der Dotter-technik. Dtsch Med Wochenschr 1974; 99:2502–5.

3. Johnston KW, Rae M, Hogg-Johnston SA, et al. Five-year results of a prospective study of percutaneous transluminal angioplasty. Ann Surg 1987;206:403–13.
4. White RA, White GH: Laser angioplasty: is it a useful tool or a hoax? In Veith FJ (ed): Current Critical Problems in Vascular Surgery, St. Louis: Quality Medical Publishing, Inc., 1989, chap. 32.
5. Whittemore AD. Endovascular atherectomy devices. In Veith FJ (ed): Current Critical Problems in Vascular Surgery. St. Louis: Quality Medical Publishing, 1989, chap. 38.
6. Strandness DE Jr. Angioplasty devices will not prevent restenosis. Cardio 1988;5:116–9.
7. Rutherford RB, Patt A, Kumpe DA: The current role of percutaneous transluminal angioplasty. In Greenhaugh RM, Jamieson CW, Nicolaides AN (eds): Vascular Surgery: Issues in Current Practice. New York: Grune & Stratton, 1986.
8. Bernhard VM. Current status of vascular endoscopy. In Veith FW (ed): Current Critical Problems in Vascular Surgery. St. Louis: Quality Medical Publishing, 1989, chap. 36.
9. Johnston KW. Indications and late results of percutaneous transluminal angioplasty: a surgeon's evaluation. In Veith FJ (ed): Current Critical Problems in Vascular Surgery, St. Louis: Quality Medical Publishing, 1989, chap. 30.
10. Clowes AW. Pathobiology of arterial healing. In Strandness DE Jr, Didisheim P, Clowes AW, Watson JT (eds): Vascular Diseases: Current Research and Clinical Applications. New York: Grune & Stratton, 1987:351–63.

2 Noninvasive Evaluation of Peripheral Vascular Disease

Riccardo Di Segni, M.D.

The evaluation of peripheral vascular disease (PVD) is a complex problem that comprises different diagnostic methods. The role of noninvasive vascular techniques in the diagnosis of PVD is to confirm the diagnosis, define the extent of disease, and help decide among the different therapeutic modalities. The results of treatment, either medical, surgical, or percutaneous revascularization, need to be evaluated. Follow-up examinations should be ideally simple, noninvasive, objective, and easily repeatable. In the last few years, important technical developments have occurred in the diagnostic methods, both invasive and noninvasive. These new methods are contributing to define the exact role of the different revascularization techniques in respect to the individual clinical problem, thus avoiding the use of procedures of limited usefulness, and at the same time are helping to limit the use of the invasive procedures only when necessary. The information provided by noninvasive studies further improves the quality of the examinations by focusing the study on specific arterial segments. The technologic improvements have also influenced the way medicine is practiced. For example, the association of ultrasound real-time imaging of vessels with the Doppler examination in the same unit has transformed an examination previously considered as a physiologic evaluation performed by clinicians into an imaging/physiologic study more closely related to the diagnostic imaging area.

In noninvasive studies of PVD, the assessment of the blood vessels can be done by evaluating the arterial wall anatomy, pressures, limb volume changes during circulatory cycle, tissue oxygenation, and flow dynamics. There are now several techniques available that selectively focus on one or more of these aspects.

The purpose of this chapter is to provide basic information on these techniques, with particular attention to their indications and drawbacks.

NONINVASIVE RADIOLOGIC STUDIES

Radiologic studies without intra-arterial or intravenous injection of contrast medium may be included in the initial assessment of peripheral vascular disease. Those studies (namely, plain films of the abdomen and lower limbs) may be considered relatively "noninvasive" even if they are based on ionizing radiations, as long as they do not include invasive maneuvers. The most important information these studies offer is to show the presence, severity, and extension of vascular calcification from the abdominal aorta to the vessels of the feet. In order to detect calcification, special projections are required to avoid overlapping of bones. Plain films may also give information on other possible diseases involving mainly bones and joints, which may coexist, worsen, and sometimes mimic the painful symptomatology of arterial diseases. This is particularly the case of radicular compression, which may require further radiologic studies, such as computed tomography and myelography. In advanced arterial occlusions with gangrenous complications, plain films are necessary to show involvement and extension of the disease to soft tissues and bones.[1]

MAGNETIC RESONANCE IMAGING

Magnetic resonance imaging (MRI), which employs magnetic fields and computer manipulations, has an important and, by this time, definite role in vascular evaluation, particularly of large vessels such as the aorta and its major branches. A possible role of magnetic resonance to the anatomic study of the small vessels of the lower limbs offers a promising perspective, but is still far from clinical practice.[2,3] Magnetic resonance is mainly an anatomic imaging system, but there are also important applications to the study of blood flow. Salles-Cunha et al[4] showed that blood flow studies with MRI before and after percutaneous revascularization techniques provide hemodynamic data of diagnostic and prognostic significance. For example, in patients with ankle-arm indexes before percutaneous transluminal angioplasty of less than 0.80, either the direct measurement of pressures or MRI flow measurements can corroborate the results of the revascularization procedure, whereas if the ankle-arm index is greater than 0.80, MRI flow measurements are most likely to substantiate changes in peripheral hemodynamics.

SYSTOLIC PRESSURE MEASUREMENT

Systolic pressure measurement is a simple and quite reliable method of preliminary assessment. In this method, the arterial systolic pressures are measured at various levels of the limbs and then compared with the brachial systolic pressure, which is used as reference, being approximately equal to the aortic root pressure.

Pressure measurements in the lower limbs are obtained with the same principles and systems as the brachial artery measurements, with pneumatic cuffs. For each leg, two cuffs are placed below the knee and one or two above the knee. The four-cuff method is preferable. Automatic computerized systems are available, which make the procedure faster and safer. The cuffs are inflated at a systolic pressure higher than the patient baseline, then slowly deflated to detect the pulse. This may be done with a strain gauge or more commonly with a Doppler probe. When the Doppler acoustic or graphic signal appears, the systolic pressure is recorded. A Doppler probe is preferred to the common stethoscope, since it is more sensitive and accurate (Fig. 2-1). In the brachial artery, measurements are taken in both arms and, if there is a difference, the higher level is taken as reference. For the ankle, the posterior tibial and the dorsalis pedis pulses are recorded. The higher of the two readings is considered as reference for the ankle.

In normal persons the high thigh pressure is slightly (20 to 30 mmHg) higher than the brachial pressure due to a technical artifact of the cuff; above the knee, the pressure should be less than at the thigh, but still more elevated than the brachial pressure. From that level down to the ankle, there is a slow decrease, but the normal pressure at the ankle is still normally higher (10 to 20 mmHg) than the brachial pressure.

The basic principle underlying this method is that caliber reductions in the vessels, caused by stenosis or obstructions, decrease the amount of flowing blood and cause a pressure drop below the obstruction.[5–7]

The measured values are evaluated in both their absolute and reciprocal relationships. The first value to be considered is that of the ankle. Values less than brachial pressures are indicative of obstructive disease; if, on the contrary, ankle pressure is elevated more than 40 mmHg over the brachial pressure, it is a sign of loss of elasticity of the lower limb

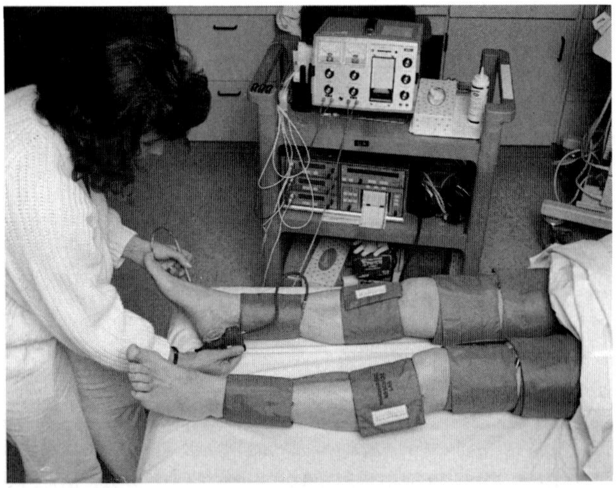

Figure 2–1. Segmental pressure measurement. In each leg four pressure cuffs are placed, two above the knee and two below. A Doppler probe is positioned over the posterior tibial artery or the dorsalis pedis (where the pressure is higher). Each cuff is inflated separately, and the value at which the pulse is heard during deflation is taken as the pressure value reference of that segment.

arteries.[5] The relationship of the ankle pressure to the brachial pressure is commonly expressed in the form of an index, the ankle-brachial index, which gives a simple and standardized measure that can be repeated over time (Fig. 2-2).

The normal values of the ankle-brachial index are equal to or slightly greater than 1; below the unity, there are two main groups: an index equal to or inferior to 0.5 is indicative of severe occlusive disease and an index from 0.6 to 0.9 is correlated with a clinical situation of claudication.[5]

The ankle-brachial index gives an important score on the status of occlusive disease. Since it is noninvasive and easily repeatable, it is very frequently used in the long-term follow-up of peripheral vascular disease after therapeutic interventions to assess efficacy and to detect early recurrences.[8,9] Ankle pressure by itself is also used as a predictive value for the healing of distal lesions. It is considered positive when it is above 55 mmHg and 80 mmHg in nondiabetic and diabetic patients, respectively.[8,9]

Ankle pressure by itself or as an index is, however, of generic value. The site of involvement is better evaluated with other segmental pressure measurements. At the level of the high thigh, a low pressure in comparison with the brachial pressure may indicate stenotic or occlusive disease at any site between the abdominal aorta and the common femoral artery, as well as disease involving both the superficial femoral and the profunda femoris arteries.

For this reason, a low pressure of the upper thigh by itself is nonspecific. This is an important limitation of this method. More reliable and sensitive information is provided by the comparison of the pressures between the various levels of the lower limb, starting with the upper thigh. The gradient is abnormal when it exceeds 20 to 30 mmHg; it will be slightly elevated above this level in the case of stenosis, and progressively higher with increasing degrees of stenosis. The site of the gradient points to the diseased artery. If it is detected between the two levels in the thigh, it means that the superficial femoral artery is involved (an isolated occlusion of the profunda femoris cannot be detected). Between the two levels of the knee, the distal superficial femoral artery or the popliteal artery is involved; between the upper calf and the ankle any of the three vessels may be involved. Specific pressures are to be measured (anterior tibial, posterior tibial) for precise definitions.

When multiple disease involving several segments is present, the exact definition of the site may be obscured, since the more proximal lesion may conceal distal lesions.

Symptomatic patients with a normal or borderline ankle-brachial index, as well as patients with a slightly low index, should be further evaluated with stress testing or reactive hyperemia testing in order to assess the real vascular status. By reducing the peripheral resistance, there is a more physiologic increase of flow, which makes it possible to make apparent a significant pressure gradient that is otherwise obscured at rest. On the contrary, simple exposure to cold (which may happen during the clinical examination)

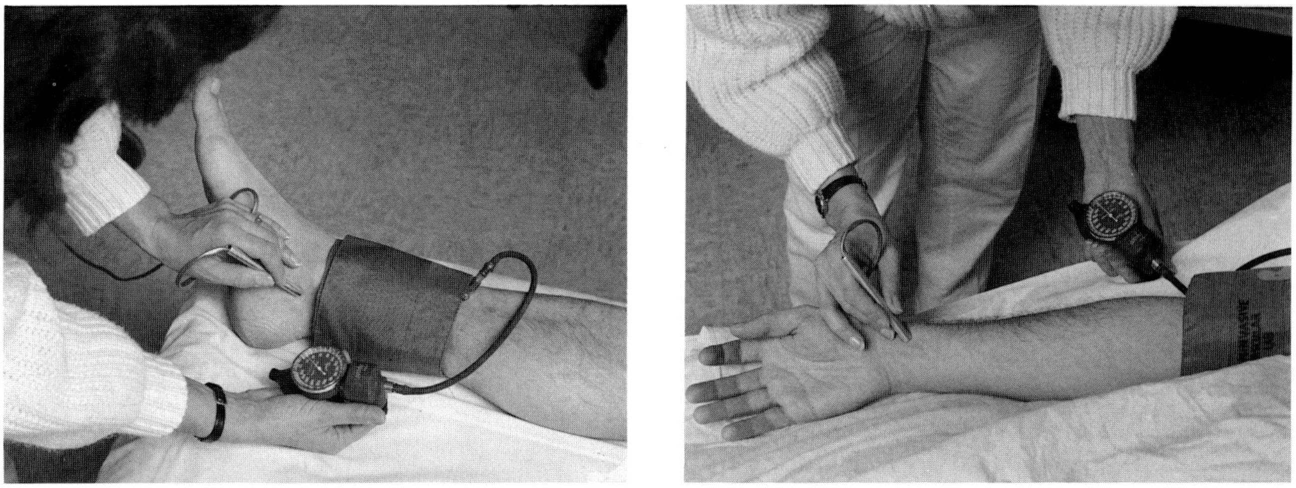

A B

Figure 2–2. Ankle-brachial index measurement. **A:** A pressure cuff is inflated over the ankle. A Doppler probe is positioned over the posterior tibial artery at the ankle; the cuff is slowly deflated and the pressure at which the pulse reappears is registered. The procedure is repeated over the dorsalis pedis artery. The highest of the two values is the reference for the ankle pressure. **B:** The procedure is repeated in both the arms, with the cuff above the elbow and the probe over the radial artery. The higher value registered is taken as the brachial pressure. Ankle-brachial index is given by the relationship of the two values.

may produce an increase of peripheral resistance, thus obscuring the pathophysiologic effects of the disease. Operators should be aware of this and be prepared to warm the exposed surfaces. Increase of flow as a consequence of reactive hyperemia may be obtained by blocking the circulation on the foot by inflating a pressure cuff for 3 to 5 minutes, then deflating the cuff.[5]

A physiologic drop of pressure occurs after the release of the cuff, but in normal subjects the value at the ankle will not drop below 35% of the previous value and will return to this value within 1 minute. This simple testing is reserved for patients who cannot undergo more tiresome studies, such as stress testing. The most common stress test is the treadmill. Pressures are taken at the ankle during and after the exercise, until they return to the base value. In normal subjects, ankle-brachial indexes do not change with exercise, whereas in patients with arterial disease there is a drop in the ankle pressure with a more or less slow recovery to the baseline in relation to the severity of the illness.[5,10] Electrocardiographic monitoring during the examination is not only a safety precaution, but it has also a screening and predictive value, since it is necessary to identify patients with asymptomatic but potentially dangerous coronary disease that may be manifested only during increased flow conditions, but prone to occur after successful revascularization procedures.[6]

Pressure measurement methods are limited by several drawbacks: by detecting the pulse with a Doppler probe, the reading can be altered by adjacent pulsatile veins (as in congestive heart failure); adjacent vessels or collateral arterial flow may reduce the selectivity of the study; and calcified vessels give falsely elevated values.[5,6] Because of the possible variables in equipment (mainly the cuff) and operator experience, the techniques should be standardized in the same laboratory, and the pressure measurements obtained with noninvasive methods should be compared whenever possible with the values detected during invasive procedures.

Toe pressure measurement is done with plethysmographic methods and will be discussed in the next section.

PLETHYSMOGRAPHY

Plethysmography is a technique of measurement of volume changes in a part of the body.[11] *Plethysmos* in Greek means increase and *graphein,* to write. It is a very old technique, its principle having been formulated more than 2 centuries ago.

In the earliest methods, the body was immersed in water and the displacement of the fluid was directly measured. This principle is still applied in more sophisticated instruments (water-filled plethysmography).

Other systems measure the volume variation indirectly, by recording the compression of air in a closed system (air-filled plethysmographs). A recently developed system is the pulse-volume recorder.[12] Other systems, such as the mercury strain gauge, measure the variation of electrical resistance in a silicone rubber tube filled with mercury; this tube is wrapped around the part of the body to be studied and changes its length, and then its electric resistance, with blood flow variations.[13] Impedance plethysmography measures the variations of electrical impedance within a segment of a body; in a certain volume of body, impedance is inversely proportional to its total fluid content, and therefore blood flow will change the impedance. In modern instruments a four electrode system is used; two electrodes are placed in external positions, which deliver a high frequency, low current; two inner electrodes measure the voltage changes.[5,14,15] In all those systems, a pulse wave form is obtained and registered.

In photoplethysmography, a photoelectric cell measures changes in blood cutaneous content; it is not strictly a volume change measurement, but its pulse wave form (digit pulse wave form) is quite similar to the recordings obtained by other methods. Very commonly, photoplethysmography is also employed to measure the toe systolic pressure; the photocell is placed over the plantar surfaces of the toe, together with a 2.5 mm pneumatic cuff wrapped around the toe; the cuff is inflated over the level of the brachial pressure, then deflated, and the time of pulse reappearance represents the toe pressure. Normal toe pressures are between 60% of values greater than the ankle pressure.[5] A reactive hyperemia test is also performed by measuring the time of pulse reappearance (normally 1 second) after 5 minutes of occlusion. The pressure in the great toe can also be measured with mercury strain gauge plethysmography.[13] This value has a recognized prognostic significance for skin lesion healing.

With any of these plethysmographic systems, a wave form is obtained. In normal conditions, the pulse contour is characterized by a sharp systolic upstroke with a narrow peak followed by a slow drop-off toward the baseline, interrupted by a dicrotic wave.

The pathologic findings distal to an occlusion are easily recognized: the wave becomes rounded, its amplitude is reduced, and the upswing is more gradual. Erratic wave form may appear, due to collateral flow. The dicrotic notch and wave are not discernible. In total occlusion the wave form is flat. From the analysis of the wave forms, the hemodynamic significance of an obstruction and its approximate site can be detected. These results are easily obtained with low-cost equipment.

It has to be stressed that normal plethysmographic values in resting conditions may not be reliable because of the capacity of the arterial bed to compensate; reactive hyperemia and exercise testing are therefore necessary for an adequate assessment.[10–12]

In clinical practice, the technique may be used instead of or in association with Doppler studies in the assessment of arterial insufficiency, to study arterial compliance, and to determine healing prognosis. Even if Doppler analysis is considered more reliable and superior in quantitative analysis, plethysmography has some advantages, such as in diabetic patients with calcified arteries that cannot be compressed by a pressure cuff.[7,12–15]

Digital pressure recording is used also to assess sympathetic reactivity. Pressure recording is done during several respiratory cycles and under deep inspiration and expiration maneuvers. Sympathetic response may be altered in diabetic and Raynaud's disease patients; it is important to assess sympathetic reactivity, before sympathectomy.[3,7]

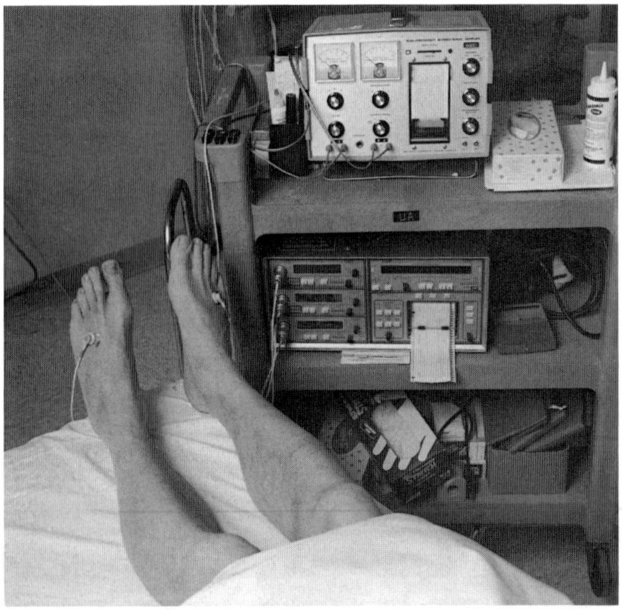

Figure 2–3. Transcutaneous oxygen pressure ($TcPO_2$) measurement. For the $TcPO_2$ measurement, two probes are placed in each dorsum of the foot, and two other over the chest skin. The probes are connected to an automatic measurement system.

TRANSCUTANEOUS OXYGEN TENSION MEASUREMENT

Transcutaneous oxygen pressure ($TcPO_2$) monitoring is a useful method of detection and quantification of arterial insufficieny in PVD. It is a recent method, which appears to be very useful, especially in predictive evaluations. In a resting supine position, the normal absolute value range is approximately 53 to 67 mmHg. Occlusive arterial disease is expected to reduce the tissue oxygenation in the involved segment. A greater part of the variable that may affect the method's reliability is avoided by measuring the relationship between the limb and chest $TcPO_2$. Either calf or foot values can be measured (Fig. 2-3): normal values range, respectively, from 0.9 to 1 and from 0.8 to 1. In analogy with the previously described methods, the accuracy of the test at rest is enhanced by measuring the limb-chest $TcPO_2$ ratio under stressful conditions, especially in doubtful or borderline situations by a treadmill technique.[16–18]

As an alternative, the $TcPO_2$ recovery half-time can be measured without requiring any effort by the patient. This parameter is defined as the time required to recover half the decrease in the limb-chest $TcPO_2$ ratio produced by temporary limb ischemia. In normal subjects, this time is 1.5 minutes or less; this time increases in relation to the severity of the disease.[19]

Another simple method of evaluation is the change in $TcPO_2$, which normally increases when assuming an erect posture from the supine position. A failure to increase the absolute $TcPO_2$ reading at the foot by at least 15 mmHg on the standing position is a valuable index of poor prognosis for arterial reconstruction in patients with advanced occlusive disease in that foot.[20]

ULTRASOUND: REAL-TIME IMAGING, DOPPLER, DUPLEX SCANNING

There are two main possibilities of arterial studies by means of ultrasound: real-time imaging and Doppler scanning. Each of the two methods has its advantages and drawbacks. Recently, significant technologic advances have occurred that have improved the diagnostic capabilities of each of the two techniques, but the most important innovation has been the combination of the two methods in a single piece of equipment, called, for that reason, "duplex."[21–26]

In the real-time component, one of the main problems was the possibility of having a range of different frequency transducers capable of penetrating any depth within the body. The more superficial the structure to be examined, the higher the frequency required. The study of vessels that are directly beneath the skin have to be performed with 7.5 to 10 MHz transducers. The quality of the images is decidedly better with an adequate choice of frequency. Technologic improvement also includes new forms of scanners, such as annular-array transducers. Real-time ultrasound imaging of vessels by itself may give important information on the vessel's anatomy: caliber of the lumen, thickness of the walls, and possible calcification. Normally, arteries are distinguished from the adjacent veins on the basis of such criteria as a known anatomic relationship in certain segments, a relatively smaller caliber and a thicker wall, the presence of pulsatility, and a poor compressibility in comparison with the veins. However, the recognition of the different structures and the detection of possible abnormalities may be impossible even for the most trained examiners due to particular anatomic situations; moreover, it could be impossible to distinguish between a thrombosed or patent vessel only on the basis of lumen caliber criteria. The simultaneous study of the flow, which is performed with Doppler scanning, may reduce and often eliminate many of these limitations. In the Doppler component, the ultrasound emission is used to evaluate the velocity of flow in the scanned area. Doppler effect means the change of frequency of a sound when it interacts with a moving structure. When an ultrasound beam is directed over a vessel in which blood is circulating, the change of frequency is proportional to the velocity of the blood and to the cosine of the angle between the transducer and the direction of the blood flow. The velocity parameter is essential in arterial pathophysiology. When the caliber of a vessel is reduced by stenosis, the increase in velocity at the site of the lesion is the physiologic response to equilibrate the system. On the other hand, distal to the stenotic or occluding lesion, the overall velocity of the system will be reduced.

There are several ways of ultrasound emission and recording of the Doppler signal. The most simple is a continuous wave audible sound that employs a little inexpensive hand-held unit. It is the system used in pressure measurements. The frequency of the perceived sound increases with the velocity and therefore with the degree of stenosis. There are two main limitations of this system. First, it is an almost "blind" examination, which scans in a nonselective way a relative wide body segment, where more than one vessel, either arterial or venous, may be present. Second, the assessment of the degree of a lesion depends on the subjective capacities of the examiner and may not be objectively quantified.

The selectivity of the system is sensibly enhanced with a pulsed rather than continuous emission of ultrasound and by gating the reception of the signal. It is thus possible to select, within the area investigated by the acoustic beam, a definite segment to examine. When this is done in the duplex system, the choice of the vessel is directed by its real-time images. Thus, the two methods take reciprocal advantage; the Doppler study will be focused on each distinct vessel of interest, whereas the problems of identification of the structures shown in real-time imaging will be solved by the detection of typical flow signals. The problem of an objective documentation of velocity changes was solved before the development of the duplex technology, and the technologic improvement has been transferred to this system.

The Doppler signal is elaborated by a computer with complex mathematic calculations (mainly fast Fourier transformation) and then displayed on the screen.[26] In normal conditions, a typical wave form is obtained. Pathologic changes are easily recognized with direct visual interpretation of wave form; objective data are obtained with measurement of certain parameters of the wave form.

The Doppler wave form is a graphic display of the blood velocity (which is represented in the vertical axis) over time (horizontal axis). The normal wave form has three main components: a rapid systolic upslope followed by a rapid downward slope in the opposite direction, with negative values, and a new forward slope, with positive values lower than 1. The first slope corresponds to the systole, during which the blood flow reaches its maximal velocity; the following deflection below the zero baseline is due to flow in reversed direction, which occurs in early diastole because of the elastic recoil of arterial walls previously distended; the third component corresponds to the late diastole when the energy of arterial recoil is dissipated, and the flow starts again in the forward direction toward the arterioles. An increased resistance in the arterial system will cause an obstacle to flow, with a consequently increased back-flow in the early diastolic phase and a reduction of velocity (height of the peak) in the third phase.

The pathologic changes in the Doppler wave form are quite typical. At the site of a stenosis, the increase in velocity will appear as an elevated first slope. Beyond a stenosis, there will be several changes due to the systolic velocity reduction. The systolic downward slope will be prolonged; the negative flow of the early diastolic phase will also be markedly reduced or lost. Forward flow of the diastolic phase will be visible when peripheral vessels are dilated. According to the severity of the lesions, the curve will be more flattened in the first peak and will lose the diphasic pattern, showing a slow decrease after the early systolic peak. At the maximal level of obstruction, there will be only a flattened irregular succession of small waves (Figs. 2-4, 2-5).

The simplest objective evaluation of the wave form is given by the height of the peaks. A useful parameter is the pulsatility index, given by the relationship of the maximum vertical excursion of the wave form with the mean value throughout the cardiac cycle. More sophisticated methods include the principal component analysis or the evaluation, by means of the Laplace transform method, wave form damping, arterial elasticity, and peripheral resistance.[25]

With the duplex system, following the course of the arteries of the lower limbs, it is possible to detect changes in flow velocity indicative of stenotic or occlusive disease with relative precision on the exact site of the lesion. The limits of the system are given by the accessibility to certain segments by both the real-time and Doppler components: in the iliac segment, the arteries cannot always be shown, and therefore a distal change in the flow has an important screening value, but requires further investigation for the exact localization of the lesion; in the calf, also, the arteries cannot be directly demonstrated and the changes are only indirectly detected. Furthermore, the reliability of the system is reduced by calcified arteries. Nevertheless, the quality of information given by a duplex analysis is essential, and, as a consequence, arteriographic studies are more precisely directed over the affected area (Figs. 2-6 through 2-10).

Duplex studies for their simplicity and repeatability are

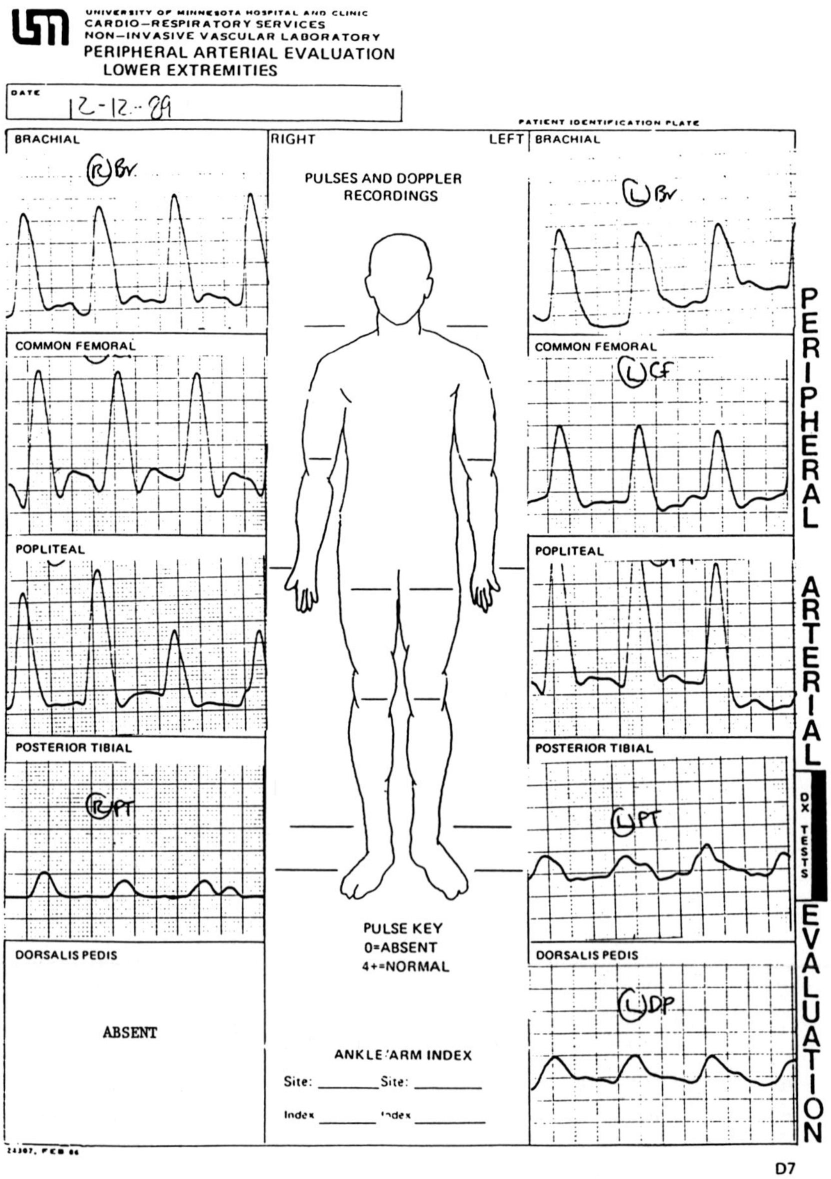

Figure 2–4. Doppler wave form study of the leg. Wave form registered at different levels are arranged in preformed sheaths. In this case, there is evidence of bilateral obstruction below the popliteal artery.

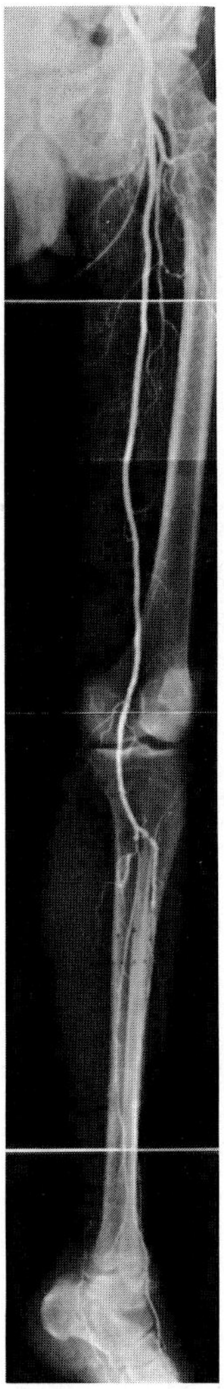

Figure 2–5. Angiogram of the left leg confirms the Doppler diagrams showing total occlusion of the posterior tibial artery and occlusion of large segments of the anterior tibial artery.

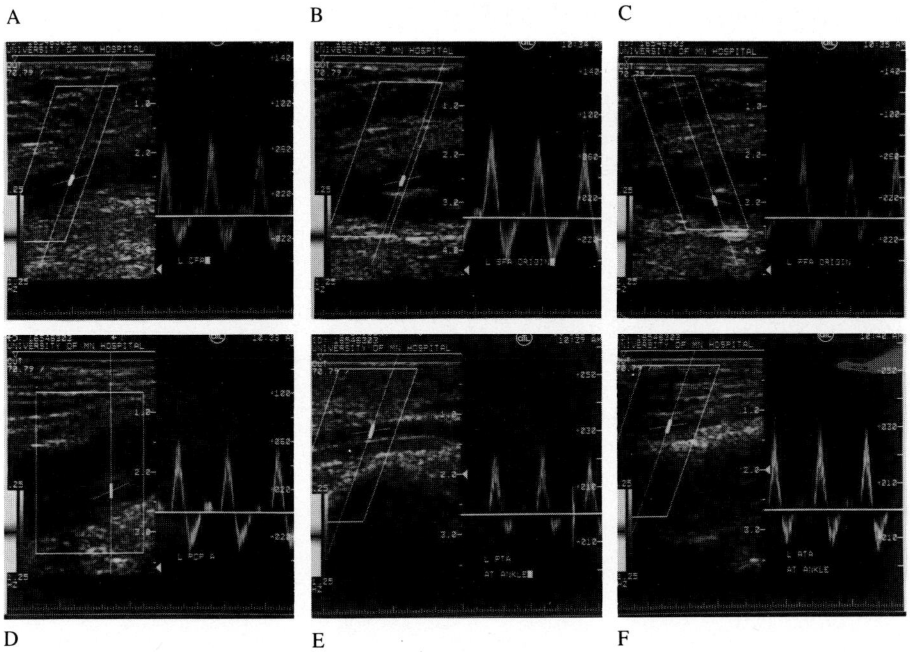

Figure 2–6. Duplex study in a normal lower extremity arterial tree. Real-time ultrasound images in longitudinal sections are shown together with Doppler wave forms at various levels. **A:** Common femoral artery. **B:** Superficial femoral artery at the origin. **C:** Profunda femoris artery at the origin. **D:** Popliteal artery. **E:** Posterior tibial artery at the ankle. **F:** Anterior tibial artery at the ankle.

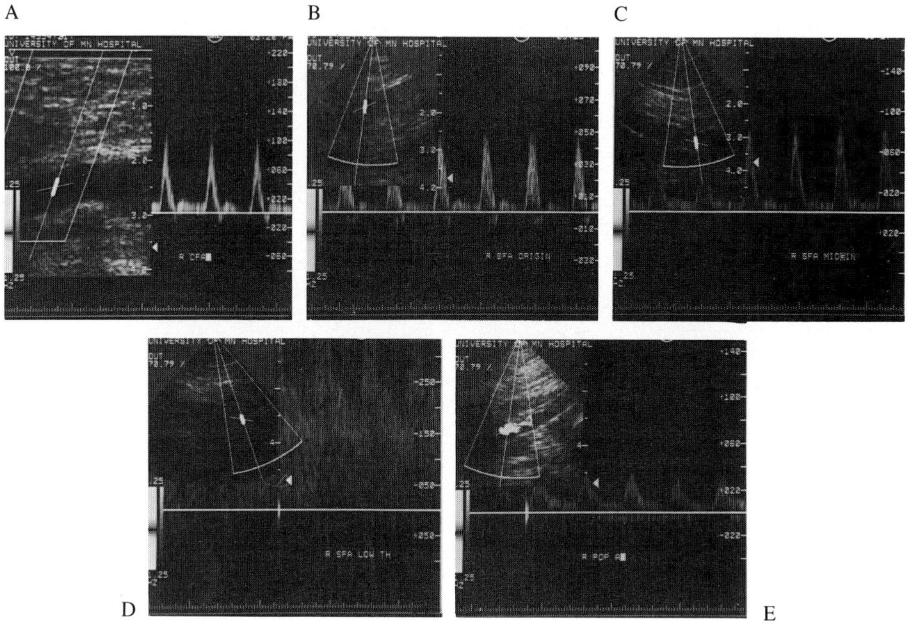

Figure 2–7. Duplex study in a case of severe stenosis of distal superficial femoral artery. Real-time ultrasound and wave form are normal in the common femoral **(A)** and in the superficial femoral artery **(B)** up to the midthigh **(C)**; wave form is altered due to turbulence at the level of the stenosis **(D)**; the height of the wave form is significantly reduced in the popliteal artery **(E)**.

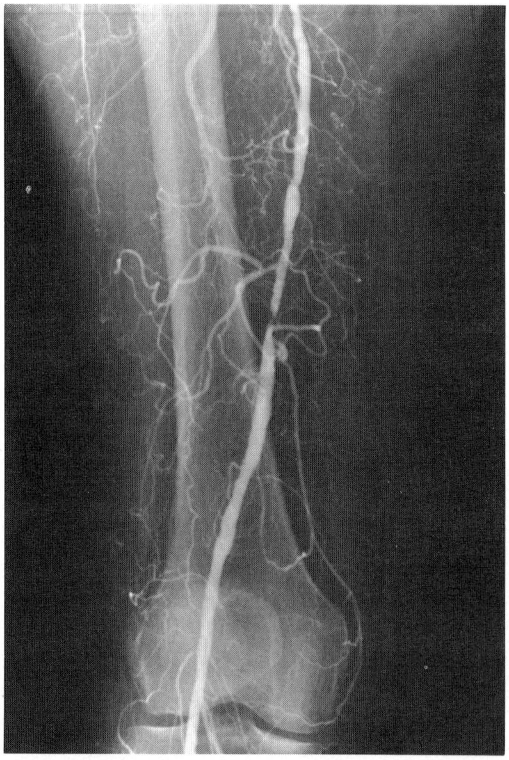

Figure 2–8. Angiogram of the same patient showing the lesion at the level of the distal superficial femoral artery.

A 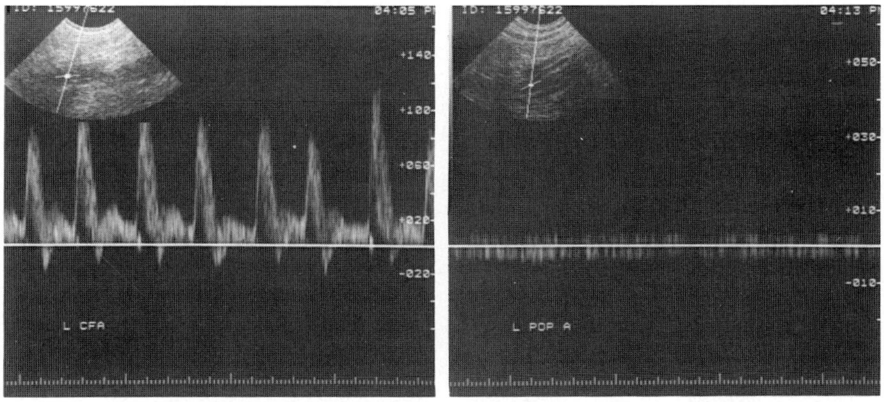 B

Figure 2–9. Duplex study in a case of acute occlusion of the left superficial femoral artery. **A:** Real-time ultrasound image in longitudinal section and Doppler wave form at the level of the common femoral artery. Wave form is normal. **B:** At the popliteal level, the Doppler signal is definitely altered, which is indicative of proximal total occlusion.

now the simplest method for objective assessment in several vascular conditions, including the screening of arterial disease, even in presymptomatic stages in larger groups of population, and the planning and follow-up of percutaneous revascularization procedures. Duplex studies are also useful in more specific problems, such as in the detection of aortoiliac stenosis in candidates for distal bypass grafts, in whom the surgical success is threatened and conditioned by a proximal stenosis that can be easily treated by transluminal angioplasty before the major surgery.

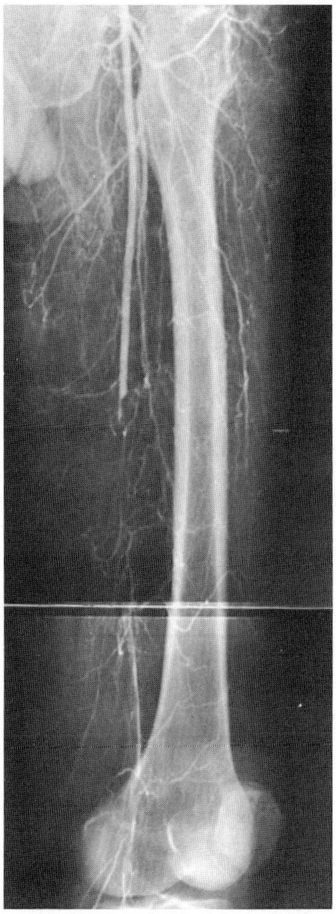

Figure 2–10. Angiogram in the same case as Figure 2–9 shows a total occlusion of the lower half of the superficial femoral artery due to thrombosis.

A further decisive improvement in diagnostic capabilities has been recently achieved by the development of color Doppler systems. These allow the superimposition on the real-time vascular bidimensional image of a color documentation of the flow in the examined area. The color may vary in a range selected by the examiner showing the different velocities and directions of the flow. The technologic improvement related to the development of these new systems has led to more sensitive equipment. Thus, color Doppler has several advantages over the conventional duplex systems. It makes the localization of vessels, especially the small ones, easier, faster, and more reliable. Localization of stenosis is easier without laborious searches; venous mapping and localization of side branches is also facilitated.[27,28]

REFERENCES

1. Patton T. Soft tissues. In Grainger RG, Allison DJ. Diagnostic Radiology, vol. 2. Edinburgh: Churchill Livingstone, 1986: 1509–22.
2. Underwood R, Firmin D. An Introduction to Magnetic Resonance of the Cardiovascular System. London: Current Medical Literature, 1988.
3. Alfidi RJ, Masarik TJ, Haacke EM, et al. Magnetic resonance angiography in peripheral, carotid and coronary arteries. In Taveras JM, Ferrucci JT. Radiology Diagnosis-Imaging-Intervention, vol. 2. London: JB Lippincott, 1988, chap. 139.
4. Salles-Cunha SX, Andros G, Dulawa LB, et al. Changes in peripheral hemodynamics after percutaneous transluminal angioplasty. J Vasc Surg 1989;10:338–42.
5. Gerlock AJ, Giyanani VL, Krebs C. Applications of Noninvasive Vascular Technique. Philadelphia: WB Saunders, 1988:283–380.
6. Barnes RW. Noninvasive evaluation of peripheral vascular disease: recent advances and future implications. South Med J 1986;79:55–9.
7. Kempczinski RF. Clinical application of noninvasive testing in extremity arterial insufficiency. In Kempczinski RF, Yao JST (eds): Practical Noninvasive Vascular Diagnosis. Chicago: Year Book Medical Publishers, 1982:350–7.
8. Breslaw PJ, Van Soest M, Janevski B, et al. Hemodynamic evaluation of transluminal iliac artery balloon dilatation. Neth J Surg 1985;37:145–7.

9. Rees CR, Palmaz JC, Garcia O, et al. Angioplasty and stenting of completely occluded iliac arteries. Radiology 1989;172: 953–9.
10. Fronek A. Pressure, flow velocity and reactive hyperemia. In Nicolaides AN, Yao JST (eds): Investigation of Vascular Disorders. New York: Churchill Livingstone, 1981:229–48.
11. Sumner DS. Volume plethysmography in vascular disease: an overview. In Bernstein EF (ed): Non-invasive Diagnostic Techniques in Vascular Disease. St. Louis: CV Mosby, 1982:67–86.
12. Raines JK. The pulse volume recorder in peripheral arterial disease. In Bernstein EF (ed): Non-invasive Diagnostic Techniques in Vascular Disease. St. Louis: CV Mosby, 1982:360–9.
13. Sumner DS. Mercury strain-gauge plethysmography. In Bernstein EF (ed): Non-invasive Diagnostic Techniques in Vascular Disease. St. Louis: CV Mosby, 1982:117–35.
14. Golden JC, Miles DS. Assessment of peripheral hemodynamics using impedance plethysmography. Phys Ther 1986;66: 1544–7.
15. Anderson FA. Impedance plethysmography in the diagnosis of arterial and venous disease. Ann Biomed Eng 1984;12:79–102.
16. Byrne P, Provan JL, Ameli FM, et al. The use of transcutaneous oxygen tension measurements in the diagnosis of peripheral vascular insufficiency. Ann Surg 1986;200:159–65.
17. Cina C, Katsamouris A, Megerman J, et al. Utility of transcutaneous oxygen tension measurement in peripheral arterial occlusive disease. J Vasc Surg 1984;1:1362–71.
18. Franzek UK, Talke P, Bernstein EF, et al. Transcutaneous PO_2 measurements in health and peripheral arterial occlusive disease. Surgery 1982;91:156–62.
19. Kram HB, Appel PL, White RA, et al. Assessment of peripheral vascular disease by postocclusive transcutaneous oxygen recovery time. J Vasc Surg 1984;1:628–34.
20. Oh PIT, Provan JL, Ameli FM. The predictability of the success of arterial reconstruction by means of transcutaneous oxygen tension measurements. J Vasc Surg 1987;5:356–62.
21. Strandness DE. Duplex scanning and the vascular surgeon. J Cardiovas Surg 1987;28:235–42.
22. Jonnart LE. Non-invasive assessment of blood vessels. Acta Cardiol 1989;44:1–6.
23. Jäger K, Bollinger A, Siegenthaler W. Duplex-Sonographie in der Gefässdiagnostik. Dtsch Med Wochenschr 1986;111: 1608–13.
24. Grant EG. Duplex ultrasonography: its expanding role in noninvasive vascular diagnosis. Radiol Clin North Am 1985;23:563–82.
25. Bruce Campbel W. Doppler waveform analysis in the management of lower limb arterial disease. Ann R Coll Surg Engl 1986;68:103–6.
26. Zuech PE, Cobbold RSC, Johnston KW, et al. Spectral analysis of Doppler flow velocity signals. Assessment of objectives, methods and interpretation. Ann Biomed Eng 1984;12:103–16.
27. Switzer DF, Nanda NC. Doppler color flow mapping. Ultrasound Med Biol 1985;11:403–16.
28. Landwehr VP, Nicolas V, Dölken W, et al. Farbdopplersonographie: Nicht-invasive Möglichkeiten der morphologischen und funktionellen Gefässdiagnostik. Fortschr Rontgenstr 1988;148:1–7.

3 Angiographic Evaluation of Peripheral Vascular Disease

Tony P. Smith, M.D.

Angiography of the lower limb is one of the most commonly performed angiograms in radiology departments today. Although Doppler and duplex examinations have improved greatly, the gold standard remains the angiogram. The future, however, may lie in sonography, magnetic resonance imaging, and other forms of noninvasive studies. At present, the performance of excellent quality angiography is still essential prior to endovascular or surgical therapy.

ANATOMY

The initial step in angiography is to study the inflow vessels, that is, the pelvic vessels to the level of the inguinal ligament (Fig. 3-1). The aortic bifurcation as well as the iliac arteries must be well visualized. There is considerable variation in the branching pattern of the internal (hypogastric) arteries. Prior to any endovascular therapeutic procedure in the pelvis, the anatomy should be thoroughly reviewed and there are excellent textbooks available.[1]

The external iliac artery extends from the bifurcation of the common iliac artery to the inguinal ligament, which is represented by a line between the anterior superior spine of the ilium and the symphysis pubis. It is at this point that the external iliac artery becomes the common femoral artery. The common femoral artery is contained within the femoral sheath accompanied by the femoral vein, nerve, and lymphatics. Approximately 2 to 5 cm below the inguinal ligament, the common femoral artery divides into the deep (profunda) femoral artery and the superficial femoral artery. The deep femoral artery consists mostly of perforating and muscular arteries, as well as the femoral circumflex branches. The superficial femoral artery continues its course through the thigh giving only small muscular branches until just proximal to the adductor canal (Hunter's canal, named for a Scottish surgeon). The descending genicular artery usually arises from the superficial femoral artery just prior to the vessel entering the adductor hiatus. At the lower end of the adductor canal, the vessel continues as the popliteal artery. The popliteal artery is contained within the popliteal fossa, where it is held in close proximity to the popliteal vein by dense connective tissue. The popliteal artery gives rise to several muscular and genicular branches. At approximately the level of the lower end of the popliteus muscle, the popliteal artery bifurcates into an anterior tibial artery and a posterior tibial-peroneal trunk. The anterior tibial artery passes anteriorly between the two heads of the tibialis posterior muscle and lies in close association to the medial neck of the fibula. The artery then descends on the anterior surface of the interosseus membrane, gradually approaching the tibia until it lies on the anterior surface of the tibia at the ankle joint. The anterior tibial artery continues into the foot, past the ankle joint as the dorsalis pedis artery. Approximately 2 to 5 cm below the bifurcation of the popliteal artery, the posterior tibial-peroneal trunk bifurcates, giving rise to the posterior tibial and peroneal arteries. The peroneal artery courses toward the fibula and runs along the tibiofibular syndesmosis and terminates in calcanean branches. The posterior tibial artery descends from its origin obliquely downward in the posterior compartment of the calf, to lie behind the tibia in the lower portion of the leg. The posterior tibial artery continues into the foot, giving rise to a smaller medial and larger lateral plantar arteries. The formation of the plantar arch in the foot is from a deep plantar branch of the dorsalis pedis and the lateral plantar artery of the posterior tibial.

The typical anatomic distribution of pelvic and lower extremity arterial anatomy just described is demonstrated in Figure 3-1. All who perform lower extremity angiography should be intimately familiar with this pattern, as well as typical variations that exist. In addition, well-known collateral pathways have been well outlined in other sources and should be familiar to all angiographers.[2]

TECHNIQUE

The technique for performance of lower extremity angiography should be dictated by the disease process and proposed endovascular or surgical treatment (Table 3-1). Such disease processes as trauma, tumors, or limb salvage require only single leg angiography. However, inflow disease or severe involvement of both limbs requires bilateral leg angiography. For arterial occlusion, noninvasive evaluation such as segmental limb pressures will roughly determine the location of disease prior to angiography.

The initial evaluation is most important for the site of arterial access, which is also determined by the proposed treatment. The common femoral artery is the most commonly used arterial access. It can be safely utilized if attention is paid to anatomic landmarks. Punctures above the inguinal ligament, that is, into the distal external iliac artery, have been associated with retroperitoneal hemorrhage, and lower puncture sites, that is, into the superficial femoral or profunda arteries, have been associated with a higher percentage of complication (including pseudoaneurysm and

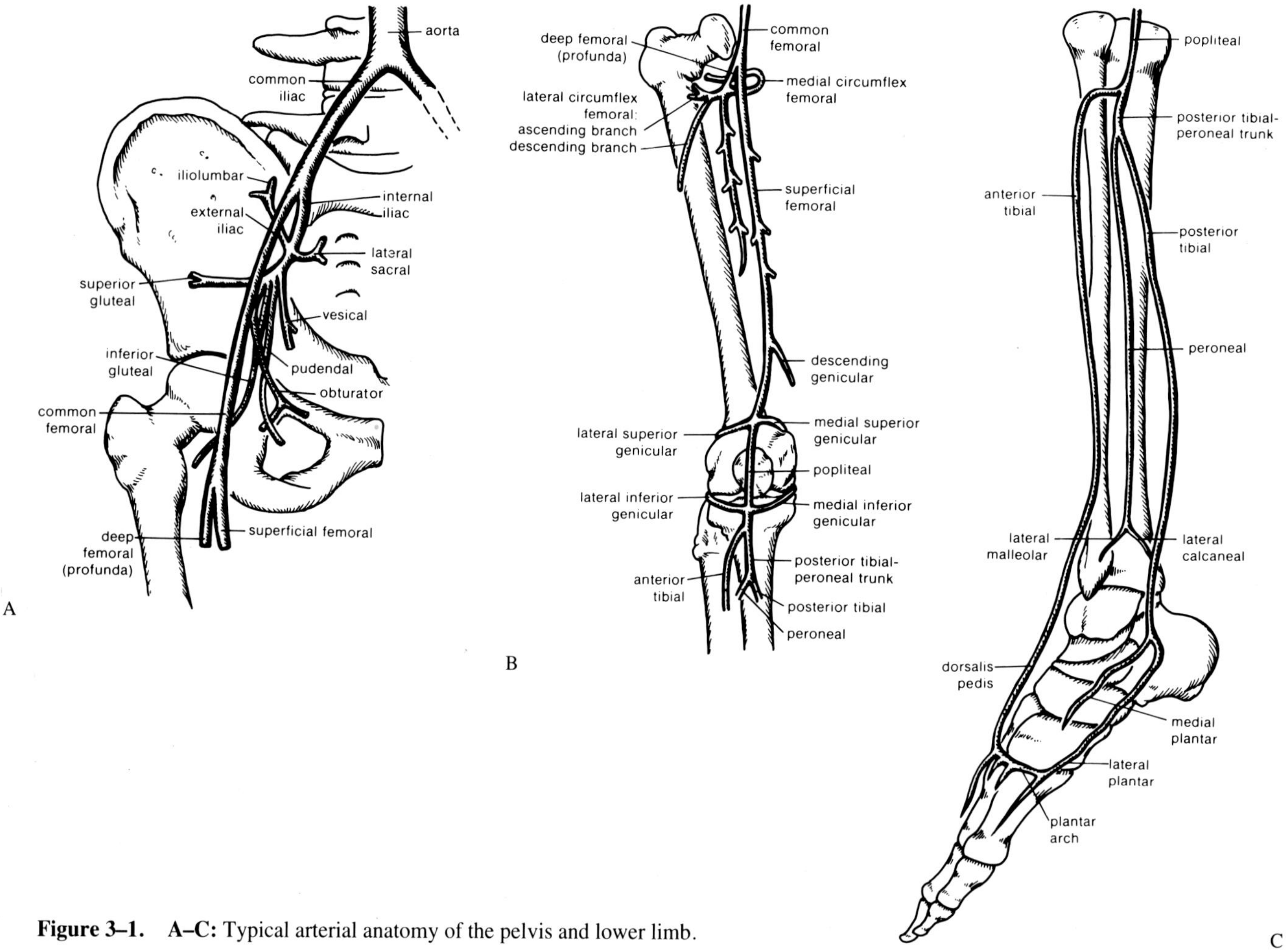

Figure 3–1. **A–C:** Typical arterial anatomy of the pelvis and lower limb.

arteriovenous fistulas).[3,4] Even prosthetic femoral grafts can be safely used for arterial access.[5] For bilateral angiography, it is obviously best to approach the side with the more normal, palpable femoral pulse. Depending on femoral pulses, the ipsilateral common femoral artery is probably easiest in the absence of inflow disease and if single leg angiography is to be performed.[6] However, this approach precludes an easy antegrade approach if required in the same sitting. The contralateral arterial approach allows excellent diagnostic angiography and an easier antegrade approach (even using fluoroscopic contrast guidance from the contralateral catheter) if necessary. Axillary approaches allow diagnostic and interventional techniques to the lower limbs from the same access, but have higher puncture site complications.[7] The translumbar approach permits diagnostic angiography given lower aortic occlusions, but is of virtually no use as a therapeutic access.

Table 3–1. Arterial Abnormalities of Lower Limb That Could Necessitate Endovascular Therapy

Arterial occlusion
Atherosclerosis
Embolization
Thrombosis
Trauma
Arteriovenous malformation
Hemangioma
Tumors
Bone
Soft tissue
Extrinsic disease
Foreign bodies
Bypass grafts

Most lower extremity angiography is performed using a pigtail catheter that is placed at the aortic bifurcation or even at the level of the renal arteries where 60 to 80 ml of contrast material is injected.[8] Although the resulting study is usually adequate for inflow and thigh vessels, this technique often produces suboptimal visualization of the lower leg and foot vessels. Patent distal vessels, including the plantar arch in the foot, have been well correlated with distal graft patency and therefore their visualization at arteriography is essential.[9] In fact, some have advocated the necessity of intraoperative angiography to visualize such vessels due to the usually poor opacification of standard preoperative angiograms.[10,11]

Higher contrast volumes (100 to 150 ml) can be successfully employed, although when severe unilateral lower extremity disease is present, vessel opacification still tends to be very poor with aortic injections.

Unilateral angiography utilizing contrast injection below the internal iliac artery, particularly with higher contrast volumes (60 ml), is very effective for single limb angiography.[12] If single limb angiography is all that is clinically required, inflow vessels should be first evaluated followed by lower limb angiography performed from the level of the external iliac artery. Catheters can be placed even more distally into the superficial femoral artery for contrast injection and have been shown to provide excellent visualization of small vessels[13] (Fig. 3-2).

Balloon occlusion angiography also produces excellent lower extremity angiograms.[14] Such angiography is based on the occlusion of arterial inflow by a small balloon catheter followed by contrast material injection through a separate lumen that is located distal to the site of balloon occlusion. Balloon occlusion temporarily prevents washout of contrast material by arterial inflow. The balloon can then be released, allowing the contrast material to travel in a bolus down the extremity. Film timing is therefore usually less critical. Although there have been reports of complications with occlusion balloons in early animal work, newer products now allow these procedures to be performed without difficulty.[15,16]

Angiography is obtained in most centers using screen-film technique and either a translating (step) table or a long-leg changer. Both of these devices can produce excellent quality angiograms if attention is paid to technical details. Film timing is somewhat more difficult using the translating table, although theoretically it produces films with less scatter and is less expensive to purchase and less cumbersome to use when compared with the standard long-leg changer. Film timing is best set on an individual patient basis, depending on the rate of blood flow, amount of contrast material injected, and type of filming device used.

Digital subtraction angiography (DSA) has improved greatly in quality since its inception. Intravenous DSA is used in most centers only as a screening technique, but intra-arterial DSA is often being used as the primary angiographic study. Particularly when angiography is performed from an aortic injection, DSA is utilized to visualize the lower leg and foot arteries, which are not well visualized on the initial conventional angiogram. There is, however, some controversy as to the resolution of current DSA units when compared with their film-screen counterparts, and until further evidence is generated, it is probably best to use even intra-arterial DSA only in an adjunctive fashion to the best film-screen angiogram obtainable.[17–19]

For lower leg angiography, especially where there is major vessel occlusion, every effort should be made to increase blood flow distally. A blood pressure cuff placed on the ankle and inflated to suprasystolic levels for at least 5 minutes has proven to increase blood flow by virtue of reactive hyperemia.[20] This technique is safe and convenient because it does not require the injection of medication and is available in virtually all radiography departments. Temperature elevation also has been shown to increase arterial flow by a peripheral vasodilation.[21]

The remaining techniques to increase arterial flow are pharmacologic in nature. The most commonly used vasodilating drugs are papaverine (30 to 60 mg), lidocaine (50 to 100 mg), and tolazoline (50 mg).[22,23] The administration of any such pharmacologic agent should be done with care and the angiographer must possess a thorough understanding of the medication's actions and adverse effects.

Lower limb angiography has been a notoriously painful procedure. The introduction of low osmolality contrast agents has significantly decreased the pain and use of these agents should be routine.[24,25] In addition to lower osmolality agents, analgesia or sedation serve to relieve patient anxiety and increase patient tolerance. Many centers prefer to give the patient preoperative medications prior to their arrival for the angiogram. Agents such as morphine or meperidine, particularly combined with diazepam, are effective; however, patients must be monitored closely, including during transport to the radiology department. Intravenous sedation alone is usually adequate when administered in the angiography suite. As with premedication, a combination of a narcotic such as morphine or fentanyl citrate when combined with diazepam or midazolam have proven to be extremely effective.[26,27] Again, close physiologic monitoring including electrocardiography, vital signs, and pulse oximetry are mandatory. Finally, many have advocated the use of intra-arterial lidocaine, either before contrast injection or mixed with the contrast material to alleviate pain.[28,29] Although effective, intra-arterial lidocaine is probably unnecessary given the lower osmolality agents now available.

Outpatient angiography has recently become commonplace. Diagnostic angiography can be safely performed and most patients discharged on the same day, usually 4 to 6 hours following the procedure.[30,31] It is obviously essential that patients be closely monitored following the procedure and inpatient facilities must be available if patients cannot be released.

COMPLICATIONS

The complications of angiography are extremely low and have been shown to be inversely related to the number of procedures performed.[32,33] Complications consist mostly of contrast-related problems (renal insufficiency, reactions) and catheterization-related problems (puncture site, arterial thrombosis).

Contrast reactions are quite rare, occurring in approximately 2.5% of the patients undergoing intra-arterial contrast injections and fatal reactions occur in less than 0.008%.[34] The rate of postarteriographic contrast-induced renal insufficiency, 7.1% in a large series, depends on preexisting renal

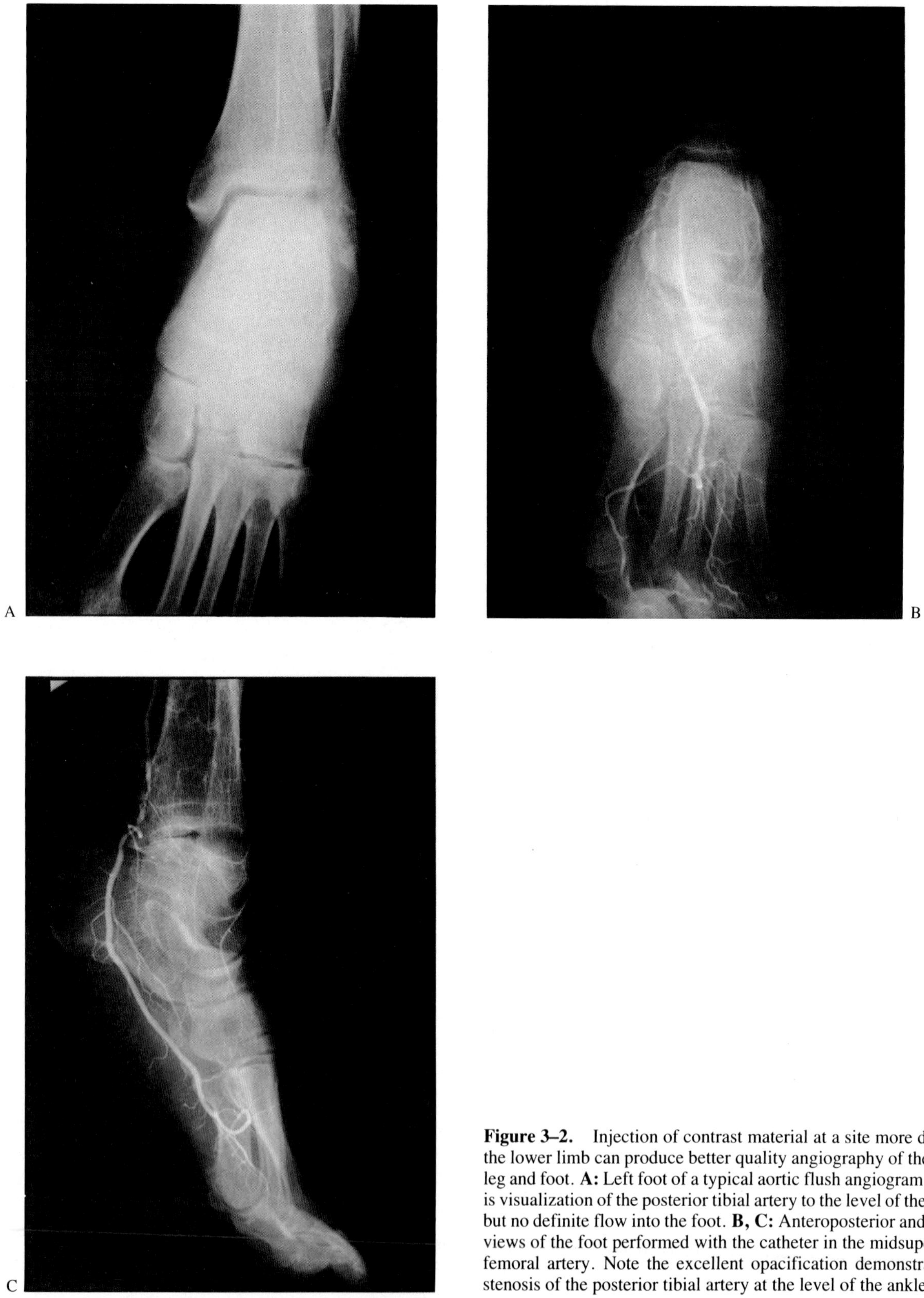

Figure 3–2. Injection of contrast material at a site more distal in the lower limb can produce better quality angiography of the lower leg and foot. **A:** Left foot of a typical aortic flush angiogram. There is visualization of the posterior tibial artery to the level of the ankle, but no definite flow into the foot. **B, C:** Anteroposterior and lateral views of the foot performed with the catheter in the midsuperficial femoral artery. Note the excellent opacification demonstrating a stenosis of the posterior tibial artery at the level of the ankle.

disease, advanced age, the volume of contrast material used, type of study performed, diabetes, and coexisting heart disease.[35] The state of patient hydration did not figure into the frequency of acute renal dysfunction. For both contrast reactions and renal insufficiency, the newer low osmolality agents are probably superior, although this has not been determined at the time of this writing.

Puncture site complications vary according to the access site. In a large series, both translumbar (2.89%) and axillary (3.29%) accesses had higher rates than the femoral (1.73%) route.[33] Although hematoma is the most frequent complication, arterial dissection may occur at the puncture site or within vessels being selectively catheterized. Distal embolization can also occur, most often representing thrombus, but rarely cholesterol embolization can occur in patients with severe atherosclerotic disease.[36,37]

All complications can be minimized by complete evaluation of the patient prior to and meticulous technique during angiography.

REFERENCES

1. Clemente CD. Anatomy of the Human Body. Philadelphia: Lea & Febiger, 1985:748–87.
2. Quiring DP. Collateral Circulation. Philadelphia, Lea & Febiger, 1949:72–82, 124–129.
3. Kaufman JL. Pelvic hemorrhage after percutaneous femoral angiography. AJR 1984;143:335–6.
4. Rapoport S, Sniderman KW, Morse SS, et al. Pseudoaneurysm: a complication of faulty technique in femoral arterial puncture. Radiology 1985;154:529–30.
5. Wade GL, Smith DC, Mohr LL. Follow-up of 50 consecutive angiograms obtained utilizing puncture of prosthetic vascular grafts. Radiology 1983;146:663–4.
6. Owens AP, Logan H, MacErlean DP, et al. Simplified peripheral arteriography. Clin Radiol 1987;38:425–6.
7. Molnar W, Paul DJ. Complications of axillary arteriotomies: an analysis of 1,762 consecutive studies. Radiology 1972;104: 269–76.
8. Bron KM. Femoral arteriography. In Abrams HL (ed): Abrams Angiography. Boston: Little, Brown, 1983:1843.
9. O'Mara CS, Flinn WR, Neiman HL, et al. Correlation of foot arterial anatomy with early tibial bypass patency. Surgery 1981;89:743–52.
10. Scarpato R, Gembarowicz R, Farber S, et al. Intraoperative prereconstruction arteriography. Arch Surg 1981;116:1053–5.
11. Flanigan DP, Williams LR, Keifer T, et al. Prebypass operative arteriography. Surgery 1982;92:627–33.
12. Smith TP, Cragg AH, Berbaum KS, et al. Techniques for lower limb angiography: a comparative study. Radiology 1990;174:951–55.
13. Kozak BE, Bedell JE, Rosch J. Small vessel leg angiography for distal vessel bypass grafts. J Vasc Surg 1988;8:711–5.
14. Cardella JF, Smith TP, Darcy MD, et al. Balloon occlusion femoral angiography prior to in-situ saphenous vein bypass. Cardiovasc Intervent Radiol 1987;10:181–7.
15. Burgener FA, Gutierrez OH, Logsdon GA. Complications and hazards with angiographic occlusion balloon catheters. Radiology 1981;140:647–50.
16. Vincent RN, Hawkins LE, Pelech AN, et al. Balloon occlusion angiography. Can J Cardiol 1987;3:52–9.
17. Garvey CJ, Wilkins RA, Lewis JD. Peripheral vascular disease: prospective study of intraarterial digital subtraction angiography using a 9-inch intensifier. Radiology 1986; 159:423–7.
18. Skau T, Bolin T, Karner G. Digital subtraction angiography versus standard contrast arteriography in evaluation of peripheral vascular disease. Int Angiol 1988;7:42–5.
19. Hol PK, Heldaas J, Skjennald A. Demonstration of pedal arterial arcades in occlusive arteriosclerotic disease. Acta Radiol 1989;30:61–3.
20. Hishida Y: Peripheral arteriography using the reactive hyperemia. Jpn Circ J 1963;27:349–56.
21. Rosch J, Antonovic R, Porter JM. The importance of temperature in angiography of the hand. Radiology 1977;123:323–6.
22. Cohen MI, Vogelzang RL. A comparison of techniques for improved visualization of the arteries of the distal lower extremity. AJR 1986;147:1021–4.
23. Jacobs JB, Hanafee WN. The use of priscoline in peripheral arteriography. Radiology 1967;88:957–60.
24. Dotter CT, Rosch J, Erlandson M, et al. Iopamidol arteriography: discomfort and pain. Radiology 1985;155:819–21.
25. Sacks BA, Ellison HP, Bartek S, et al. A comparison of hexabrix and renografin 60 in peripheral arteriography. Invest Radiol 1984;19:S320–2.
26. Holmes CM, Galletly DG: Midazolam/fentanyl: a total intravenous technique for short procedures. Anaesthesia 1982; 37:761–5.
27. Miller DL, Wall RT. Fentanyl and diazepam for analgesia and sedation during radiologic special procedures. Radiology 1987;162:195–8.
28. Gordon IJ, Westcott JL. Intra-arterial lidocaine: an effective analgesic for peripheral angiography. Radiology 1977; 124:43–5.
29. Widrich WC, Singer RJ, Robbins AH. The use of intra-arterial lidocaine to control pain due to aortofemoral arteriography. Radiology 1977;124:37–41.
30. Rogers WF, Moothart RW. Outpatient arteriography and cardiac catheterization: effective alternatives to inpatient procedures. AJR 1985;144:233–4.
31. Saint-Georges G, Aube M. Safety of outpatient angiography: a prospective study. AJR 1985;144:235–6.
32. Lang EK. A survey of the complications of percutaneous retrograde arteriography. Radiology 1963;81:257–61.
33. Hessel SJ, Adams DF, Abrams HL. Complications of angiography. Radiology 1981;138:273–81.
34. Shehadl WH, Toniolo G: Adverse reactions to contrast media. Radiology 1980;137:299–302.
35. Gomes AS, Baker JD, Martin-Paredero V, et al. Acute renal dysfunction after major arteriography. AJR 1985;145:1249–53.
36. Barnes RW, Slaymaker EE, Hahn FJY. Thromboembolic complications of angiography for peripheral arterial disease: prospective assessment of doppler ultrasound. Radiology 1977;122:459–61.
37. Lonni YG, Matsumoto KK, Lecky JW. Postaortographic cholesterol (atheromatous) embolization. Radiology 1969; 93:63–5.

4 Pharmacologic Manipulation in Transluminal Angioplasty of Peripheral Vascular Disease: Spasm Control

Riccardo Di Segni, M.D., Wilfrido R. Castañeda-Zúñiga, M.D.

Pharmacologic management has an important role in the success of percutaneous transluminal angioplasty (PTA) that is much more relevant than its role in any other cardiovascular and interventional procedure. This is due to the complex response induced in the arterial wall and circulating blood by the injury provoked by the balloon inflation or by the changes induced by other revascularization procedures, such as lasers, atherectomy, and stents.

There are many factors involved in this response, with complex relationships and mechanisms that still need to be clarified. Understanding and controlling these processes is a current focus of research on PTA, since the success of these procedures in the immediate, short term, and long term is thought to be decisively conditioned by the chain of events started by the arterial wall injury. Manipulation of these changes during and after the procedure is thought to be an important factor in affecting the long-term outcome of these procedures.

Vasospasm is certainly one of the main factors involved. Spasm may occur in two different set-ups during or after the procedure. In the first of the two situations, it is not specifically related to the dilating procedure; it is an event directly related to the catheterization itself and for this reason has been well known since long before the beginning of angioplasty. Catheter-induced vasospasm may occur even in presumed rigid and thick-walled arteries; it is more common in the external iliac artery, and very frequent in smaller vessels, such as the popliteal or tibioperoneal arteries.[1,2] The consequences of this type of spasm are that catheter manipulations are made difficult and sometimes risky; the flow is reduced and this predisposes to a subsequent thrombosis. In addition, the real extension of a lesion can be overestimated.[1,3] Treatment of this eventuality, whenever present or suspected, is necessary; prophylactic medication in selected patients, such as those undergoing angioplasty of small vessels, is advisable.

The second type of vasospasm is more specifically related to the balloon dilation itself. It may occur in as many as 25% of cases in PTA of renal arteries, in spite of premedication.[4] Even transient vasospasm has relevant consequences in critical vascular beds.[5] Moreover, vasospasm is thought to be, together with intimal dissection, thrombosis, and elastic arterial recoil, an important contributing factor to the immediate failure of PTA, with acute vascular occlusion.[6–8] It is also suspected to be a possible contributor to restenosis,[9–11] but there is no agreement on this point; in some reviews vasospasm is not even mentioned.[12]

Studies in vitro have shown that spontaneous vasospasm after PTA is related to the dilating force; moderate dilation enhances the vasospastic response, whereas greater dilation forces attenuate the vasospastic response. This explains why vasospasm is most likely to occur at the margins of dilated segments, where the dilating pressure is less.[6] Vasospasm is probably a multifactorial effect. Factors to be considered among the possible mechanisms are: a neurogenic input; vasoactive substances (mainly thromboxane A_2 and serotonin) released from platelets that adhere to the injured arterial wall;[10,13,14] a consequence of thrombosis, either indirect due to induced platelet activation or directly related to vasoactive products of the coagulation chain released following local fibrin deposition, such as fibropeptides and fibrin split products;[5] loss of endothelial vasodilators such as prostacyclin and the endothelium-derived relaxant factor;[5,15] and release of endothelially derived contractile factor, probably a cyclooxygenase-derived product.[16]

The dreaded consequences of vasospasm, either clearly demonstrated or reasonably suspected, impose pharmacologic prophylaxis and treatment. This can be done by two different means: either by directly treating the arterial contraction or by indirectly controlling the possible etiologic cause, namely, platelet aggregation and fibrin deposition. In this review, the principal drugs considered in clinical practice are discussed.

DIRECT ANTISPASM THERAPY

Nitrates and Nitrites: Nitroglycerin

Nitroglycerin (glyceryl trinitrate) is considered the premier of the group of nitrate and nitrite vasodilators. It is a very selective drug; its action is directed almost exclusively to the smooth muscle cells, thus relaxing the vascular wall. In the vascular system, the dilation is relatively less in arterioles and precapillary sphincters. In common clinical practice, nitroglycerin is used in the treatment of angina pectoris. Its specific action in this case is not due to direct coronary dilation, but to a reduction of the ventricular preload because of peripheral venous dilation. The liver has a high capacity to inactivate the drug. When directly injected into an artery, the vessel dilates and spasm is prevented or relieved if present.

With the sublingual route, there is a rapid onset of action (1 to 2 minutes); the effect lasts for a short period of time, not more than 20 to 30 minutes.[17]

Nitroglycerin is therefore used in peripheral angioplasty whenever arterial spasm is present or suspected in relation to catheter and wire manipulations.[1,8] Its use is suggested immediately before balloon angioplasty in order to prevent undesired spastic reactions during the procedure.[3] The preferred route of administration is intra-arterial, directly above the area of interest; the normal dose is 100 μc, which can be repeated at will if a more prolonged effect is desired.[1] Caution has to be taken, since a hypotensive reaction or reflex tachycardia can occur.[8,17] The sublingual route is less desirable, being considered as less selective. Transdermal administration is recommended by some authors for a longer duration of action.[1]

Calcium Antagonist Drugs: Nifedipine and Verapamil

These drugs act by blocking transmembrane calcium influx, which is responsible for normal reflex tone and contractile responses. This group of drugs is clinically used in the treatment of many conditions, including hypertension, angina pectoris, and cardiac arrhythmias.[17]

The calcium antagonist drugs differ in their cardiovascular effect; verapamil and diltiazem decrease atrioventricular conduction, whereas nifedipine does not affect it. Therefore, although verapamil is contraindicated in bradyarrhythmias, reflex tachycardia in response to hypotension is most likely to occur with nifedipine, thus precipitating an anginal attack. The negative inotropic effect of these drugs may worsen congestive heart failure, but the arteriolar dilating effect of nifedipine balances this drawback, making, in this case, nifedipine preferable to verapamil.[8,17]

The prophylactic use of calcium antagonists to prevent vasospasm in angioplasty is recommended. Patients already receiving calcium antagonists do not need further medications. The drug of choice is usually nifedipine, with a careful consideration of possible cardiac effects. It may be given orally with a dose of 10 to 30 mg/day, or by the sublingual route immediately before the procedure[1,3] (by puncturing the capsule and squeezing the liquid under the patient's tongue).[8] In this way, the effect starts in 10 to 15 minutes and lasts for 4 to 6 hours.

Experimental studies on efficacy of verapamil showed that this drug prevented vasospasm only in the presence of heparin.[5] Studies on the long-term effects of prolonged (6 weeks to 6 months) use of nifedipine after angioplasty showed no benefit on prevention of restenosis.[18] This suggests that restenosis may not be due to spasm.[19]

INDIRECT ANTISPASM THERAPY

Antispastic effect may be achieved by blocking the two components of thrombus formation, namely, platelet aggregation and fibrin deposition, since fibrin split products and platelet derivations have a vasospastic effect.

Antiplatelet Aggregation

In platelet aggregation, arachidonic acid is released and transformed to endoperoxides by cyclooxygenase enzyme. Endoperoxides may be transformed in different metabolites; for example, platelets help transform endoperoxides in thromboxane A_2, a powerful stimulator of platelet aggregation and vasospasm; on the contrary, endothelial cells help in the transformation of endoperoxides into prostacyclin, which has the opposite effect of thromboxane.

Platelet aggregation by itself is considered an undesired effect of angioplasty for its probable role in restenosis; antiplatelet therapy is therefore thought to be an important means of preventing restenosis; however, clinical results are controversial.[11,20]

The problem is particularly complex in relation to possible antispastic effects. Aspirin, one of the most common drugs in antiplatelet therapy, acts by blocking the cyclooxygenase; as a consequence, a nonspecific effect may result, since not only the platelet vasospastic metabolites could be inhibited, but also the endothelial vasodilating products.[6,8,11]

In clinical experience, an antiaggregant effect is obtained with low doses of aspirin, but the opposite happens at higher doses. This could also be due to individual absorption variations. There is no agreement therefore on the use of aspirin in angioplasty. Some prescribe it indefinitely, others only for very short terms, and others do not include it in the pharmacologic therapy.[6,8]

More selective goals in antiplatelet—and therefore antispasm—therapy could be achieved, on the one hand, with more selective inhibitors or, on the other hand, with the administration of synthetic prostacyclin.[6,21] The antiplatelet adhesion properties of dextran could be used,[11] but caution is required due to the risk of severe anaphylactic reactions with consequent severe vasospasm.[22]

Antifibrin Deposition

The undesired effect of fibrin deposition can be controlled by heparin, which interferes in this process by accelerating the neutralization of several clotting factors. Inhibition by heparin of acute platelet and fibrinogen deposition is dose dependent.[23] Heparin is the most commonly used drug in the clinical practice of angioplasty. It is generally given with a systemic infusion of 2500 to 10,000 U immediately before the dilation procedure. Heparin's action is twofold: direct on fibrin deposition and indirect over platelet accumulation. Consequently, less thromboxane A_2 is released, and, in this way, a powerful stimulation of vasospasm is blocked.[5,8]

Heparin administration may be limited to a single bolus injection, or continued for 24 hours or more in particular conditions, such as in below-knee angioplasty or when the surface of the dilated segment is long or looks irregular, with careful monitoring of the coagulation parameters.[1] The half-life of heparin is basically 1 hour, but it may vary in patients with kidney and liver dysfunctions and is also dose dependent.

After heparin administration, the introducer sheaths used for balloon introduction should not be removed immediately, due to the risk of prolonged bleeding and hematoma formation at the puncture site. The sheath itself is infused with a very small dose of heparin (5 to 20 U/hour) to prevent thrombus formation within it. If necessary, intravenous protamine can be used to reverse the heparin effect.[7]

As an alternative to heparin, the use of polysulfate of pentosan has been proposed;[24] in animal experiments, hirudin proved to be more effective than heparin in preventing thrombosis, probably because of a more specific and potent inhibition.[23]

REFERENCES

1. Schwarten DE. Aortic, iliac and peripheral arterial angioplasty. In Castañeda-Zúñiga WR, Murthy Tadavarthy S (eds): Interventional Radiology. Baltimore: Williams & Wilkins, 1988:268–97.
2. Zeitler E, Grüntzig A, Schoop W (eds). Percutaneous vascular recanalization: Technology, application, clinical results. Berlin: Springer-Verlag, 1978.
3. McDermott JE, Crummy AB, Voeglli DW, et al. Complications of transluminal angioplasty. (Letter.) Radiology 1987;162:286–7.
4. Beinart C, Sos TA, Saddenklni S, et al. Arterial spasm during renal angioplasty. Radiology 1983;149:97–100.
5. LeVeen RF, Wolf GL, Biery D. Angioplasty-induced vasospasm in rabbit model. Mechanism and treatment. Invest Radiol 1985;20:938–66.
6. Zollikofer CL, Cragg AH, Hunter DW, et al. Mechanism of transluminal angioplasty. In Castañeda-Zúñiga WR, Murthy Tadavarthy S (eds): Interventional Radiology. Baltimore: Williams & Wilkins, 1988:207–65.
7. Gardiner GA, Meyerovitz MF, Harrington DP. Complication of transluminal angioplasty. (Letter.) Radiology 1987;162: 287–8.
8. Becker GJ, Katzen BT, Dake MD. Noncoronary angioplasty. Radiology 1989;170:921–60.
9. Hallman J, Austin GE, Grüntzig AR, et al. Coronary artery spasm at the site of angioplasty in the fist 2 months after successful percutaneous transluminal coronary angioplasty. J Am Coll Cardiol 1983;2:1039–45.
10. Wilentz JR, Sanborn TA, Haudenschild CC, et al. Platelet accumulation in experimental angioplasty time course and relation to vascular injury. Circulation 1987;75:636–42.
11. Pope CF, Ezkovitz MD, Smith EO, et al. Detection of platelet deposition at the site of peripheral balloon angioplasty using indium-111 platelet scintigraphy. Am J Cardiol 1985;55: 495–7.
12. Cox JL, Gottlieb AJ. Restenosis following percutaneous transluminal angioplasty: clinical, physiologic and pathologic features. Can Med Assoc J 1986;134:1129–32.
13. Lam JYT, Chesebro JH, Steele PM, et al. Is vasospasm related to platelet deposition? Relationship in a porcine preparation of arterial injury in vivo. Circulation 1987;75:243–8.
14. Vanhoutte PM, Houston DS. Platelets, endothelium, and vasospasm. Circulation 1985;72:728–31.
15. Vallance P. EDRF and microvascular constriction after angioplasty. Lancet 1989;1:1139.
16. Fischell TA, Nellessen V, Johnson DE, et al. Endothelium-dependent arterial vasoconstriction after balloon angioplasty. Circulation 1989;79:899–910.
17. Katzung BG, Chatterjee K. Vasodilators and the treatment of angina pectoris. In Katzung BG (ed): Basic and Clinical Pharmacology. Norwalk: Appleton & Lange, 1987:125–37.
18. Whitworth HB, Roubin GS, Hollman J, et al: Effect of nifedipine on recurrent stenosis after percutaneous transluminal coronary angioplasty. J Am Coll Cardiol 1986;8:1271–6.
19. Kemp HG: Coronary angioplasty and the persistent problem of restenosis. J Am Coll Cardiol 1986;8:1277–8.
20. Minar E, Eringer H, Ahmad R, et al. Platelet deposition at angioplasty sites and its relation to restenosis in human iliac and femoropopliteal arteries. Radiology 1989;170:767–72.
21. Riess H, Höfling B, vonArnin T, et al. Thromboxane receptor blockade versus cyclooxygenase inhibition: antiplatelets effects in patients. Thromb Res 1986;42:235–45.
22. Klugmann S, Salvi A, Valente M, et al. Coronary artery spasm after administration of dextran 40: implications concerning percutaneous transluminal coronary angioplasty. Am Heart J 1986;1202–6.
23. Heras M, Cheseko JH, Penny WJ, et al. Effects of thrombin inhibition on the development of acute platelet-thrombus deposition during angioplasty in pigs. Circulation 1989;79:657–65.
24. Menanteau B, Gausserand F, Marcus C, et al. Le polysulfate de pentosane, traitement adjuvant de l'angioplastie transluminale des artères des membres inférieurs. Presse Med 1986;15:213.

5 Transluminal Angioplasty of Peripheral Vascular Disease: Aggregation Inhibitors

Reingard Sörensen, M.D., Soraya Wenig, M.D.

Successful percutaneous transluminal angioplasty (PTA) causes a split of the arteriosclerotic plaque, the intima, and the media of the vascular wall.[1–8] A deep intimal injury and an underlying localized dissection of the media is necessary to produce immediate and long-term improvement of narrowed or occluded vascular segments. Stretching of the media is another important mechanism.[1] Irreversible overstretching of the vascular wall, however, results in disruption of the intercellular junctions of the medial smooth muscle cells and is followed by necrosis of the myocytes. Histologic studies on vascular walls of dogs following the acute injury of angioplasty showed pyknotic cell nuclei of the smooth muscle cells.[9] In spite of those lacerations, several weeks after the injury there was removal of the necrotic debris by macrophages and evidence of a neointima. Additional therapy during and following the procedure of percutaneous transluminal angioplasty can help to maintain vascular patency and may prevent recurrent disease.

THROMBOGENESIS

The injury to the endothelium causes close contact of blood and the subendothelial structures. Subendothelial structures are mainly collagen fibers. Collagen induces platelet adhesion and aggregation. The platelets interact with the protein of the thrombocyte membrane and the subendothelial collagen and platelet adhesions, especially of Factor VIII. Platelet adhesions induce platelet aggregation. The alpha granules of the thrombocytes produce adenosine diphosphate (ADP), platelet factor 4, beta globulin, and platelet-derived growth factor. Together with the activation of the platelet membrane phospholipase complex, thromboxane A is created. Thromboxane A and ADP activate the circulation of platelets.[10–16] Fibrin receptors at the surface of aggregated platelets capture fibrinogen. In the presence of calcium and these aggregates fibrin becomes stable. Thrombin mainly has an influence on the growth of a thrombus, because very small amounts of thrombin at the surface of the platelets activate the coagulation system. The amount of thrombin increases during this process. Thrombin splits fibrinogen into fibrin. A network of fibrin finally stabilizes the thrombus.[14,15,17–21]

MECHANISM OF PERCUTANEOUS TRANSLUMINAL ANGIOPLASTY AND RESTENOSIS

According to Harker,[15] there is evidence from animal studies that the proliferative intimal lesion formed in arteries after mechanical or endothelial denudation is platelet dependent. The loss of endothelium and the consequent adherence, aggregation, and release of platelets are followed by migration of smooth muscle cells from the media into the intima and by proliferation of those cells in response to released mitogens. Besides angioplasty, other mechanically induced endothelial injuries produce arterial stenosis and occlusion (endarterectomies, vascular grafts, indwelling catheters, vascular stents). Several growth factors have the potential to induce smooth muscle cell proliferation within the intima of human arteries. Growth factors are released from platelets. They are released in high concentrations at the sites of vascular injury and platelet deposition.[2,9,12,15,20–36] Despite a significant increase in the primary success of PTA, restenosis has complicated the long-term cure rate. This is particularly true for percutaneous transluminal coronary angioplasty, where restenosis has been reported in as many as 30% of patients. The factors responsible for restenoses and its prevention are not known.

AGGREGATION INHIBITION

The effect of antiplatelet agents to prevent restenosis has been studied. In 25 New Zealand rabbits bilateral iliac stenoses were created by balloon deendothelialization and a cholesterol diet. After creation of atherosclerosis, angioplasty was performed. An average increase in luminal diameter of 81% could be established. Seven rabbits received aspirin plus dipyridamole; nine received sulfinpyrazone, and nine served as controls. Following 4 weeks of drug therapy and continuation of the diet, angiography was repeated and the rabbits were sacrificed for histologic examination. At angiography, the diameter of the vascular lumen was similar for these groups. Four weeks later, however, the vascular diameter was significantly larger in both the aspirin plus dipyridamole and the sulfinpyrazone groups when compared with the control rabbits ($p < 0.05$). Histologically, intraluminal clots were seen in four of nine controls and in none of the drug-treated rabbits. The authors concluded that the use of antiplatelet agents in clinical angioplasty is to be recommended.[27–29,31,33–39]

If platelet aggregation following angioplasty is not treated, there would always be a thrombus at the site of vascular injury. Thrombi form by sequential accretion of alternating layers of fibrin and platelets. Therefore it is important to limit those aspects during PTA. In both platelets and endothelial cells, the metabolism of prostaglandin endoperoxides has a profound regulatory impact on this process. In platelets arachidonic acid is mobilized from the cell membranes by the action of the enzyme phospholipase A_2. This mobilization also occurs in endothelial cells. Cyclooxygenase converts arachidonates to endoperoxides. In endothelial cells, endoperoxides are converted by the action of prostacyclin synthesis to prostacyclin (PGI_2). PGI_2 prevents platelet aggregation, disaggregates platelet clumps, and is a potent vasodilator. In platelets, endoperoxides are converted by the action of thromboxane synthesis to thromboxane A_2 (TXA_2). TXA_2 induces platelet aggregation and constricts arterial smooth muscles. Although TXA_2 has a very short half-life and is rapidly metabolized to TXB_2, its extremely potent effects in its environment demand that it should be inhibited during PTA. Although aspirin is a nonspecific inhibitor of cyclooxygenase, small doses cause acetylation of cyclooxygenase, a reduction of TXA_2, and thereby a tipping of the endoperoxide metabolic balance in favor of PGI_2 predominance and away from TXA_2. Although the clinical manifestation of impaired platelet function is prolongation of the bleeding time, the desired effect is decreased by platelet activation and aggregation during and after PTA.

Once aggregation and adhesions have occurred, the release of platelet factors such as ADP, thromboxane, and platelet growth factors may promote aggregation, clot formation, vasospasm, and smooth muscle cell proliferation. This may be the pathway through which platelet adhesion could promote atherosclerosis. This is still unknown. Nevertheless, platelets apparently play an important role in the progress of atherosclerosis. Aspirin plus dipyridamole can inhibit platelet aggregation. There are, however, potentially important differences in their pharmacologic action. Aspirin blocks platelet cyclooxygenase. At high doses, it may also reduce the formation of PGI_2 from the vascular wall. PGI_2 is a potent inhibitor of platelet adhesion and function. Dipyridamole inhibits platelet phosphodiesterase, and thereby may increase cyclic adenosine monophosphate (cAMP) levels. It is postulated that the increase in cAMP may reduce platelet function. In experimental studies, the combination of low-dose aspirin and dipyridamole has potentiated the inhibitory effect of each other on platelet aggregation. Sulfinpyrazone blocks cyclooxygenase reversibly, but it does not block PGI_2. Neither aspirin nor sulfinpyrazone appear to prevent platelet adhesion. In addition, sulfinpyrazone may have a stabilizing effect on damaged endothelial cells as well as lengthening shortened platelet survival. Baumgartner et al[10,29] showed less neointimal thickening in rabbits treated with sulfinpyrazone than in those treated with aspirin or dipyridamole.[39–42] These factors may be important after PTA, when the denuded endothelium needs time to regenerate. The results of this study do not show a significant difference between these two regimens, and both are effective in preventing intraluminal thrombosis. There is, however, the suggestion in different publications that rabbits treated with sulfinpyrazone have less intimal thickening than those treated with aspirin plus dipyridamole, as is evident from a slightly larger luminal diameter at 4 weeks. The difference is not statistically significant.[40,43–48]

Studies of antiplatelet drugs in the prevention of intimal thickening in coronary bypass grafts yielded findings similar to those of previous studies. Aspirin plus dipyridamole reduced intimal thickening in dogs who had vein grafts placed.[49] More recently, the benefit of aspirin plus dipyridamole in patients was reported by Chesebro et al.[34] Sulfinpyrazone has been reported to reduce vein graft occlusion in patients who have undergone coronary artery bypass grafts. Those forms of injury appear to be compatible with the response to the hypothesis of injury of atherosclerosis.[50]

The results of animal experiments are unlike human atherosclerosis in many respects. Human lesions are more necrotic and fibrotic and may respond differently to these agents. In addition, the doses of sulfinpyrazone used in these studies exceed the usual doses used in human beings. The doses of aspirin plus dipyridamole are more appropriate. Finally, antiplatelet drugs are used in clinical angioplasty, but restenosis occurs despite the use of these agents. Additional mechanisms or more potent drugs are necessary to prevent restenosis in man.[14,15,35]

THERAPEUTIC TRIALS

Pharmacologic modification of platelet behavior has been shown to reduce vascular occlusion. The indications for clinical use, however, are not clear. There is a lack of knowledge of the precise pathogenesis of this process, a lack of suitable pharmacologic agents for definitive clinical testing, and a lack of adequately controlled clinical studies.

In cerebrovascular atherosclerotic disease, aspirin has been shown to reduce stroke or death in men with transient ischemic attacks. There was no additional benefit by combining aspirin with dipyridamole and sulfinpyrazone. No benefit was found using sulfinpyrazone, dipyridamole, or sulfinpyrazone alone.[52–55]

In coronary atherosclerotic disease, six studies have assessed the efficacy of aspirin alone in patients after acute myocardial infarction. Five studies, incorporating a range of doses from 300 to 1500 mg daily, reported trends in favor of aspirin. In contrast, the Aspirin Myocardial Infarction Study demonstrated no effect of aspirin. A subsequent analysis, in which the results of all the aspirin trials were combined, suggested that there may be a benefit of aspirin. The pooled estimate of risk reduction with aspirin was 16% ($p < 0.01$); for the outcome of first infarctions, fatal or nonfatal, the pooled estimate of risk reduction was 21% ($p < 0.001$). As a result, the present evidence for a beneficial effect of aspirin therapy in the prevention of myocardial infarction is inconclusive. Additionally, the efficacy of sulfinpyrazone alone was not established. In contrast to the inconclusive results in acute myocardial infarction, aspirin (324 to 1300 mg daily) clearly reduces myocardial infarction or cardiac death in patients with unstable angina. The efficacy of aspirin in patients with unstable angina parallels the beneficial results with aspirin in patients with transient cerebral ischemia and suggests the possibility of similar mechanisms.[51–56]

In coronary bypass grafting using autogenous saphenous veins, over 90% of patients can be expected to have improvement or absence of symptoms of angina for at least 1 year after surgery. Graft patency rates are reported to be about 90% at 2 weeks and 65 to 85% at 1 year. The major factors to vein graft occlusion are thrombosis and intimal proliferation within the graft. It is believed that early vein graft occlusion occurs secondary to thrombosis and later graft occlusion is related to intimal proliferation. The combined regimen of aspirin and dipyridamole in bypass graft surgery prevents both early and late graft occlusion. The capacity of the aspirin and dipyridamole to synergistically normalize platelet survival has been proven in animal models of arterial thrombosis. Although previous investigators reported less or no benefit using this combination, none had initiated antiplatelet therapy before bypass graft surgery. However, the relative importance of drug combination compared with either agent used singly was not addressed by this study. In a smaller study, a significant antithrombotic effect of low-dose aspirin was reported for patients undergoing coronary artery bypass surgery. To resolve the question of relative efficacy for the various regimens reported to show benefit, the Veterans Administration Cooperative Group had organized a double blind, randomized multicenter clinical trial. Patients are being randomly assigned to one of five treatment groups (aspirin 325 mg once daily; aspirin 325 mg three times daily; aspirin 325 mg plus dipyridamole 75 mg three times daily; sulfinpyrazone 267 mg three times daily; placebo). Results are pending.

The effect of platelet-modifying drugs on the progression of peripheral vascular disease has recently been assessed angiographically in the first controlled trial reported. The 240 patients were randomized into one of three treatment groups (aspirin 330 mg, dipyridamole 75 mg plus aspirin 330 mg, and placebo, all three times daily). Treatment was maintained for 2 years. Arteriography was performed at the entry into the study and at 2 years or earlier if deterioration was observed; 199 patients completed the study. Paired arteriograms were assessed in a blinded manner both qualitatively, by means of simple comparative viewing, and semiquantitatively using an objective scoring system. Progression of the disease was most pronounced in the placebo-treated group, less in the aspirin-treated group, and least in the dipyridamole and aspirin groups. In the paired comparisons the difference between the patients receiving the aspirin-dipyridamole combination and the placebo group was statistically significant ($p < 0.001$). The difference between the patients receiving the combination versus aspirin-only treatment was also statistically significant ($p < 0.001$) in favor of the combination. There was no significant difference between the aspirin and the placebo groups. The results of this study show that the natural course of peripheral atherosclerotic disease may be slowed by long-term treatment with a combination of dipyridamole and aspirin. Combined treatment with dipyridamole and aspirin is superior to the use of aspirin alone. This report requires independent confirmation.

Vascular grafts have been successfully used in large human blood vessels for a long time. Indium-111 platelet imaging studies have shown platelet deposition continuing for many years. This technique has also been used to assess the capacity of antiplatelet therapy to reduce platelet deposition. Whereas combination therapy with aspirin and dipyridamole is known to reduce platelet deposition in patients with femoropopliteal grafts, no other drug has been reported to be effective. Smaller caliber prosthetic vascular grafts may fail because of occlusive thrombosis or embolization from their thrombogenic surface. The anastomosis of a graft and the vascular wall is particularly prone to thrombus formation, due to the endothelial injury together with the narrowing by intimal proliferation. Despite improved material and antiplatelet agents, vascular grafts with an internal diameter less than 5 mm become occluded. Biomaterial with little reactivity to flowing blood and with characteristics that promote endothelial coverage or those that inhibit anastomotic initimal stenosis will be required for successful grafting of small vessels. Because the effect of antiplatelet agents on the long-term patency of prosthetic grafts is inconclusive, no general recommendation can be made at present.[51–61]

SIDE EFFECTS

The side effects of aspirin therapy are well documented in the literature. They are dosage dependent except for allergic reactions.[44,62–70] Common complications include gastrointestinal symptoms and signs in 5 to 25% (abdominal discomfort, gastric pain, vomiting, hematemesis, gastric ulcers, melena.[58,61,67,68,71–85]) May[85] reported a cumulative study from the United States. Gastric symptoms with and without gastric ulcerations were found in 22 to 48%, and in 10 to 25% treatment had to be terminated. In almost all patients mucosal erosions could be seen endoscopically.[58] An adaptation of the gastric mucosa in patients receiving long-term treatment of aspirin can be expected after 1 to 9 weeks. This is dose dependent. The gastrointestinal blood loss increases with the increasing dose.[58]

Especially in children but also in adults there is a syndrome called "salicylism" in patients receiving aspirin over a long period of time.[82,85] This is actually an intoxication by accumulation of aspirin. Symptoms include neurologic signs such as dizziness, headache, hyperventilation, convulsions; acidosis, dehydration, hypopotassemia with reduced alkaline reserve.[82] In the United States more than 10,000 salicylate intoxications are reported, including deaths. Allergic reactions to aspirin are rare.

DOSAGE

Oral anticoagulants are suitable for the delay of progression of arteriosclerosis. The therapeutic effect is bound to the stability of the hypocoagulation with values of thromboplastin time between 15 and 20%. There is a high risk of thrombosis after discontinuation of this therapy. Of the inhibitors of thrombolytic function, acetylic acid preparations are antithrombotically effective. The controversies of dosages, high (1500 mg daily) or low (20 to 30 mg daily), are opposed by the concept of individual dosages.

Acetylsalicylic acid is the most common aggregation inhibitor. There is an antithrombotic effect by the drug itself as well as by the salicylate created by fast hydrolysis. There is acetylation not only of the thrombus creating platelet enzymes, but there is also a uniform effect on the proteins and enzymes of different localization and function. The antithrombotic and antiatherosclerotic effects of aspirin are: (1) inhibition of cyclooxygenase with decreased aggregation creating thromboxane; (2) loss of chemotaxis of the macrophages; and (3) hypothetically, the inhibition of the platelet growth factor with inhibition of the proliferation of the smooth muscle cells, the morphologic nucleus of atherosclerosis.

Salicylate is a preserving factor against inhibition of prostacyclin synthesis. It has an antiarrhythmic effect and is responsible for the fibrinolytic activity of aspirin.[63,64] Unfortunately, high doses of aspirin may have the opposite effect. The problem is that the rate of absorption of aspirin from the gastrointestinal tract varies with gastric pH and the presence or absence of food. The plasma concentration of salicylate depends on the volume of distribution.[1,37,38] The inhibition of platelet function may obtain the desired effect with one baby aspirin in some patients (81.25 mg daily), whereas in others little effect derives from the same dose. Although individualized dose regimens based on in vitro platelet function studies may seem ideal, this approach is not feasible. For all these reasons, the "ideal" dose does not exist. There has been a dose identified that is the best for most people. Therefore most physicians who perform PTA have decided to prescribe either one baby aspirin per day or one adult aspirin per day. Some prescribe aspirin only around the time of PTA, and others prescribe it indefinitely.[1,37–43]

There is an interesting study published by Norden and Heine[63,64] concerning the necessity to find an individual dose (standard dose, 20 to 1500 mg). This dose should be calculated according to the aspirin test and the disaggregation rate. This test is able to discover aspirin-resistant patients, and such patients should be treated with a different drug. There is also the possibility of using a therapy-free interval to calculate the initial dose. Of the patients in the study, 29% are nonresponders. Of the responders, 45% need only a dose up to 250 mg, 38%, up to 500 mg, 14%, up to 1000 mg, and 3% need more than 1000 mg as indicated by the therapy-free intervals of 1, 2, or 3 days. It cannot be ruled out that some patients need only 20 to 30 mg daily. The minimal possible dose and the ministandard dose show a decrease of side effects. Concerning the length of treatment with aspirin, no clinical studies have been described in the literature. In comparison with anticoagulant therapy, it is assumed that a delay in the progression of the atherosclerotic process can only be achieved under continuous treatment with aspirin.

EFFECTIVENESS OF ASPIRIN THERAPY

In 1988 a study was published in the *British Medical Journal*[55] describing the effectiveness of all aggregation inhibitors in 29,000 patients with transient ischemic attacks, nonhemorrhagic brain infarcts, variant angina pectoris, or myocardial infarction. The results of the study showed a decrease of the lethality of vascular disease in 15% and a decrease of the amount of nonlethal brain and myocardial infarcts of 30%. There was no difference in the effectiveness of high-dose (900 to 1500 mg) and low-dose (300 to 325 mg) therapy with aspirin. There was also no difference when compared to the treatment of aspirin alone and aspirin in combination with dipyridamole. This study does not include the individual doses of aspirin. Another study by Norden and Heine[63,64] showed that under the treatment of 30 mg aspirin per day the frequency of reinfarction was 6.7% in comparison with 15.9% under treatment with 1500 mg aspirin.[63,64]

The efficacy of acetylsalicylic acid and dipyridamole for prevention of recurrence of femoral and popliteal arterial lesions following PTA has been studied in a randomized and double blind trial in three groups: 156 patients were given placebo, 100 mg aspirin plus 75 mg dipyridamole, and 330 mg acetylsalicylic acid alone three times daily, starting 1 to 2 hours after PTA. There was no significant difference among the groups.[75]

CONCLUSION

We know that anticoagulation therapy can prevent myocardial infarction. There has been a reduction of 20% (8 to 15% for acetylsalicylic acid) concerning lethality and 50% (20 to 25% for acetylsalicylic acid) concerning reinfarction. Acetylsalicylic acid is the most important aggregation inhibitor.

REFERENCES

1. Becker GJ, Katzen BT, Dake MD. Noncoronary angioplasty. Radiology 1989;170:921–40.

2. Block PC, Fallon JT, Elmer D. Experimental angioplasty: lessons from the laboratory. AJR 1980;135:907–12.
3. Block PC. Mechanism of transluminal angioplasty. Am J Cardiol 1984;53(suppl C):69C–71C.
4. Castañeda-Zúñiga WR, Formanek A, Tadavarthy M. The mechanism of balloon angioplasty. Radiology 1980;135:565–71.
5. Cragg AH, Einzig S, Rysavy JA, et al. The vasa vasorum and angioplasty. Radiology 1983;148:75–80.
6. LeVeen RF, Wolf GL, Turco MA. Morphometric changes in normal arteries and those undergoing transluminal angioplasty. Invest Radiol 1983;18:63–7.
7. Wolf GL, LeVeen RF, Ring EJ. Potential mechanisms of angioplasty. Cardiovasc Intervent Radiol 1984;7:11–7.
8. Zollikofer CL, Redha FH, Bruhlmann WF, et al. Acute and long-term effects of massive balloon dilatation on the aortic wall and vasa vasorum. Radiology 1987;164:145–9.
9. Castañeda-Zúñiga WR, Amplatz K, Laerum F. Mechanics of angioplasty: an experimental approach. Radiographics 1981; 1:1–14.
10. Baumgartner HR, Muggli R. Adhesion and aggregation: morphological demonstration and quantitation in vivo and in vitro. In Gordon JL (ed): Platelets in biology and pathology. New York: Elsevier, 1976:23–39.
11. Berndt MC, Philips DR. Platelet membrane proteins: composition and receptor function. In Gordon JL (ed): Platelets in biology and pathology. New York: Elsevier, 1981:43–75.
12. George JN, Nurden AT, Philips DR. Molecular defects in interactions of platelets with the vessel wall. N Engl J Med 1984;311:1084–98.
13. Gerard JM, White JG. Prostaglandins and thromboxanes: "middlemen" modulation platelet function in hemostasis and thrombosis. Prog Hemost Thromb 1982;4:87–125.
14. Harker LA, Ross R, Slichter SJ, Scott C. Homocystine-induced arteriosclerosis: the role of endothelial cell injury and platelet response in its genesis. J Clin Invest: 1976;58:731–41.
15. Harker LA: Role of platelets and thrombosis in mechanism of acute occlusion and restenosis after angioplasty. Am J Cardiol 1987;60:20B–28B.
16. Zucker MB. The functioning of blood platelets. Sci Am 1980;242:86–103.
17. Bowen-Pope DF, Ross R. Platelet derived growth factor. II. Specific binding to cultured cells. J Biol Chem 1982; 357:5161–71.
18. Bowen-Pope DF, Ross R. Is epidermal growth factor in human blood? Alteration of EGF binding specificity in the radioreceptor assay. Biophys Res Commun 1983;114:1036–41.
19. Deuel TF, Senior RM, Huang JS, Griffin GL. Chemotaxis of monocytes and neutrophils to platelet-derived growth factor. J Clin Invest 1982;69:1046–9.
20. Friedman RJ, Stemerman MB, Wenz B, et al. The effect of thrombocytopenia on experimental arteriosclerotic lesion formation in rabbits. Smooth muscle proliferation and re-endothelialization. J Clin Invest 1977;60:1191–202.
21. Fuster V, Bowie JW, Lewis JC, et al. Resistance to arteriosclerosis in pigs with von Willebrand's disease. J Clin Invest 1981;61:722–30.
22. Heldin CH, Westerkark B, Wasteson A. Platelet-derived growth factor: purification and partial characterization. Proc Natl Acad Sci USA 1979;76:3722–6.
23. Heldin CH, Westermark B, Wasteson A. Specific receptors for platelet derived growth factor on cells derived from connective tissue and glia. Proc Natl Acad Sci USA 1981;79:3664–3668.
24. Ross R, Raines EW, Bowen-Pope DF. The biology of platelet-derived growth factor. Cell 1986;46:155–69.
25. Ross R. The pathogenesis of atherosclerosis an update. N Engl J Med 1986;314:488–500.
26. Seppa H, Grotendorst G, Seppa S, et al. Platelet-derived growth factor is chemotactic for fibroblasts. J Cell Biol 1982;92:584–8.
27. Steele PM, Chesebro PM, Stanson JH, et al. Balloon angioplasty. Natural history of the pathophysiological response to injury in a pig model. Circ Res 1985;57:105–112.
28. Lam JYT, Chesebro JH, Steele PM, et al. Deep arterial injury during experimental angioplasty. Relationship to a positive 111 indium-labeled platelet scintigram, quantitative platelet deposition, and mural thrombus. J Am Coll Cardiol 1986;8:1380–6.
29. Baumgartner HR, Sakariassen KS. Factors controlling thrombus formation on arterial lesions. Ann NY Acad Sci 1985;454:162–77.
30. Sanborn TA, Faxon DP, Haudenschild C, et al. The mechanism of transluminal angioplasty: evidence for formation of aneurysms in experimental atherosclerosis. Circulation 1983; 68:1136–40.
31. Houdijk WPM, Sakariassen KS, Nievelstein PFEM, Sixma JJ. Role of factor VIII—von Willebrand's factor—and fibrinectin in the interaction of platelets in flowing blood with monomeric and fibrillar human collagen types I and III. J Clin Invest 1985;75:531–540.
32. Schneider E, Grüntzig A, Bollinger A. Langzeitergebnisse nach perkutaner transluminaler Angioplastie (PTA) bei 882 konsekutiven Patienten mit iliakalen und femoral-poplitealen Obstruktionen. Vasa 1982;11:322–6.
33. Faxon DP, Sanborn TA, Haudenschild CC, Ryan TJ. Effect of antiplatelet therapy on restenosis after experimental angioplasty: Am J Cardiol 1984;53(suppl C):72–6.
34. Chesebro JH, Lam JYT, Badimon L, Fuster V. Restenosis after arterial angioplasty: a hemorrheologic response to injury. Am J Cardiol 1987;60(suppl B):10–16.
35. Hanley SP, Bevan J. Inhibition by aspirin of human arterial and venous prostacyclin synthesis. Prostaglandins Leukotrienes Med 1885;20:141–9.
36. Eckstein HH, Müller-Bühl U, Zimmermann R, Diehm C. Bedeutung der Acetylsalicylsäure in der Sekundärprevention der peripheren arteriellen Verschlußkrankheit. Dtsch Med Wochenschr 1988;113:822–7.
37. Davi G, Pinto A, Palumbo MG, et al. Dipyridamole and aspirin in arteriosclerosis obliterans of the lower limbs. Adv Prostaglandin, Thromboxane, Leukotriene Res 1985;13:271–5.
38. Goodman L, Gilman A. The Pharmacologic Basis of Therapeutics. New York: Macmillan, 1980.
39. Hess H, Müller-Faßbender H, Ingrisch H, Mietschk A. Verhütung von Wiederverschlüssen nach Rekanalisation obliterierter Arterien mit der Kathetermethode. Dtsch Med Wochenschr 1978;103:1994–7.
40. Hess H, Mietaschk A, Deichsel G. Drug-induced inhibition of platelet function delays progression of peripheral occlusive arterial disease. A prospective double blind arteriographically controlled trial. Lancet 1985;1:415–9.
41. Schneider E, Brunner U, Bollinger A. Medikamentöse Rezidivprophylaxe nach femoro-poplitealer Arterienrekonstruktion. Angiology 1979;2:73–7.
42. Gordon JL, Pearson JV. Effect of sulfinpyrazone and aspirin on prostacyclin synthesis by endothelial cells. Br J Pharmacol 1978;62:481–7.
43. Zeitler E, Reichold J, Schoop W, Loew D. Einfluß von Acetylsalicylsäure auf das Frühergebnis nach perkutaner Rekanalisation arterieller Obliterationen nach Dotter. Dtsch Med Wochenschr 98;1973:1285–8.
44. Lorenz R. Prophylaxe mit Thrombozytenaggregationshemmern bei kardiovaskulären Indikationen. Internist 1989; 30:315–21.
45. Kretschmer G, Wenzl E, Wagner O, et al. Influence of

anticoagulant treatment in preventing graft occlusion following saphenous vein bypass for femoropopliteal occlusive disease. Br J Surg 1986;73:689–92.
46. Kretschmer G, Wenzl E, Piza F, et al. The influence of anticoagulant treatment on the probability of function in femoropopliteal vein bypass surgery: analysis of a clinical series (1970–1985) and interim evaluation of a controlled clinical trial. Surgery 1987;102:453–9.
47. Horvath L. Percutaneous transluminal angioplasty: importance of anticoagulant and fibrinolytic drugs. AJR 1980;135:951–4.
48. Erikson SE. Enteric-coated acetylsalicylic acid plus dipyridamole compared with anticoagulants in the prevention of ischemic events in patients with transient ischemic attacks. Acta Neurol Scand 1985;71:485–93.
49. Metke MD, Lie JT, Fuster M, et al. Reduction of intimal thickening in canine coronary bypass vein grafts with dipyridamole and aspirin. Am J Cardiol 1979;43:1144–8.
50. Ross R, Glomset J, Kariya B, Harker LA. A platelet dependent serum factor that stimulates the proliferation of arterial smooth cells in vitro. Proc Natl Acad Sci USA 1974;71:1207–10.
51. Cairns JA, Gent M, Singer J, et al. Aspirin, sulfinpyrazone, or both in unstable angina. Results of a Canadian multicenter trial. N Engl J Med 1885;313:1369–75.
52. Pfisterer M, Jockers G, Regenass S, et al. Trial of low-dose aspirin plus dipyridamole versus anticoagulants for prevention of aorto-coronary vein graft occlusion. Lancet 1989;70:1–7.
53. Brewer ML, Kinnison ML, Perler BA, White RI. Blue toe syndrome: treatment with anticoagulants and delayed percutaneous transluminal angioplasty. Intervent Radiol 1988; 166:31–36.
54. Gershlick AH, Lyons JP, Wright JEC, et al. Long term clinical outcome of coronary surgery and assessment of benefit obtained with postoperative aspirin and dipyridamole. Br Heart J 1988;60:111–6.
55. United Kingdom transient ischaemic attack (UK-TIA) aspirin trial: Interim results. Br Med J 1988;296:316–31.
56. AMIS: Aspirin Myocardial Infarction Study Research Group: a randomized, controlled trial of aspirin in persons recovered from myocardial infarction. JAMA 1980;243:661–669. Final results. Circulation 1980;62:79–84.
57. Marshall M. Thrombozyten-Funktionshemmung und Antikoagulation bei der koronaren, zerebralen und peripheren arterieller Verschlußkrankheit. Fortschr Med 1982;14:650–5.
58. Ranke C, Creutzig A, Alexander K. Therapie mit Acetylsalicylsäure bei vaskulären Erkrankungen. Dtsch Med Wochenschr 1988;113:1158–61.
59. Bollinger A, Brunner U. Antiplatelet drugs improve the patency rates after femoro-popliteal endarterectomy. Vasa 1985; 14:272–9.
60. Bollinger A. Medikamentöse Therapie bei peripherer arterieller Verschlußkrankheit. Schweiz Med Wochenschr 1988; 118:1283–9.
61. Pfisterer M. Dipyridanol und niedrig dosiertes Aspirin bei Patienten mit aorto-coronarem Bypass—Vergleich mit der Antikoagulation. Schweiz Med Wochenschr 1987;117:1688–92.
62. Hirsh J, Fuster V, Salzman E. Dose of antiplatelet agents: the relationship among side effects and antithrombotic effectiveness. Arch Intern Med 1986;146:465–6.
63. Norden C, Heine H. Antikoagulatien und Thrombozytenfunktionshemmer zur Langzeitbehandlung der Arteriosklerose. Z Ges Inn Med 1989;44:183–6.
64. Norden C, Heine H. Arteriosklerose und Thrombose. Jena: VEB Gustav Fischer Verlag, 1988.
65. Sinzinger H, O'Grady J, Fitscher P, Kaliman J. Extremely-low-dose aspirin (1 mg/day) renders human platelets more sensitive to antiaggregative prostaglandins. N Engl J Med 1984;311:1052–5.
66. Sinzinger H, Silberbauer K, Kaliman J, Fitscher P. 20 mg aspirin daily—evidence for a clinical future of this extremely low dose in arterial disease? Vasa 1988;17:10–5.
67. Zilchner R, Weihrauch TR. Übersicht zur optimalen Dosierung von Acetylsalicysäure (ASS). Part I. Med Klin 1989;84: 43–51.
68. Zilchner R, Weihrauch TR. Zur optimalen Dosierung von Acetylsalicylsäure (ASS). Part II. Med Klin 1989;84:110–5.
69. Altman R, Scazziota A, Cordero Funes J. Why single daily dose of aspirin may not prevent platelet aggregation. Thromb Res 1988;51:259–66.
70. Minar E, Ehringer H, Jung M, et al. Lack of influence of low-dose acetylsalicylic acid (100 mg daily) on platelet survival time, β-thromboglobulin and platelet factor 4 in patients with peripheral arterial occlusive disease. Thromb Res 1988;52:219–26.
71. Veith FJ, Gupta SK, Samson RH, Scher LA, Fell SC, Weiss P. Progress in limb salvage by reconstructive arterial surgery combined with new improved adjunctive procedures. Ann Surg 1981;194:386–401.
72. Simrock R, Rehders K, Spahn H, et al. Plasma drug and antiplatelet profiles of the original acetylsalicylic acid preparations used in the AMIS, PARIS and German-Austrian trials for secondary prevention of myocardial infarction. Eur J Clin Pharmacol 1988;33:541–7.
73. Thornton MA, Grüntzig A, Hollman J, et al. Coumadin and aspirin in the prevention of recurrence after transluminal coronary angioplasty: a randomized study. Circulation 1984;69:721–7.
74. Lejeune A, Fattet M, Degos JD. Aspirin dose, bleeding time, platelet adhesion and aggregation in cerebral thrombosis. Int J Clin Pharmacol Ther Toxicol 1988;26:237–42.
75. Heiß HW, Mathias K, Beck AH, et al. Rezidivprophylaxe mit Acetylsalicylsäure und Dipyridamol nach perkutaner transluminaler Angioplastie der Beinarterien bei obliterierender Arteriosklerose. CorVas 1987;1:25–32.
76. Hess H, Mietschk A, Deichsel G. Drug-induced inhibition of platelet function delays progression of peripheral occlusive arterial disease. Lancet 1985;1:415–9.
77. Schoop W, Levy B, Schoop B, Gaentsch A. Experimentelle und klinische Studien zu der sekundäreren Prävention der peripheren Arteriosklerose. In Bollinger A, Rhyner K (ed): Thrombozytenfunktionshemmer. Stuttgart: Thieme, 1983:49.
78. Albert JP, Regensburger D, Rudolf I, et al. Rezidivprophylaxe operativ korrogierter Arterienverschlüsse der unteren Extremitäten. Med Welt 1982;3:64–8.
79. Merz B. Multicenter study indicates one aspirin can do the job in preventing stroke. JAMA 1987;257:2134–5.
80. Britton M, Helmers C, Samuelsson K. High dose acetylsalicylic acid after cerebral infarction: a Swedish cooperative study. Stroke 1987;18:325–34.
81. Vogel G, Fischer C, Huyke R. Prevention of reinfarction with acetylsalicylic acid. In Breddin K, Loew D, Ueberla K, Marx R (ed): Prophylaxis of venous, peripheral, cardiac, and cerebral vascular disease with acetylsalicylic acid. Stuttgart: Schattauer Verlag, 1981:123–8.
82. Gross R. Wie hoch dosiert man Aspirin? Dt Ärztebl 1990;24:1409–14.
83. Weksler BB, Tack-Goldman K, Subramanian VA, Gay WA. Cumulative inhibitory effect of low-dose aspirin on vascular prostacyclin and platelet thromboxane production in patients with atherosclerosis. Circulation 1985;71:332–40.
84. Graham DY, Smith L. Aspirin and the stomach. Ann Intern Med 1986;104:390–6.
85. May B. Arzneimittelinduzierte peptische Läsionen im oberen Gastrointestinaltrakt. Arzneimittelforschung 1988;35:1–3.

6 Guide Wire Technology

George P. Teitelbaum, M.D.

HISTORICAL PERSPECTIVE

Guide wire design and function have played a vital role in percutaneous transluminal angioplasty (PTA) since the initial report of this technique by Dotter and Judkins.[1] The original antegrade femoral technique employed 0.05 inch (1.27 mm) spring coil guide wires to traverse femoropopliteal stenoses. These guide wires lacked the steerability, variable taper, and low-friction coatings that greatly enhance the utility of present-day guide wires. However, even in the earliest developmental stages of PTA, Dotter recognized the importance of these spring coil guide wires in establishing access across a stenosis and in preventing "periatheromatous" or subintimal passage of his telescoping catheter system.

In the succeeding years, the quality and versatility of guide wires for diagnostic angiography improved greatly with smaller wire diameters, decreased fragility, newer tip designs, variable tapers, spring coil sheaths made with flat wires, and the addition of heparin and Teflon coatings.

Although Grüntzig's initial balloon catheter designs included a leading wire tip,[2] it soon became obvious that greater control in crossing and dilating obstructive vascular lesions could be obtained with an over-the-wire system. This would allow more effective manipulations across stenoses and occlusions with a guide wire and catheter combination. Over-the-wire balloon systems also afforded "safety" wire access across a dilated arterial segment, eliminating the risk of vessel dissection and acute closure due to manipulations to recross a lesion (should additional balloon dilations be necessary).

A major advance was the development of digital substraction angiography (DSA), which afforded the opportunity of roadmap imaging of irregular, stenotic vascular segments. This imaging technique has greatly reduced the risk of subintimal wire passage or vessel perforations during attempts to negotiate diseased vessels with guide wires. This amplified the need for torque control guide wires capable of accurate, atraumatic maneuvering through irregular vascular channels. The Wholey wire was an important development in this regard.[3] Many refinements in torque-control guide wires have been made during the development of coronary angioplasty, including high visibility, atraumatic platinum tips, and smaller wire diameters.[4] These thin, flexible tip guide wires have been adapted for use in peripheral angioplasty, particularly in smaller calf and renal artery branches. Their stiffer mandrel portion has allowed excellent tracking of newer, low-profile balloon angioplasty catheters designed for peripheral use.[5] In addition, they have allowed for multiple techniques employing dual guide wires placed through the same vascular access sheath or guiding catheter, including the protection of sidebranch vessels during balloon angioplasty.[6]

A major breakthrough in guide wire technology has been the development of steerable hydrophilic polymer guide wires (Glidewire, Medi-tech, Watertown, MA).[7] Their low-friction coating affords superior catheter trackability and can allow negotiation of the tightest stenoses.

A number of coaxial devices are now available for infusion of thrombolytic and antispasmotic agents as well as DSA contrast injections. These include injectable guide wires (Sos wire, USCI; Cragg wire, Medi-tech),[8] which have been important adjuncts to PTA, especially in terms of thrombolytic therapy.[9]

Finally, wire devices have been developed that are designed to effect recanalization of long arterial occlusions and dilation of arterial stenoses.[10]

BASIC GUIDE WIRE DESIGN

Fixed-core guide wires (Fig. 6-1) have usually consisted of a Teflon-coated outer spring coil sheath with a mandrel core. The distal mandrel tip may possess varying degrees of taper. Distally, the mandrel may be soldered or welded to the wire tip, or it may terminate proximal to the wire tip. The latter case would result in a wire with increased distal floppiness but requires the presence of a minute safety wire running the length of the guide wire and joined to both proximal and distal tips. This safety wire avoids uncoiling of the spring coil sheath and detachment of a distal portion of sheath. Fixed core guide wires may have either straight or "J" tips.

Movable core guide wires (Fig. 6-1) also possess a Teflon-coated spring coil sheath, mandrel core, and safety wire. However, the mandrel may be withdrawn in varying lengths from the spring coil sheath in order to create the desired degree of distal floppiness. Movable core guide wires are also produced in straight and "J"-tip varieties.

Spring coil sheaths have generally been produced using round (in cross-section) wire. However, there are several advantages in using flat wires for sheath production (Fig. 6-1).[11] Use of a flat wire affords a greater inner sheath diameter. This allows larger mandrel cores to be used, resulting in increased stiffness for working and exchange wires (viz., Amplatz Extra- and Super-Stiff guide wires). The increased inner sheath diameter provides more room for movement of mandrel cores, resulting in greater ease of core withdrawal and advancement.

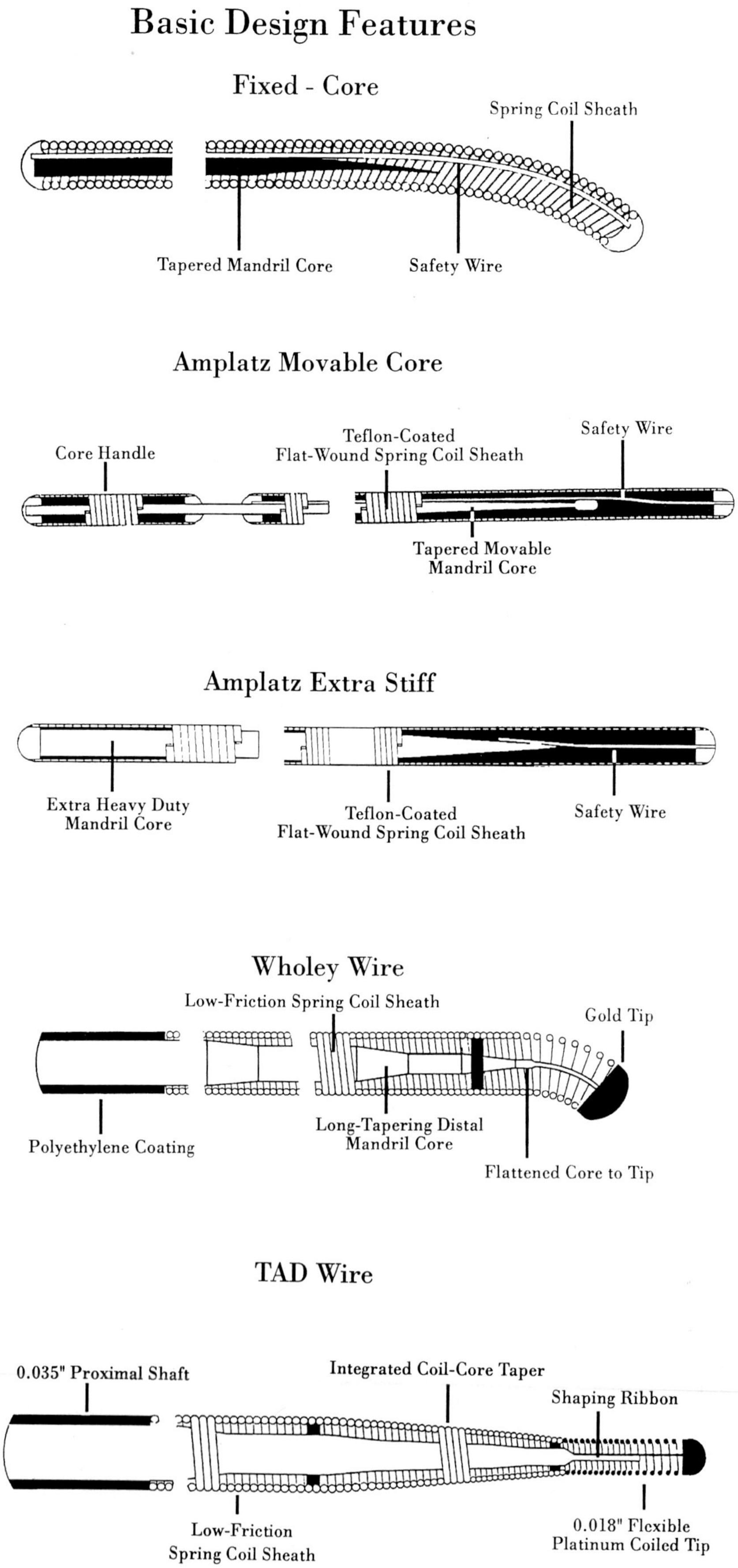

Figure 6–1. Basic design features of various guide wires.

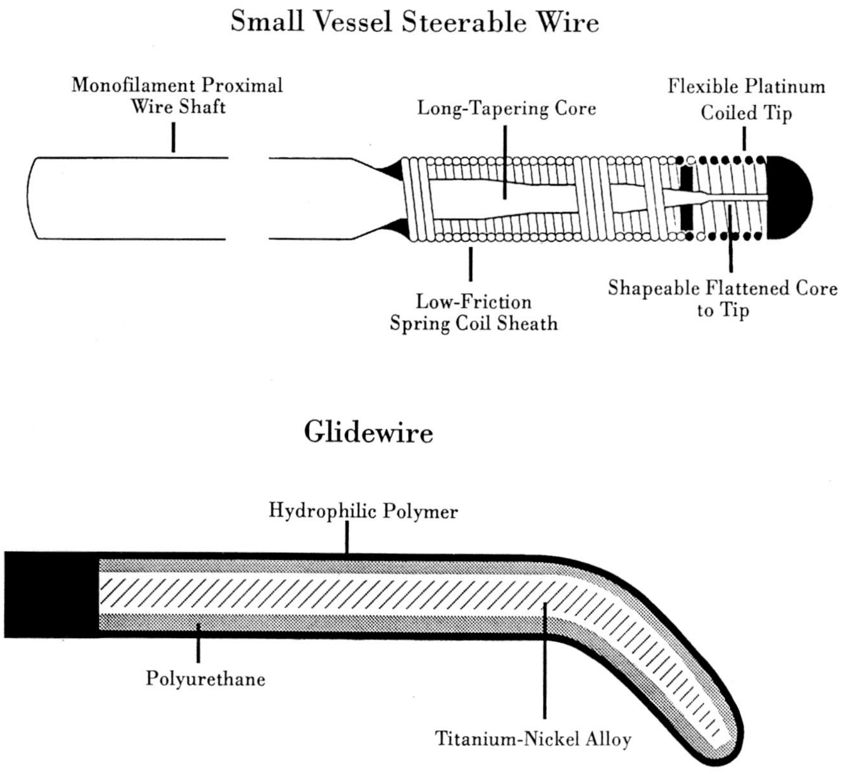

Figure 6–1. (Continued).

SUPER MOVABLE GUIDE WIRE

This is similar to flat-wound design of the Amplatz movable core guides except that an outer Teflon tubing layer obviates the need for an internal safety wire. Available in 145 cm length, 0.032 to 0.038 inch diameter, 7 cm taper length, and either straight or 3 mm "J" tips (Schneider). Used for negotiating tortuous vessels or may be used to provide a variable taper straight wire for vessel recanalization.

Fixed-Core Working and Exchange Wires

AMPLATZ EXTRA- AND SUPER-STIFF WIRES

Produced by Cook and Medi-Tech, respectively, these Teflon-coated flat-wound wires with heavy-duty mandrels are available with taper lengths of 6 to 15 cm, total wire lengths of 145 to 260 cm, and either straight (Fig. 6-2) or "J" tips. The most useful diameters are 0.035 and 0.038 inch. These wires are valuable in providing guide wire access across atherosclerotic tortuous iliac arteries (e.g., in advancing 4 F and 5 F catheters into the aorta or into the femoral arteries via a contralateral femoral approach) and in providing antegrade femoral guide wire access into calcified, diseased arteries (especially in obese patients). The flat wire design, stiffness, and special Teflon coating allow improved catheter tracking. The LT and LLT versions of these wires (Cook) are suitable for vessel recanalization.

ROSEN (EXCHANGE) WIRE

This firm wire, possessing a 1.5 mm "J" tip with 2 cm of distal taper, is produced by Cook and USCI (Bard Interventional) in lengths of 145 to 260 cm. The most useful diameters are 0.035 and 0.038 inch. In its shorter length, it may be used in conjunction with a Van Andel catheter to recanalize occluded arterial segments (Fig. 6-2). In its longer length, it is a suitable exchange wire, particularly for renal angioplasty. Care must be taken not to over-advance this wire into small renal arteries because this might result in vessel spasm or dissection. The tight "J" tip should not be pulled back across a balloon dilated arterial segment but rather should first be straightened by withdrawal into a catheter before removal from the angioplasty site.

Torque-Control Wires

WHOLEY WIRES

These wires are available in Hi-Torque-Modified "J," Floppy, and Standard varieties (ACS) and provide differing degrees of distal tip flexibility (Fig. 6-1, 6-3). All three types come in 145 cm length and 0.035 inch wire diameter. A

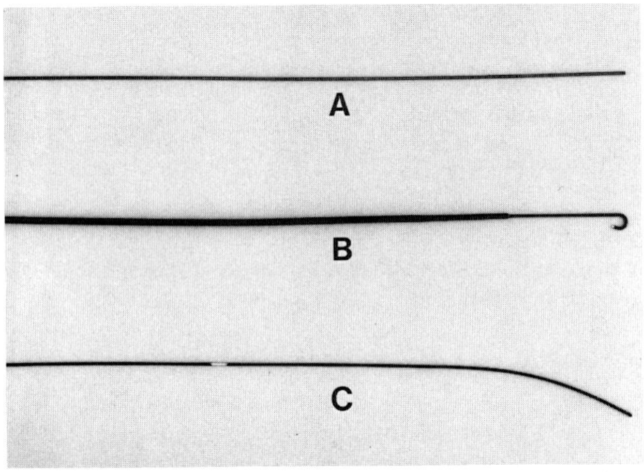

Figure 6–2. Distal portions of several fixed-core guide wires. **A:** A 0.035 inch Bentson wire. **B:** A 0.035 inch 1.5 mm "J" wire placed through a 6 F Van Andel catheter. **C:** A 0.035 inch Amplatz extra-stiff straight wire.

steering device is used with these wires to negotiate tortuous, irregular vascular lumina and stenoses. Once these wires have been positioned in their desired location, they can be converted to exchange guide wires by the attachment of a LOC guide wire extension (ACS). The extension device has a length of 115 cm to give a total exchange wire length of 260 cm.

AMPLATZ TORQUE WIRE

This wire is available in 145 cm length and 0.035 and 0.038 inch diameters (Medi-Tech) and provides many of the same functions as the Wholey wire (see before).

TAD II TAPERED WIRE

This wire is available in 145 cm length with a shaft diameter of 0.035 inch that tapers to 0.018 inch distally (ACS) (Fig. 6-1, 6-2). This device provides a flexible, thin, highly radiopaque distal tip that is preferred for gaining access to smaller, shorter, spasm-prone vessels (e.g., within the renal arteries). This is coupled to a stiffer, larger proximal wire shaft that provides better trackability for low-profile balloon catheters. Like the Wholey wires, the TAD II wire can be converted to a 260 cm exchange wire by attachment of the LOC extension device. The TAD wire's flexible tip may be somewhat fragile for use as the primary recanalization wire in calcified, occluded extremity vessels.

TAPERED TORQUE WIRE

This wire provides many of the same design and function features as the TAD II wire (see before). The tapered torque wire is available in a 145 cm length, a 3 cm platinum tip, and proximal and distal wire diameters of 0.035 and 0.018 inch (Medi-Tech). Torque control is afforded by attachment of a steering device.

Small Vessel/Coronary Torque-control Wires

These devices are well suited for cannulating smaller, more spasm-prone arteries in the extremities and kidneys. Their high torque response and low-friction coating aids in negotiating tight stenoses and complex vascular anatomy. The relatively stiff proximal mandrel promotes ease of catheter insertion (Fig. 6-1, 6-3). Straight 5 F Kifa catheters (Cook) and newer low-profile Schwarten (ACS), ProFlex (ACS), and Ultrathin (Medi-tech) balloon catheters will frequently follow 0.016 and 0.018 inch varieties of such wires over the aortic bifurcation and into the renal arteries (Fig. 6-3B). When two of these wires are used through the same 6 F vascular sheath, they permit side-branch protection during angioplasty of lower extremity branchpoint stenoses using a single arterial puncture. In addition, smaller vessel guide wires can be used as a safety wire through a dilated arterial segment. Postangioplasty contrast injection can be performed easily around these wires using a vascular sheath or through a catheter fitted with a Tuohy Borst adapter or rotating hemostatic valve. Care must be taken during use to prevent damage to the fragile tips of these guide wires. The tips can usually be shaped easily, to provide better steerability, by gently passing the wire tip between one's thumb and the edge of a slat of a 10 ml plastic syringe's plunger.

ACS WIRES

Hi-Torque Floppy varieties are available in 0.018 and 0.014 inch diameters in 175 cm length and with Microglide coating (Fig. 6-3). These wires can be converted to 320 cm exchange guide wires by attachment of LOC extension devices. Hi-Torque, intermediate, and standard varieties are also available that provide somewhat less distal flexibility and increased pushability.

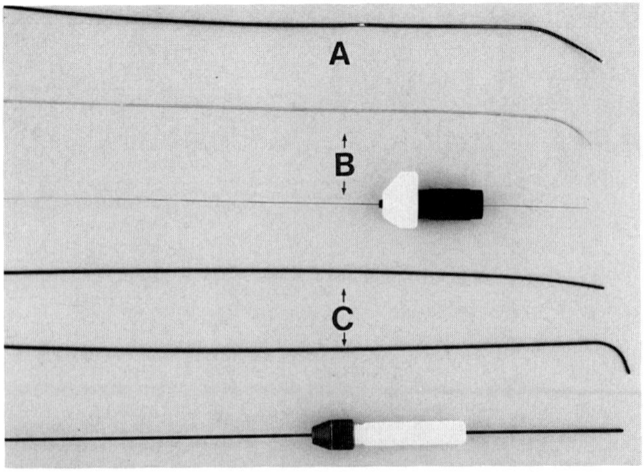

Figure 6–3. Torque-control guide wires. **A:** A 0.035 inch Wholey wire. **B:** A 0.018 inch small vessel or coronary artery wire with USCI steering device attached to its proximal end. **C:** A 0.035 inch curved and straight Glidewires with PGS steering device attached to proximal portion of wire.

USCI

A variety of Teflon-coated platinum-tip small diameter guide wires are available in sizes of 0.014 to 0.018 inch. All are steerable using an attachable torque device. Standard, Flex, and VeriFlex "J" tip varieties provide increasing degrees of distal wire floppiness in the 0.014 inch diameter wires. The 0.016 inch wires are available in Standard and Flex "J" tips. These wires possess a 25 cm distal spring coil sheath and an overall length of 180 cm, which is extensible to 300 cm with use of an attachable Stertzer/Myler extension wire (applied with a crimping tool). An 80 cm 0.018 inch platinum tip wire is also available.

MEDI-TECH

A 0.015 inch diameter 145 cm long wire is available. There is a 25 cm distal floppy portion and a platinum tip. Torque control is provided by attachment of a steering device. Straight and angled 0.018 inch Glidewires are also available in lengths of 150 to 180 cm (see later).

TARGET THERAPEUTICS

Taper-16 and Taper Flex-Tip steerable guide wires are available with a proximal diameter of 0.016 inch and a distal diameter of 0.013 inch. The maximum available length is 175 cm. The distal 12 cm of both is a bendable radiopaque platinum coil tip. These highly supple wires are designed for use with Tracker-18 catheters (Target Therapeutics). These wires have only a moderate torque response. However, they pass quite easily into distal portions of highly tortuous vessels, and the Tracker-18 catheter displays excellent trackability over this wire. In certain instances a Tracker-18 catheter and Taper wire combination can act as a guide wire for a larger catheter capable of accepting a 0.038 inch wire (e.g., 5 F straight Kifa).

Torque/Steering Devices

PERIPHERAL SYSTEMS GROUP

Torque device is designed for wire sizes of 0.032 to 0.038 inch. A smaller wire model is also available. The device is particularly well suited for use with Glidewires.

USCI

Steering handle models are available for 0.014 to 0.018 and 0.035 to 0.038 inch wires.

MEDI-TECH

Torque vise is adjustable to fit 0.025 to 0.038 inch wire sizes.

TARGET THERAPEUTICS

Torque device has a pin vise for use with Taper and Seeker wires.

HYDROPHILIC WIRES

Glidewires (Terumo/Medi-Tech) are available in either straight or angled varieties in lengths of 120 to 180 cm and in diameters of 0.018 to 0.038 inch (Figs. 6-1, 6-3). A 260 cm version is available in both the 0.035 and 0.038 inch sizes. Torque control is best effected using either a Peripheral Systems Group Torque Device or a Medi-tech Torque Vise. The wire must be completely wetted and catheter flushed before the device is used in order to prevent the wire from sticking within the catheter. This exceptionally slippery wire is useful in a number of situations: negotiating tortuous vascular anatomy, attaining access through very tight stenoses, recanalizing vascular occlusions, and providing superior catheter trackability through irregular, atherosclerotic arteries. Although the 0.035 and 0.038 inch diameter wires have adequate visibility, smaller wire sizes may be difficult to see fluoroscopically. A newer 0.018 inch version with a more radiopaque tip is now available. This device should not be used as the primary access wire during arteriography, nor should it be inserted or withdrawn through a needle or metal cannula. These maneuvers might result in stripping of the polymer coating from the central metal wire. Once the guide wire has been advanced into a tortuous vessel, it may have the tendency to recoil rapidly out of the selected artery or vein. For this reason, it is a poor exchange wire. However, during maneuvers to advance a catheter into such a vessel over a Glidewire, recoil can be counteracted with constant forward force applied to the wire by means of an attached steering device. The Glidewire may be used through a Sidewinder catheter in order to cross a highly stenotic renal artery lesion. In addition, the angled wire may be used to attempt immediate recrossing of a balloon-dilated iliac or femoropopliteal arterial segment. Using roadmap imaging, the Glidewire is gently advanced through the angioplasty segment while twirling or torquing the angled tip at a moderate rate. Although this device may appear to pass with ease through highly diseased arterial segments, caution should be exercised to avoid using the Glidewire with excessive antegrade force in order to prevent vessel dissections or perforations.

Injectable Wires and Coaxial Systems

SOS WIRE

This device is available in a 145 cm length in 0.035 and 0.038 inch diameters (USCI/Bard Interventional) (Fig. 6-4). The removable central core is available in either a long taper or standard version. Injection is made following core removal, using an attachable Luer lock hub. Contrast, saline, or other fluid injection through this device is facilitated using a 3 cc or smaller syringe. A power infusion pump is necessary for infusion of a urokinase solution through the Sos wire. The device can be directed into a desired vessel by means of a coaxially placed torque-control small vessel guide wire. A 0.014 inch coronary wire passes through the 0.035

inch Sos wire. A 0.016 inch wire is compatible with the 0.038 inch Sos wire. During removal of an injectable Sos wire, either the core wire or an appropriately sized coronary guide wire should be reinserted to prevent dehiscence or breakage of the device's spring coil sheath.

CRAGG WIRE

Available in 0.038 inch diameter and 145 cm length (Medi-tech). Injection is made following central core removal by attaching a proximal Luer lock hub. Maximum flow rate is 6.2 ml/sec at 750 psi. This device will accept a central coaxial guide wire of up to 0.025 inch diameter.

T3 AND N3 CATHETER

A 3F Teflon catheter is generally used in an 80 cm length (Cook) (Fig. 6-4). It will accept up to 0.021 inch wire. Also useful as a coaxial infusion device and as a catheter for DSA contrast injection. Directionality can be achieved with concurrent use of a steerable coronary wire. Disadvantages include its poor visibility and stiffer distal end (compared with Tracker catheters). The newer 3F nylon N3 catheter (Cook) is less stiff, has a distal radiopaque marker, and is more trackable. It is available in lengths of 100-150 cm and accepts a 0.025 inch wire. T3 and N3 catheters are compatible with a guiding catheter that will accept a 0.038 inch guide wire.

TRACKER-18 CATHETER

This catheter is available in lengths of 60 to 150 cm with a distal floppy segment length of 12 to 18 cm (Target Therapeutics) (Fig. 6-4). Its proximal outer diameter is 3 F; distally, it tapers to a 2.2 F size. It passes through any catheter that accepts a 0.038 inch guide wire, including 4 F Novoste, 5 F Cook Kifa straight, and 5.5 F Cook Hi-Flow catheters. The Tracker-18 is designed to be used with 0.016 inch (0.013 inch distally) Taper guide wires (Target Therapeutics), although frequently the catheter can be easily advanced (with only flow directionality) without use of a guide wire. An advantage of the Tracker-18 over the T3 catheter is its flexible tip with a radiopaque marker. Before a wire is inserted into the Tracker-18, all contrast must be flushed thoroughly from the catheter using saline (in a 1 to 3 cc syringe) to prevent wire adhesion within the catheter lumen. Hand injection of contrast for DSA is best performed using a 1 to 3 cc syringe. Although the Tracker-18 is most suitable as a coaxial infusion device, it is more expensive than the Sos and Cragg wires and the N3 and T3 catheters. Also, care must be taken not to advance forcefully the highly flexible Tracker catheter against hard vascular obstructions in order to avoid catheter kinking, breakage, and knotting.

STRAIGHT KIFA CATHETER

This 5 F catheter (Cook) accepts up to a 0.038 inch guide wire (package states that maximum acceptable wire size is 0.035 inch). It is not only useful as a guiding catheter for coaxial infusion devices, but it is also valuable as an exchange catheter (Fig. 6-4). Since this supple catheter will usually follow 0.035 inch Bentson and 0.016 to 0.018 inch coronary wires over the aortic bifurcation and into the renal arteries, the Kifa catheter can be used to replace these guide wires with stiffer 0.035 to 0.038 inch exchange wires.

Balloons on a Wire

TEG WIRE

This wire is available in usable lengths of 100 cm and proximal shaft diameter of 0.035 inch (Medi-tech). All have a 4 cm distal, steerable platinum tip (tapers down to 0.018 inch diameter). Available balloon diameters include 3, 4, 5, and 6 mm in either 2 or 4 cm lengths (Fig. 6-5). Maximum recommended inflation pressure is 6 atm (88 psi). The 3 and 4 mm balloon sizes require an introduction catheter or sheath of at least 0.051 inch (4 F) inner diameter (owing to the deflated balloon profile). This figure increases to 0.075″ (5.8 F) for the 5 and 6 mm balloons. The device's torque control, flexibility, and small diameter allow it to both cross and dilate tight stenoses in smaller peripheral arteries. This device is probably best suited for distal femoropopliteal dilations performed via a small diameter antegrade femoral sheath. The Teg wire is not recommended for use over the aortic bifurcation. A newer version is now available with a shorter, steerable tip for renal arteries.

HARTZLER LPS AND ACS MINI BALLOONS

Both types of devices have overall lengths of 135 cm with available tip lengths of 1, 2, and 3 cm. The radiopaque tips are steerable. Balloon sizes include 1.3 (ACS Mini), 1.5,

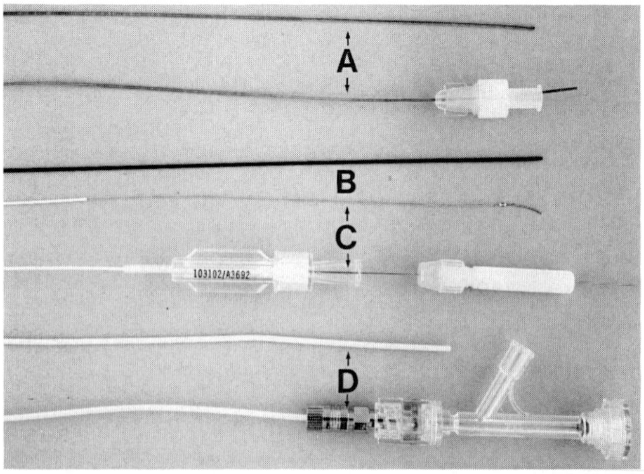

Figure 6–4. Coaxial systems. **A:** A 0.035 inch Sos injectable wire with proximal Luer lock hub. **B:** A 3 F T3 Teflon catheter. **C:** Tracker-18 catheter with coaxially placed 0.016 inch (0.013 inch distally) Taper guide wire. Torque vise is attached to the proximal portion of this wire. **D:** A 5 F straight Kifa guiding and exchange catheter (with proximally attached rotating hemostatic valve) which will accept devices shown in Figures **A** through **C.**

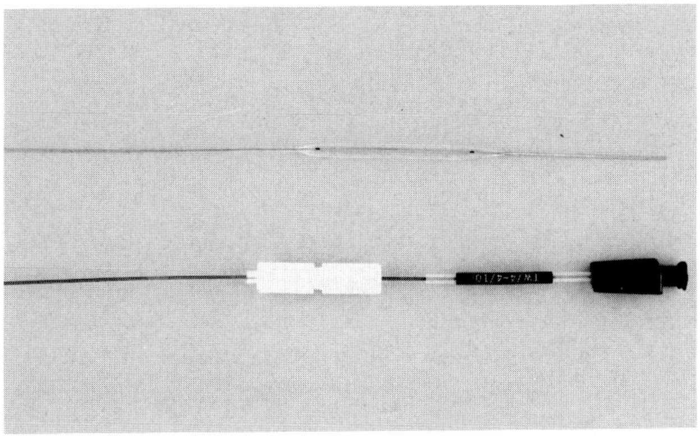

Figure 6–5. Teg wire balloon angioplasty device (with torque vise attached proximally).

Table 6–1. Diameter Conversions

INCHES	MILLIMETERS	FRENCH
0.013	0.33	1.00
0.014	0.36	1.08
0.015	0.38	1.15
0.016	0.41	1.23
0.018	0.46	1.38
0.021	0.54	1.62
0.025	0.64	1.92
0.026	0.67	2.00
0.032	0.82	2.46
0.035	0.90	2.69
0.038	0.97	2.92
0.039	1.00	3.00
0.053	1.35	4.00
0.066	1.67	5.00
0.078	2.00	6.00

2.0, 2.5, 3.0, 3.5, and 4.0 mm (Hartzler LPS). All balloons are 2 cm in length. The largest of the balloons requires for insertion a guiding catheter or sheath of a 4.3 F (0.056 inch) inner diameter. Both types of devices are coated with a friction-reducing polymer. These devices may prove to be useful in treating stenoses of the popliteal trifurcation or calf arteries.

CONCLUSION

Multiple new guide wire devices are now available that draw on technologic advancements from multiple fields and medical specialties. These wires have greatly increased the ease with which vessel recanalizations and balloon dilations can be performed. In so doing, these newer devices have expanded the scope of and indications for peripheral PTA.

REFERENCES

1. Dotter CT, Judkins MP. Transluminal treatment of arteriosclerotic obstruction: description of a new technique and a preliminary report of its application. Circulation 1964;30:654–70.
2. Grüntzig A. Die perkutane transluminale Rekanalisation chronischen arterieenverschlusse mit einem neuen doppellumigen Dilatations kateter. Fortschr Rontgenstr 1976;124:180–6.
3. Wholey MH. A newly designed directionally controlled guidewire. Cathet Cardiovasc Diagn 1986;12:66–70.
4. Meyerovitz MF, Levin DC, Boxt LM. Superselective catheterization of small-caliber arteries with a new high-visibility steerable guide wire. AJR 1985;144:785–6.
5. Schwarten DE, Cutcliff WB. Arterial occlusive disease below the knee: treatment with percutaneous transluminal angioplasty performed with low-profile catheters and steerable guide wires. Radiology 1988;169:71–4.
6. Teitelbaum GP, Joseph GJ, Matsumoto AH, Barth KH: Double-guide-wire access through a single 6-F vascular sheath. Radiology 1989;173:871–3.
7. Kikuchi Y, Graves VB, Strother CM, et al. A new guidewire with kink-resistant core and low-friction coating. CVIR 1989;12:107–9.
8. Sos TA, Cohn DJ, Srur M, et al. A new open-ended guidewire/catheter. Radiology 1985;154:817–8.
9. Matsumoto AH, Barth KH, Teitelbaum GP, Kremers PW. Self-contained, coaxial delivery system for intraarterial infusion of thrombolytic agents. Radiology 1990;174:1056-7.
10. Wholey MH, Jarmolowski CR: New reperfusion devices: the Kensey catheter, the atherolytic reperfusion wire device, and the transluminal extraction catheter. Radiology, RSNA-SCVIR Special Series 1989;172:947–52.
11. Smith TP, Derauf BJ, Darcy MD, et al. Movable core guide wire: evaluation of improved model. Radiology 1986; 159:552–3.
12. Robinson JD, Hunter DW, Castañeda-Zúñiga WR, Amplatz K: A new torque guide wire. Radiology 1987;165:572–3.

7 Peripheral Angioplasty Balloon Technology

Alan H. Matsumoto, M.D., Klemens H. Barth, M.D.

Although Dotter and Judkins first described the technique of percutaneous transluminal angioplasty (PTA) using coaxial Teflon dilators in 1964,[1] the procedure did not gain widespread popularity until 1976, when Grüntzig described his double lumen balloon catheter.[2] This catheter incorporated a rigid balloon that could be inflated to a predetermined diameter at relatively high pressures and could be directly advanced over a guide wire. This type of balloon dilation system facilitated the performance of PTA on larger vessels such as iliac arteries, while using smaller diameter catheters (7 F to 8 F). Since 1976, a number of technologic and design changes have been made to improve the performance of balloon catheters. The current status of balloon catheter materials and design, and future development considerations will be reviewed.

BASIC PHYSICAL PRINCIPLES

The radial or outward force that is exerted against a stenotic lesion to enlarge a vessel's lumen is called the dilating force. The dilating force is dependent on a number of factors, including balloon diameter, balloon inflation pressure, compliance of the balloon, balloon length, and length of and degree of stenosis.[3,4]

According to the law of Laplace, the tension (T) exerted on the wall of an inflated balloon is directly proportional to the pressure (P) within the balloon and the radius (R) of the balloon ($T = P \times R$). Therefore a balloon with twice the radius of a smaller balloon will produce twice the wall tension for a given inflation pressure. If the diameter of the balloon is kept constant, the tension on the wall of the balloon will increase linearly with increases in inflation pressure. Since tension on the balloon wall translates into the dilating force, the dilating force generated by a balloon is directly proportional to the balloon diameter and inflation pressure.

Compliance is a measure of how much a balloon will stretch beyond a predetermined diameter when a force is applied to it. Since all balloon materials are elastic, each balloon will have some degree of compliance, depending on the material from which it is constructed. A totally noncompliant balloon will not stretch. It will maintain its profile and shape with repeated inflations and will have a very predictable diameter. If the balloon material is compliant (stretches at low pressures), the balloon will deform in the region of a stenosis. This prevents the dilating force from being concentrated in the region of the stenosis. Therefore a noncompliant balloon will generate a greater amount of dilating force in a lesion than a compliant one. The length of the balloon also has an effect on the dilating force but is also dependent on the balloon material. Compliant balloons will continue to increase in diameter and deform with increasing inflation pressures. Therefore a shorter compliant balloon, which has less surface area than a longer one, will exert more of a concentrated dilating force. In contrast, the dilating force generated by a balloon constructed from a noncompliant material does not decrease with increasing balloon length.

Since a longer stenosis has more total area than a shorter one, the dilating force created by a balloon will be greater in a longer lesion. In addition, more dilating force will be generated in a tight, high-grade stenosis than a shallow stenosis. This relationship is almost linear in that the dilating force generated in a lesion is directly proportional to the degree of stenosis, given a fixed balloon diameter and inflation pressure. The principle is governed by the so-called "clothesline effect," that is, the radial force vector diminishes as the circumference of the balloon at the stenosis increases.[3]

BALLOON MATERIAL

Most balloons are currently being made from one of four basic classes of plastic polymers: polyvinyl chloride (PVC), polyethylene (PE), polyethylene teraphthalate (PET), or reinforced polyurethane (PU). PVC is a class of material that was used in Grüntzig's original balloon design[2] and is still being used in several currently available balloon catheters. PVC frequently contains an additive that can vary its characteristics. Traditionally, balloons constructed from PVC have shown some degree of compliance, even at recommended working pressures. In vitro studies have demonstrated that balloon diameters can increase from the first to the second inflation by 5 to 17% and by as much as 33% after six inflations.[5,6] PVC balloons can also deform and elongate with increasing pressures,[7] and larger diameter PVC balloons are more compliant than smaller ones. Since most balloons made from PVC demonstrate some degree of compliance, the dilating force generated by their inflation is much less than that generated by less compliant balloons of the same diameter.[3,4] Furthermore, PVC balloons rupture at significantly lower inflation pressures when compared with balloons constructed from other materials.[3,5] More recently, balloons manufactured in Europe from a PVC derivative have shown better compliance characteristics (Schneider/Meditag, Zurich, Switzerland).

PE is a relatively inert plastic that contains no additives. This material can be specially treated so that its properties can be altered. In general, balloons constructed from PE are less compliant than those made from PVC. PE balloons have shown only minor increases in diameter (less than 2%) and minimal deformity when inflated to suggested working pressures,[5,7] although the thin-walled PE balloons used with the newer low-profile catheters have demonstrated slightly more compliance (5 to 10% increases in diameter at maximum recommended inflation pressures). PE balloons generate almost twice as much dilating force as the same size PVC balloon and also have higher burst pressures than PVC balloons.[3,6]

PET, a polyester derivative, has been developed for use with some of the so-called low-profile (Table 7-1) and small vessel balloon catheters. Balloons made from this material have demonstrated less compliance and higher burst pressures than both PVC and PE balloons. Initial clinical experience with PET balloons suggests that they have more of a tendency to rupture when used in calcified lesions, when compared to balloons made from PVC and PE.

Balloons constructed from polyurethane (PU) reinforced with a nylon mesh are relatively noncompliant. PU balloons inflated to recommended inflation pressures increase their diameters less than 2.5% and have radial dilating forces similar to PE balloons. In addition, nylon reinforced PU balloons have comparatively high burst pressures (greater than 12 atm).[5]

CATHETER DESIGN

Grüntzig's first double-lumen balloon catheter was actually a coaxial catheter design in which both the catheter shaft and the balloon were constructed from PVC.[2] The catheter shaft was surrounded by a thin tube of PVC with an expandable end, which corresponded to the balloon (Fig. 7-1). The inner catheter had a longitudinal groove along its outer surface,

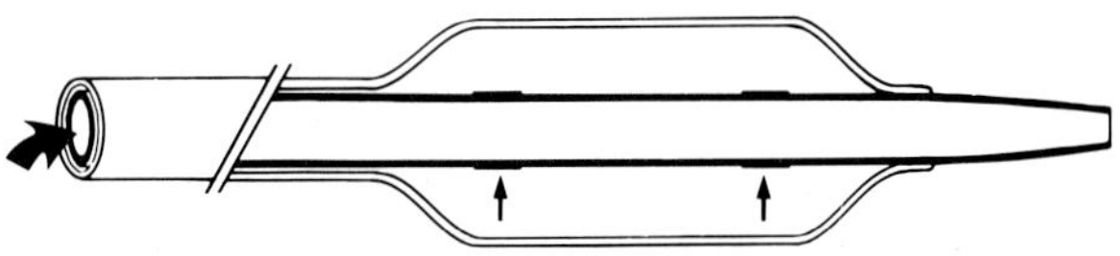

Figure 7–1. Coaxial catheter design (similar to Grüntzig's original catheter). Straight arrows: tantalum markers indicating balloon segment; curved arrow: central lumen for guide wire.

which connected to the sideport and served as a channel for inflating and deflating the balloon. The inner and outer catheters were bonded together with heat. This coaxial catheter design has become less popular because of the suboptimal compliance characteristics of PVC and the concern for overexpansion of the outer lumen at higher inflation pressures, causing compression of the inner lumen.[5,7] One putative advantage of coaxial catheters is that balloon deflation times are better than comparably sized double-lumen balloon catheters. At present, catheters of this design are primarily limited to small vessel balloon catheters (Table 7-2), where, according to the law of Laplace, compliance is less of a problem.

Most current balloon catheters utilize a true double or triple lumen catheter design (Fig. 7-2). The shaft of the catheter is usually composed of a polyester, polyethylene, nylon, or polyamide derivative. The balloon is attached to the catheter shaft using some combination of an adhesive and thermal bonding. The outer, smaller lumen, which communicates with the sideport, is used to inflate and deflate the balloon. The shape of the lumen that communicates with the balloon varies and may be round, crescentic, or a half-circle, depending on the manufacturing company.

A third type of catheter design involves the use of sliding coaxial catheters[8] (Fig. 7-3A,B). The inner catheter is made

Table 7–1. Low-Profile Balloon Catheters*

NAME	SHAFT SIZE†	BALLOON DIAMETER (mm)	BALLOON MATERIAL	MAXIMUM INFLATION PRESSURES (atm)	CATHETER DESIGN	INTRODUCER SHEATH	1992 COST (U.S. DOLLARS) (approx.)	MANUFACTURER
Bard 5F	5 F	4,5,6,7,8,9	PET	10	Triple lumen‡	6 F	180–190	Bard, Cardiosurgery
Accent DG	5 F	4,5,6,7,8	PE	7–10	Double lumen	6 F	165	Cook
Ultrathin	5 F	4,5,6,7,8,9,10	PET	12	Double lumen	5 F, 6 F, 7 F§	180–225	Medi-Tech
PE-MT5	5 F	4,5,6,7,8	PE	4–6	Double lumen	6 F, 7 F‖	175	Medi-Tech
TEG Wire	0.035 inch	4,5,6	PET	6	Balloon on a wire	4 F, 5 F¶	395	Medi-Tech
Proflex	5.3 F	4,5,6,7,8	PE	6	Double lumen	6 F, 7 F‖	250	Peripheral Systems Group
Stellar 535	5 F	4,5,6,7,8	PE-60	6	Double lumen	6 F	200	Peripheral Systems Group
Olbert No Profile	5.8 F	4,5,6,7,8	PU	10–12	Sliding coaxial	6 F, 7 F‖	180	Meadox/Surgimed
Match-35	5 F	4,5,6,7,8	PET	6–10	Coaxial	6 F	180–195	Schneider
Total Cross	4.3 F	4,5,6,7,8	PET	9–10	Coaxial	5 F, 6 F#	195	Schneider

*F: French; PE: polyethylene; PET: polyethylene teraphthalate; PU: polyurethrane reinforced with a nylon mesh.

†All balloon catheter shafts accept an 0.035 inch guide wire, except the TEG wire and the Total Cross (0.021 inch lumen).

‡Two lumina for balloon.

§Ultrathin, 4 to 7 mm balloons (5 F sheath), the 8 mm balloon (6 F sheath), and the 9 and 10 mm balloons (7 F sheath).

‖PE-MT5 8 mm balloon, Olbert 8 mm balloon and Proflex 7 mm and 8 mm balloons use 7 F sheaths.

¶TEG wire 5 mm and 6 mm balloons (5 F sheath).

#Total Cross 7 mm and 8 mm balloons use a 6 F sheath.

Table 7–2. Small Vessel Balloon Catheters*

NAME	SHAFT SIZE	BALLOON DIAMETER (mm)	BALLOON MATERIAL	CATHETER DESIGN	GUIDE WIRE ACCEPTED (inches)	INTRODUCER SHEATH	MAXIMUM INFLATION PRESSURES (atm)	1992 COST (U.S. DOLLARS) (approx.)	MANUFACTURER
Low Profile	4.3 F	2,3,4	PVC	Double Lumen	0.016†	6 F	6–8	300	Bard Cardiosurgery
OMG 4	4.0 F	2–4.5‡	PE	Double Lumen	0.018	5 F	6–8	165	Cook
OMG 4.5	4.5 F	2–4.5‡	PE	Double Lumen	0.028	6 F	6–8	165	Cook
SUB-4	3.8 F	2–6.0‡	PE	Double Lumen	0.018	4 F, 5 F§	8–10	295–315	Medi-Tech
TEG Wire	0.035 inch	2–4‡,5,6	PET	Balloon on a wire	—	4 F, 5 F§	6	395	Medi-Tech
Schwarten LP	4.3 F	2–3.5‡	PE	Coaxial	0.018	5 F	6–8	275	Peripheral Systems Group
Schwarten LP	4.7 F	4,4.5,5	PE	Coaxial	0.018	5 F, 6 F‖	6–8	275	Peripheral Systems Group
Advanced 418	4.3 F	3–5‡,6	PE	Double Lumen	0.018	5 F, 6 F‖	8	300	Peripheral Systems Group
No Profile	4.8 F	3,4,5,6	PU	Sliding coaxial	0.025	5 F	10	275	Meadox/Surgimed
Total Cross	4.3 F	2–4‡,5,6	PET	Coaxial	0.021	5 F	10–16	195	Schneider

*PE: polyethylene; PET: polyethylene teraphthalate; PVC: polyvinyl chloride; PU: polyurethrane reinforced with a nylon mesh.

†The 2 mm balloon catheter has an 0.014 inch guide wire lumen.

‡Contiguous sizes at 5 mm increments.

§SUB-4 4.5 to 6 mm balloons and TEG wire 5 mm and 6 mm balloons require 5 F introducer sheaths.

‖Schwarten LP 4.7 F 4.5 and 5.0 mm balloons and advanced 418 6 mm balloon require 6 F introducer sheaths.

from PE and the outer catheter is made from Teflon. The balloon is constructed of polyurethane reinforced with a nylon mesh and glued distally to the inner catheter and proximally to the outer catheter. The space between the two catheters communicates with the balloon lumen. When the balloon is inflated, the inner catheter moves backward in relation to the outer catheter. On deflation, the inner catheter is fully extruded and the balloon returns to a "no profile" contour without any folds.

A relatively recent development has been the balloon on a guide wire (Fig. 7-4).[9] The current design consists of a Teflon-coated, braided, stainless steel guide wire with a hollow core that communicates with a PET balloon. The 20 cm segment immediately adjacent to the balloon has been constructed in a fashion that makes it more flexible than the more proximal portion of the guide wire shaft. Distal to the balloon, there is a variable length platinum-coated or polyamide wire tip that tapers from 0.025 to 0.018 inch. A centrally positioned safety wire is continuous with the distal wire tip, making this a highly torqueable system. In contrast to other balloon catheter designs, the balloon on a wire does not require insertion over a guide wire. In theory, this provides a steerable, low-profile balloon system, which can be inserted directly through an introducer sheath or guiding catheter and eliminate several steps in the angioplasty procedure.

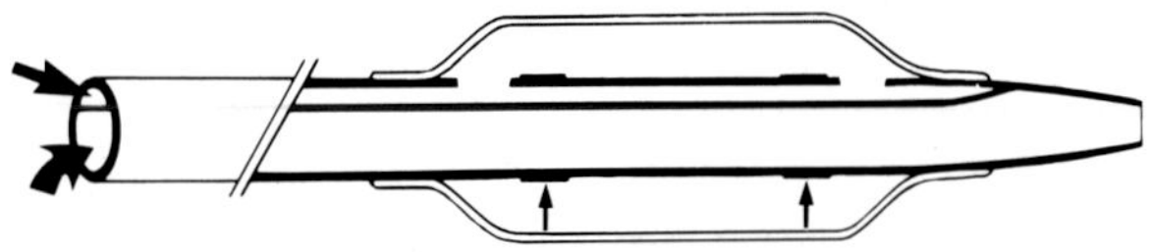

Figure 7–2. True double-lumen catheter design: Most manufacturers use a design similar to this one. Straight arrows: tantalum markers indicating balloon segment; curved arrow: larger, central lumen for the guide wire; larger straight arrow: smaller, side lumen that communicates with the balloon.

NEWER DEVELOPMENTS

A variety of balloon catheters have been developed to expand our armamentarium in the application of balloon angioplasty to new vessels. These include catheters with sideholes proximal[10] and distal[11] to the balloon, a preshaped catheter with a balloon,[12] catheters with larger balloons for aortic or valvular angioplasty,[13] and high-pressure balloon catheters. Perhaps the most significant advancement in peripheral vascular balloon catheter technology has been the development of the so-called low-profile balloon catheters (Table 7-1).

Applying the progress made in the field of polymer chemistry in the food industry to balloon and catheter technology, proprietary formulations of polyethylene derivatives have been used to construct very low-profile, pliable balloons that have working inflation pressures of 4 to 12 atm. The balloon profile is essentially the same as the shaft of the catheter so that the balloon catheter can be inserted directly through the arteriotomy site with usually no bleeding occur-

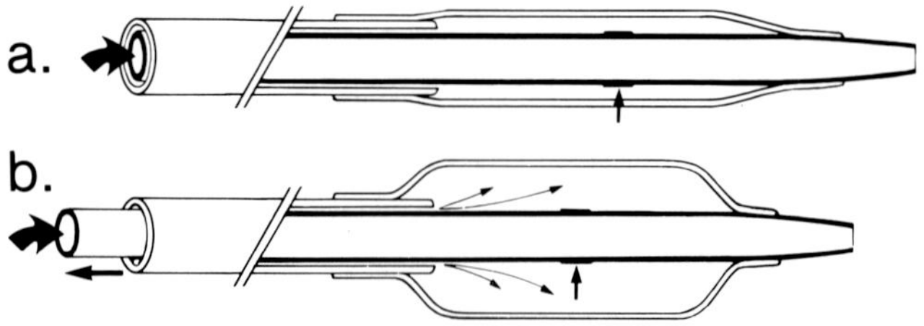

Figure 7–3. **A:** Sliding coaxial catheter with the balloon deflated. **B:** Sliding coaxial catheter with the balloon inflated. Smaller straight arrow: tantalum marker defining the center of inflated balloon; larger curved arrow: central lumen for the guide wire; larger straight arrow: indicates inner catheter moving retrograde relative to the outer catheter with balloon inflation; smaller curved arrows: space between the two catheters communicating with the balloon.

ring around the catheter during the angioplasty procedure. These balloons are mounted on thin-wall, flexible 4.3 F to 5.8 F catheter shafts. They are available with balloon diameters of 4 through 10 mm and can be advanced or withdrawn through 5 F to 7 F sheaths (Table 7-1). The flexibility of these low-profile balloon catheters enhances their trackability over the guide wire and despite the small diameter of the shafts, these catheters demonstrate satisfactory pushing characteristics. These tapered catheters can be easily advanced around the aortic bifurcation, through tortuous vessels, and through tight stenoses. The lumen communicating with the balloon is also large enough to allow for satisfactory inflation and deflation times. Therefore, they can be utilized in a variety of vessels (iliac, femoral, popliteal, tibial, renal, visceral, and brachiocephalic).

Further refinements in technology have led to the development of smaller caliber balloon catheters for use in the dilation of infrapopliteal and renal artery branch vessels.[14–17] They are available on 3.8 F to 4.8 F shafts and are compatible with any of the 0.014 to 0.018 inch steerable guide wires. Balloon diameters range from 2.0 through 6.0 mm (Table 7-2). These flexible, small caliber systems minimize undesirable axial shear forces and intimal damage that can be seen with larger, stiffer and less tapered balloon catheters.

Lastly, the balloon on a steerable guide wire, which has been described earlier in this chapter, represents the next step in the evolution of the angioplasty balloon[9] (Fig. 7-4; Tables 7-1 and 7-2). This balloon system eliminates several steps in the angioplasty procedure and its flexibility and small profile allows it to be advanced through tight stenoses and through small, tortuous vessels relatively atraumatically.

FUTURE DIRECTIONS

As the field of polymer chemistry continues to evolve, further refinements in balloon catheter technology will lead to more flexible, miniaturized, and less traumatic balloon dilation systems.[9,14,15] Hydrophilic polymers or silicon derivatives will also be used more extensively to coat the balloons and catheters to increase their lubricity and decrease their coefficient of resistance.[18] This, in combination with further miniaturization of balloon dilation systems, will reduce intimal damage and vascular spasm; minimize the resistance in advancing balloon catheters through small, tortuous vessels or tight stenoses; improve trackability; and diminish the trauma at the puncture site.

The concept of "controlled compliance" of the angioplasty balloon is also being evaluated. In theory, if the balloon material allowed for reproducible changes in balloon diameter and shape with graduated increases in inflation pressures, the angiographer would have some degree of subjective control of the angioplasty procedure. This would allow the angiographer the ability to continue balloon expansion in tiny, controlled increments, in order to optimize the dilation of a lesion with a single balloon. Although interesting, this concept needs further evaluation because we know that compliant balloons deform more in lesions and expand more outside the lesion.

Although balloon compliance can be objectively compared from balloon to balloon, other balloon catheter characteristics, such as catheter taper, flexibility, trackability, pushability, and lubricity, are described somewhat arbitrarily. As manufacturers work to create an optimal balloon catheter, a system of standards will need to be devised to allow for the objective evaluation and description of these important features. This would provide the angiographer a standard set of criteria so that as new balloon catheters became available, their performance characteristics could be objectively compared.

Ultimately, the ability to characterize a lesion before, during, and after a procedure and identifying the factors that lead to the development of restenosis will contribute most to the advancement of PTA. Visualizing the intraluminal surface of arteries using either angioscopy[19,20] or intravascular ultrasound[21,22] may facilitate better characterization of atheromatous lesions. This may help in determining which lesion will respond to balloon dilation alone and which lesion will require adjunctive therapy with an atherectomy device,[23,24] laser ablation,[25–27] or a vascular stent.[28,29] As we begin to understand the factors that stimulate smooth muscle and fibrous intimal hyperplasia,[30–34] pharmacologic agents can potentially be developed that inhibit myointimal hyperplasia.[4,35] Whether the addition of thermal energy directly to an inflated balloon can cause "welding" of the angioplasty-induced intima-media dehiscence and reduce myointimal hyperplasia is also being assessed.[36–39]

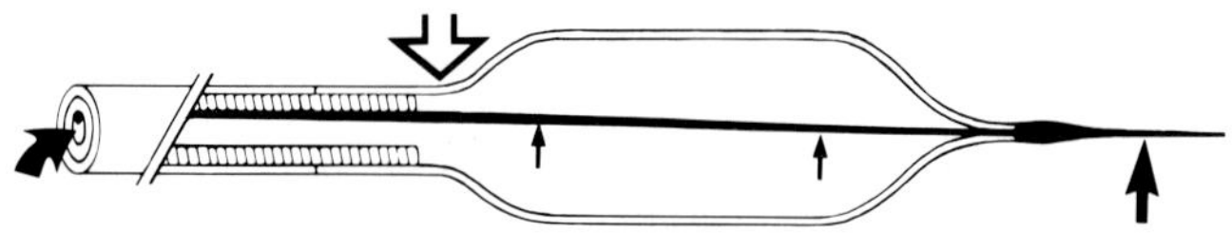

Figure 7–4. Balloon on a guide wire design. Curved arrow: central lumen which communicates with the balloon; smaller straight arrow: 0.010 inch safety wire; larger straight arrow: variable-length tip of wire that tapers from 0.025 inch proximally to 0.018 inch distally; open arrow: 20 cm flexible segment, not drawn to scale.

SUMMARY

The current goal in balloon catheter design is to develop a dilation system that is low in profile, is flexible, has a low coefficient of resistance, demonstrates good trackability, has a noncompliant, high pressure balloon, is relatively atraumatic, and is easy to use. As this goal is rapidly being approached, further technologic advancements will be directed toward combining balloon catheters with various thermal energy sources, imaging and atheroablative devices, stents, and possibly pharmacologic agents.

REFERENCES

1. Dotter CT, Judkins MP. Transluminal treatment of arteriosclerotic obstruction. Circulation 1964;30:654–70.
2. Grüntzig A. Die Perkutane rekanalization chronischer arterieller verschlusse (Dotter-Prinzip) mit einem neuen Dilatations Katheter. Rofo 1976;124:80–6.
3. Abele JE. Balloon catheters and transluminal dilatation: technical considerations. AJR 1980;135:901–6.
4. Zollikofer CL, Cragg AH, Hunter DW, et al. Mechanism of transluminal angioplasty. In Castañeda-Zúñiga WR, Tadavarthy SM (eds). Interventional radiology. Baltimore: Williams & Wilkins, 1988, p: 236–65.
5. Zollikofer CL, Salomonowitz E, Bruhlmann WF, et al. Dehungs-Verformungs und Berstungs-Charakteristika haufig verwendeter Balloon-Dilatation-Katheter: in vitro Untersuchungen (Teil 1). Rofo 1986;144:40–6.
6. Gerlock AJ, Regen DM, Shaff MI. An examination of the physical characteristics leading to angioplasty balloon rupture. Radiology 1982;144:421–2.
7. Zollikofer CL, Salomonowitz E, Bruhlmann WF, Castañeda-Zúñiga WR, Amplatz K: Dehungs-Verformungs und Berstungs-Charakteristika haufig verwendeter Balloon-Dilatation-Katheter: in vivo Untersuchungen an Hundegefassen (Teil 2): Rofo 1986;144:189–95.
8. Olbert F, Hanecka L. Transluminal vascular dilatation with a modified dilatation catheter. In Zietler E, Grüntzig A, Schoop W (eds). Percutaneous vascular recanalization. Berlin: Springer-Verlag, 1978:32–8.
9. Tegtmeyer CJ. Guide wire angioplasty balloon catheter: Preliminary report. Radiology 1988;159:253–4.
10. Ricketts HJ. Side-hole balloon-angioplasty catheters. AJR 1985;144:123–6.
11. Barth KH. A modified catheter for transluminal angioplasty of the femoropopliteal artery. Radiology 1984;149:571–2.
12. Levin DC, Murray P, Harrington D. New curved catheter for renal angioplasty. AJR 1982;138:359–60.
13. Mitchell SE, White RI, Kan J, Tolkoff J. Improved balloon catheters for large vessel and valvular angioplasty. AJR 1984;142:571–2.
14. Schwarten DE, Cutcliff WB. Arterial occlusive disease below the knee: treatment with percutaneous transluminal angioplasty performed with low-profile catheters and steerable guide wires. Radiology 1988;169:71–4.
15. Brown KT, Schoenberg NY, Moore ED, Saddekni S. Percutaneous transluminal angioplasty of infrapopliteal vessels: preliminary results and technical considerations. Radiology 1988;169:75–8.
16. Cassarella WJ. Percutaneous transluminal angioplasty below the knee. New techniques, excellent results. Radiology 1988;169:271–2.
17. Tegtmeyer CJ, Sos TA. Techniques of renal angioplasty. Radiology 1986;161:577–86.
18. Wholey MH. The design and clinical application of a new #5 French angioplasty catheter. Cathet Cardiovasc Diag 1987; 13:347–51.
19. Rees MR, Gehani AA, Ashley S, Davies A. Percutaneous video angioscopy in peripheral vascular disease. Clin Radiol 1989;40:347–51.
20. Rees MR, Gehani AA, Ashley S, Brooks S. Angioscopy in the evaluation of dynamic angioplasty. Semin Intervent Radiol 1989;6:123–8.
21. Tobia J, Mallery J, Gessert J, et al. Intravascular ultrasound cross-sectional arterial imaging before and after balloon angioplasty in vitro. Circulation 1989;80:873–82.
22. Isner JM, Rosenfield K, Losordo DW, et al. Percutaneous intravascular US as an adjunct to catheter-based interventions: preliminary experience in patients with peripheral vascular disease. Radiology 1990;175:61–70.
23. Simpson JB, Selmon MR, Robertson GC, et al. Transluminal atherectomy for occlusive peripheral vascular disease. Am J Cardiol 1988;61(suppl G):96–101.
24. Wholey MH, Jarmolowski CR. New reperfusion devices: the Kensey catheter, the atherolytic reperfusion wire device, and the transluminal extraction catheter. Radiology 1989;172:947–52.
25. Cragg AH, Gardiner GA Jr, Smith TP. Vascular applications of laser. Radiology 1989;172:925–35.
26. Sanborn TA, Cumberland DC, Greenfield AJ, Welsh CL, Guben JK. Percutaneous laser thermal angioplasty; initial results and 1 year follow-up in 129 femoropopliteal lesions. Radiology 1988;168:121–5.
27. Becker GJ. Intravascular stents: general principles and status of lower-extremity arterial applications. Circulation 1991;83 (suppl I):I-122–36.
28. Palmaz JC, Richter GM, Noeldge G, et al. Intraluminal stents in atherosclerotic iliac artery stenosis: preliminary report of a multicenter trial. Radiology 1988;168:727–32.
29. Strecker EP, Berg G, Schneider B, et al. A new vascular balloon-expandable prosthesis: experimental studies and first clinical results. J Intervent Radiol 1988;3:59–62.
30. Faxon DP, Sanborn TA, Weber VJ, et al. Restenosis following transluminal angioplasty in experimental atherosclerosis. Arteriosclerosis 1984;4:189–95.
31. Austin GE, Ratliff NB, Hollman J, et al. Intimal proliferation of smooth muscle cells as an explanation for recurrent coronary artery stenosis after percutaneous transluminal angioplasty. J Am Coll Cardiol 1985;6:369–75.
32. Becker GJ. Advances in angioplasty: theoretical and practical. Categorical Course in Interventional Radiology Syllabus. RSNA Meeting, 1991:127–40.
33. Consigny PM. Vascular smooth muscle contraction and relaxation: pathway and chemical modulation. J Vasc Intervent Radiol 1991;2:309–17.
34. Roeren T, LeVeen RF, Villanueva T, Reisman J. Restenosis and successful angioplasty: histologic-radiologic correlation. Radiology 1989;172:971–7.
35. Pepine CJ, Hirschfield JW, MacDonald RG, et al. A controlled trial of corticosteroids to prevent restenosis after coronary angioplasty: M-HEART Group. Circulation 1990;81:1753–61.
36. Gleason TJ, Cragg AH, Smith TP, Landas SK, De Jong SC. Thermal balloon angioplasty in a canine model: preliminary results. J Vasc Intervent Radiol 1990;1:121–6.
37. Spears JR. Percutaneous transluminal coronary angioplasty restenosis: potential prevention with laser balloon angioplasty. Am J Cardiol 1987;60(suppl B):61–4.
38. Becker GJ, Lee GI, Waller BF, et al. Potential of radiofrequency balloon angioplasty: weld strengths, dose-response relationship, and correlative histology. Radiology 1990; 174:1003–8.
39. Anand RK, Sinclair N, Jenkins RD, et al. Laser balloon angioplasty: effect of constant temperature versus constant power on tissue weld strength. Lasers Surg Med 1988;8:40–4.

8 Intravascular Ultrasound

Christopher E. Engeler, M.D., Joseph W. Yedlicka, Jr., M.D.

EQUIPMENT AND METHODS

Instrumentation

Miniaturization of ultrasonic transducers has recently been achieved with crystal thicknesses under 0.1 mm. Accordingly, feasible transducer frequencies are in the range of 10 to 30 MHz. Axial resolution can be expected to be very high. Lateral resolution will depend on focusing of the ultrasonic beam. However, depth of field is limited because tissue penetration decreases with higher frequency.

Such high-frequency ultrasound transducers have been mounted on catheters for intraluminal imaging and are now commercially available. Either a linear array arrangement or mechanical scanning is possible.[1] In the linear array transducer, there are no moving parts. However, the volume of the transducer increases with the number of crystals mounted at the catheter tip. With mechanical scanning, the crystal is rotated 360° to accumulate 8-mode data for axial display. Both types of transducers have been introduced.

The illustrations in this chapter are from a rotating type transducer with a crystal frequency of 20 MHz. Mounted on a long flexible shaft, the transducer is rotated at 1800 rpm within a catheter. Real-time images are thus obtained.

Introduction and Guidance

The shaft with the transducer tip is introduced into a sterile catheter filled with water, which provides internal acoustical coupling. This assembly can then be advanced through any vascular sheath of at least 7 F diameter. A coaxial guide wire may aid in positioning and provide exchange capabilities with interventional catheters. Current limitations include catheter stiffness, which results in poor torque control as well as the relatively short catheter length (100 cm). Maneuverability is also limited at the present time by the inability of the current catheter to be passed over a guide wire. Nevertheless, access to most major arterial or venous systems is possible by using directional sheaths. Even transvenous advancement through the right heart chambers into pulmonary artery branches has been accomplished.

Display and Imaging Recording

Real-time images are projected on the monitor of the ultrasound machine. The time gain compensation setting is critical to proper image interpretation. Due to the high frequency of the ultrasound beam, significant scattering from cellular blood components is observed.[2] It is important to reduce these echoes as much as possible. Once the appropriate settings have been selected, the images may then be displayed on videotape or on film.

ENDOSONOGRAPHY OF VASCULAR DISEASE

Pathologic Overview

Figure 8-1 summarizes the spectrum of arteriosclerosis. The normal arterial wall consists of three layers: intima, media, and adventitia. Intimal edema, thickening, and proliferation are early responses to endothelial injury. Atherosclerosis is characterized by the accumulation of lipids in the intima. Atheromatous disease may progress to fibrous plaques, cholesterol deposition, and calcification. Complications include hemorrhage and ulceration. Specific degeneration of the tunica media is known as Mönckeberg's sclerosis. In large and medium-sized muscular arteries, characteristic calcification of the media is seen in some of these patients; these vessels are radiographically visible and may be clinically palpable.

Sonography of Intimal Hyperplasia

It is possible with high-resolution ultrasonography to differentiate the layers of the arterial wall as they demonstrate characteristic morphologic changes. Intimal hyperplasia is particularly evident in vascular grafts when veins have been employed as arterial conduits for long periods of time. In the lower extremities, in situ grafts utilizing the saphenous vein are common surgical procedures. Progressive luminal narrowing leads to recurrent arterial insufficiency. Intimal hyperplasia in a 15-year-old saphenous vein graft is demonstrated sonographically in Figure 8-2.

Sonography of Atheromatous Lesions

Simple atheromas are echogenic due to the deposition of lipids in the tunica intima. The size of atheromatous lesions and the degree of echogenicity vary considerably. An increased fibrous component is expected to decrease echogenicity, whereas cholesterol deposits likely increase echogenicity. Early investigators have correlated histologic and magnetic resonance findings with images from a prototype high-resolution intravascular ultrasound unit in vitro.[3] Calcification of an atheroma is obvious when there is reflection of the ultrasound beam with distal acoustic shadowing. Figures 8-3 and 8-4 show variations of atheromatous disease.

Sonography of Medial Sclerosis

Atheromatous disease and medial sclerosis may overlap in many patients. With advanced disease, there is circumferential involvement of the affected artery. Ultrasound waves are

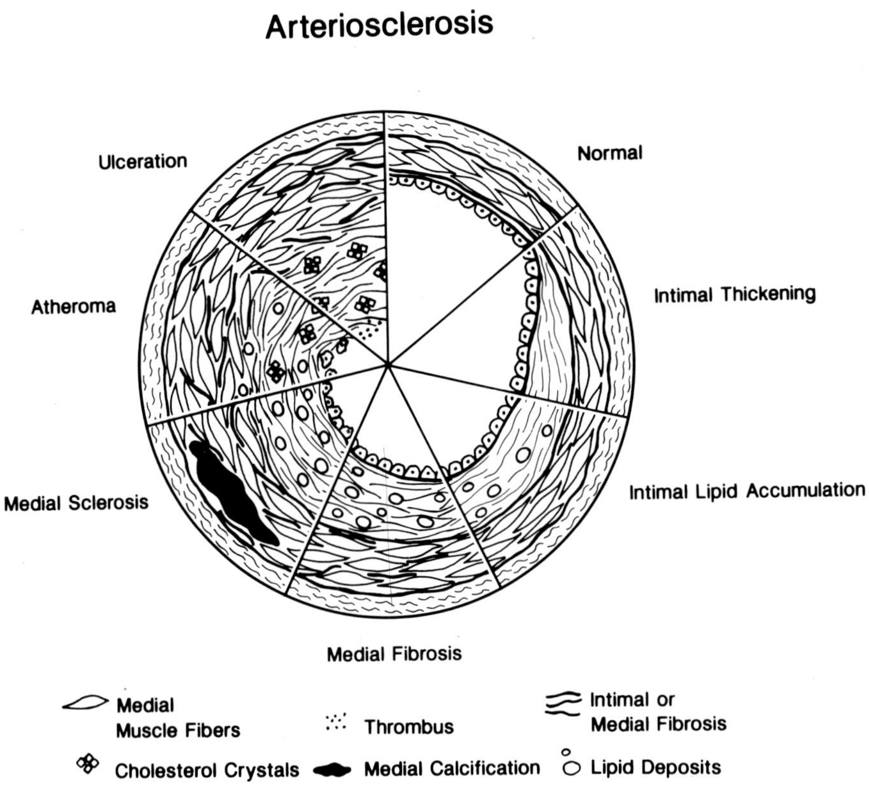

Figure 8–1. The pathologic spectrum of arteriosclerosis.

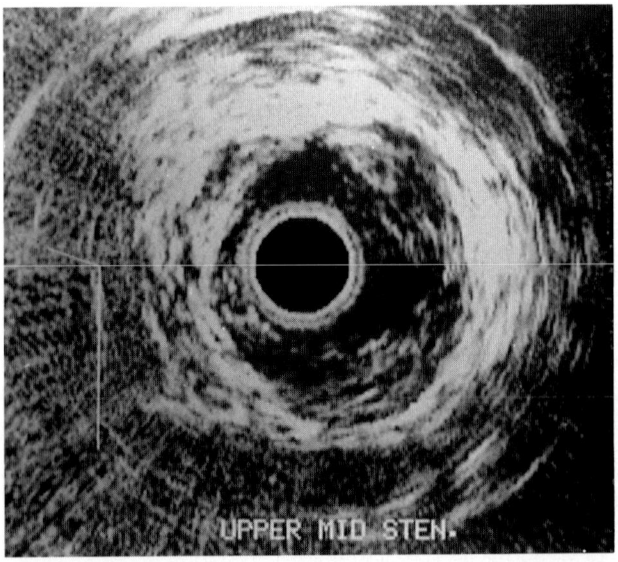

Figure 8–2. Severe intimal hyperplasia in a saphenous vein graft after partial atherectomy.

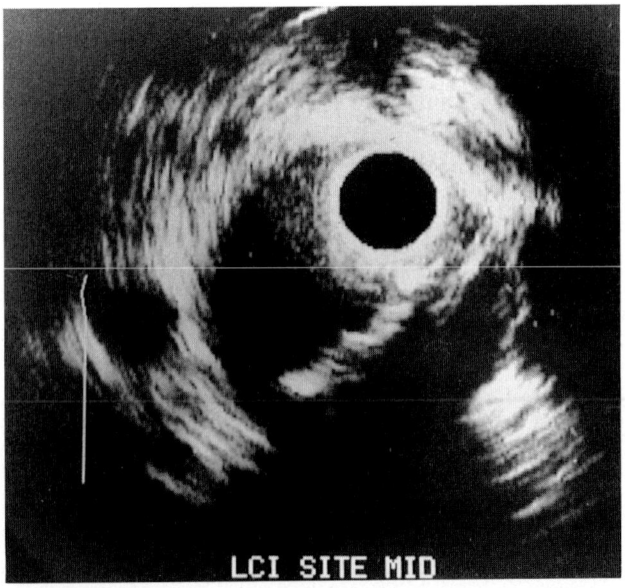

Figure 8–3. Large calcified intimal flap after iliac angioplasty.

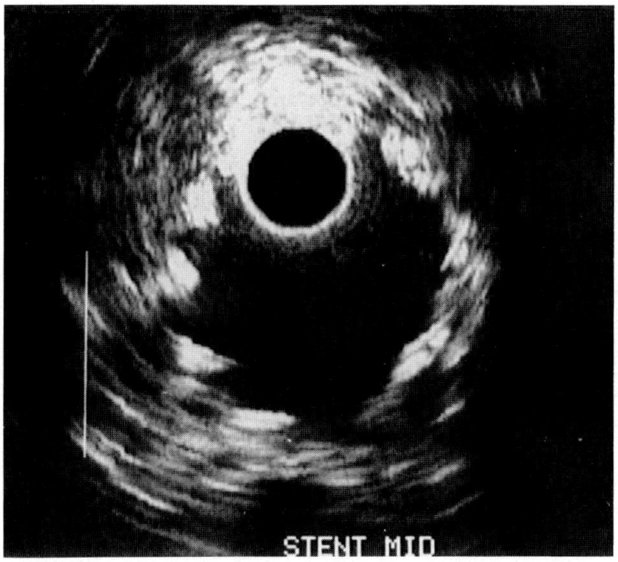

Figure 8–4. Palmaz stent in iliac artery.

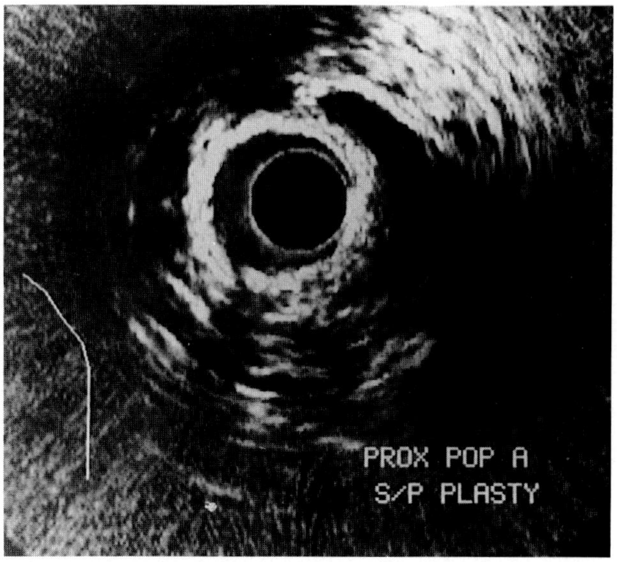

Figure 8–5. Angioplasty bursting of medial sclerosis in a popliteal artery.

then unable to pass beyond the tunica media. The calcifications of medial sclerosis and other arteriosclerotic pathologic states can be differentiated sonographically. Figure 8-5 demonstrates a case of severe medial sclerosis in a popliteal artery.

INTRAVASCULAR ULTRASOUND OF REVASCULARIZATION PROCEDURES

Methods

Adequate access to the diseased vessel is established for both the introduction of interventional catheters and the ultrasound probe. For the latter, a 7 F or greater sheath size is required. Characterization of the general degree of arteriosclerosis and the specific local vascular disease is accomplished angiographically and sonographically. The locations of the stenotic areas are marked on the drape covering the patient for future reference. The progress of the revascularization procedure can be intermittently monitored without contrast by using intravascular ultrasound to assess the degree of any residual stenosis. Further technical advances may lead to coaxial procedures in which the ultrasound probe is used to monitor directly the effects of intervention. This could be achieved when, for example, the balloon is mounted around the probe itself.

Angioplasty: Assessment by Intravascular Ultrasound

Various success rates for immediate and long-term results of angioplasty have been reported. Obviously, the nature of the lesion and the immediate effect of dilation are both critical variables in the eventual result. Intravascular ultrasound can both characterize the diseased vessel and confirm the effect of angioplasty.

The cross-sectional image furnished by intravascular ultrasound can be used to calculate the area and flow through a vessel. This information is similar to that obtained by measuring pressure gradients and is probably more accurate in situations with impaired runoff or distal occlusions. Breaks in the vessel wall, either in the intima or media, may be visualized, particularly if this occurs in a calcified lesion. Intimal flaps are commonly encountered after angioplasty, but may not be evident angiographically. Such flaps increase the risk of restenosis at the site of angioplasty. Intravascular ultrasound has proved to be of great value in recognizing these complications, thus allowing for treatment of these complications and hopefully improving the long-term outcome (Figs. 8-3, 8-5).

Atherectomy: Assessment by Intravascular Ultrasound

The goal of atherectomy is to remove pathologic deposits or accumulations that are obstructing vessels. A cutting device such as the Simpson atherectomy catheter is used. Large amounts of material can be extracted. Atherectomy can be used to supplement angioplasty and vice versa. As a secondary procedure, the atherectomy device is capable of removing intimal flaps after angioplasty. Its role as a primary procedure is currently under investigation. Intravascular ultrasound characterizes arterial disease by demonstrating the thickness and composition of the wall. Although further experience is necessary, it is becoming evident that the larger the pathologic deposit, the greater the relative merits of atherectomy over angioplasty (i.e., severe intimal hyperplasia and large intimal flaps). Figure 8-2 illustrates such a case in a diseased saphenous in situ graft. In some cases of severe calcific arterial disease, atherectomy was able to remove enough material to allow for successful angioplasty.

STENTS: ASSESSMENT BY INTRAVASCULAR ULTRASOUND

Both arterial and venous stents are coming into widespread clinical use. They are designed to overcome the inherent elasticity of vessels that causes them to collapse. The true lumen of a stent cannot be established on a conventional basis without multiple radiographic projections. With intravascular ultrasound, it is possible to measure directly the cross-sectional area of a stented vessel as well as establish the relationship of the stent to adjacent structures, including normal and abnormal vessels as well as masses (Fig. 8-4).

Intravascular Lasers: Role of Intravascular Ultrasound

Vascular recanalization with lasers is a potential alternative to other techniques already described. At the present time, the risk of perforation and lack of guidance limit its clinical applications severely. Intravascular ultrasound delivers essential information on the exact location of the native vessel wall and may serve as a guide to the laser beam.[4] The technical challenge lies in mounting the ultrasound transducer near the tip of the laser catheter.

CONCLUSIONS

Intravascular ultrasound provides interesting new insights into vascular disease and interventional radiographic procedures. The information it gives to the interventionalist has greatly increased with the availability of the new catheter-based units. With further experience, it is hoped that the relative indications and results of different revascularization procedures may be better defined by intravascular ultrasound. Direct guidance and real-time monitoring of interventional procedures will become possible with further technical advances.

REFERENCES

1. Bom N, ten Hoff H, Lancee CT, Gussenhoven WJ, Bosch JG. Early and recent intraluminal ultrasound devices. Int J Card Imaging 1989;4:79–88.
2. Zagzebski JA. Physics and instrumentation in Doppler and B-mode ultrasonography. In Zwiebel WJ (ed): Vascular ultrasonography. Orlando: Grune & Stratton, 1986:21–51.
3. Meyer CR, Chiang EH, Fechner KP, et al. Feasibility of high-resolution, intravascular ultrasonic imaging catheters. Radiology 1988;168:113–6.
4. Borst C, Rienks R, Mali WPTM, van Erven L. Laser ablation and the need for intra-arterial imaging. Int J Card Imaging 1989;4:127–133.

9 Clinical Applications of Angioscopy in Cardiovascular Disease

Jacob Segalowitz, M.D., Warren Grundfest, M.D., Frank Litvak, M.D.

During recent years, angioscopy has allowed for improved in vivo assessment of the vascular endothelial surface. Due to the advances of new intravascular techniques, such as atherectomy, laser ablation, stents, and use of thrombolysis, there may be a need to visually characterize the disease process and monitor the effects of these interventions. The ability to obtain real-time imaging provided by flexible fiberoptics may yield important information during and following intravascular procedures and allow for direct inspection to help direct diagnosis and therapy. In this chapter, we will describe the technology, technique, and clinical application of angioscopy in the coronary and peripheral arteries.

HISTORY AND DEVELOPMENT OF ANGIOSCOPY

The use of fiberoptics for cardiovascular applications emerged from early attempts to perform cardioscopy during cardiotomy procedures. As reported by Cutler et al[1] in 1924, Rhea and Walker in 1913 were the first to employ a rigid tube connected to an external illumination source to visualize intracardiac structures during thoracotomy. Further development was reported by Allen and Graham[2] in 1922, who employed a convex-shaped lens at the distal end of the tube for better visualization and manipulation within the internal cardiac cavity. In 1941 Keith and Wappler were the first to use a fiberoptic device that displaced blood with a bubble effect in order to clear the inspected field. Reported by Harken and Glidden[3] in 1932, the optical system was modified and housed within a glass tube carrying a thin, inflatable plastic balloon at the distal end of the tube. However, when inserted through the heart's atrium for inspection of cardiac chambers, it caused obstruction of blood flow.[3] In Japan, Sakakibara[4] developed a cardioscope in 1936 that permitted ejection of Ringer's solution under pressure to clear the blood field in front of the distal lens of a cardioscope. Subsequent Japanese experience employed a rigid, curved scope for inspection of valvular disease in left heart cardioscopy. Intraventricular inspection of stenotic mitral valves was reported by Murray[5] in 1950 as an adjunct to selection of resection site and inspection of stenotic cardiac valves. Butterworth[6] in 1951 and Bolton et al[7] in 1954 further used homogenous plastic cardioscopes with external light sources for inspection of atrial septopexy. In 1961, Carlens and Silander[8] used a 90° angled rigid scope of 4 mm in diameter fitted with a distal end inflatable balloon. With this device good quality images of intracardiac anatomy were first obtained. Greenstone et al[9] in 1966 reported the use of fiberoptic endoscopy in animals and humans using a 7.0 mm modified choledochoscope. Gamble and Ennis,[10] in 1967, were able to develop a flexible fiberoptic catheter with a distal inflatable latex balloon. This was the first catheter inserted through a peripheral artery that was able to clear the inspected visual field.[10]

In the early 1980s, highly flexible, ultrathin angioscopes, 3.3 to 1.8 mm in diameter, became available, along with advanced fiberoptics technology for improved spatial resolution, videocamera adaptation, and high-resolution monitoring equipment. At that time, our group at Cedars-Sinai Medical Center employed angioscopy intraoperatively in the coronary and peripheral arteries to evaluate the inner anatomy and to study in vivo morphologic appearance of cardiovascular disease.[11] Extensive collaboration with industry led to further development of smaller angioscopes (Fig. 9-1). By 1984, 0.85 mm diameter angioscopes were available for intraoperative application and by 1987, 0.5 mm diameter angioscopes were developed for percutaneous inspection of coronary arteries.

Recently, efforts have focused on refinement of percutaneous use of angioscopy in peripheral and coronary arteries. Several companies (Olympus, NY; Advanced Interventional Systems, CA; Vascucare, MI; Baxter-Edwards, CA; Intramed, CA; Nihon Koden, CA) have developed 0.5 to 0.7 mm diameter highly flexible angioscopes suitable for percutaneous angioscopy. To date, the smallest available angioscope contains 3000 fibers in 0.3 mm diameter imaging bundle. However, further improvement in adjunctive catheter design is necessary in order to optimize coaxialization of delivery systems for intravascular tractability and steerability of angioscopes.

TECHNOLOGY OF ANGIOSCOPY

Progress in the communication industry has led to significant improvement of fiberoptic "tools" used in medicine. At present, individual fibers as small as 1.6 μm in diameter are available. Glass fibers, or fiberoptics, are capable of conducting light from one point to another and around curves. The light transmitting material has two components: an inner core that delivers light from the distal to the proximal end of the fiberoptic and an exterior cladding portion that keeps the light within the inner core material (by different indices of refraction).

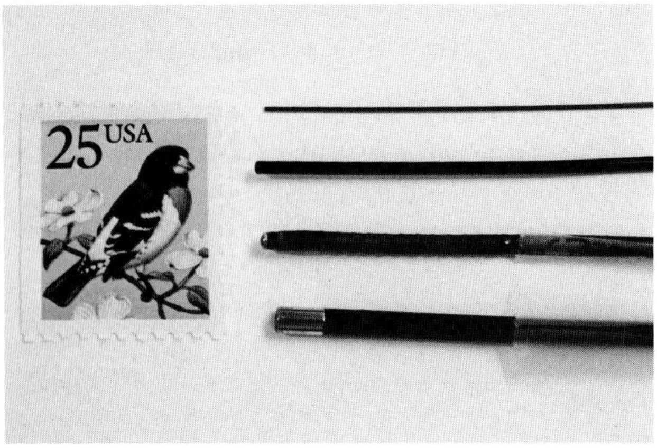

Figure 9–1. Distal end tips of ultrathin angioscopes of various sizes: 0.8, 1.4, 2.2, and 2.8 mm (from top to bottom).

Individual fiberoptics can be assembled into a coherent fiberoptic bundle, creating a close array. Each fiberoptic obtains one area point (pixel) image of the distal inspected visual field and the complete image at the proximal view portion is created by the sum of the fiberoptic bundle pixels presented through a videocamera on a high-resolution television monitor. Lenses are incorporated at the distal end of the fiberoptic bundle to enhance focusing of the vessel's intraluminal light into the imaging fiber bundle. Recent developed technology permits assembly of 0.45 mm diameter angioscopes with 0.35 mm diameter lenses integrated at the distal end of the imaging bundle (Fig. 9-2). For optimal image quality, these distal lenses are wide angled (i.e., 90°) and provide a short focal length (i.e., 0.5 mm). To enable intraluminal vessel inspection, it is necessary to provide light into the field of inspection. For this purpose, relatively large illumination fibers, ranging in size from 25 to 50 μm are concentrically arranged, surrounding the imaging bundle to provide uniform lighting in front of the distal end of the angioscope. These illumination fibers conduct the light from an external light source (300 W Xenon) connected to the proximal end of the angioscope. Higher image resolution with sharper picture are obtained by incorporating a greater number of fibers within the imaging bundle. Spatial resolution of current angioscopes ranges from 200 to 20 μm at 5 mm.

The development of pressure-controlled irrigation pumps has further improved image quality and enhanced simplicity of the angioscope system operation. With this pump, pressure-controlled irrigation fluid provides a clear-from-blood inspection field in proximity to the distal end of the angioscope. These rotary irrigation pumps can deliver up to 400 ml/min irrigation fluid through the coaxially positioned irrigation catheter or the irrigation channel as incorporated within the angioscope. Currently, several manufacturers (Olympus, Vascucare, Intramed) provide a complete angioscopic system including a rotary irrigation pump (Fig. 9-3).

Image quality improvement and ease of use further resulted with the use of charge-coupled devices (CCD) chip videocameras, which are connected on-line to high-resolution television monitors (Fig. 9-4). These CCD videocameras can be sterilized and placed on the sterile field. The latest of such devices is 1 cm in diameter and only 5 cm long (Toshiba, Japan).

To enhance intraluminal negotiation capabilities further, angioscopes were developed to have steerable deflecting distal tips (Olympus, Vascucare, Intramed). Further catheter technology housed a separate lumen within the angioscope as an irrigation channel, which eliminates the need for coaxially positioning the angioscope by and within an auxiliary irrigation catheter in order to obtain a clear-from-blood inspection field in proximity of the distal end of the angioscope. However, such adjunctive catheter technology is still required to improve subselective delivery catheters for angioscopes that are 0.5 mm in diameter or less. Such catheter delivery systems, ideally 5 to 7 F in size, can be guided by

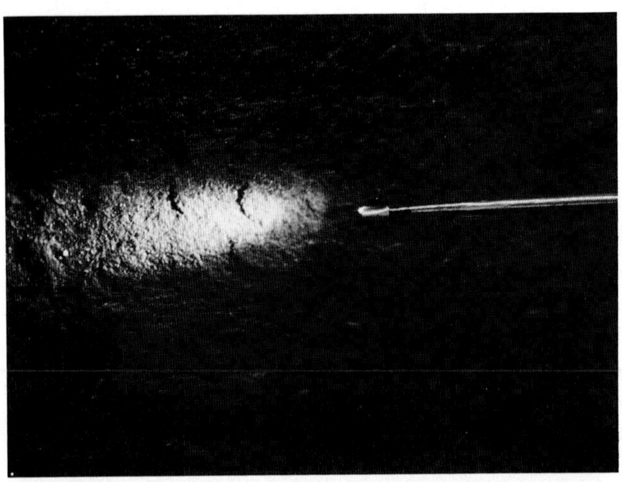

Figure 9–2. A 0.45 mm diameter prototype angioscope used for percutaneous coronary applications. This angioscope may be introduced into a 4.5 F (1.67 mm) coronary catheter that is subselectively negotiated over a guide wire (0.014 inch).

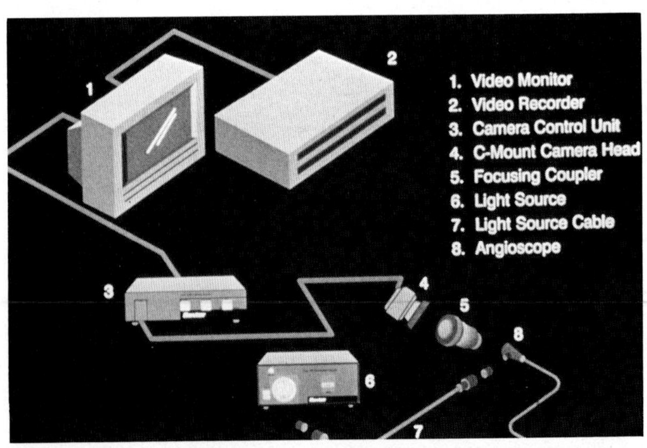

Figure 9–3. Component diagram of a complete system for angioscopy operated during intraoperative and percutaneous cardiovascular procedures.

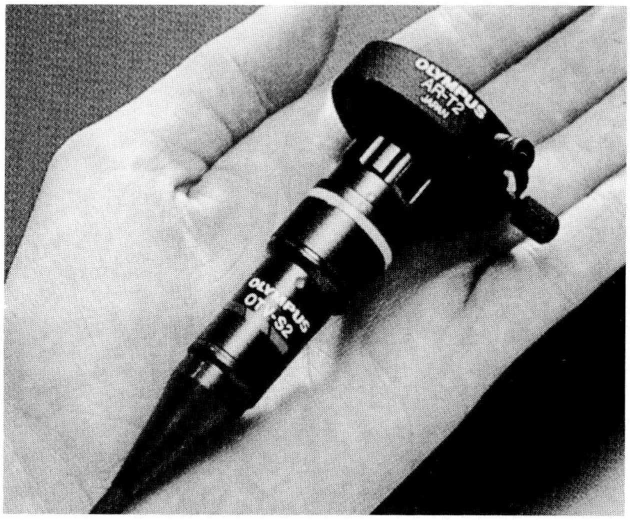

Figure 9–4. Charge-coupled device videocamera used for intraoperative and percutaneous angioscopy. This CCD high-resolution videocamera can be sterilized and placed on the sterile field.

over-the-wire technique and can be positioned coaxially within the vessel's lumen by means of a distal inflatable low-profile balloon.

TECHNIQUES OF ANGIOSCOPY

Intraoperative Angioscopy

At Cedars-Sinai Medical Center, angioscopy has been extensively employed during peripheral vascular surgery and coronary artery bypass surgery. In lower extremity vascular operations, access to the common profunda and superficial femoral artery is performed at the time of bypass or thromboembolectomy. The angioscope is introduced into the lumen of the artery or graft through a longitudinal incision for bypass or a transversal incision for thromboembolectomy at the most convenient site for inspection and guided by the surgeon to the precise area of interest by gentle anterograde advancing-rotating manipulation. Imaging in a flowing bloodstream is facilitated by the use of rotary pressure-controlled irrigation pumps that are pulsed generated and may be adjusted on demand by a remote foot switch for immediate high bolus operation or low-flow maintenance irrigation mode.

Angioscopes ranging from 0.45 to 3.3 mm in diameter are available to inspect vessels that range from 1 mm to 1 cm in diameter. Angioscopy of aortofemoral synthetic limb graft may be performed from the femoral approach with proximal inflow control by an occlusive balloon from a catheter that is held parallel to the angioscope. For iliac artery inspection, this method is relatively unsatisfactory because of collateral blood flow from the internal iliac artery and lumbar arteries.

For aortofemoral and femoral applications, we employ 2.8, 2.5, 2.3, 1.8, 1.5, and 1.4 mm outer diameter angioscopes. For popliteal, tibial, and peroneal applications, we use 0.45 to 1.5 mm outer diameter angioscopes. Irrigation quantity used during intraoperative peripheral procedure is 150 to 400 ml of normal saline solution.

Intraoperative coronary angioscopy has been relatively easier to perform than the peripheral vascular procedures. Intraoperatively, during coronary bypass surgery, there is a direct exposure of the arteries or grafts of an arrested heart with clamped aorta while the patient is supported by a cardiopulmonary bypass pump. During angioscopy, the artery may be irrigated with cold crystalloid cardioplegic solution buffered with additional sodium bicarbonate, delivered either through the aortic root or a coaxial 18-gauge catheter. Inspection may take 2 to 4 minutes. For native coronary artery inspection, the angioscope is inserted through the distal arteriotomy site and advanced in retrograde fashion.

When coronary vein grafts are inspected, the angioscope is passed through the proximal end of the graft, prior to completion of the aortic anastomosis. Further inspection of the distal native coronary artery may be performed if the angioscope is advanced beyond the distal anastomotic site. Continuous low-flow irrigation has the advantage of distending the coronary arteries, thus increasing their diameter and clearing the inspected vessel of any blood that may originate from collateral circulation.

Percutaneous Angioscopy

Percutaneous access of angioscopy requires different parameters than in the intraoperative setting. Technical difficulty during angioscopy is mainly in vessels of large diameter (more than 5 mm), since significant blood flow obscures the inspected intraluminal field. Proximal control to reduce the blood flow in these large vessels is difficult to obtain by means of a proximal accessory occlusive balloon catheter, for multiple catheter manipulation through the same single percutaneous access site is not simple. External vessel compression was found to be unsatisfactory to control blood flow volume.

In order to obtain good quality angioscopic images in these peripheral vessels of large diameter, it is also necessary to use 2.3 to 2.8 mm (7 to 9 F) diameter angioscopes, which often are too large to fit into a standard peripheral percutaneous introducer sheath. To facilitate practicality and ease of use, percutaneous angioscopy is used in conjunction with balloon catheter technologies, slightly refined and adapted for this application.

Percutaneous access is performed with Seldinger technique. A guide wire is inserted to access the common femoral or external iliac artery. A dilation catheter is then inserted over the guide wire to widen the arteriotomy, followed by insertion of a 7 or 8 F introducer sheath having a proximal port valve for angioscope or guide wire insertion and a side port for fluid irrigation pumping or contrast solution injection. Specifically, a catheter-shaped, highly flexible angioscopic delivery system of 4 to 7 F in size fits through the introducer catheter. The delivery catheter is approximately 90 cm in length and carries an occlusion balloon positioned at the distal end, the tip of which when inflated occludes the inspected vessel. At a firm position, the catheter's distal balloon may be inflated to occlude intraluminal blood flow. Visualization is obtained when the angioscope is advanced antegrade through the distal open end of the delivery catheter. The position of the angioscope's distal tip may be monitored by fluoroscopy.

During the last decade, percutaneous transluminal coronary angioplasty (PTCA) has achieved refinements in technique and catheter design that were used to overcome most of the previously mentioned difficulties. Ultrathin and highly flexible fiberoptic bundles were incorporated into catheters that track over steerable guide wires and enable selection of any major coronary artery for angioscopic inspection. Intraluminal coaxial positioning has been a most challenging problem and ability to manipulate the catheter tip yet requires further modifications and improvement.

Percutaneous coronary angioscopy has resulted from clinical research that demonstrated that thrombosis and endothelial lesions are key factors in the development of unstable angina and acute myocardial infarction. Access to a coronary artery must be obtained via femoral artery or brachial artery guiding catheters. In the nonarrested heart, the coronary arteries are in constant motion and the potential inspection site must be cleared from blood flow. Preferably, no occluding balloon should be used to reduce blood flow in the coronary artery during irrigation, since distal myocardial ischemia may occur. Relatively small amounts of flushing fluid (1 to 8 ml/sec) may be sufficient to displace the blood flow from the inspected field. Continuous pressure-controlled rotary pump irrigation, channeled within the fiberoptic catheter, may be used to clear the visual field.

Percutaneous coronary angioscopy was first performed by Spears et al using 1.8 mm angioscope[12] (Olympus). Inoue et al[13] used a 1.0 mm angioscope that contained 3000 fibers in an imaging bundle that fit through an 8 F coronary guiding catheter. Susawa et al[14] used a 1.2 mm angioscope (Olympus Corp.) through an 8.3 F guiding catheter to observe intracoronary thrombus information. Further experience by Susawa et al[29] employed a 0.75 mm diameter angioscope (Fukada Denshi Co.) to study intracoronary thrombolysis. Uchida et al[15,16] used successfully a 1.3 mm angioscope (Olympus) through a 9 F guiding catheter employing coaxial irrigation to clear the inspected field.

The use of a double guiding catheter system to assist intraluminal positioning of an angioscope has been reported by Morice et al.[17] A 1.0 mm angioscope (American-Edwards) was used inside a 4 F catheter inserted through a 9 F coronary guiding catheter following thrombolysis therapy and PTCA.

Kuwaki et al[18] performed angioscopy during heart catheterization using a 0.75 mm angioscope coaxialized within a 5 F guiding catheter, which was then introduced into an 8 F outer guiding catheter.

Late advances have been reported using steerable wire-guided angioscopes for better negotiating capability in the coronary vasculature. A steerable angioscope (Advanced Cardiovascular Systems) used by Ramee et al[19] consists of a fiberoptic channel incorporated into a 1.4 mm diameter PTCA balloon catheter having a lumen for insertion of a 0.014 to 0.016 inch steerable PTCA guide wire or contrast media injection. The angioscope was advanced over the guide wire and a clear inspection field was obtained with minimal irrigation of lactated Ringer's solution (1 to 5 ml) and 15 to 30 seconds balloon inflation. Further experience was reported in Germany by Hoeher et al[20] using 1.2 or 1.8 mm diameter angioscope (Olympus) modified to be negotiated over a guide wire and introduced through a 9 F coronary guiding catheter.

Mitzuno et al.[21] reported the use of a 1.1 mm diameter angioscope negotiated over a 0.014 inch guide wire through a catheter with tip angulation mechanism and no distal occluding balloon, which allowed precise coaxial positioning of the angioscope in the coronary artery.

CLINICAL APPLICATIONS OF ANGIOSCOPY

Angioscopy During Peripheral Vascular Surgery

Our experience with angioscopy suggests that direct real-time imaging of the arterial or graft lumen during reconstructive peripheral procedures provides the surgeon with an improved method of assessing luminal morphology and completeness of the surgical procedure than angiography alone. Angioscopy does not replace preoperative angiography, which remains essential to delineate the location and extent of stenosis or occlusion. However, angiography is limited to detailing the extent of intraoperative changes made or the morphologic nature and appearance of the lesion. Angioscopy, which decreases dye load, can be performed concurrent with the surgical procedure and is more sensitive to the presence of thrombus and luminal obstruction than angiography.[22]

In 1987, we first reported on a large clinical experience regarding routine intraoperative peripheral vascular angioscopy.[23] Our experience demonstrated improved ability to detect intimal flaps, misplaced sutures of anastomosis, atherosclerotic debris, residual thrombi, neointimal flaps, retained venous valves and sclerotic vein segments (Fig. 9-5). Correction of these abnormalities, not identified by completion angiogram, improved graft patency and limb salvage rate (Fig. 9-6). This initial series of 86 patients yielded 118 angioscopic inspections with 15% failure rate to obtain good angioscopic images. Our study reported that changes in intraoperative management based on angioscopic findings were significant: revision of 5 of 37 (14%) anastomoses, deletion of 4 of 31 (13%) completion angiograms, revision of 8 of 17 (47%) in situ vein grafts, and repeated thrombectomy in six of seven procedures. In 22 of 73 (30%) cases, potential

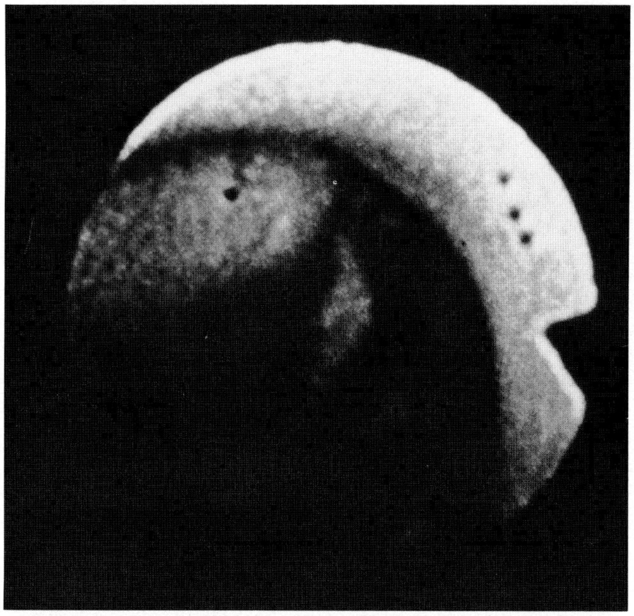

Figure 9–5. Angioscopic image obtained in a Gore-Tex bypass graft of suprageniculate popliteal artery. A large vertical intimal flap is seen obstructing the distal outflow tract.

causes of graft pathologic changes were identified by angioscopy.

Since 1988, angioscopy has been performed in additional 75 peripheral vascular procedures; 61 intraoperatively and 14 during percutaneous intravascular interventions. In 75 patients, high-quality diagnostic angioscopic images were obtained in 74 cases (99%), including 32 anastomoses, 40 vein grafts, 31 thromboembolectomies, and 13 valvulotomies. Angioscopic information was the basis of intraoperative changes in 12 of 32 anastomoses (38%), 4 of 40 vein grafts (10%), and in all 13 valvulotomy inspections. In this second series angioscopy permitted deletion of completion angiogram in 11 procedures.

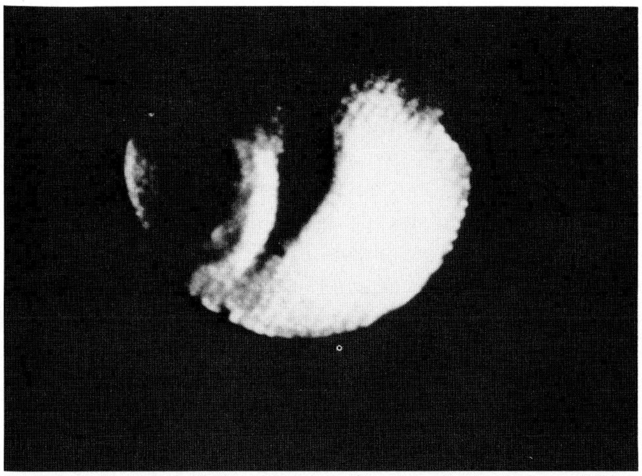

Figure 9–6. An angioscopic image obtained during inspection following thrombectomy in femoropopliteal in situ bypass graft demonstrates an intimal flap obstructing the intraluminal outflow.

Additional clinical experience by our group suggests that direct visualization during thromboembolectomy procedures provides a more reliable method of assessing intraluminal morphology than angiography alone. We inspected 32 grafts (seven aortobifemoral, 18 infrainguinal bypasses, and seven dialysis access fistulas) in 32 patients. Angioscopy following standard catheter thromboembolectomy revealed significant amounts of retained thrombus or neointima in all thrombectomies. Angioscopic information from 18 patients with infrainguinal bypass graft led to graft revision in six cases and placement of a new graft in ten cases. In five of the six cases, graft replacement was initiated on the basis of angioscopic findings. One limb of seven aortobifemoral grafts was replaced and multiple repeat thrombectomies were performed to extract intraluminal debris in the remaining six cases. Repeated graft thrombectomy was also performed in all dialysis access fistulas.

Intraoperative Coronary Angioscopy

At Cedars-Sinai Medical Center, we performed angioscopic examination of the coronary arteries during coronary artery bypass graft procedures in 139 patients, who have had chronic stable angina, accelerated angina, unstable rest angina, or were postmyocardial infarction, post-thrombolytic therapy, and post acute failed balloon angioplasty (Fig. 9-7).

Our experience suggests the direct relationship between endothelial pathologic states as seen by angioscopy and clinical symptoms.[24,25] Patients with stable angina, as seen by angioscopy, have a smooth atheroma in a single coronary artery (Fig. 9-8). Large smooth lesions are localized and eccentric. The plaque is partially obstructive with yellow-white surface color.

The finding that differentiates acute from stable coronary syndromes, as observed[32] angioscopy, is endothelial ulceration. As endothelial surface of atheroma ulcerate, immediately induced platelet aggregation and release of coronary

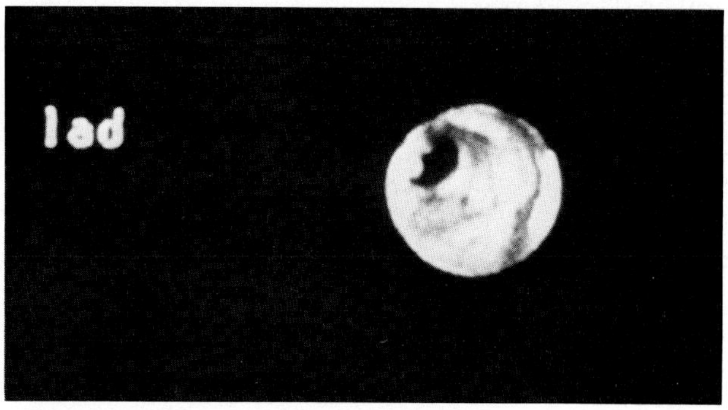

Figure 9–7. Mild stenotic atherosclerosis observed in left anterior descending coronary artery during coronary artery bypass surgery. The endothelial surface is seen ragged with multiple light reflections resulting from fresh occlusive material.

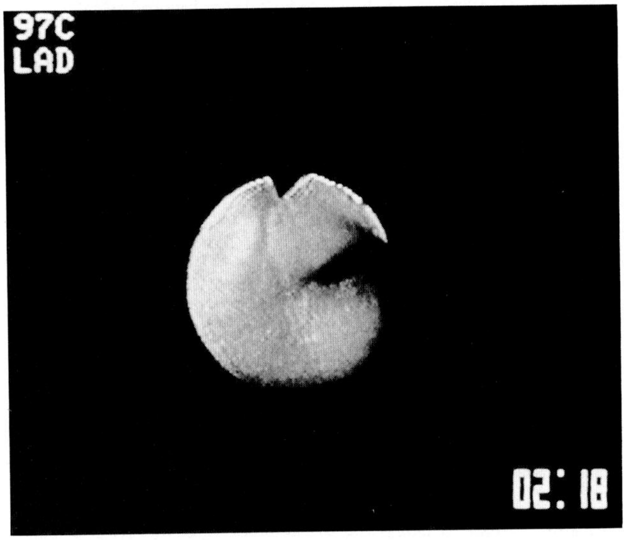

Figure 9–8. An angioscopic image of a left anterior descending coronary artery stenotic lesion in a patient with chronic stable angina. The intimal surface is smooth and white-yellow in color. No ulceration or thrombus is seen.

vasoconstrictors cause accelerated angina[26] (Fig. 9-9). Based on our data, we have suggested that endothelial ulceration is the cause of acute coronary syndromes. Platelets that aggregate at the ulcerated plaque may form a thrombus that causes unstable rest angina if it is partially obstructive or myocardial infarction if it completely obstructs the coronary lumen (Fig. 9-10). Emboli may originate from the ulcerated

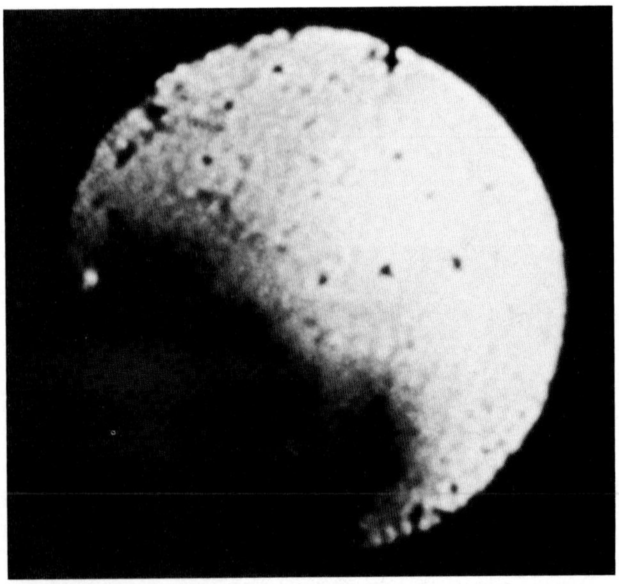

Figure 9–9. A moderate eccentric thrombotic occlusion in left anterior descending coronary artery seen during coronary artery bypass surgery. The distal portion of the arterial lumen is seen at the 8 o'clock position.

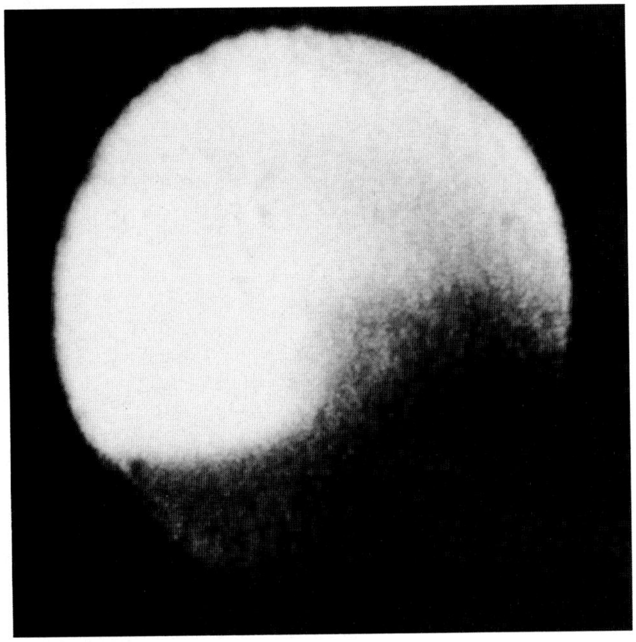

Figure 9–10. Angioscopic image obtained during coronary artery bypass graft surgery in a patient with acute ischemic event. A subtotal thrombotic occlusion is seen extending from 3 to 8 o'clock.

plaque and cause ventricular arrhythmias that may lead to sudden cardiac death.

Endothelial injury is frequently the trigger of atheroma formation, by macrophage activity and smooth muscle cell response that cause localized progressive accelerated stenosis. Our angioscopic data led to conclusions that both stable and unstable coronary syndromes accelerated stenosis that results from endothelial ulceration and that coronary disease is cyclical, characterized by long stable periods peaked by sudden fatal events.

Angioscopic Observation of Interventional Procedures

We have employed angioscopy to evaluate coronary arterial wall surface following failed PTCA (Fig. 9-11). Angioscopy proved to be more sensitive than angiography in detecting thrombus formation and postprocedure dissection.[27] Onset of ischemic syndromes postangioplasty was related to acute intraluminal pathologic changes that resulted from intimal flaps, thrombi, or endothelial ulcer formation. By precisely delineating morphologic pathologic events, angioscopy may assess decision of proper therapy.

Fiberoptic technology was also employed to visualize directly 308 nm excimer laser ablation of atherosclerotic vascular tissue in aortocoronary saphenous vein grafts obtained at repeated coronary artery bypass graft surgery. Angioscopic observation before, during, and following excimer laser ablation showed precise pulsed contact tissue removal without thermal injury to the surrounding tissues.[28]

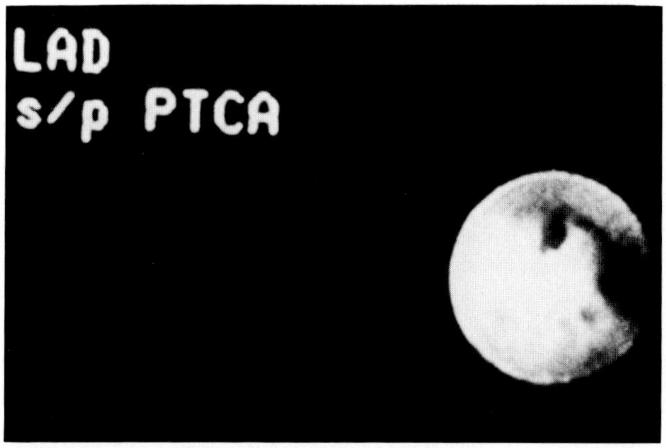

Figure 9–11. Angioscopic image obtained in a patient after percutaneous transluminal coronary angioplasty. The left anterior descending coronary artery is seen during coronary artery bypass graft surgery. A large endothelial tear is seen extending from 4 to 10 o'clock. No thrombotic formation was observed.

We further used angioscopy to inspect pre- and postballoon angioplasty directly in coronary vein grafts. Quantitative angioscopy was performed and images were planimetered, showing relatively small increases in luminal diameter of the vein grafts with creation of intimal flaps and dissections.

CONCLUSION

Intraoperative angioscopy is now a well-refined technique. Intraoperative peripheral angioscopy, and to a lesser extent coronary angioscopy, are adjunctive tools of the cardiovascular surgeon. Angioscopy has been useful in vascular surgery to delineate quality and completeness of anastomosis, thrombectomy, valve stripping, and angioplasty. Percutaneous angioscopy of the peripheral and coronary arteries remains, at this time, developmental. This technique, which demonstrates in real-time the morphologic correlation of clinical syndromes, has provided valuable information describing the pathogenesis of stable and unstable ischemic syndromes. As angioscope design and quality are improved so as to allow percutaneous application in a wider variety of patients, further information with respect to in vivo findings on patients with unstable ischemic syndromes, ischemic cardiomyopathy and who have had interventional procedures should be possible. Furthermore, percutaneous angioscopy may play a role in the choice of the appropriate interventional device in this era of multiple device development.

REFERENCES

1. Cutler EC, Levine SA, Beck CS. The surgical treatment of mitral stenosis: experimental and clinical studies. Arch Surg 1924;9:689–821.
2. Allen DS, Graham EA. Intracardiac surgery; a new method. JAMA 1922;79:1028–30.
3. Harken DE, Glidden EM. Experiments in intracardiac surgery. J Thorac Surg 1932;12:566–72.
4. Sakakibara T. Cardioscope. Rinsho igaku (Clin Med) 1941;29:548–562.
5. Murray G. Cardioscope. Angiology 1950;1:334–6.
6. Butterworth RF. A new operating cardioscope. J Thorac Surg 1951;22:319–22.
7. Bolton HE, Bailey CP, et al. Cardioscopy: simple and practical. J Thorac Surg 1954;27:323–9.
8. Carlens E, Silander T. Method for direct inspection of the right atrium: experimental observation in the dog. Surgery 1961;49:619–624.
9. Greenstone SM, Shore JM, et al. Arterial endoscopy (arterioscopy). Arch Surg 1966;93:811–2.
10. Gamble WJ, Ennis RE. Experimental intracardiac visualization. N Engl J Med 1967;276:1397–1403.
11. Grundfest WS, Litvack F, Lee M, et al. High resolution intraoperative angioscopy of peripheral and coronary arteries in man. Surg Forum 1984;35:423–5.
12. Spears JR, Spokojny AM, et al. Coronary angioscopy during cardiac catheterization. J Am Coll Cardiol 1985;6:93–7.
13. Inoue K, Kuwaki K, et al. Angioscopy guided coronary thrombolysis. (Abstr.) J Am Coll Cardiol 1987;9(suppl A):62A.
14. Susawa T, Yui Y, et al. Directo observation of coronary thrombus using a newly developed ultrathin flexible angioscope. (Abstr.) J Am Coll Cardiol 1987;9(suppl A):197A.
15. Uchida Y, Fukuse A, et al. Percutaneous coronary angioscopy using a novel balloon guiding catheter in patients with ischemic heart diseases. (Abstr.) Circulation 1987;76(suppl IV):185.
16. Uchida Y, Tomaru T, et al. Percutaneous coronary angioscopy in patients with ischemic heart disease. Am Heart J 1987; 114:1216–22.
17. Morice M, Marco J, et al. Percutaneous coronary angioscopy before and after angioplasty in acute MI. Preliminary results. (Abstr.) Circulation 1987;76 (suppl IV):282.
18. Kuwaki K, Inoue K, et al. Percutaneous transluminal coronary angioscopy during cardiac catheterization: the results of experiences in the first 30 patients. (Abstr.) Circulation 1987; 76(suppl IV):186.
19. Ramee SR, White CJ, et al. Percutaneous coronary angioscopy using a steerable microendoscope. (Abstr.) J Am Coll Cardiol 1988;2(suppl A):173A.
20. Hoeher M, Hombach V, et al. Percutaneous coronary angioscopy during cardiac catheterization. (Abstr.) J Am Coll Cardiol 1988;2(suppl A):65A.
21. Mitzuno K, Arakawa K, et al. A serial observation of coronary thrombosis in-vivo by a new angioscope. (Abstr.) J Am Coll Cardiol 1988;2(suppl A):30A.
22. White GH, White RA, et al. Angioscopic thromboembolectomy: preliminary observations with a recent technique. J Vasc Surg 1988;7:318–25.
23. Grundfest WS, Litvack F, Glick D, et al. Circulation 1988;78 (suppl I):I-13–7.
24. Forrester JS, Litvack F, et al. A perspective of coronary disease seen through the arteries of living man. Circulation 1987;75:505–13.
25. Sherman CT, Litvack F, et al. Coronary angioscopy in patients with unstable angina pectores. N Engl J Med 1986;315:913–9.
26. Willerson JT, Hillis LD, et al. Speculation regarding mechanisms responsible for acute ischemic syndromes. J Am Coll Cardiol 1986;8:245–50.
27. Hickey A, Litvack F, et al. In-vivo angioscopy following balloon angioplasty. Circulation 1986;74 (suppl II):II-458.
28. Segalowitz J, Litvack F, et al. Direct angioscopy observation of plaque ablation by excimer laser. (Abstr.) Circulation 1988;80:89.
29. Susawa T, Yui Y, Hattori R, et al. Direct observation of coronary thrombus using a newly developed ultrathin (1.2 mm) flexible angioscope (Abstr.). J Am Coll Cardiol 1987;9 (suppl A):197.

10 Transluminal Angioplasty of the Aorta and Iliac Arteries

Riccardo Di Segni, M.D.

Percutaneous transluminal angioplasty (PTA) is acquiring more and more acceptance as an effective recanalizing procedure in arterial occlusive disease. As an alternative to surgery, PTA appears to be simpler, faster, and less expensive, with less complications, more easily repeatable, and better tolerated by the patients.[1]

Experience in the last years has shown that success in these procedures is determined not only by the skillful adequate use of the technique, but also by the correct choice of lesions to be treated. Each arterial segment has its unique problems of approach and management. In this chapter the problems related to PTA of the infrarenal aorta and iliac vessels will be discussed.

AORTA

In comparison with other arterial segments, PTA of the infrarenal aorta seems to be a technique less commonly used. However, the number of reports on aortic PTA is slowly increasing,[2–14] thus allowing a reasonable evaluation of the benefits of this technique. Probably one of the reasons for the initial reluctance to use PTA in aortic lesions was the concern about complications, not only regarding the vessel itself, but also its major branches. This concern was also theoretically supported by Laplace's law. According to Laplace's law, the force at the surface of a cylinder is proportional to its radius; consequently, a small increase of the dilating pressure at the balloon diameters that are needed for aortic dilation could result in stretching of the vessel beyond its elastic tolerance.[12,13] In common clinical practice, this concern still imposes a very careful choice of the lesions to be treated with respect to the extent of disease present, vicinity of major branches, and the optimal choice of balloon catheters.

Indications

The ideal lesion for aortic angioplasty is a focal, concentric, distal abdominal aortic stenosis, of atherosclerotic origin. More proximal or eccentric lesions, as well as nonatherosclerotic obstructions, are considered by some as relative anatomic contraindications.[2] However, good results have been recently reported in the dilation of eccentric, calcified stenosis[12,13] and of proximal aortic lesions.[14]

In the first reports, generally short stenosis (mean 8 mm) were dilated, with very few cases of long stenosis.[7,8] In more recent series, short stenoses (less than 2 cm) still prevail, but there are also successful reports on treatment of longer segments (up to and over 4 cm).[12,13]

A special group of treatable aortic lesions is found in relatively young patients, usually female smokers, with small distal aortas, who are more susceptible to focal aortic stenosis and are poor candidates for reconstructive surgery because of the small vessel size.[14] Hypoplastic aortas with superimposed stenosis are also included among the indications.[11]

Total occlusion of the lower abdominal aorta and of the aortic bifurcation due to atherosclerosis with associated thrombosis is the cause of the well-known Leriche syndrome. The first case of Leriche syndrome was treated with PTA in 1980,[3] and this vessel is still patent after 9 years[15] (Fig. 10-1). Following this initial report, other cases of Leriche and pre-Leriche syndromes have been treated with PTA.[5–7,10,16]

Success in the treatment of abdominal aortic stenosis due to nonatherosclerotic diseases such as Takayasu's arteritis[17] and aortitis[18] has been recently reported.

TECHNIQUE

The noninvasive evaluation includes ankle-brachial index measurement, Doppler studies, and pulse volume recording.[3,5,8–11,14,17] A preliminary angiographic assessment of the lesion is essential in order to plan the procedure. Angiography is also important after PTA to verify its results immediately. In the short- and long-term follow-up there is no need to repeat the angiographic study except in specific cases in which there is clinical evidence of worsening.[2]

Digital subtraction angiography is useful to reduce the total dose of contrast medium. This is particularly important when multiple projections are required. Road mapping techniques are useful for guiding the revascularization procedure.[1,15] In the follow-up, intravenous digital subtraction angiography can be used to obtain graphic minimally invasive documentation. There are no printed reports of the possible use of magnetic resonance imaging in the follow-up of aortic angioplasty, with the exception of the report by Tadavarthy et al[15] (Fig. 10-1). The utility of this technique should be carefully evaluated, since it offers a very valid and at the same time noninvasive demonstration of the aortic anatomy.

Intravascular pressure measurements are done immediately before the dilatation procedure, preferably after the

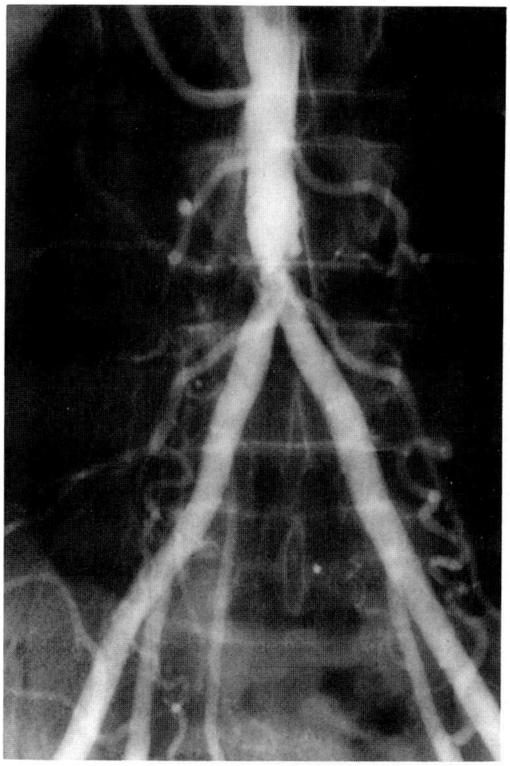

A

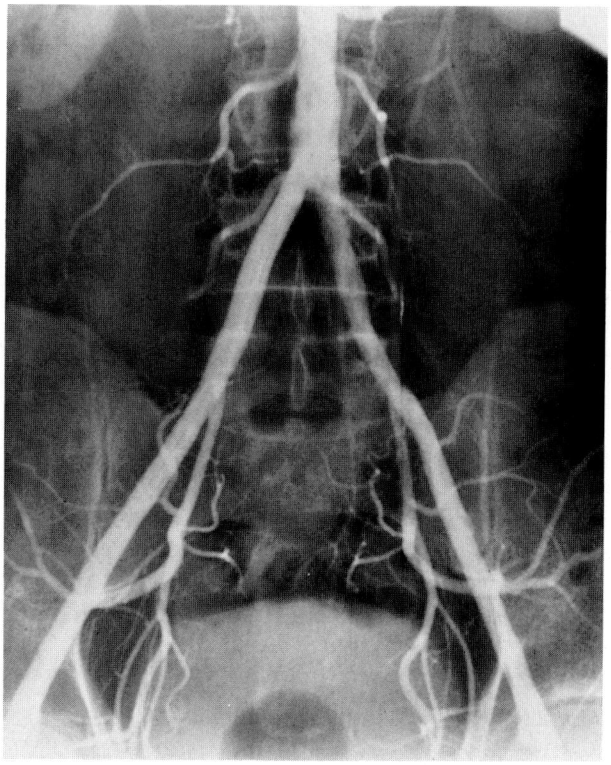

B

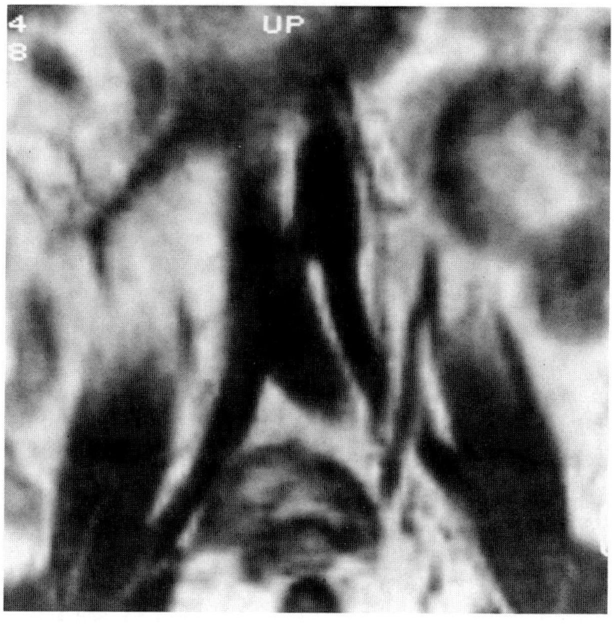

C

Figure 10–1. **A:** Pelvic angiogram: severe narrowing of the distal abdominal aorta. **B:** Following balloon angioplasty with kissing balloon technique. Observe marked increase in diameter. **C:** Magnetic resonance imaging of distal lumbar aorta showing patency of the lumen 9 years after the angioplasty. (Reprinted with permission from Tadavarthy et al.[15])

injection of vasodilating drugs. Pressure measurements are repeated after the angioplasty to verify the hemodynamic result;[2,10] the presence of a pressure gradient over 20 mmHg means that the dilating procedure was not successful and needs to be repeated.

In transluminal angioplasty, the diameter of the inflated balloon should match the caliber of the normal vessel either proximal or distal to the lesion; the technical limitation in aortic angioplasty at its beginning was the relatively small size of the commercially available balloons in relation to the size of the aorta.

This problem was solved in two different ways: initially with the simultaneous use of two or three balloons[3] and later with the development of larger balloons. Current aortic

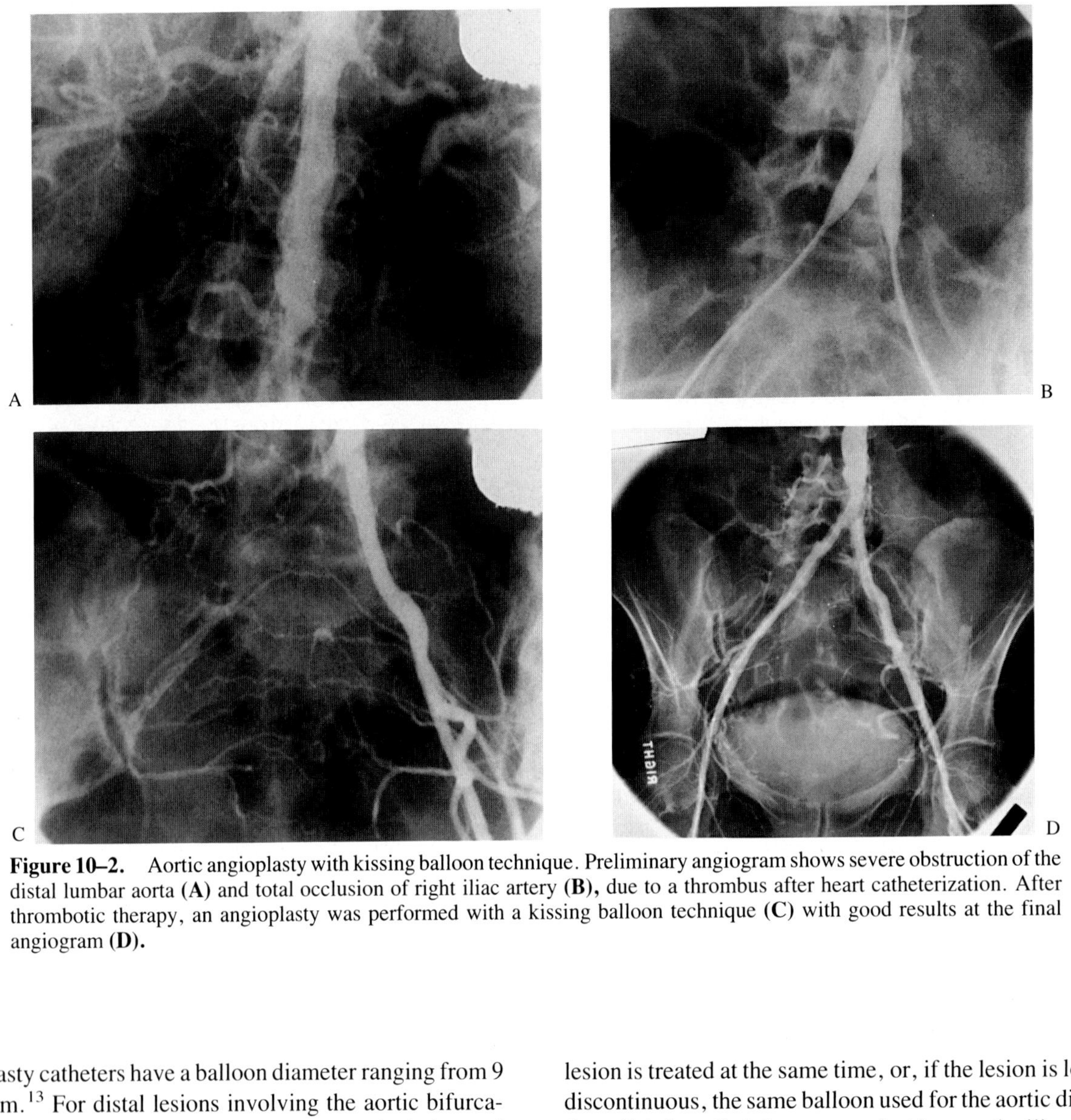

Figure 10–2. Aortic angioplasty with kissing balloon technique. Preliminary angiogram shows severe obstruction of the distal lumbar aorta **(A)** and total occlusion of right iliac artery **(B),** due to a thrombus after heart catheterization. After thrombotic therapy, an angioplasty was performed with a kissing balloon technique **(C)** with good results at the final angiogram **(D).**

angioplasty catheters have a balloon diameter ranging from 9 to 15 mm.[13] For distal lesions involving the aortic bifurcation, two or three catheters are advanced up to the lesion and are inflated simultaneously. When using a two-balloon technique, each catheter is introduced through a femoral artery. This technique is commonly known as the "kissing balloon" technique (Fig. 10-2).[3,6,7] When a third catheter is employed, it is introduced with a left axillary puncture. For example, a dilation size of 18 mm was achieved in the past with three 6 mm balloon catheters. The axillary approach is potentially more risky, and the two-catheter technique is preferable whenever possible.[2]

The double balloon or kissing balloon technique was proposed specifically for the dilation of distal lesions, to avoid the possible risk, when using a single balloon catheter, of contralateral displacement of plaque with the consequent iliac artery occlusion or distal embolization.[3] This technique is preferred for the distal lesions also because they are often associated with or extended into the iliac arteries. One advantage of the kissing balloon technique is that in lesions extending from the aorta into the iliac arteries, the entire lesion is treated at the same time, or, if the lesion is longer or discontinuous, the same balloon used for the aortic dilation is then slightly pulled down on each side over the iliac stenosis and again inflated for another treatment.[5,7]

The two balloons are inflated simultaneously, for 30 to 40 seconds, then deflated, and the procedure is repeated two or three times.[7] Single balloon technique is preferred in higher discrete lesions of the aorta, at a safe distance from the iliac arteries,[12–14] which must not be dilated by the balloon used for the aorta. A sequential dilation technique may be performed, using first a smaller catheter, and then a larger one.[9]

The principles of pharmacologic treatment do not differ from those used for other arterial angioplasties and are discussed in other chapters of this book. When the presence of a thrombus is suspected or known, as in total occlusions, angioplasty should not be performed without previous thrombolysis to prevent the risk of distal embolization of thrombus. In these cases, after the preliminary angiography, a catheter is left in place for thrombolytic infusion. Once there is evidence of a successful thrombolysis, angioplasty can be attempted.

RESULTS AND COMPLICATIONS

Data are now available for more than 144 patients.[4,7,8,10,11,13,14,16] A meaningful analysis is not possible due to the different criteria of evaluation and methods of reporting; in any case, a series of observations may be reached from the analysis of these data.

The postangioplasty pressure gradient ranged from mean values of 1.9 to 13 mmHg. Relatively higher residual gradients and less satisfactory postdilation angiographic results are more likely to occur in patients with eccentric stenosis.[14] In a follow-up to 5 years, with a mean value between 8 months to 3 years, only 11 cases of recurrence have been reported. The longest follow-up reported is 9 years.[15] Only seven cases of immediate failure were reported.

There have been only a few complications of aortic angioplasty reported. The more relevant seems to be an aortic rupture with a retroperitoneal hemorrhage, successfully treated by surgery.[19] In another major complication that also required surgery, the catheter was in a subintimal position, with a subsequent thrombosis of the iliac artery and embolization of thrombus into the ipsilateral superficial femoral artery.[7] Other cases of thrombosis in common iliac and iliofemoral arteries have been described.[8,10] The first was pharmacologically lysed, and the second required an operation. Minor complications include one case of mild spasm in the iliac arteries,[7] two cases of hematoma at the puncture site,[7,8] one case of small peripheral embolism,[8] and one case of a small pseudoaneurysm.[7] These minor complications were promptly controlled and did not require surgery. In the Takayasu's arteritis group two failures were reported in nine patients; one was due to aortic dissection and the other to thrombosis of the femoral artery.[17]

PTA of the aorta is an attractive alternative to aortofemoral bypass grafting or thromboendarterectomy. Both these surgical techniques are associated with numerous complications; even if the morbidity of the thromboendarterectomy is minor in comparison with that of aortofemoral bypass, there are some specific limitations of this technique, such as the higher (11 to 30%) percentage of postoperative impotence and the difficulty of performing the procedure in long segments.[15] The high success rate of aortic angioplasty, together with a relative minor frequency of complications, makes aortic angioplasty the treatment of choice, at least in the short distal aortic and bifurcation lesions.

ILIAC ANGIOPLASTY

The iliac arteries appear to be the arterial segment where the highest number of PTA procedures has been performed. Almost 2700 cases are included in a recent review,[7] and hundreds of cases are reported in other series.[20–25] This is due to several factors, such as the easy approach, a relatively less complicated technique, satisfactory results, and its combination with surgical revascularization. PTA of an iliac stenosis is frequently associated with a distal surgical bypass as a combined reconstructive procedure.[26]

INDICATIONS

Clinical indications for iliac angioplasty are the same as for surgical reconstruction, from intermittent claudication to rest pain and gangrene.[1,27] In selected patients, it has proved to be useful in the management of vascular impotence.[28]

In the iliac vessels, the more frequent cause of stenosis and occlusion is atherosclerosis. Another possible cause is fibromuscular dysplasia (FMD), which is diagnosed on the basis of the characteristic "corkscrew" or "beaded" angiographic appearance. Severe FMD lesions are generally treated surgically, but there are some recent reports of successful treatment with PTA.[21,29,30]

In relation to the anatomic situation, the ideal lesion to be treated is a short (1 to 2 cm) concentric stenosis, at some distance from a major bifurcation, whereas longer, eccentric, heavily calcified, or near bifurcation lesions are considered as less ideal indications.[2] Total occlusions, initially included among the contraindications, are now considered as treatable lesions.[31–34]

A classification of the severity of the lesion as a guideline for selection of cases for PTA has been proposed. It comprises four grades: the first is "ideal" for angioplasty and includes iliac stenosis less than 5 cm; the second is considered reasonable for angioplasty, and includes iliac stenosis of 5 to 10 cm or occlusion less than 5 cm; the third category is considered possible for angioplasty, but better treated by other means, and includes iliac stenosis more than 10 cm and iliac occlusion of 5 to 15 cm. More extensive disease (fourth grade) is considered completely unsuitable for angioplasty.[35]

TECHNIQUE

Criteria for the functional assessment and follow-up after the treatment are the same as those commonly employed in aortic dilations. A particular problem arises when iliac lesions are associated with superficial femoral artery occlusions. In this case, a precise demonstration of the hemodynamic improvement cannot be achieved by indirect ankle pressure measurements, and intra-arterial pressure measurements are mandatory.[35] Intra-arterial pressure measurements are particularly important when the angiographic appearance of a lesion does not correlate with its clinical significance, since in the absence of a gradient, angioplasty should not be performed. Some authors perform postangioplasty intra-arterial pressure measurements only when the angiographic result is not convincing.[2]

The pharmacologic manipulations are the same as those described in previous chapters; it is to be mentioned, however, that an intra-arterial injection of nitroglycerin (usually 100 μg) may be required for relief of spasm and to assess the exact extent of the lesion.[2]

The technique is generally very simple, but in some cases, there are particular difficulties that require special maneuvers. In the simplest lesions, PTA is performed with an ipsilateral femoral puncture. A contralateral approach may be used when the ipsilateral puncture is difficult, as, for example, for the presence of heavy calcifications or surgical bypass graft, or when the other side has been punctured for the diagnostic study and there is no special need for a new puncture. The contralateral iliac artery may be reached in different ways: by simply placing the pigtail catheter used for the diagnostic study at the aortic bifurcation and gently pulling it down until its tip is open in the contralateral iliac artery. Then a floppy tip guide wire is carefully advanced through the catheter into the contralateral iliac artery, and the pigtail catheter is advanced over the guide wire. Once the lesion is passed by the catheter, the floppy wire is exchanged for a stiff one and the pigtail is removed and replaced by the balloon catheter (Fig. 10-3). As an alternative to the use of the pigtail catheter, a sidewinder catheter can be used; the catheter needs to be reshaped in the aortic arch to reform its curve and is then carefully pulled down until the tip is in the contralateral iliac artery. The floppy wire is then advanced and the procedure proceeds as described before. A bilateral approach with simultaneous inflation of balloons on both sides is advisable when the lesion is close to the orifice of the common iliac artery.[2]

Particular problems arise when the lesion is not easily passed by a standard guide wire. The maneuver is made easier with the use of special wires, like the steerable or tapered guide wires, or by manipulating a floppy tip guide wire together with a small caliber JB1 or hockey-stick catheter. Digital road mapping may be very useful in handling the different individual anatomic situations.[2] Ipsilateral approach may be possible even in total iliac occlusion. The femoral artery can be localized and punctured even in the absence of a pulse;[23,31] under fluoroscopy, the artery is generally located over the medial border of the femoral head.[31] Ultrasound guidance could also be employed. The arterial occlusion is almost never totally due to the atherosclerotic process, but it is precipitated by the presence of a superimposed thrombus.[31] Chronic occlusions can be carefully negotiated by a guide wire and a catheter. As in total aortic occlusions, preliminary thrombolysis is requested in these cases to avoid the risk of distal embolization. In total occlusions, balloon angioplasty may be employed as the first step of a stenting procedure; data from the clinical series are promising.[34]

RESULTS

Results of iliac PTA are very definitely satisfactory, with a mean of 92% for the technical success and initial patency. The 2-year patency is 81%, with a 5-year patency of 72%. These data, corresponding to a large series of 2697 cases,[7] have been generally supported by data from other series.[20–25] Critical review of these data mandates some changes, however, of the percentages reported. For example, the 90% values given for technical success have to be lowered when the angiographic results are correlated with pressure gradient measurements. If gradients over 20 mmHg persist, the procedure cannot be considered a technical success, and the overall percentage drops to 75%. The reported patency rates of 80% after 2 years also need to be evaluated with respect to patient groups. Higher patency rates are to be expected in patients with claudication, whereas strikingly lower patency rates occur in patients with rest pain or tissue loss.[36]

In relation to the anatomic lesion, it appears that shorter (less than 5 cm) stenoses respond better to PTA than diffuse lesions.[36] The decrease of the patency rate in the long term is mainly related to restenosis, which appears to be the most relevant limitation of PTA. Restenoses are classified as acute, early, and late. Some of the causes of acute restenosis

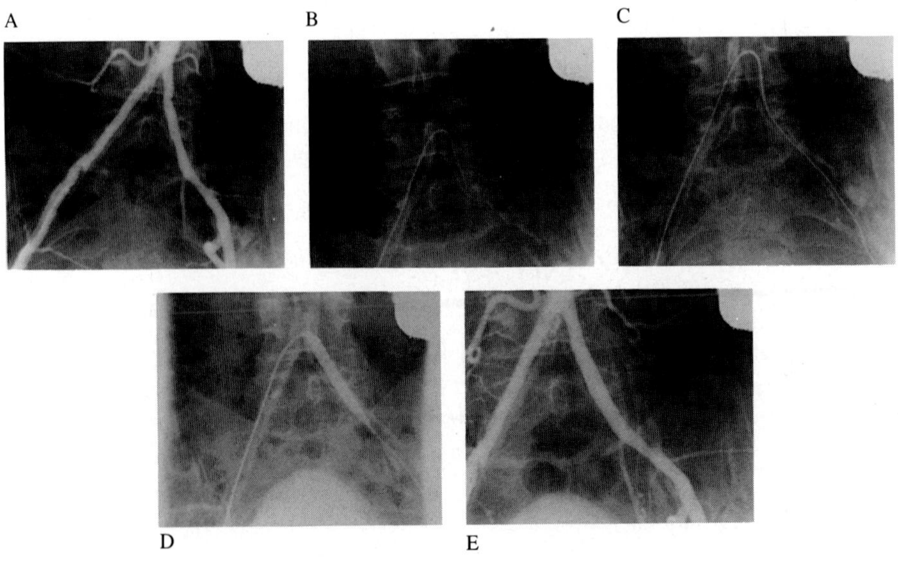

Figure 10–3. Iliac angioplasty with a contralateral approach. **A:** An aortoiliac angiogram shows stenosis of left common iliac artery. **B:** The pigtail catheter is pulled over the aortic bifurcation and it has been hooked over to the contralateral iliac artery. **C:** The pigtail catheter is advanced into the contralateral iliac artery over a Bentson guide wire. **D:** The Bentson wire is then replaced with a stiff wire and the pigtail catheter replaced by an angioplasty catheter that is inflated over the lesion. **E:** Postangioplasty angiogram shows disappearance of the stenosis.

can be managed with aggressive pharmacologic therapy to prevent vasospasm and thrombosis.[4] Complex strategies for the solution of the various other causes are under development; they are discussed in other chapters of this book.

COMPLICATIONS

The frequency of complications ranges in different series between 2 to 25%.[37,38] Complications may be classified according to their severity in minor and major problems. Minor clinical complications are mainly hematoma, thrombus, pseudoaneurysms, and nerve damage at the puncture site.[20,23,38]

Major clinical complications include distal embolization, septic symptoms, reversible or irreversible renal insufficiency, occlusion of the iliac or adjacent vessel,[38] and four cases of iliac artery rupture.[39–41] One unusual case of distal bowel infarction has also been reported; this was probably a result of a thromboembolic event occurring in a patient with a compromised mesenteric arterial tree because of previous radiation therapy.[42]

The possibility of these complications mandates careful execution of the procedures by well-trained interventionalists in well-equipped angiographic suites with vascular surgical backup. Nevertheless, when comparing the results of PTA with those obtained by surgical procedures, it is evident that iliac PTA has doubtless some major advantages: it may be performed under local anesthesia, in a short hospital admission, and with a very low discomfort for the patient.[27] An early or late failure in PTA does not preclude or compromise subsequent surgical management.[43] Moreover, angioplasty can be repeated. It is therefore clear that in iliac stenosis, particularly of short segments, a carefully and correctly performed PTA is the procedure of choice.

REFERENCES

1. Becker GJ, Katzen BT, Dake MD. Noncoronary angioplasty. Radiology 1989;170:921–940.
2. Schwarten DE. Aortic, iliac and peripheral arterial angioplasty. In Castañeda-Zúñiga WR, Murthy Tadavarthy S (eds): Interventional radiology. Baltimore: Williams & Wilkins, 1988:268–97.
3. Velasquez G, Castañeda-Zúñiga WR, Formanek A, et al. Nonsurgical angioplasty in Leriche syndrome. Radiology 1980;136:359–60.
4. Heeney D, Bookstein J, Daniels S, et al. Transluminal angioplasty of the abdominal aorta. Radiology 1983;148:81–3.
5. Bean WJ, Rodan BA, Thebut AL. Leriche syndrome: treatment with streptokinase and angioplasty. AJR 1985; 144:1285–6.
6. Marty AT, Penkava R, Whitehead D, et al. Kissing balloon therapy for Leriche syndrome. Ind Med 1985;78:288–9.
7. Tegtmeyer CJ, Kellum CD, Kron IL, et al. Percutaneous transluminal angioplasty in the region of the aortic bifurcation. Radiology 1985;157:661–5.
8. Charlebois N, Saint-George G, Hudon G. Percutaneous transluminal angioplasty of the lower abdominal aorta. AJR 1986;146:369–71.
9. Walstra BRJ, Janevski BK. Sequential PTA of abdominal aorta. Fortschr Rontgenstr 1987;146:446–9.
10. Morag B, Rubinstein Z, Kessler A, et al. Percutaneous transluminal angioplasty of the distal abdominal aorta and its bifurcation. Cardiovasc Intervent Radiol 1987;10:129–33.
11. Courthéoux P, Théron J, Alachkar F, et al. L'angioplastie endoluminale per-cutanée dans le traitement des sténoses athéromateuses de l'aorte abdominale terminale. Ann Radiol 1987;30:37–41.
12. Yakes WF, Kumpe DA, Parker SH, et al. Angioplasty of the infrarenal abdominal aorta. Semin Intervent Radiol 1989; 6:129–37.
13. Yakes WF, Kumpe DA, Brow SB, et al. Percutaneous transluminal aortic angioplasty: techniques and results. Radiology 1989;172:955–70.
14. Odurny A, Colapinto RF, Sniderman KW, et al. Percutaneous transluminal angioplasty of abdominal aortic stenoses. Cardiovasc Intervent Radiol 1989;12:1–6.
15. Tadavarthy AK, Albert Sullivan W, Nicoloff D, et al. Aorta balloon angioplasty: 9-year follow-up. Radiology 1989; 170:1039–41.
16. Wholey M. Advances in balloon technology and reperfusion devices for peripheral circulation. Am J Cardiol 1988;61:87G–95G.
17. Gu ZM, Lin G, Yi JR, et al. Transluminal catheter angioplasty of abdominal aorta in Takayasu's arteritis. Acta Radiol 1988;29:509–13.
18. Khalilullah M, Tyagi S, Lochan R, et al. Percutaneous transluminal balloon angioplasty of the aorta in patients with aortitis. Circulation 1987;76:597–600.
19. Berger T, Sorensen R, Konrad J. Aortic rupture: A complication of transluminal angioplasty. AJR 1986;146:373–6.
20. Henriksen LO, Jorgensen B, Holstein PE, et al. Percutaneous transluminal angioplasty of infrarenal arteries in intermittent claudication. Acta Chir Scand 1988;156:573–6.
21. Simonetti G, Bonomo L, Falappa PG, et al. PTA of iliac arteries. Ann Radiol 1985;28:159–62.
22. Simonetti G, Urigo F, Guazzarion M, et al. Iliac artery lesions: a comparison between PTA and surgery. Ann Radiol 1986; 29:127–9.
23. Blankensteijn JD, van Vrounhover TJ, Lampmann L. Role of PTA in aorta-iliac reconstruction. J Cardiovasc Surg 1986; 27:466–8.
24. Cormier E, Laissy JP, Bernier J, et al. Angioplastie endoluminale des oblitérations iliaques. Résoultats immediats et perméabilité cumulée a 2 ans chez 23 patients. J Radiol 1988; 69:571–6.
25. Van Andel G, van Erp WFM, Krepel UM, et al. PT dilatation of the iliac artery: Long-term results. Radiology 1985; 156:321–3.
26. Zeitler E, Raithel D, Gailer H, et al. PTA combined with surgical vascular operations in iliac and femoral obstruction. Ann Radiol 1987;30:142–6.
27. Reidy JF. Angioplasty in peripheral vascular disease. Postgrad Med J 1987;63:435–8.
28. Valji K, Bookstein JJ. Transluminal angioplasty in the treatment of arteriogenic impotence. Cardiovasc Intervent Radiol 1988;11:245–52.
29. Wilms G, Nevelsteen A, Ballt AZ. Dysplasie fibromuscolaire de l'artère iliaque externe. Traitement per angioplastie endoluminale. J Radiol 1988;69:549–51.
30. Parnell AP, Loose HW, Chamberlain J. Fibromuscular dysplasia of the external iliac artery: treatment by PTA. Br J Radiol 1988;61:1080–2.
31. Colapinto RF, Stronell RJ, Johnston WF. Transluminal angioplasty of complete iliac obstructions. AJR 1986;146:859–62.
32. Kroogi Y, Takahashy M. Percutaneous transluminal angio-

plasty of totally occluded iliac arteries in high-risk patients. Br J Radiol 1986;59:1167–70.

33. Rubinstein ZJ, Morag B, Peer A, et al. Percutaneous transluminal recanalization of common iliac artery occlusions. Cardiovasc Intervent Radiol 1987;10:16–20.
34. Rees CR, Palmaz JC, Garcia D. Angioplasty and stenting of completely occluded iliac arteries. Radiology 1989;172: 953–9.
35. Campbell WB, Higgins JRA, Barker CS, et al. Grading for angioplasty. Clin Radiol 1988;39:516–8.
36. Breslau PJ, van Soest M, Janevski B, et al. Hemodynamic evaluation of transluminal iliac artery balloon dilatation. Neth J Surg 1985;37:145–7.
37. Cambria RP, Faust G, Gusberg R, et al. PTA for peripheral arterial occlusive disease. Arch Surg 1987;122:283–7.
38. Weibull H, Bergquist D, Jonsson K, et al. Complications after PTA in the iliac femoral and popliteal arteries. J Vasc Surg 1987;5:581–6.
39. Simonetti G, Rossi P, Passariello R, et al. Iliac artery rupture: a complication of transluminal angioplasty. AJR 1983; 140:989–90.
40. Jensen JR, Vopegeli BR, Crummy AB, et al. Iliac artery rupture during transluminal angioplasty: treatment by embolization and surgical bypass. AJR 1985;165:381–2.
41. Villarica J, Gross RC. Treatment of angioplasty-related iliac-artery rupture without bypass surgery (case report). AJR 1986;147:389–90.
42. Bennett IC, Downes MO, Collins REC. Distal bowel infarction following angioplasty of the internal iliac artery. Br J Radiol 1989;62:489–90.
43. Fletcher JP, Kershaw LZ. Outcome in patients with failed PTA for peripheral vascular disease. J Cardiovasc Surg 1988; 29:733–5.

11 Transluminal Angioplasty of the Popliteal and Tibial-Peroneal Arteries

Donald E. Schwarten, M.D.

The percutaneous management of aortoiliac atherosclerotic occlusive disease has become a widely accepted treatment.[1] Primary anatomic success, immediate clinical improvement, and long-term patency rates make aortoiliac balloon angioplasty the treatment of choice in atherosclerotic occlusive disease in patients who are clinically and anatomically suitable.[2] The percutaneous management of atherosclerotic occlusive disease of the superficial femoral and deep femoral arteries is less widely accepted as an alternative to traditional surgical procedures.[3] It is possible to achieve a high primary technical success rate even in long segments of disease of the superficial femoral artery.[4] Infrainguinal percutaneous interventions for atherosclerosis are plagued by relatively high recurrence rates and therefore in most institutions the percutaneous treatment of superficial femoral artery atherosclerotic disease is reserved for patients with relatively focal disease, or patients whose symptoms are not severe enough to warrant surgery.

Initial reports of angioplasty of the distal popliteal artery and tibial-peroneal arteries indicate relatively poor primary anatomic success and limb salvage rates.[5] Prior to 1983, physicians attempting to manage percutaneously patients with atherosclerotic occlusive disease in the tibial and peroneal arteries were hampered by the fact that the patients who were submitted were frequently not ideal subjects anatomically and the fact that catheters designed to treat atherosclerosis in the small caliber vessels were large and somewhat primitive. Most reports described using a series of tapered catheters placed sequentially across the occlusive lesion, in effect performing a "mini-Dotter" procedure. Van Andel type catheters were also employed.[6] The excessive sheer forces generated by these non-balloon catheter systems frequently caused extensive intimal trauma that led to aggressive myointimal hyperplasia and, often within months, a failed procedure. Since the development of angioplasty systems designed to treat coronary artery disease, the natural fallout for the interventionalist interested in managing limb-threatening distal popliteal and tibial peroneal disease has been the availability of catheters identical to, or derived from, those designed for percutaneous coronary angioplasty. With these more delicate tools available, significantly improved results have been reported.[7,8]

SELECTIONS OF PATIENTS FOR DISTAL POPLITEAL AND TIBIAL-PERONEAL ANGIOPLASTY

Candidates for distal popliteal and tibial-peroneal angioplasty should have a threatened limb; ischemic rest pain, ulceration, or gangrene should be present. Arterial insufficiency should be confirmed and documented by noninvasive laboratory testing. Most patients who have a limb threatened because of arterial insufficiency have multilevel disease. It is rare for a patient presenting with calf or foot claudication to have isolated, focal disease suitable for angioplasty in the tibial-peroneal trunk, peroneal artery, or posterior tibial artery. It will therefore be rare to consider tibial or peroneal angioplasty for claudication. The patient who presents with claudication as the only symptom and does not have hemodynamically significant proximal disease and who desires intervention must be made aware of the possible consequences of a failed percutaneous procedure. If three-vessel runoff is present, and only the posterior tibial artery origin is diseased, a successful procedure may relieve the claudication. A failure would probably not have catastrophic results requiring a more distal bypass graft for limb salvage. In the patient who presents, however, with claudication, no hemodynamically significant proximal disease, an occluded anterior tibial artery with a small peroneal artery, and a focal lesion in the proximal posterior tibial artery, a complication, if it occurs, may result in an acutely threatened limb requiring distal bypass grafting for salvage. Balloon angioplasty for claudication is the exception in our community and not the standard of practice.

If the principal clinical indication for angioplasty of the distal popliteal and tibial-peroneal vessels is limb salvage, then, obviously, a nonischemic limb is, at least, a relative contraindication to angioplasty. An additional contraindication to percutaneous angioplasty below the knee is the presence of acute ischemia. It may be possible to identify angiographically that the pathology appears to be atherosclerotic disease with a superimposed thrombosis. It may be possible to perform thrombolysis and reestablish flow and then perform balloon angioplasty, all in a time frame that will be short enough so that complications of a delayed revascularization for an acutely ischemic limb will not develop. It is incumbent on the angiographer to be aware of the potential problems of delayed revascularization and to know when there is not enough time to wait for thrombolysis instead of proceeding with direct surgical intervention.

Besides clinical indications and contraindications, there are anatomic indications and contraindications to angioplasty of the distal popliteal artery and tibial-peroneal arteries. Short focal stenoses are the ideal, but not usually the only lesion. Multiple lesions are generally present. We have somewhat arbitrarily decided to limit angioplasty to fewer than five lesions in any single vessel. An occluded segment of vessel longer than 4 cm is considered less than optimal for angioplasty and if a suitable vessel is present distally for bypass grafting, then angioplasty will not be attempted, unless there is a compelling reason to avoid the risk of operative intervention.

Patients with a threatened limb who present for angiography are studied from a contralateral common femoral artery whenever possible. Percutaneous transluminal angioplasty of the distal popliteal and tibial-peroneal arteries should be performed via an ipsilateral antegrade puncture. By performing the diagnostic arteriogram from the contralateral side, it may be possible, if contrast limits would not be exceeded, to perform the angioplasty as an extension of the diagnostic study. Alternatively, if the angioplasty is to be deferred, there is no risk that a hematoma would be present that would make the ipsilateral antegrade puncture more difficult.

PHARMACOLOGIC ADJUNCTS

Prior to obtaining vascular access for distal popliteal or tibial-peroneal angioplasty, our patients are premedicated with 10 to 20 mg of nifedipine. This may be administered orally prior to transporting the patient to the angiographic suite or, alternatively, it may be administered by puncturing the gelatin capsule and squeezing the viscous fluid into the patient's mouth. We instruct our patients to swallow the nifedipine fluid rather than to attempt to hold it in the sublingual position. It will be as rapidly absorbed by the gastric mucosa as it would be by the sublingual. Swallowing the nifedipine reduces the tendency toward excessive salivation and the coughing and gagging it stimulates, which we find makes performing a quick antegrade puncture a bit more difficult.

Our patients are placed on antiplatelet therapy, salicylates, 80 to 325 mg orally daily. During, and sometimes after the procedure, our patients are systemically heparinized for 24 to 48 hours. Patients maintained on heparin postprocedure are those who are deemed to have particularly "slow flow" or have an unusually large intimal-medial cleft that may threaten to occlude abruptly.

Peripheral vasodilation is essential to maximize flow and to prevent vasospasm. We find nitroglycerin to be not only the most effective agent in preventing or abating vasospasm, but the most benign as well. Nitroglycerin is employed in 100 to 200 μg boluses; it is used liberally throughout the procedure as long as hypotension does not develop. Nitroglycerin paste may be applied as a patch at the conclusion of the procedure to help maintain peripheral vasodilation and maximum flow.

Verapamil is a calcium antagonist that can be used parenterally to obtain peripheral vasodilation. Its use is contraindicated in the presence of bradyarrhythmias or congestive heart failure. If verapamil is given too rapidly, or in too large a dose, it can induce severe bradyarrhythmias. We do not use verapamil to treat catheter-induced vasospasm.

MECHANICAL EQUIPMENT FOR DISTAL POPLITEAL AND TIBIAL-PERONEAL ANGIOPLASTY

Distal popliteal and tibial-peroneal angioplasty is performed through a sheath. A 5 or 6 F sheath is of adequate size to permit easy passage of the angioplasty catheters. The flush port of the sheath also allows the angiographer to inject small volumes of contrast material to localize the angioplasty system within the vessels. The guide wires used through the angioplasty catheter are of 0.014 or 0.018 inch diameter. The first of these wires available to us were usually "liberated" from the adjacent Cardiology Interventional Laboratory. The "coronary wires" had rather long floppy segments that were fine for gaining access to and having a catheter track over the wire into the posterior tibial and peroneal arteries, but would not allow a catheter to track a High Torque Floppy (ACS, Mountain View, CA) guide wire into the anterior tibial artery. The Flex-T (ACS) guide wire is a modification that maintains an excellent torque control, but has a shorter distal floppy segment and becomes stiff enough so that with only a moderate length of guide wire into the tibial artery, a catheter will almost always easily track over the wire into the anterior tibial artery.

The angioplasty catheters are made by most manufacturers approximately in a 90 cm length. A 145 cm guide wire is not long enough to permit a catheter exchange while maintaining guide wire tip position distal to a lesion in a tibial or a peroneal artery. We routinely use 175 cm guide wires. These are long enough to permit catheter exchange while maintaining guide wire tip position distally and yet are not so long as to be cumbersome.

In selected instances (usually total occlusions) 0.025, 0.028, or 0.035 inch guide wires have a place in angioplasty of the tibial-peroneal arteries.

CATHETERS

The balloon angioplasty catheters used for tibial-peroneal angioplasty range from 4.3 to 4.7 F. Balloon diameters are available up to 5.0 mm. The most commonly used balloon sizes range from 2.0 to 4.0 mm. We rarely use balloons longer than 2 cm in length. Balloon size is selected based on matching the size of the vessel of interest, measured from analog films without correction for magnification. In selected circumstances, a straight non-balloon or a gently curved 5 F catheter is used as part of an angioplasty procedure of the tibial-peroneal arteries.

TECHNIQUE OF ANGIOPLASTY OF THE DISTAL POPLITEAL AND TIBIAL-PERONEAL ARTERIES

Vascular access is achieved via an ipsilateral antegrade puncture. A 5 or 6 F sheath is advanced over a soft-tipped guide wire into the proximal superficial artery. Once access has been achieved, the patient is heparinized through the sheath, and a 100 to 200 μg nitroglycerin bolus "chaser" is administered through the sheath.

TECHNIQUE FOR STENOSES

The angioplasty guide wire system is prepared by back-loading the guide wire through the end hole of the angioplasty catheter so that the soft platinum tip of the guide wire is retracted just inside the end hole of the catheter. The catheter is introduced through the hemostatic valve of the sheath and into the distal portion of the sheath where the guide wire is then advanced 6 to 8 cm beyond the catheter tip. The guide wire and catheter can be advanced through the superficial femoral and popliteal arteries as a unit. When the popliteal artery level has been reached, the fluoroscope is positioned so that both the tip of the guide wire and the area of pathologic interest are included in the field. A single hand injection of contrast is made and a roadmap is acquired. The roadmap image is then superimposed on the live fluoroscopic image and the catheter and guide wire are advanced into the stenosis and angioplasty is performed. The catheter is then retracted over the guide wire, with the guide wire left with its tip distal to the angioplasty site, and a concluding angiogram is acquired. If the anatomic result is acceptable, the angioplasty procedure itself is considered complete (Figs. 11-1, 11-2). If the result is unacceptable, a longer inflation time may be tried, or a slightly larger balloon may be used.

Atherosclerosis tends to occur at bifurcations. When balloon angioplasty is performed at a bifurcation lesion, if only one of the vessels harbors significant disease extending into its orifice, the "normal" vessel is at approximately a 20% risk of being occluded by a non-colinear intimal-medial cleft. If both vessels have disease extending into their origins and if one is not protected by a guide wire to permit the catheter access, it has approximately a 40% risk of occluding as a result of angioplasty of the adjacent branch. We routinely place guide wires in both vessels when a bifurcation lesion is encountered and perform angioplasty of the bifurcation and one vessel. If the other branch vessel is, as a result of the procedure, compromised, the balloon catheter is removed,

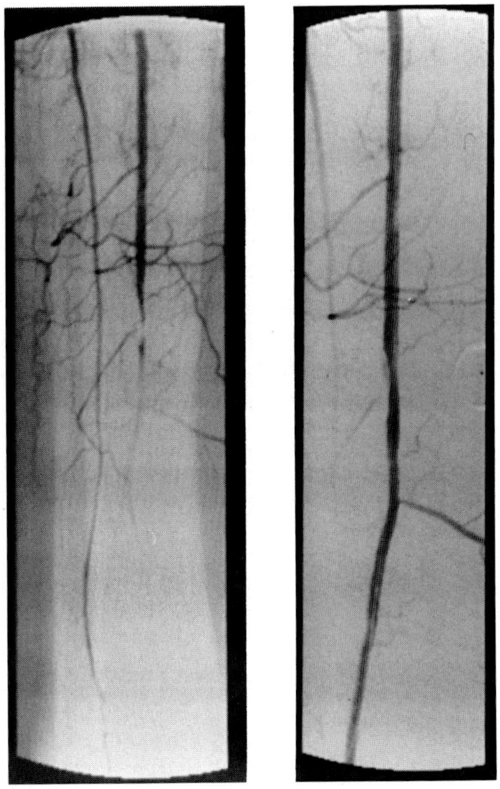

A B

Figure 11–1. **A:** High-grade midperoneal stenosis with slow flow. **B:** Postangioplasty study (guide wire position has been maintained).

and either it or a catheter with a different size balloon is advanced over the other guide wire into the adjacent branch vessel, and a balloon dilation of the orifice of that vessel is performed to restore a widely patent lumen (Fig. 11-3).

TECHNIQUE FOR OCCLUSION

The delicate 0.014 or 0.018 inch guide wires used to negotiate stenoses rarely will cross a chronic occlusion in the distal popliteal, tibial, or peroneal arteries. We therefore, in order to recanalize the occluded segment, pass a 4 or 5 F diagnostic catheter over a 0.025 inch guide wire (usually a hydrophilically coated guide wire) and attempt to gain access to the distal true lumen. Once catheter position in the distal true lumen has been confirmed with a small volume of contrast material, the recanalizing catheter is removed over a 0.018 inch guide wire and exchanged for an angioplasty catheter, and a balloon angioplasty procedure is performed. We believe that dilation is accomplished primarily by the radial force of the balloon catheter rather than the radial and shear forces generated by the recanalizing catheter (Fig. 11-4).

RESULTS

Since 1983, we have employed the technology described in the preceding text to achieve primary anatomic success in all

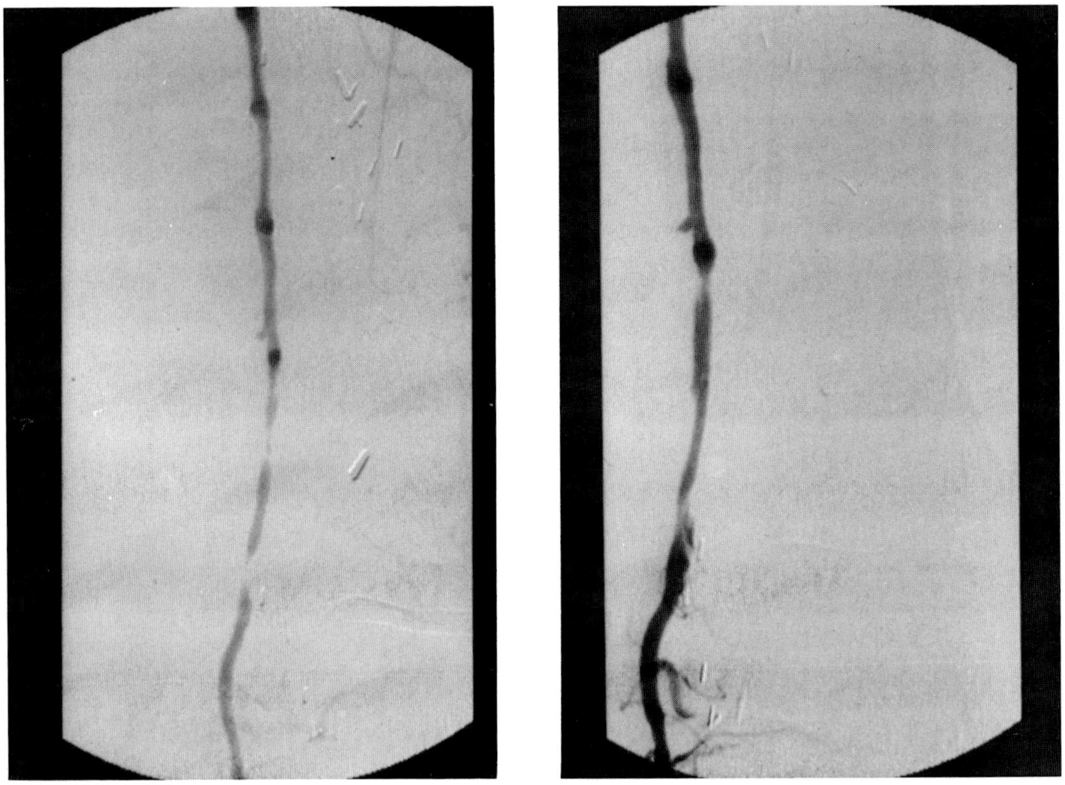

A B

Figure 11–2. **A:** Multiple high-grade stenoses in a vein graft to a posterior tibial artery. The medial malleolus and ankle mortise are faintly visible. **B:** Postangioplasty study.

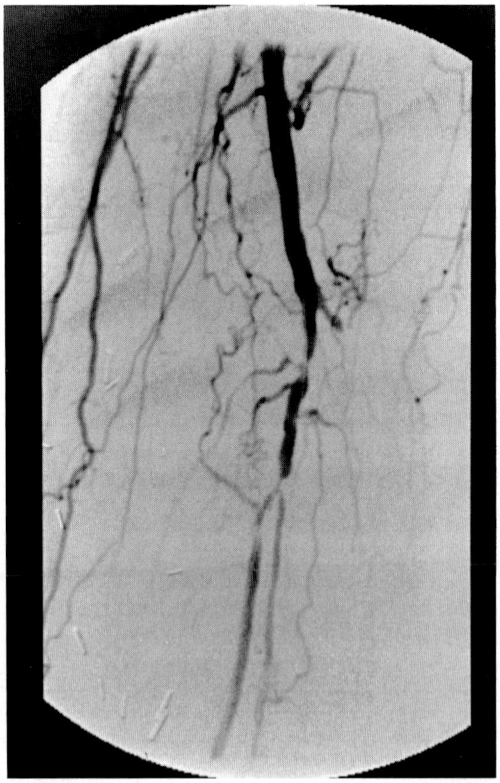

A

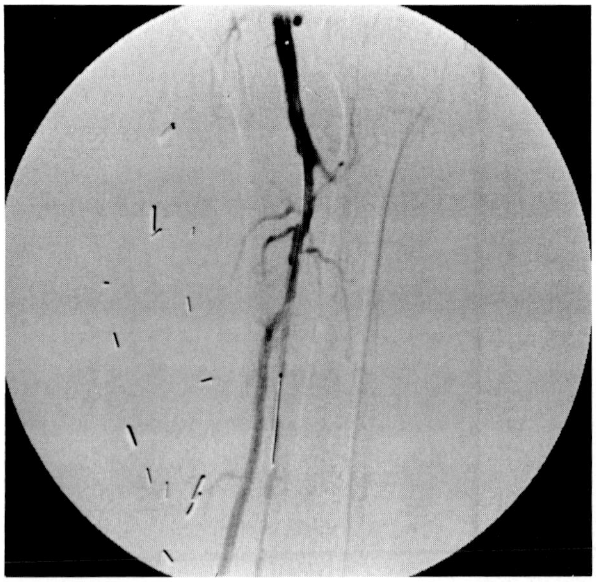

B

Figure 11–3. **A:** Diffuse tibial-peroneal trunk, posterior tibial and peroneal disease. **B:** After percutaneous transluminal angioplasty, the guide wire position is maintained in the peroneal artery.

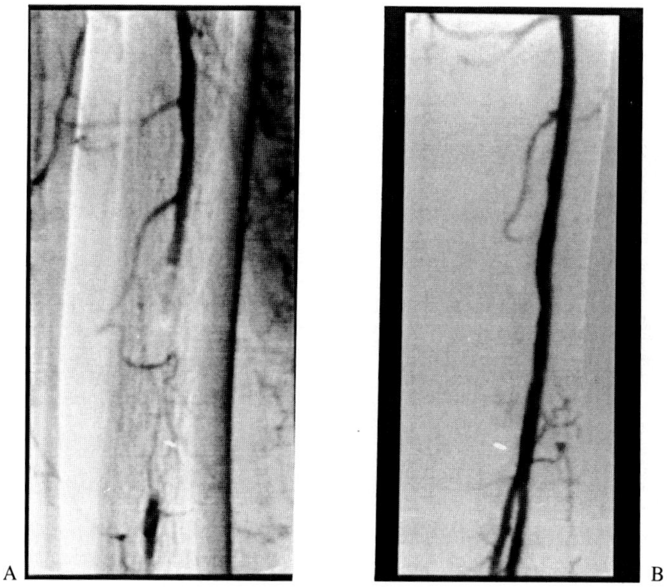

Figure 11–4. **A:** Isolated peroneal artery occlusion. **B:** After recanalization followed by balloon angioplasty.

patients who exhibited stenotic disease amenable to balloon angioplasty and in 87% of patients who had occluded vessels below the knee and who were considered to be suitable for balloon angioplasty. Our overall primary anatomic success rate in over 175 vessels is 97%. The long-term results in regard to limb salvage have been gratifying: at 2 years, 84% of our patients had pain-free viable extremities. This compares favorably to high-quality surgical series.[9,10]

COMPLICATIONS

Four complications have occurred and one required surgical intervention. In two instances (both anterior tibial angioplasty) thrombosis of the angioplasty site with extension of a long segment of the anterior tibial artery resulted in acute ischemia. In each instance, a concentrated bolus of 250,000 U of urokinase in 5 cc of fluid was administered in a pulsed bolus fashion along the length of the anterior tibial artery. Surgical intervention was requested immediately on recognition of the complication, but in each instance, the 30 to 45 minutes it took to have surgical assistance ready, complete lyses had occurred and the acute ischemia resolved. There was one instance of a large groin hematoma that did not require intervention and one instance of a large groin hematoma with a dissection into the retroperitoneum that did require surgical intervention.

CONCLUSION

Percutaneous balloon angioplasty for limb salvage in patients with angiographically suitable anatomy involving the distal popliteal artery or the tibial or peroneal arteries can be as effective, or nearly as effective, as the best surgical procedures with obviously less morbidity and a significantly lower cost. The patient with a chronically ischemic foot will be likely to have multilevel disease. It behooves the interventionalist to assess carefully, in consultation with a surgeon capable of doing high-quality distal bypass procedures, the status of the deep femoral artery, any lesions in the superficial femoral artery, or above the inguinal ligament. When it has been decided that a percutaneous procedure is in the patient's best interest, the interventionalist angiographer should plan carefully to deal with the anatomy to permit resolution of the ischemic signs and symptoms and not merely to meet a technical challenge.

With care, and proper patient selection, the percutaneous management of popliteal and tibial-peroneal atherosclerotic occlusive disease may help preserve the saphenous vein for use when other options are not available.

REFERENCES

1. Becker GJ, Katzen BT, Dake MD. Noncoronary angioplasty. Radiology 1989;170:921–40.
2. Casarella WJ. Noncoronary angioplasty. Curr Probl Cardiol 1986;11:138–74.
3. Veith FJ, Gupta SK, Samson RH, et al. Progress in limb salvage by reconstructive arterial surgery combined with new or improved adjunctive procedure. Ann Surg 1981;194:386.
4. Krepel VM, Van Andel GJ, Van Erp WFM, et al. Percutaneous transluminal angioplasty of the femoropopliteal artery: initial and long term results. Radiology 1985;156:325–8.
5. Sprayregen S, Sniderman KW, Sos TA, et al. Popliteal artery branches: percutaneous transluminal angioplasty. AJR 1980;135:945–50.
6. Tamura S, Sniderman KW, Beinart C, Sos TA. Percutaneous transluminal angioplasty of the popliteal artery and its branches. Radiology 1982;143:645–8.
7. Schwarten DE, Cutcliff WB. Arterial occlusive disease below the knee: treatment with percutaneous transluminal angioplasty with low profile catheters and steerable guidewires. Radiology 1988;169:71–4.
8. Brown KT, Schoenbert NY, Moore ED, Saddekni S. Percutaneous transluminal angioplasty of infrapopliteal vessels: preliminary results and technical considerations. Radiology 1988;169:75–8.
9. Buchbinder D, Rolins DL, Jerta MJ, et al. Early experience with in site saphenous vein bypass for distal arterial reconstruction. Surgery 1986;99:350–6.
10. Taylor LM Jr, Phinney ES, Proter JM. Present status of reversed vein bypass for lower extremity revascularization. J Vasc Surg 1986;3:28–97.

12 Vasa Vasorum Changes Following Angioplasty and Stenting

João Martins Pisco, M.D., Miguel Correia, M.D., José A. Esperança Pina, M.D., Luis Aires de Sousa, M.D.

Vasa vasorum are the small vessels that supply the vessel wall. The first observation of the vasa vasorum is attributed to Wills in 1757 (cited by Clarke[1]). Several other authors later studied the vasa vasorum using different methods. Woodruff[2] injected the aorta of animals with India ink and concluded that the vasa vasorum arose from the collateral branches of the aorta. Winternitz[3] injected diluted India ink into the abdominal aorta and by the Spalteholz method revealed vascular patterns in the outer media of the human and animal arterial wall. He demonstrated intimal vascularization in atheromatous plaques.

Celestino da Costa[4] studied the abdominal aorta of the dog with stained fat. He mentioned that in the majority of cases the arterial wall is irrigated by the vasa vasorum only in its outer layers, the inner ones being dependent on diffusion of plasma. The degree and extent of irrigation by the vasa vasorum and the diffusion of plasma differs with the species and with the individual. Geiringer[5] found that the innermost layer of the arterial wall derives its nutrient directly from the main lumen. The arterial wall is vascularized only beyond some thickness of the inner layers, a "critical depth" that is variable with different arteries and species. The thickness of the avascular zone of the abdominal aorta in the different mammals is 0.5 mm. However, in man that thickness is 0.7 mm and is probably a reason for the high incidence of atherosclerosis in the abdominal aorta of humans. Ayres de Sousa and Alvares[6] studied the vasa vasorum with microangiography after opacification with Micropaque. They described the distribution of the vasa vasorum as arising from aortic collaterals and forming an adventitial network.

We studied the distribution of the vasa vasorum of the abdominal aorta of the dog, pig, and atherosclerotic abdominal aorta of human cadavers. We also investigated the changes that occurred following angioplasty of experimental stenosis in the abdominal aorta of the dog (Fig. 12-1) and experimental atherosclerosis of the abdominal aorta of the pig. Following that, we studied the changes after stent placement in the aorta of the dog (Fig. 12-2). Although we used the Spalteholz method, microangiography, histologic studies, and scanning electron microscopy, the Spalteholz method was the one that gave better information concerning the morphology and is the one used in the different illustrations shown.

DISTRIBUTION OF THE VASA VASORUM OF THE ABDOMINAL AORTA

The vasa vasorum arise from branches of the abdominal aorta, particularly from the lumbar arteries, and have a caliber of 0.35 mm. The initial trunk has an extension of 4 mm and is situated in the connective tissue of the peripheral adventitia of the aorta. The trunk divides into two secondary branches that supply the aorta superiorly and inferiorly. These secondary vessels measure approximately 0.15 mm and they anastomose with vessels from both sides. Thus, a polygonal or true plexus with branches measuring 0.2 to 0.1 mm is formed in the adventitia. From the inner surface of that plexus arise arterioles whose caliber is between 0.1 and 0.03 mm. These arterioles penetrate and reach the media of the aorta and form an incomplete arch of 90° to 120°. From the inner surface of those arterioles arise precapillary arterioles whose caliber is 0.03 to 0.01 mm and are situated in the junction of the external and middle third of the media (Fig. 12-3).

The pattern of the vasa vasorum of the abdominal aorta of the pig was similar to that observed in the dog. In the pig in which atherosclerosis was induced, we observed vasa vasorum proliferation particularly at the level of the plaques.

In the atherosclerotic abdominal aorta of human cadavers, the distribution of the vasa vasorum was similar to that of the aorta of the dog. However, at the level of the plaques, there was more vascularization and the vasa vasorum reached the inner third of the media and sometimes the subintima (Fig. 12-4).

VASA VASORUM CHANGES CAUSED BY ANGIOPLASTY AND STENTING

The first study of the effect of angioplasty on the microcirculation of the dilated arteries was performed by Cragg et al[7] in animals. They demonstrated significant hyperemia of vessel walls, although no morphologic changes could be found. Zollikofer[8] found disruption of the vasa vasorum in dilated atherosclerotic human cadaver vessels. Zollikofer et al[9] overdilated canine aortic segments to more than 100% over normal size to investigate the acute and long-term

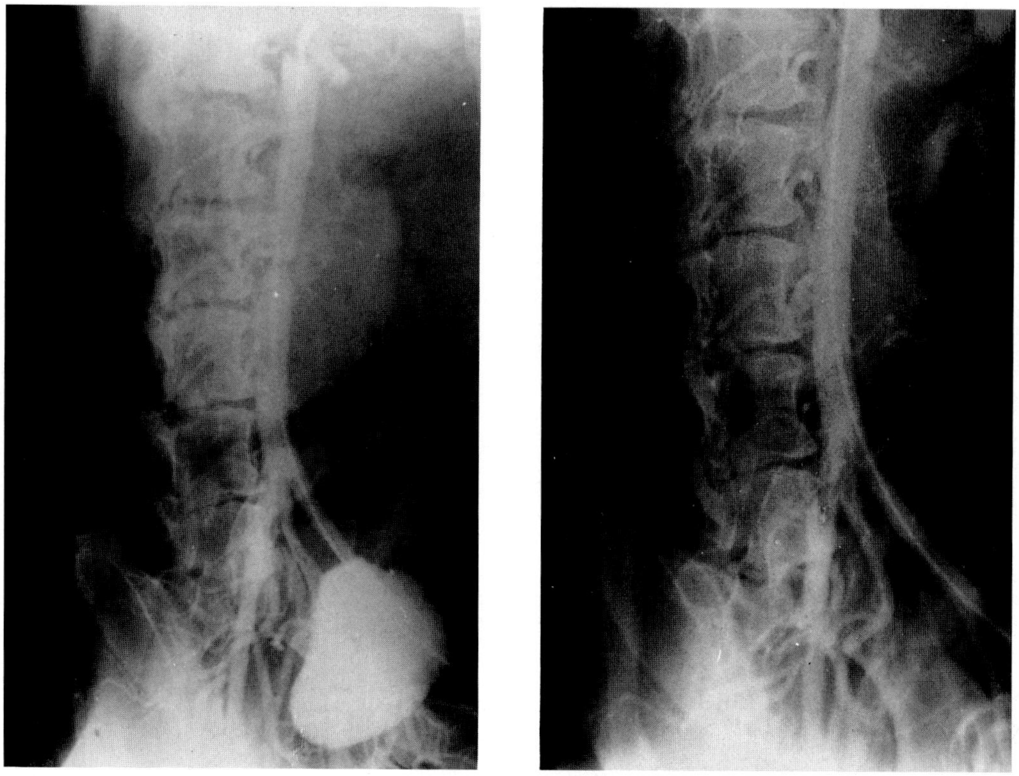

A B

Figure 12–1. **A:** Aortography before angioplasty. **B:** Aortography following angioplasty.

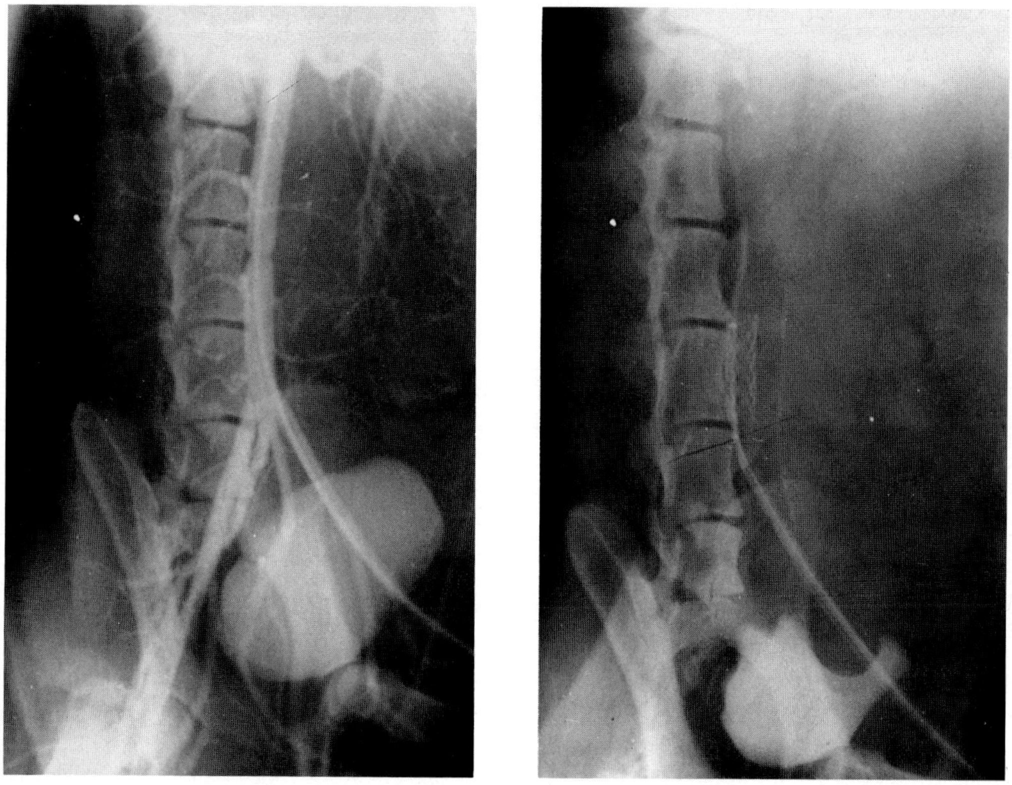

A B

Figure 12–2. **A:** Aortography of the abdominal aorta of the dog; experimental stenosis. **B:** Plain film of the abdomen following stent placement.

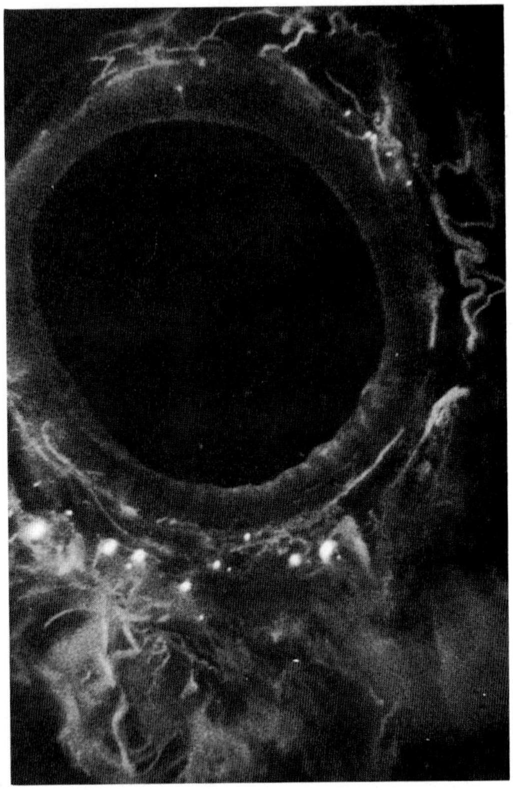

A

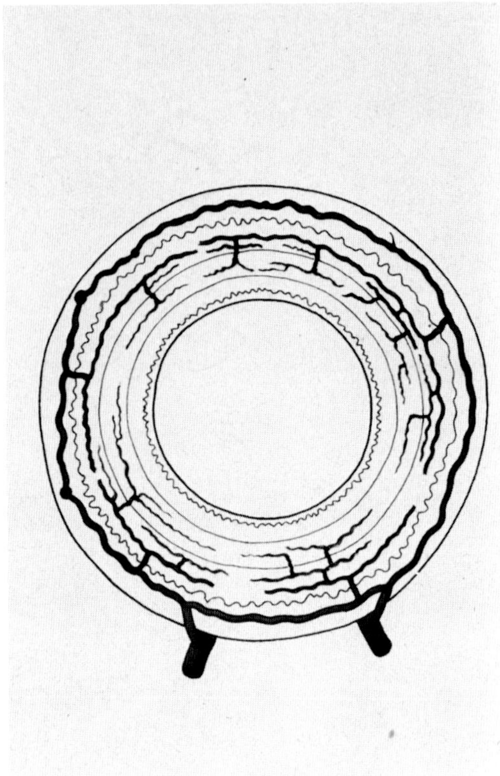

B

Figure 12–3. **A:** Transverse cut of the abdominal aorta of the dog. Normal distribution of the vasa vasorum in the abdominal aorta. **B:** Corresponding diagram.

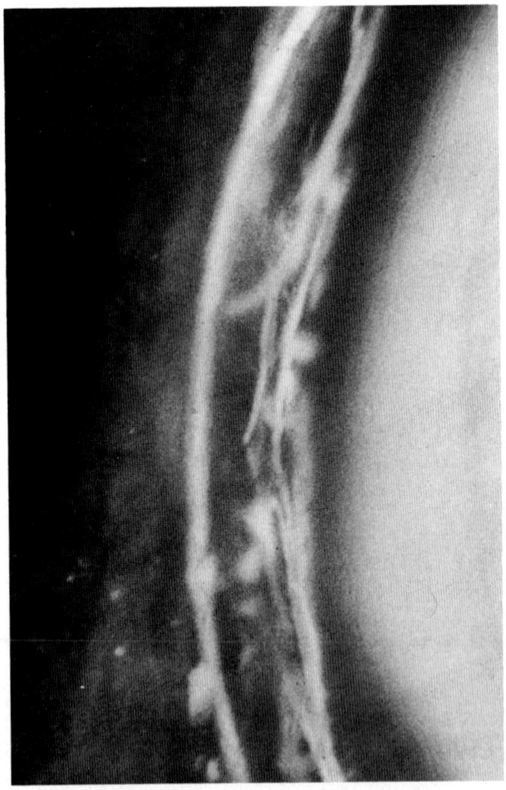

Figure 12–4. Transverse cut of the abdominal aorta of the man: atherosclerotic plaque. Vasa vasorum reach the subintima.

effects on the vasa vasorum. In the acute study they found rupture and stretching of the vasa vasorum. In the chronic study proliferation of the vasa vasorum was found.

Changes of the vasa vasorum by angioplasty on stenotic arteries have not been studied.

To evaluate the effect of angioplasty on the microcirculation of the dilated artery, we studied the morphology of the vasa vasorum before and after angioplasty. For that purpose, we selected the aorta of the dog and pig because those arteries are rich in vasa vasorum and their distribution is similar to that in man.[10] Research was performed in the abdominal aorta, because it is one vessel in which atherosclerosis occurs most frequently.

In the pig, we induced atherosclerosis following a lipid diet and denudation of the endothelium. In the dog, experimental stenosis was produced with catgut sutures in order to develop lesions similar to fibromuscular dysplasia.[11,12] Twenty-four hours following angioplasty, there was rupture of the precapillary arterioles, with a caliber of 0.03 to 0.01 mm, situated at the junction of the external and middle third of the media (Fig. 12-5). At 3 weeks, there was partial reabsorption of the hemorrhage, reorganization, and revascularization with new vasa vasorum formation (Fig. 12-6). At 6 weeks, there was complete reabsorption of the hemorrhage, reorganization, and revascularization with formation of a rich plexus of new vasa vasorum. Those vessels were precapillary arterioles (Fig. 12-7) and postcapillary venules

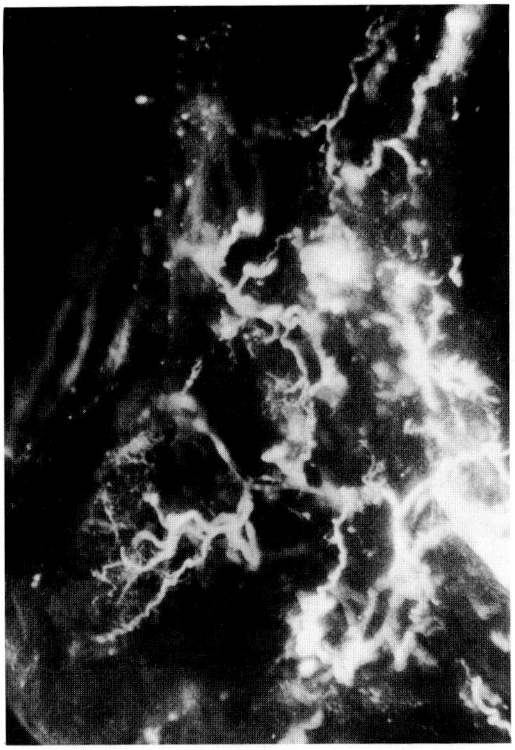

Figure 12–5. Transverse cut of the abdominal aorta of the dog, 24 hours following angioplasty of an experimental stenosis; extravasation of contrast material due to rupture of precapillary arterioles in the media.

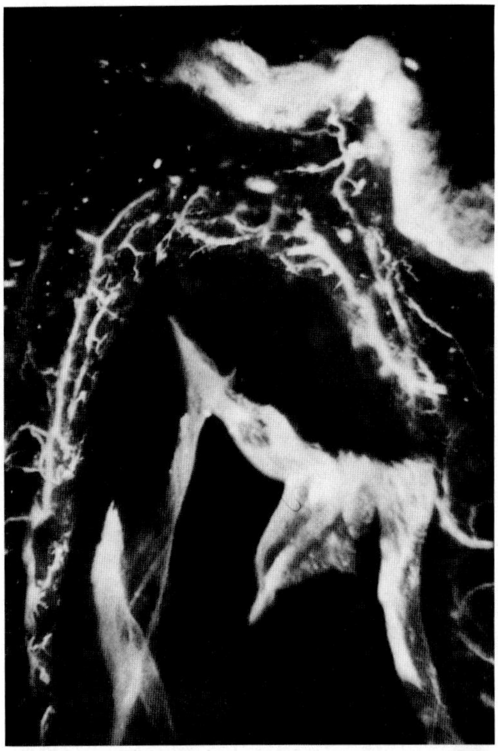

Figure 12–7. Transverse cut of the abdominal aorta of the dog, 6 weeks following angioplasty of an experimental stenosis; total reabsorption of the contrast material. Many new arterioles in the media; rupture of the intima.

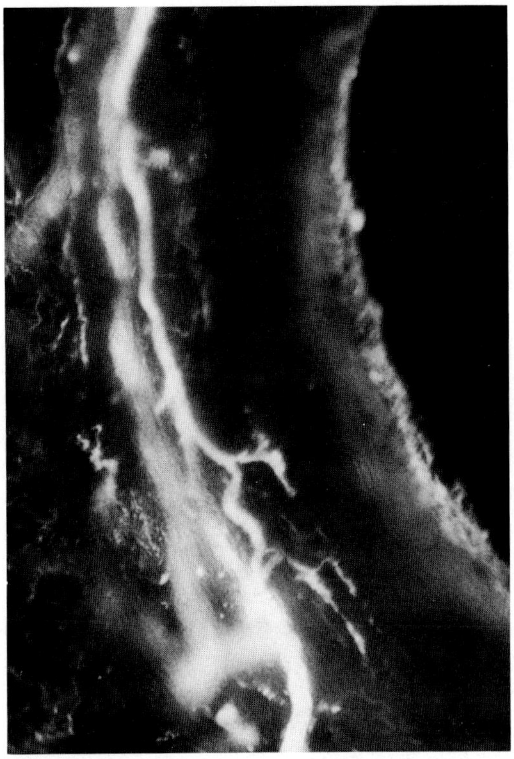

Figure 12–6. Transverse cut of the abdominal aorta of the dog, 3 weeks following angioplasty of an experimental stenosis; partial reabsorption of the contrast material. New vasa vasorum formation at the precapillary level in the media.

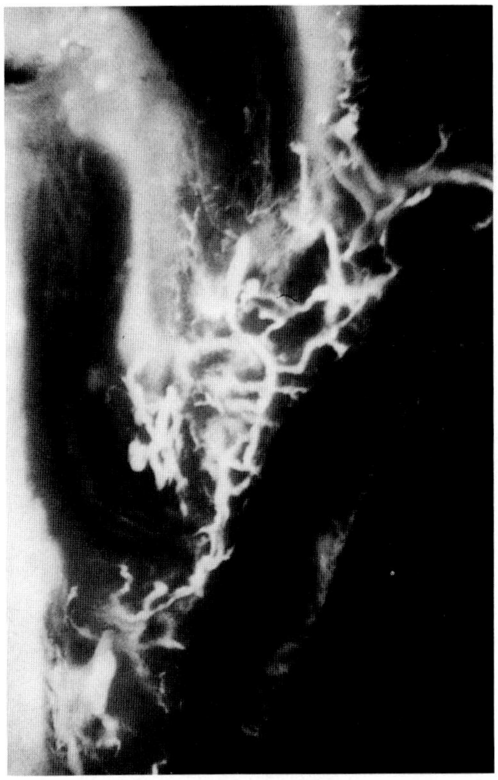

Figure 12–8. Transverse cut of the abdominal aorta of the dog, 6 weeks following angioplasty of an experimental stenosis; many new venules at the media.

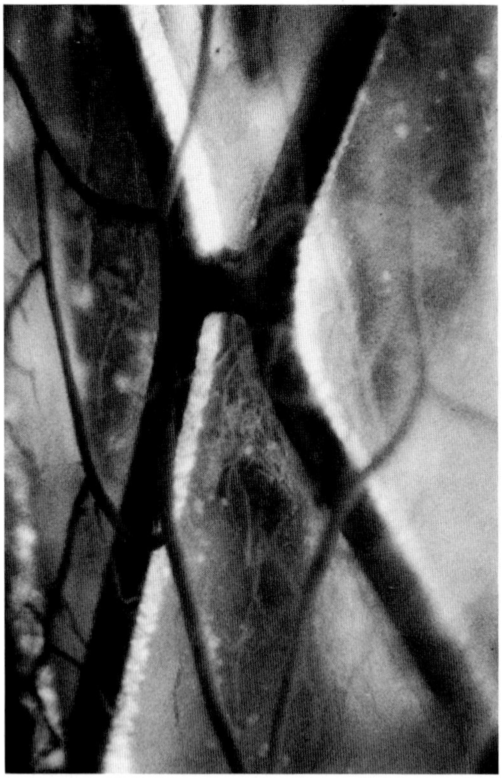

Figure 12–9. Sagittal cut of the abdominal aorta of the dog, 4 months following stent placement; new vasa vasorum around the stent.

(Fig. 12-8). They were located at the junction of the external and middle third of the media. At 10 months, the new revascularization was still larger and the vasa vasorum crossed all the media and reached the subintima.

The changes following angioplasty of the atherosclerotic aorta of the pig were the same as those observed in the dog. Therefore it is possible that the vascular changes after angioplasty in man are similar.

Four months following stent placement in experimental stenosis in the abdominal aorta of the dog, there was proliferation of the precapillary arterioles, which was more extensive than following angioplasty (Fig. 12-9). The precapillary arterioles invaded the inner third of the media with their ramification. At 10 months following stent placement, the new arterioles formed at precapillary levels were more extensive (Fig. 12-10). At this time, there was formation of a new venular plexus, whose vessels arose from the intima and drained to a trunk that ended at the subintimal plexus.

The new vessel formation following angioplasty and stent placement may be the result of the wall anoxia caused by damage of the vasa vasorum and by the temporary compression by the balloon or by permanent compression by the stent. The intimal and medial hyperplasia also causes increased oxygen demand and stimulates the proliferation of the vasa vasorum.

The plexus formed following stent placement infiltrated more media and was richer in small, new vessels, probably due to the permanent anoxia as a result of compression of the vasa vasorum.

It seems that the new vascularization changes from angioplasty and stenting cause either the arterioles or the venules to contribute to a better irrigation and venous return from the arterial wall. These changes may have a role in long-term patency.

REFERENCES

1. Clarke JA. The vasa vasorum of normal human lower limb arteries. Acta Anat 1965;61:481–7.
2. Woodruff CE. Studies on the vasa vasorum. Am J Pathol 1926; 2:567–9.
3. Winternitz MC, Thomas RM, Le Compte PM. The biology

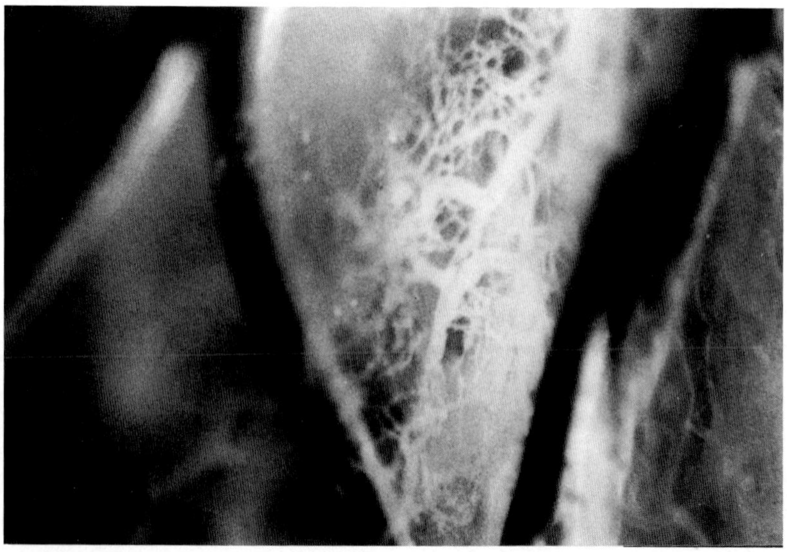

Figure 12–10. Sagittal cut of the abdominal aorta of the dog, 10 months following stent placement; much more new vasorum around the stent than at 4 months.

of arteriosclerosis. Springfield, IL: Charles C Thomas, 1938:3–9.
4. Celestina da Costa J. A parede arterial. Dissertaçäo de doutoramento F. M. L., 1945.
5. Geiringer E. Intimal vascularisation and atherosclerosis. J Pathol Bacteriol 1951;63:202–11.
6. Ayres de Sousa A, Alvares L. Microangiographic study of the vasa vasorum of the thoracic aorta. Radiology 1960;75:91–6.
7. Cragg AH, Einzig SP, Rysavy JA, et al. The vasa vasorum and angioplasty. Radiology 1983;148:75–80.
8. Zollikofer CL. Experimental basis of PTA. Front Euro Radiol 1987;5:51–135.
9. Zollikofer CL, Redha FH, Bruhlmann WF, et al. Acute and long-term effects of massive balloon dilation on the aortic wall and the vasa vasorum. Radiology 1987;164:145–9.
10. Schlichter J, Harris R. The vascularization of the aorta II. A comparative study of the aortic vascularization of several species in health and disease. Am J Med Sci 1949;218:610.
11. Ekelund L, Gerlock J, Chocharenco V, Novak G. Balloon catheter dilatation of renal artery stenosis in the dog. Eur Urol 1978;4:298–302.
12. Stridbeck H, Jonsson N, Lindstedt E, Ekelund L. Experimental fibrous renal artery stenosis dilated by balloon catheter. Acta Radiol Diagn 1982;23:177–84.

13 Biochemistry and Pharmacology of Fibrinolytic Therapy

Robert W. Holden, M.D., John T. Mail, M.D.

The fibrinolytic and coagulation enzyme systems promote circulatory fluidity in normal conditions and coagulation in the presence of vascular injury and life-threatening hemorrhage. This chapter emphasizes the dynamic changes brought about in this physiologic equilibrium by the administration of exogenous plasminogen activators. To promote an understanding of the effects of plasminogen activation, we describe the natural fibrinolytic system, examine available exogenous enzymes, and describe the known responses of this equilibrated enzyme system. The physiologic response to exogenous fibrinolysis is the mobilization of contrary force mechanisms such as coagulation, plasminogen activator inhibitors, and plasmin inhibitors. To understand plasminogen activator therapy, let us begin with an examination of the elemental components of the fibrinolytic system.

PLASMINOGEN AND PLASMIN

The conversion of plasminogen to plasmin is the pivotal process of the fibrinolytic system. Plasminogen activators enzymatically produce hydrolysis of a single protein bond (560–561) in the one-chain amino acid plasminogen molecule (Fig. 13-1A). Plasminogen circulates in plasma as a zymogen (inert form) and activation splits the molecule into an active two-chain form—plasmin, the only enzyme known to degrade fibrin as its main substrate. Despite the single-chain splitting, the newly formed two chains circulate conjoined by a single disulfide bond.

Plasminogen exists in two forms, Glu and Lys. Glu-plasminogen, so-called because of a glutamic acid in its N-terminus, and Lys-plasminogen, a plasmin-modified form so entitled due to a lysine in the altered N-terminus. Glu-plasminogen is the natural inactive circulating form of plasminogen and Lys-plasminogen is the conformationally altered form found bound to receptor surfaces on platelets, endothelial cells, and fibrin. A conformational change of Glu- to Lys-plasminogen occurs with plasmin exposure in the area of forming fibrin and membrane receptor surfaces.

Plasmin is a nonspecific serine (CH_2OH-CH_2-NH_2-COOH) protease that, if not neutralized (by fibrin degradation, partial plasminogen degradation, or alpha$_2$-antiplasmin), degrades circulating plasma proteins, i.e., fibrinogen, Factors V and VIII, and alters the procoagulant platelet membrane receptor functions. This enzymatic nonspecificity is unusual and the physiologic response to the circulatory presence of this nonspecific protease is extremely rapid and efficient. Alpha$_2$-antiplasmin neutralizes circulating plasmin in the fastest known protein-protein interaction and, thus, homeostasis is preserved as long as there is sufficient plasma circulating alpha$_2$-antiplasmin. However, the circulating molecular stores of plasminogen far exceed the equimolar supplies of alpha$_2$-antiplasmin. Thus, the administration of exogenous plasminogen activator therapy carries the potential of excessive plasmin production, degradation of clotting factors, and induction of a systemic lytic state.

Physiologic plasminogen activation usually does not take place in circulating plasma, but instead is highly regulated by the adsorption and binding of plasminogen to the surfaces of activated platelets, damaged cells, and fibrin—all of which in biochemical parlance may be considered to be cofactors. The importance of surface receptors in the maintenance of this equilibrium is demonstrated by the 10-second half-life of plasmin created while bound to fibrin compared with the 100 msec half-life of plasmin formed in circulating plasma.[1]

FIBRINOGEN AND FIBRIN

During initiated coagulation, thrombin cleaves fibrinopeptides A and B from soluble circulating fibrinogen. Fibrinogen, manufactured by the hepatocyte, is a large inactive soluble protein molecule that on loss of the fibrinopeptides is converted to a self-polymerizing fibrin molecule. The polymers form in a half-staggered overlapping pattern in two-stranded protofibrils that with further assembly form fibrin fibers to provide a foundation for forming thrombus. Additionally, thrombin activates fibrin-stabilizing factor, which in turn produces the following three major changes in fibrin: covalent bond formation, side chain cross-linkages, and irreversible binding of alpha$_2$-antiplasmin.[2]

Once fibrin is stabilized, several stages are required for plasmin dissolution to effect soluble degradation products. In the earliest stages, fibrin is partially lysed; however, the covalent bonds prevent the release of soluble fragments. With this early partial digestion, a strong plasminogen binding site is exposed that binds additional plasminogen. Thus, a continuously replenishing source of plasminogen is provided for activation by the exogenous plasminogen activator. Continued plasmin digestion of fibrin produces the large soluble fibrin degradation fragments entitled X and Y. Interestingly, the X fragment is a very strong anticoagulant and the Y fragment interrupts fibrin polymerization. Further plasmin degradation of these large fragments produces the smaller D and E fragments.

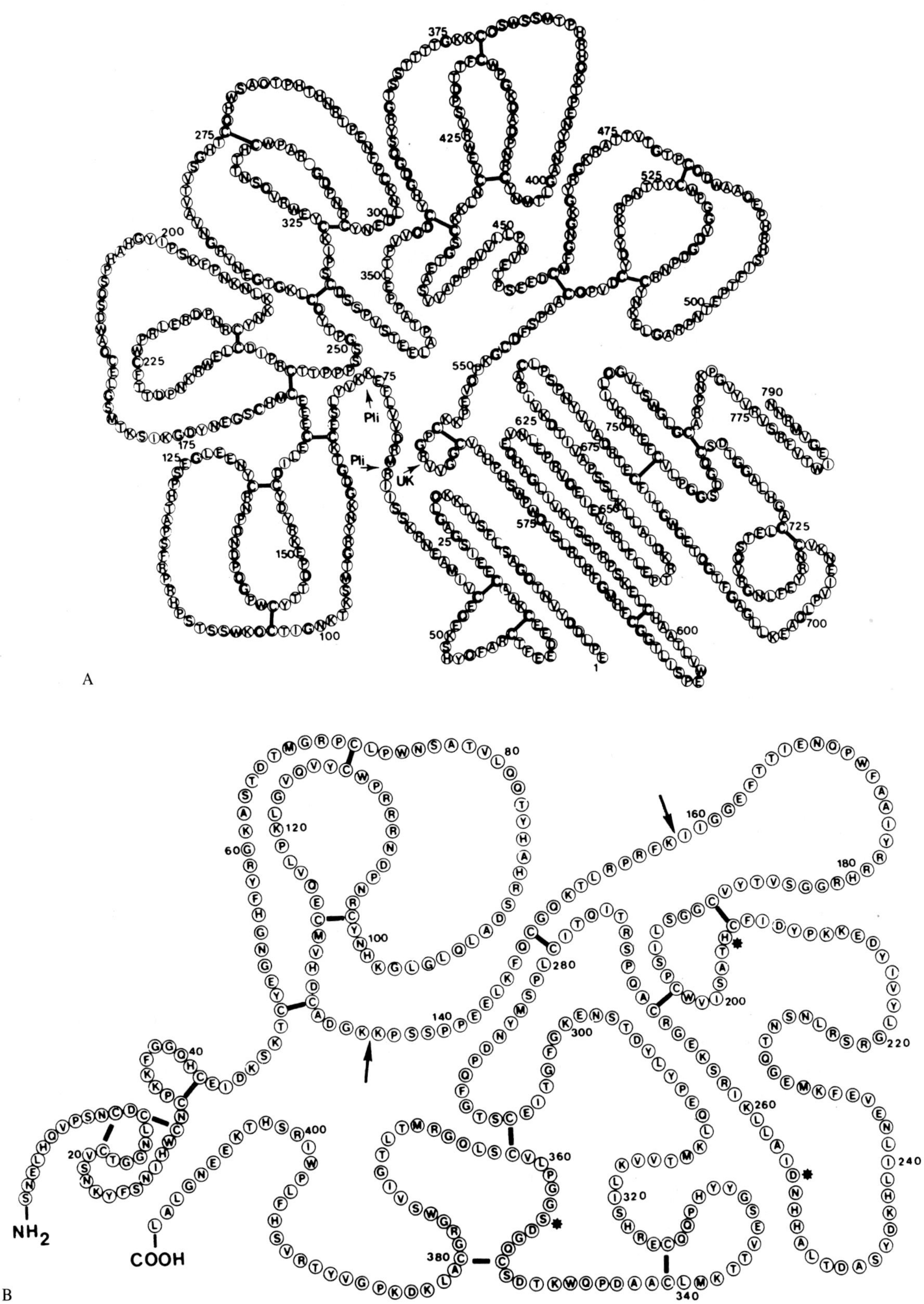

Figure 13–1. **A:** Note the polypeptide structure of plasminogen. The circled letters denote specific amino acids in the primary sequence and numbers in small print indicate specific positions in the primary sequence. The heavy bars represent disulfide bonds, Pli denotes two areas either of which when cleaved by plasmin creates Lys-plasminogen, and UK designates the Arg_{560}-Val_{561} peptide bond that when hydrolyzed converts single-chain plasminogen to two-chain plasmin. **B:** Single-chain urokinase plasminogen activator (scu-PA). Asterisks mark amino acids composing the catalytic sites. Arrows denote two cleavage sites. Hydrolysis of the Lys_{158}-Ile_{159} peptide bond produces high molecular weight two-chain urokinase (UK) and cleavage at the Lys_{135}-Lys_{136} bond produces low molecular weight two-chain UK.

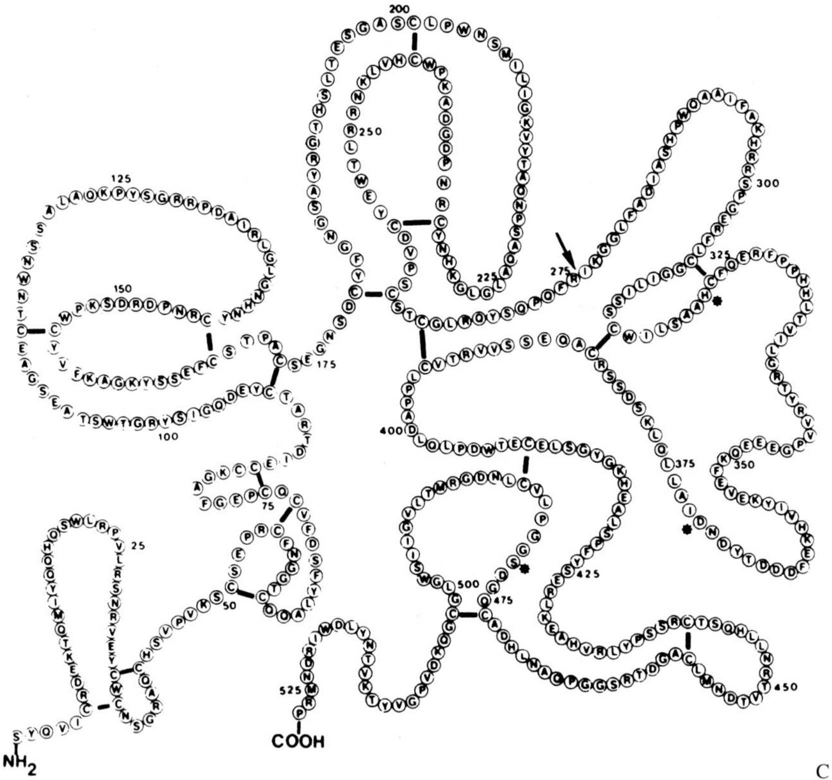

Figure 13–1 (continued) C: Single-chain tissue-type plasminogen activator (t-PA). Arrow denotes the Arg_{275}-Ile_{276} peptide bond that when hydrolyzed results in the conversion of single-chain t-PA to two-chain t-PA. Asterisks mark the amino acids containing the catalytic sites. (Reprinted with permission from Verstraete et al.[18])

C

Ritchie et al[3] have described a hepatocyte stimulating factor (HSF). Leukocyte exposure to the small fibrin degradation fragments (D and E) results in concentration and time-dependent HSF production. Exposure of hepatocytes to increasing concentrations of HSF results in increased production of fibrinogen. Following exposure to HSF, hepatocyte cell cultures demonstrate initiated fibrinogen production at 4 hours and a linear time-mediated increased production through 16 hours. These data suggest that hepatic production of fibrinogen is dependent on circulating small fibrin degradation products that, mediated by leukocytes, stimulate increased hepatic production of fibrinogen. For interventional radiology, this feedback mechanism is extremely slow and unable to correct bleeding encountered in the lytic state promptly.

PLATELETS

Vascular injury produces hemorrhage, which is controlled by platelet adhesion and aggregation at the exposed subendothelial surfaces. These platelet events activate coagulation and result in fibrin deposition. Originally, platelets were believed to be only procoagulant in function; however, recent in vitro studies have shown platelets to be multipotential. Platelets can enhance plasmin production, inhibit the generation of plasmin, and neutralize active plasmin. Thus, the platelet has both profibrinolytic and antifibrinolytic abilities that are mediated by plasmin exposure. In vitro studies demonstrate that the platelet's activities are responsive to the duration and concentration of plasmin bathing the cells. Thus, the platelet is a multipotential cell whose principal function is to maintain a circulatory homeostasis. This varying potential may account for preliminary reports of thrombi rich in platelets being resistant to enzyme therapy as well as explain the platelet's role in the hemorrhagic diathesis associated with thrombolytic therapy.[4]

PLASMINOGEN ACTIVATORS

Currently, five plasminogen activators are in either investigational or clinical use. It is important to note that currently utilized naturally occurring exogenous enzyme dosages exceed physiologic levels by at least 1000:1. Thus, circulatory stores of naturally occurring plasminogen activator inhibitors (PAI) are insufficient to provide any significant neutralization of the administered exogenous enzyme. Additionally, there has been no demonstration of significant cellular production of PAI to interfere with administered exogenous enzymes.

Streptokinase

Streptokinase (SK) is a foreign streptococcal nonenzymatic single-chain protein that achieves plasminogen activation after combining and undergoing a conformational change in a 1:1 equimolar ratio with a circulating plasminogen molecule. This complexed plasminogen-SK intermediate achieves nonspecific protease activity by activating a second plasminogen molecule. This mode of plasminogen activation provides no fibrin selectivity and, thus, SK indiscriminately activates both intrathrombus and circulating plasminogen. Previous beta-streptococcal infections generate antibodies to SK that must be neutralized with loading doses of SK prior to this enzyme being able to achieve effective fibrinolysis.

Anisoylated Plasminogen-Streptokinase Activator Complex

Anisoylated plasminogen activator complex (APSAC) is a chemically modified form of SK being evaluated in clinical trials. The in vitro acylation (placement of an organic radical derived from an organic acid by the removal of a carboxylic hydroxyl group) of an SK-plasminogen complex renders this activated intermediate form inactive. On in vivo administration, the complexed plasminogen molecule binds to fibrin, undergoes deacylation, and activates adjacent fibrin-bound plasminogen. This biochemical modification has prolonged 23 minute physical half-life of SK to 90 minutes for APSAC.[5] In animal models, this modified enzyme has been reported to produce significantly less fibrinogenolysis than urokinase (UK) or SK; however, it does produce more than tissue-type plasminogen activator (t-PA). An early cardiac trial, the APSAC Intervention Mortality Study (AIMS), reported APSAC to be possibly more effective than SK.[6]

Single-Chain Urokinase-Type Plasminogen Activator

Single-chain urokinase-type plasminogen activator (scu-PA), an endothelial cell produced single-chain plasminogen activator, is inactive in circulation due to competitive binding with PAI type 1 (PAI-1) (Fig. 13-1B). Although scu-PA does not significantly activate circulating plasminogen or efficiently bind to fibrin, it does preferentially activate fibrin-bound plasminogen more efficiently than circulating plasma plasminogen. The first multicenter scu-PA prospective myocardial infarction trial demonstrated a relative fibrin specificity similar to that of t-PA and achieved similar lytic efficacy. t-PA produced a 62% patency at 90 minutes versus a 50 and 65% patency at 90 minutes in differing dosage levels of scu-PA.[7]

Urokinase

Partial plasmin digestion of scu-PA converts the single-chain into a double-chain (UK) by hydrolysis of the protein bond at either the 135-136 domain for low-molecular weight double-chain UK or at the 158-159 bond for high molecular weight double-chain UK (Fig. 13-1B). Both UK forms circulate as two chains conjoined by a disulfide bond. The previously described increased specificity for bound plasminogen by scu-PA is lost in the conversion to double-chain form. Thus, UK is enzymatically a nonspecific protease without fibrin selectivity. Commercially available forms are approximately 70% low-molecular weight double-chain form. It is important to note that UK, like SK, has no fibrin selectivity; however, unlike SK, UK is a naturally occurring enzyme whose therapy is not complicated by antigenesis, anaphylaxis, or antibody formation.

Tissue Plasminogen Activator

t-PA is synthesized and secreted by endothelial cells as a single-chain protein (Fig. 13-1C). Limited plasmin hydrolysis of the 275-276 protein bond converts the single-chain to a two-chain molecule linked by one disulfide bond. In contrast to scu-PA and UK, clinical studies with one- and two-chain t-PA have demonstrated similar fibrinolytic and plasminogen activating properties. Both forms are known to be in the circulation and intravenously administered single-chain t-PA is within minutes converted to a two-chain form. The original commercial production of recombinant t-PA by Genentech utilized a fermentation process with a roller-bottle system that produced predominantly (90%) a double-chain form. Subsequently, production was changed to a suspension-culture method and the enzyme obtained became predominantly (60 to 80%) a single-chain species.[8]

t-PA is an inefficient enzyme in the absence of fibrin, but when bound to fibrin its catalytic efficiency increases 1000-fold. Kinetic data document the adsorption of t-PA and plasminogen to fibrin in a sequence that produces a ternary (three-part) complex. Fibrin increases the local plasminogen concentration by creating an additional interaction between t-PA and its substrate. The high affinity of t-PA for plasminogen in the presence of fibrin induces efficient plasminogen activation in the local environment of the clot and, thus, avoids circulating plasminogen activation. It was this fibrin specificity that promoted the commercial development of t-PA and is the unique feature distinguishing t-PA from SK and UK.

PHYSIOLOGY AND PATHOPHYSIOLOGY OF THROMBOLYSIS

The platelet and endothelial cells respond to their bathing environment as integrated biochemical units to maintain the contained fluidity of blood. Both have the ability to promote a procoagulant or anticoagulant state by cell membrane protein assembly or by production of t-PA, UK, or PAI-1 and -2. Thus, in a physiologic environment, the system works efficiently to provide an environment that allows thrombosis in injured tissue while maintaining perfusion. However, the administration of exogenous enzyme for the treatment of a thrombotic ischemic occlusion may eventuate in a release of plasmin exceeding the neutralizing capability of alpha$_2$-antiplasmin. This excess of plasmin consumes circulating coagulation Factors V and VIII, fibrinogen, and alters platelet receptor functions to induce a systemic lytic state, which may be accompanied by complicating hemorrhage.

PLASMINOGEN ACTIVATOR DOSAGE AND DELIVERY

The clinical evaluations of plasminogen activators have utilized many different dosage regimens; however, the optimal dosage of the various enzymes is yet to be established. Initially, Dotter and coworkers[9] as well as Katzen and van Breda[10] advocated low-dose SK lytic therapy. Currently, there is increasing acceptance of high-dose UK regional therapy due principally to the achievement of shorter infusion times. McNamara and Fischer[11] advocate mechanically passing the guide wire through the entire thrombus and then instilling UK at 4000 U/min for 2 hours through a catheter embedded in the occlusion. With restoration of patency, the catheter is withdrawn proximal to the remaining thrombus, and UK is infused at 1000 to 2000 U/min until complete lysis is accomplished.[11] With establishment of vessel patency and beginning antegrade flow, enzyme delivery should be continued until the runoff is sufficient to maintain adequate tissue perfusion and avoidance of reocclusion. Sullivan et al[12] demonstrated a significant reduction in infusion times (33.6 versus 10.4 hours) in two study groups treated with identical infusions by antecedent lacing of the thrombus with 230,000 U versus 52,000 U of UK. The study also demonstrated that the higher lacing dose effected a significant reduction in the total enzyme dose required to achieve clinically similar results.[12] These observations are also confirmed by the knowledge that enzymatic activation should be more efficacious with increasing concentrations and dosage.

All plasminogen activators produce an increasing hemostatic defect with increasing dosage. Cardiac trials, featuring very high-dose short infusion enzyme therapy to promote rapid reperfusion (60 to 90 minutes) of the myocardium, have demonstrated a significantly increased complication rate of intracranial hemorrhage with 90,000,000 U (150 mg) compared with 60,000,000 U (100 mg) of t-PA therapy. This lower dosage reduced the incidence of intracranial hemorrhage from 1.9% (11 of 582 patients) to 0.5% (15 of 2952 patients).[13] This report in conjunction with experience in the low-dose and high-dose regional therapy regimens and an understanding of the pathophysiology of excess plasmin production confirm that induction of the systemic lytic state is more dependent on the total enzyme dose delivered than the time span of delivery. Although the cardiac trials utilizing 1,500,000 U of SK seem consistently to demonstrate the most marked depletion of plasma clotting components, it is important to note the Second International Study on Infarct Survival trial demonstrated the addition of 160 mg of aspirin, prior to SK therapy and daily thereafter, significantly reduced reinfarction and the incidence of nonfatal stroke without significantly increasing the risk of hemorrhage (17,000 patients enrolled).[14] On this basis, it seems indicated to give 160 mg/day of aspirin during and after local thrombolytic therapy. Although controversial, the concomitant administration of heparin with maintenance of the partial thromboplastin time at 1.5 times normal is recommended.[15]

The patient undergoing therapy for the treatment of limb ischemia can usually tolerate a longer infusion time than can the patient with acute myocardial infarction; however, the occluded limb vessel or graft usually contains a significantly larger amount of thrombus compared with the coronary artery and too often the required cumulative enzyme dose in both situations may be approximately equal. Thus, the recent laboratory and clinical demonstration that lacing the clot achieves a cumulative dose reduction and shorter infusions times is extremely promising.[12,16]

The most efficient enzyme instillation will be within the thrombus, especially in the instance of a complete occlusion. If the catheter cannot be embedded within the thrombus, the most desirable infusion catheter site is in closest proximity to the target thrombus. In the instance of peripheral infusions, the nonocclusive thrombus will have a higher lysis success rate than will complete occlusions due to increased enzyme adsorption on the greater exposed surface area. Thus, complete occlusions are best treated by intrathrombic enzyme administration.

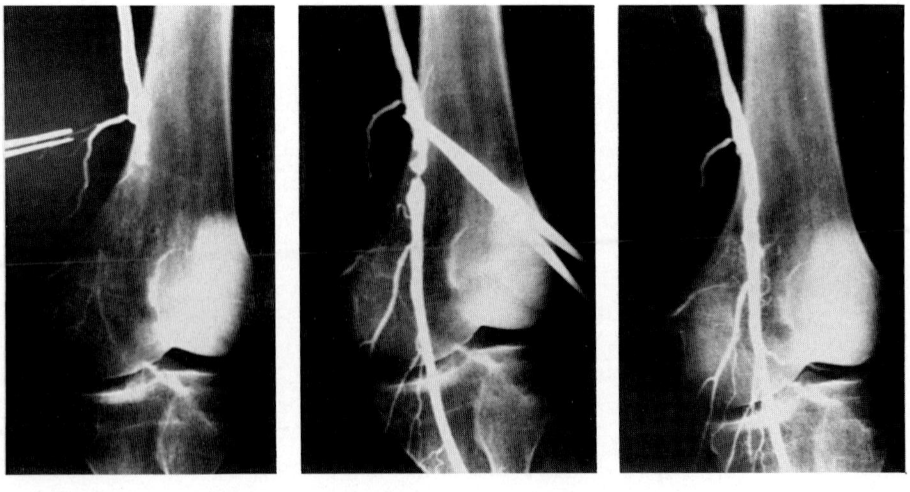

Figure 13–2. A 65-year-old man presented with one block exertional claudication of 3 months' duration. Angiogram reveals complete occlusion of the popliteal artery. Severe atheromatous stenosis was uncovered following 1,000,000 U of urokinase. Postangioplasty study reveals obliteration of stenosis.

Clinically, it is frequently difficult to determine the age of an occlusion; however, if the occlusion is suspected of being of less than 3 months' duration, one should consider a trial of fibrinolysis prior to recanalization efforts. Mechanical instrumentation of fresh thrombus may result in significant limb-threatening distal embolization. This complication can be predicted and avoided by a short trial of plasminogen activators (Fig. 13-2). Enzymatic dissolution of complete chronic occlusions is possible and, although much is not known, it appears that successful thrombolytic therapy varies inversely with the age of the thrombus.[17]

SUMMARY

The common mechanism of action for all known enzymes predicts common complications and fibrinolytic ability. General principles of plasminogen activator therapy are increasingly understood and should be applied to improve success rates and decrease complications. Despite significant advancements in our understanding of the dynamics of fibrinolytic therapy, we are still unable to predict when complications will occur by the usual and customary laboratory examinations.

REFERENCES

1. Collen D. On the regulation and control of fibrinolysis. Thromb Haemost 1980;48:294–6.
2. Doolittle R. Fibrinogen and fibrin. Annu Rev Biochem 1984;53:195–229.
3. Ritchie D, Levy B, Adams M, Fuller G. Regulation of fibrinogen synthesis by plasmin-derived fragments of fibrinogen and fibrin: an indirect feedback pathway. Proc Natl Acad Sci 1982;79:1530–4.
4. Coller B. Platelets and thrombolytic therapy. N Engl J Med 1990;322:33–42.
5. Monk J, Heel R. Anisoylated plasminogen streptokinase activator complex (APSAC): a review of its mechanism of action, clinical pharmacology and therapeutic use in acute myocardial infarction. Drugs 1987;34:25–49.
6. AIMS Trial Study Group. Effect of intravenous APSAC on mortality after acute myocardial infarction: preliminary report of a placebo-controlled trial. Lancet 1988;1:545–9.
7. Loscalzo J, Wharton T, Kirshenbaum J, et al. Clot-selective coronary thrombolysis with prourokinase. Circulation 1989; 79:776–82.
8. Loscalzo J, Braunwald E. Tissue plasminogen activator. N Engl J Med 1988;319:925–31.
9. Dotter C, Rosch J, Seaman A. Selective clot lysis with low dose streptokinase. Radiology 1974;111:31–7.
10. Katzen B, van Breda A. Low dose streptokinase in the treatment of arterial occlusions. AJR 1981;136:1171–8.
11. McNamara T, Fischer J. Thrombolysis of peripheral arterial and graft occlusions: improved results using high dose urokinase. AJR 1985;144:769–55.
12. Sullivan K, Gardiner GJ, Shapiro M, et al. Acceleration of thrombolysis with a high-dose transthrombus bolus technique. Radiology 1989;173:805–8.
13. The TIMI Study Group. Comparison of invasive and conservative strategies after treatment with intravenous tissue plasminogen activator in acute myocardial infarction. N Engl J Med 1989;320:618–27.
14. The ISIS-2 Collaborative Group. Randomised trial of intravenous streptokinase, oral aspirin, both, or neither among 17,187 cases of suspected acute myocardial infarction: ISIS-2. Lancet 1988;2:349–60.
15. Eskridge J, Becker G, Richmond B, et al. Catheter-related thrombosis and fibrinolytic therapy. Radiology 1983;149:429–32.
16. Valji K, Bookstein J. Fibrinolysis with intrathrombic injection of urokinase and tissue-type plasminogen activator results in a new model of subacute venous thrombosis. Invest Radiol 1987;22:23–7.
17. Martin M. Streptokinase in chronic arterial disease. Boca Raton, FL: CRC Press, 1982.
18. Verstraete M, Collen D. Thrombolytic therapy in the eighties. Blood 1986;67:1529–41.

14 Low-Dose Thrombolysis: Techniques, Complications, and Results

Janette D. Durham, M.D., David A. Kumpe, M.D.

The recent literature shows continued improvement in the efficacy and safety of low-dose thrombolysis for treatment of arterial occlusive disease. This chapter outlines the techniques for administration of intra-arterial thrombolytic agents, the complications of therapy, and the results of treatment of lower extremity arterial occlusive disease.

TECHNIQUES

Patient Selection

To be considered for thrombolytic therapy, the patient must be tolerating the ischemia caused by the arterial occlusion. Severe ischemia warrants surgery, and thrombolytic therapy is reserved for patients who are not facing imminent tissue necrosis. Severe loss of sensory or motor function in an extremity is a contraindication to treatment.[1,2]

Present indications for the use of thrombolytic therapy for the treatment of arterial occlusive disease include: (1) treatment of acutely ischemic limbs in patients at high risk for extensive surgical procedures; (2) conversion of a clinical situation requiring urgent or emergent surgery into one that can be treated electively; (3) treatment of small artery occlusions in the calf that cannot be treated surgically; (4) clot lysis to permit satisfactory angiographic assessment of a limb's circulation before intervention; and (5) treatment of underlying flow-limiting lesions with percutaneous techniques, as an adjunct or alternative to surgery.[3,4]

Literature on systemic treatment of deep vein thrombosis and pulmonary embolism identifies high-risk groups in whom thrombolytic therapy is contraindicated.[5] Contraindications have been classified into absolute and relative categories (Table 14-1). The increased safety margin of local versus systemic administration of fibrinolytic drugs allows some liberalization of the relative contraindications; however, if a relative contraindication exists, the risk to benefit ratio must be clearly established.

Choice of Thrombolytic Agent

Urokinase (UK) is the present drug of choice for treatment of arterial occlusive disease, because of its increased efficacy, decreased systemic thrombolytic effect, lack of circulating antibodies, and lower bleeding complication rate compared with streptokinase (SK).[6–9] The only disadvantage of UK is that it is considerably more expensive than SK; however, the actual difference in cost of treatment is less when taking into account the cost of treating complications of thrombolytic infusions, which are more frequent with SK. Data on the efficacy and safety of recombinant tissue plasminogen activator (rt-PA) has shown no superiority to UK.[10] The characteristics of SK, UK, and rt-PA are compared in Table 14-2.

Dose, Concentration, and Route of Administration

In theory, local intra-arterial administration of fibrinolytic drugs requires less of any drug compared to a systemic infusion, since more of the fibrinolytic agent activates fibrin-bound plasminogen rather than circulating plasminogen. Doses for local administration of fibrinolytic drugs have been derived from systemic doses. Initially, low doses (one twentieth of systemic doses) were utilized in an attempt to limit hemorrhagic complications.[11] Improved results, with similar or lower complication rates, were then reported using UK in higher doses.[12] This has led to a spectrum of dosage protocols, with advocates of each. In addition to the dose, the concentration of drug appears to be important in the rate of lysis. In vitro, UK has an increasing rate of lysis with increasing concentrations from 300 to 100,000 IU/ml. In contrast, the lysis rate with SK is maximum at 5000 U/ml; at higher concentrations, the lysis rate declines.[13] Optimal concentrations of UK in clinical use have not yet been established.

The initial approach to intra-arterial administration of SK and UK was infusion through a 5 or 6 F catheter embedded in

Table 14–1. Contraindications to Thrombolytic Therapy

Absolute contraindications
Active internal bleeding
Recent cerebral vascular accident or other active intracranial process*
Relative major contraindications
Recent operation of less than 10 days
Recent serious gastrointestinal bleeding
Recent major trauma
Severe hypertension
Relative minor contraindications
Recent minor trauma
Left heart thrombus
Bacterial endocarditis
Hemostatic defects, including those associated with severe renal and hepatic disease
Pregnancy
Age greater than 75 years
Diabetic hemorrhagic retinopathy

*The utility of thrombolytic therapy in treatment of stroke is currently under investigation.

Table 14–2. Characteristics of Fibrinolytic Agents

	STREPTOKINASE	UROKINASE	RECOMBINANT TISSUE PLASMINOGEN ACTIVATOR
Source	Beta-hemolytic streptococci	Fetal renal cell culture	Recombinant DNA techniques
Structure	Single-chain polypeptide (47,000 d)	Double-chain polypeptide (55,000 d)	Single-chain polypeptide (72,000 d)
Plasminogen activation	Indirect (Intermediate SK-plasminogen complex that activates circulating and bound plasminogen)	Direct (Activates circulating and bound plasminogen)	Direct (Activates circulating and bound plasminogen)
Fibrin affinity	Low	Low	High
Half-life	23 minutes	16 minutes	5 minutes
Antigenic	Yes	No	No
Cost/vial	$13 (250,000 U)	$195 (250,000 IU)	$1,127.50 (50 mg = 29,000,000 IU)
Typical dose	5000 U/hr	100,000 IU/hr	0.05–0.10 mg/kg/hr

SK: Streptokinase.

the proximal end of the clot, with advancement of the catheter as lysis occurred.[3,8,11,14] Lysis times using this technique are commonly 24 hours or greater; although this is longer than lysis times using more recent protocols, this simple approach is still useful when it is clear that overnight infusion will be necessary. UK is administered at 60,000 to 100,000 IU/hour, in concentrations of 2500 to 5000 IU/ml. SK is infused at 5000 to 10,000 U/hour.

The original high-dose UK protocol of McNamara and Fischer[12] was the administration of 250,000 IU/hour (2500 IU/ml) for up to 4 hours, periodically advancing the catheter through the thrombus, until flow has been reestablished. The dose is then decreased to 100,000 IU/hour with the catheter tip at the proximal end of the residual clot, until complete lysis has been achieved.[12] This technique frequently restores flow in less than 4 hours, with total infusion times for complete clot lysis averaging 18 hours.

The use of a coaxial catheter system for infusion has become routine in the treatment of long occlusions. This allows the simultaneous delivery of fibrinolytic drug proximally and distally within the thrombus, and distributes the lytic agent throughout the thrombus without having to advance the proximal catheter. This decreases the number of angiographic examinations required to assure that the catheter is in contact with the residual clot, decreases catheter manipulation, and decreases infusion time. In addition, the dampening effect of the proximal catheter on arterial flow is not as great as when the 5 F catheter is advanced through the clot.[4]

Sullivan et al[15] have shown that lacing the thrombus with UK prior to infusion decreases the required infusion time and the total dose of fibrinolytic agent. If the thrombus could be traversed with a guide wire and catheter, a bolus of 230,000 IU in 10 cc normal saline was injected into the thrombus before starting an infusion of 240,000 IU/hour. This technique resulted in complete clot lysis with average infusions of 10 hours and 1.26 million IU of UK.

Most recently the use of pulsed injections of highly concentrated UK directly into the clot through multi-side hole catheters (pulsed-spray technique) has been described, taking advantage of the direct delivery of the agent as well as mechanical maceration of the clot by the pulsatile jets.[16,17] Treatment requires from less than 1 to several hours to reestablish flow. A concern that these techniques might raise the incidence of embolic complications has been voiced. Although early reports do not support this concern, further investigation will be required to establish its safety.

The decision about which infusion technique to use takes into account both the clinical presentation of the patient and the practical realities of running an angiographic service.[4] In patients with critical ischemia, a high-dose, high-concentration infusion is used in order to lyse the clot quickly and relieve the severe ischemia. In patients in whom the infusion is started in the morning, a similar rapid technique is used, hoping to avoid an overnight infusion. Rapid lysis techniques require intensive physician participation during the initial stages of the infusion and occupy the angiographic suite for extended periods. If the patient's symptoms are mild, or when the infusion is started in the late afternoon, an overnight infusion at a lower infusion schedule is undertaken. The patient is returned to the angiographic suite as the first case the following morning for definition of the underlying lesion. Using current protocols, most infusions are completed in less than 24 hours.

An alternative delivery technique to infusion is the administration of repeated boluses of highly concentrated drug with rapid catheter advancement under fluoroscopy, as described by Lammer et al[18] and Hess et al.[19] This technique has been used primarily for treatment of chronic arterial occlusions prior to angioplasty. Although subintimal passage of the catheter can occur, ending the infusion prematurely, this technique can reestablish flow in hours. It is extremely physician intensive.

COMPLICATIONS

Major complication rates in recent series range from 5 to 30%, with the predominant complication being hemorrhage.[2,20] Periprocedural mortality rates of 1 to 2% have been reported in a few series.[19,21] Deaths have been related to complications of excessive blood loss, reperfusion syndrome, stroke, or severe allergic reactions.[19,21] Many of these deaths could be avoided by improved patient selection and improved management of hemorrhage.[1,2]

Bleeding complications may be local, at the catheter entry site, or remote, including retroperitoneal, intracranial, or visceral hemorrhage. Hemorrhage is often the result of disrupted vascular integrity from catheterization. Invasive procedures that may cause bleeding must be avoided during and following therapy. The risk of spontaneous bleeding is similar to that of standard heparin anticoagulation therapy using heparin.[20] The high incidence of bleeding at sites of previous vascular disruption predicts that even selective agents, such as rt-PA, will have bleeding complications. Major hemorrhagic complications range from 3 to 13%, with a trend toward higher bleeding complication rates with SK and rt-PA compared with UK.[8–10]

Extravasation of contrast through synthetic bypass grafts has been documented by several authors and is thought to occur as the result of fibrin breakdown in the neointima of the grafts.[22,23] This phenomenon is insignificant in the majority of cases, although it may result in hematoma formation. The possibility of extravasation is one reason that clotted grafts less than 6 months of age are generally treated surgically, although this complication has also occurred in grafts that are several years old.[22]

Vascular complications include pseudoaneurysm formation, pericatheter thrombus formation, and embolization. Formation of a false aneurysm, a complication of puncture technique, can generally be treated by local surgical repair. Pericatheter thrombus formation and downstream embolization may further endanger an already compromised extremity and result in limb loss. Episodes of subclinical embolization have been reported to occur in up to 48% of infusions and can be manifested by changes in the color of an extremity and pain.[24] Generally, these episodes resolve with continued infusion, and sequelae develop in only 1 to 2% of cases (Fig. 14-1). Supporters of concomitant heparin administration believe that heparin prevents thromboembolic complications associated with pericatheter thrombus formation. Activated partial thromboplastin time is kept in the range of 1.5 to 2 times normal throughout the infusion.[12] Nonsupporters fear that heparin increases hemorrhagic complications. This hotly debated issue is yet to be resolved.

The antigenic and pyrogenic nature of SK has resulted in systemic reactions that include fever, nausea, urticaria, and anaphylaxis. Serum sickness is a rare complication. Antibody formation to SK rules out its repeat administration to patients who have received SK within the previous 6 months. Although both loading doses of SK and steroids to neutralize anti-SK antibodies will help limit these reactions, their persistence has encouraged the use of alternative agents.

Reperfusion of extremities that have already developed tissue necrosis may result in a reperfusion syndrome. Manifestations include acute tubular necrosis from circulating myoglobin, respiratory failure, arrhythmias, and myocardial infarction. Compartment syndrome may also develop. These conditions are often fatal; therefore any patient who demonstrates severe motor or sensory loss in an extremity or any sign of nonviability should be excluded from thrombolytic therapy.[1]

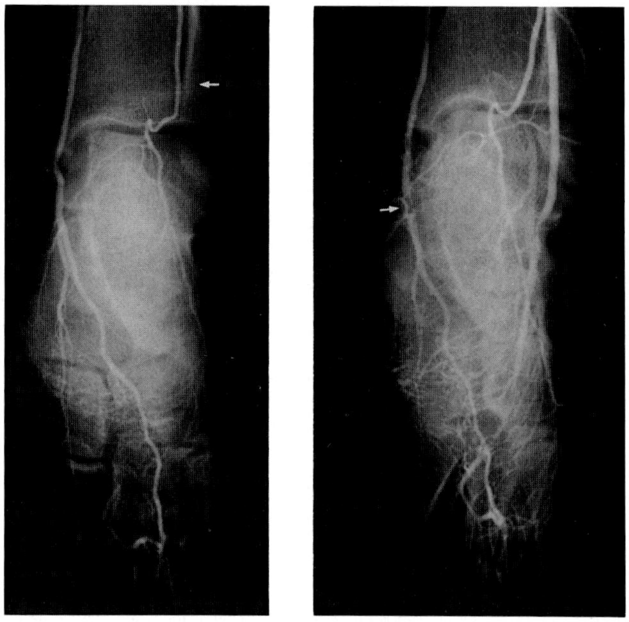

a b

Figure 14–1. Physical examination of this 20-year-old man with left great toe rest pain for several months revealed a discolored great toe with decreased sensation from midmetatarsal level to the distal toe. **A:** Arteriography reveals an occluded dorsalis pedis artery just above the ankle (arrow), with patent posterior tibial and lateral tarsal arteries. **B:** Following overnight infusion of 100,000 IU/hr of UK split between a coaxial 5 F catheter at the knee and an injectable guide wire at the ankle, the dorsalis pedis is patent with a midfoot stenosis. There is a nonocclusive embolus in the previously normal posterior tibial artery (arrow), which was incidental. Heparin had inadvertently not been given during the UK infusion. Although continued infusion and angioplasty of the dorsalis pedis resulted in little arteriographic improvement in either the posterior tibial embolus or the dorsalis pedis artery, the great toe ischemia resolved, and the patient has remained asymptomatic for 6 months.

RESULTS

The most common setting for the use of local, intra-arterial thrombolytic therapy is the treatment of either acute arterial ischemia or progressive ischemia of the lower extremities resulting from occlusion of either native arteries or bypass grafts. No prospective comparison studies of administration techniques, drug, or dose are available, and the following results reflect a compilation of data from varying protocols.

A few reports have described local thrombolysis for thromboembolic occlusions and vasospastic disorders in the upper extremities, but patient numbers are small.[25] Descriptions of local thrombolysis in the renal, visceral, and carotid arteries have been reported; however, the poor tolerance for prolonged ischemia of the end organs supplied by these arteries limit these applications.[8,11]

Native Arteries

Success rates for opening occluded native arteries in the lower extremities range from 60 to 80% (Table 14-3). Three categories of occlusion can be found: nonatherosclerotic thrombosis, embolic occlusions, and atherosclerotic thrombosis.

Nonatherosclerotic thrombosis is generally iatrogenic, related either to prior angioplasty or surgical intervention. These occlusions are recognized acutely, are ideal for infusion therapy since a catheter is often already in place, and in almost all cases can be treated successfully with short infusions of thrombolytic agents.[11,14,21]

Patients with embolic occlusions most often present shortly after the event due to profound ischemia resulting from the lack of well-developed collateral pathways. In this setting, if there is occlusion of one or several major arteries, surgical thromboembolectomy is preferred because it can most rapidly alleviate the ischemia. Surgical therapy is particularly appropriate for emboli above the inguinal ligament and when multiple emboli are present. In patients who present subacutely or with tibial artery emboli, surgical embolectomy is less successful and thrombolytic therapy is indicated. The response of acute emboli to locally administered fibrinolytic drugs has generally been favorable, with success rates with UK of 70 to 80%.[19,21] Since there is often no underlying vascular abnormality, long-term patency results are excellent. Hess et al[19] reported a 90% 2-year cumulative patency rate for treated embolic occlusions. Despite the good response of acute embolic occlusions to lytic therapy, the initial success in reopening chronic embolic occlusions (occlusions older than 6 weeks) decreases from 81 to 46%, and 2-week patency following therapy decreases from 72 to 42%.[19]

The existence of heart thrombus is evaluated with echocardiography prior to undertaking therapy. Whether the presence of heart thrombus is a firm contraindication to therapy is unclear, and a small series of 16 patients with recent myocardial infarction and left ventricular thrombi were actually treated with systemic UK, with no incidence of embolic complication. In 10 of the 16 patients the ventricular thrombus was lysed completely.[27]

Patients with atherosclerotic occlusions commonly present with subacute or chronic symptoms. These moderate symptoms permit a trial of lytic therapy prior to intervention without further compromising the limb. Increased experience with thrombolysis of long segment atherosclerotic occlusions prior to angioplasty is encouraging. Often, focal stenoses are uncovered that are easily treated with angioplasty (Fig. 14-2). Success rates range from 56 to 80% (Table 14-3). In contrast to iatrogenic or embolic occlusions, thrombolysis in atherosclerotic occlusions will unmask one or multiple stenoses that will require either percutaneous balloon angioplasty or surgical correction to maintain patency of the newly opened arterial segment. Six-month patency rates range from 70 to 90% and 2-year patency rates range from 60 to 80%.[18,19,26]

Although it is apparent that thrombus age is inversely related to the success of thrombolysis, many anecdotal cases of successfully treated occlusions that were 1 to several years old have been reported.[14,19] Success may be more related to the degree of thrombus organization than to its age. Thrombus organization can be tested by guide wire traversal prior to initiation of therapy. McNamara supports this simple test as the best predictor of successful infusion; however, some occlusions in which the guide wire will not easily pass still lyse.[12] The age of the occlusion may also affect long-term patency. Lammer et al's[18] data suggest that reocclusion occurs earlier in chronic occlusions.

McNamara and Bomberger[26] found two factors that affect long-term patency of native arterial occlusions following thrombolysis: arterial location and the persistence of a hemodynamically significant lesion following therapy. Suprainguinal (SI) lesions respond better than infrainguinal (II) lesions, with 6-month patencies of 92 versus 48%. A residual stenosis after thrombolysis and angioplasty is a grave prognostic finding, with 6-month patency data for superficial

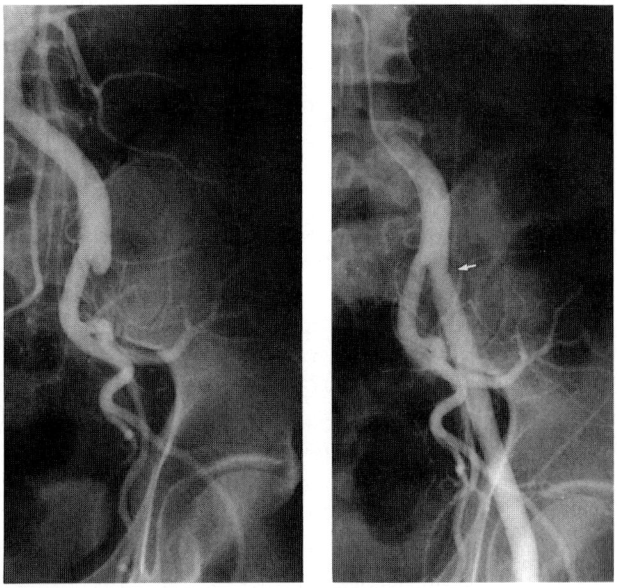

a **b**

Figure 14–2. This 40-year-old man was a long distance runner who had a recent onset of left lower extremity claudication. **A:** Arteriography revealed occlusion of the external iliac artery, with reconstitution at the common femoral level. **B:** Following overnight infusion of 100,000 IU/hour of urokinase, the external iliac was patent with a focal stenosis of the proximal vessel (arrow). This was subsequently treated with balloon angioplasty and remained patent for 1 year when reocclusion occurred. Subsequent surgery revealed cystic medial necrosis.

Table 14–3. Results of Thrombolytic Therapy in Native Arterial Occlusions

AUTHOR	# INFUSIONS	ETIOLOGY OF OCCLUSION			DRUG	HEPARIN	MEAN TIME OF INFUSION (HOURS)	SUCCESS				MAJOR COMPLICATIONS		
		Non-ASD	*EMB*	*ASD*				*Total**	*Non-ASD*	*EMB*	*ASD*	*Total*	*Hemorrhage*	*Thrombo/Embolic*
Katzen, 1984 (11)	53	7	6	40	SK	15%	26	79%	100%	50%	80%	9.1%	9.1%	0%
Graor, 1985 (14)	48	3		45	SK	No	51	58%	100%		56%	15%	13%	2%
McNamara, 1986 (26)	61			61	UK	Yes	18	79%			79%			
Lammer, 1986 (18)	136			136	SK Pulsed:90 SK-GLU-PLAS-Pulsed:14 UK-Pulsed:32	18%	1.5	78%			78%	20%	3.7%	<1%
Hess, 1987 (19)	564		92	472	SK-Pulsed UK-Pulsed	No	1.5	68%		71%	68%	7% Mort:1.6%	3%	3%
vanBreda, 1987 (9)	47				SK:24 UK:23	No	SK:14 UK:22	SK:63% UK:80%					SK:8% UK:4%	
Motarjeme, 1989 (21)	322	30	16	276	SK:14 UK:308	Yes			SK:62% UK:94%	SK:50% UK:71%	UK:80%	6% Mort:1%	4.4%	1.1%

*Success ≥ 90% Lysis

Non-ASD = Non Atherosclerotic Occlusions, EMB = Embolic Occlusions, ASD = Atherosclerotic Occlusion, UK = urokinase, SK = streptokinase, SK-GLU-PLAS = Streptokinase-GLU-plasminogen

Table 14–4. Results of Thrombolytic Therapy in Bypass Grafts

AUTHOR	# INFUSIONS	SI	II	DRUG	HEPARIN	MEAN TIME OF INFUSION (HOURS)	SUCCESS*	MAJOR COMPLICATIONS			PATENCY		
								Total	*Hemorrhage*	*Thrombo/Embolic*	*6 Month*	*1 Year*	*50% Patency (months)*
vanBreda, 1984 (3)	20	6	14	SK	No	28	60%	30%	10%	10%			
McNamara, 1986 (26)	39	11	S:28 T:28	UK	Yes	18	SI:91% II:68% T:74%				SI:70% II:25% T:41%		
Graor, 1988 (28)	22		V:10 S:12 T:22	rt-PA	No			4.5%	4.5%	0%	50%	18%	6.4
Durham, 1989 (29)	71	17	V:32 S:7 O:15 T:54	UK	34%	20	SI:88% II:59% T:75%	23% Mort:2.8%	7%	7%	48%	26%	SI:6.8 II:4.8 T:5.4
Gardiner, 1989 (30)	72	13	V:21 S:33 O:5 T:59	SK:29 UK:43	83%	SK:42 UK:22	SI:85% II:66% SK:48% UK:84% T:69%	SK:41% UK:19% T:25%	9.7%	2.8%	70%	60%	18
Belkin, 1990 (31)	35		V:35 T:35	SK:2 UK:15 rt-PA:5			60%				42%	37%	4
Meyerovitz, 1990 (10)	N:3 G:29 T:32	N:1 G:5	N:2 G:24 V:17 S:7	rt-PA:16 UK:16	Yes		rt-PA:50% UK:38% T:40%	22%	rt-PA:31% UK:13%	rt-PA:0% UK:0%			

*Success ≥ 90% Lysis

T = Total, N = Native, G = Graft, SI = suprainguinal, II = infrainguinal, S = synthetic, V = vein, O = other or unknown, UK = urokinase, SK = streptokinase, rt-PA = recombinant tissue plasminogen activator femoral lesions decreasing from 77 to 10% if a residual stenosis persists.

Arterial Grafts

Initial patency rates following infusion of thrombosed arterial bypass grafts range from 60 to 75% (Table 14-4). SI grafts respond better than II grafts with successful thrombolysis in 85 to 91% compared with 59 to 68%.[26,29,30] Successful treatment of an II graft depends on the ability to catheterize the II graft selectively. If selection of the graft is not possible, thrombolytic therapy frequently fails.[32] Initial response appears inversely related to the time of occlusion, as with native arterial occlusions.[29]

Combined 6-month patency rates for SI and II grafts are 42 to 70% and drop to 18 to 60% at 1 year.[28–31] The most important factor that influences patency is the correction of a hemodynamically significant lesion following thrombolysis. Gardiner et al[30] found an 86% 1-year patency for those grafts that had surgically or percutaneously correctable lesions following infusion, compared with a 37% 1-year patency for grafts with no correctable lesion. McNamara et al's[26] data suggest that long-term patency of SI grafts may be better than II grafts; however, this has not been shown to be a significant factor affecting long-term patency in other series.[29]

These long-term results are inferior to surgical results for reconstruction of both synthetic SI grafts and venous II grafts, although the results of thrombolysis of II grafts are similar to thrombectomy or reconstruction with synthetic material.[28,33–35] When reconstruction is not an option because of a patient's clinical condition or because of the lack of an autologous vein, thrombolytic therapy with aggressive angioplasty of any discovered stenosis is a good alternative to surgical therapy. Even when thrombolytic therapy is only partially successful or when the causative lesion cannot be corrected percutaneously, the arteriographic demonstration of the cause for occlusion and the condition of the peripheral runoff often limits and simplifies the required surgery. The unsatisfactory long-term results following either surgery or thrombolysis and angioplasty emphasize the importance of detecting failing grafts prior to thrombosis.[35]

REFERENCES

1. Lang EK. Streptokinase therapy: complications of intra-arterial use. Radiology 1985;154:75–7.
2. Hirshberg A, Schneiderman J, Garniek A, et al. Errors and pitfalls in intraarterial thrombolytic therapy. J Vasc Surg 1989;10:612–6.
3. vanBreda A, Robison JC, Feldman L, et al. Local thrombolysis in the treatment of arterial graft occlusions. J Vasc Surg 1984;1:103–12.
4. McNamara TO. The use of lytic therapy with endovascular "repair" for the failed infrainguinal graft. Semin Vasc Surg 1990;3:59–65.
5. Bell WR, Duckert FH, Fletcher AP, et al. Thrombolytic therapy in thrombosis: a National Institutes of Health consensus development conference. Ann Intern Med 1980;93:141.
6. Bell WR. Update on urokinase and streptokinase: a comparison of their efficacy and safety. Hosp Formulary 1988;23:230–41.
7. Saldinger E, Bookstein JJ. Mechanisms of fibrinolysis: native and exogenous systems. Semin Intervent Radiol 1985;2:321–30.
8. Belkin M, Belkin B, Bucknam CA, et al. Intra-arterial fibrinolytic therapy. Efficacy of streptokinase vs urokinase. Arch Surg 1986;121:769–73.
9. vanBreda A, Katzen BT, Deutsch AS. Urokinase versus streptokinase in local thrombolysis. Radiology 1987;165:109–11.
10. Meyerovitz MF, Goldhaber SZ, Reagan K, et al. Recombinant tissue-type plasminogen activator versus urokinase in peripheral arterial and graft occlusions: a randomized trial. Radiology 1990;175:75–8.
11. Katzen BT, Edwards KC, Albert AS, vanBreda A. Low-dose direct fibrinolysis in peripheral vascular disease. J Vasc Surg 1984;1:718–22.
12. McNamara TO, Fischer JR. Thrombolysis of peripheral arterial and graft occlusions: improved results using high-dose urokinase. AJR 1985;144:769–75.
13. Bookstein JJ, Saldinger E. Accelerated thrombolysis: in vitro evaluation of agents and methods of administration. Invest Radiol 1985;20:731–5.
14. Graor RA, Risius B, Denny KM, et al. Local thrombolysis in the treatment of thrombosed arteries, bypass grafts and arteriovenous fistulas. J Vasc Surg 1985;2:406–14.
15. Sullivan KL, Gardiner GA, Shapiro MJ, et al. Acceleration of thrombolysis with a high-dose transthrombus bolus technique. Radiology 1989;173:805–8.
16. Kandarpa K, Drinker PA, Singer SJ, Caramore D. Forceful pulsatile local infusion of enzyme accelerates thrombolysis: in vivo evaluation of a new delivery system. Radiology 1988;168:739–44.
17. Bookstein JJ, Fellmeth B, Roberts A, et al. Pulsed-spray pharmacomechanical thrombolysis: preliminary clinical results. AJR 1989;152:1097–100.
18. Lammer J, Pilger E, Neumayer K, Schreyer H. Intraarterial fibrinolysis: long-term results. Radiology 1986;161:159–63.
19. Hess H, Mietaschk A, Bruckl R. Peripheral arterial occlusions: a 6-year experience with local low-dose thrombolytic therapy. Radiology 1987;163:753–8.
20. Palaskas C, Totty WG, Gilula LA, Reinus WR. Complications of local intra-arterial fibrinolytic therapy. Semin Intervent Radiol 1985;2:396–404.
21. Motarjeme A. Thrombolytic therapy in arterial occlusion and graft thrombosis. Semin Vasc Surg 1989;2:155–78.
22. Rabe FE, Becker GJ, Richmond BD, et al. Contrast extravasation through Dacron grafts: a sequela of low-dose streptokinase therapy. AJR 1982;138:917–20.
23. Rosner NH, Doris PE. Contrast extravasation through a Gortex graft: a sequela of low-dose streptokinase therapy. AJR 1984;143:633–4.
24. Graor RA, Risius B, Young JR, et al. Low-dose streptokinase for selective thrombolysis: systemic effects and complications. Radiology 1984;152:35–9.
25. Tisnado J, Shao-Ru Cho, Beachley MC, Vines F. Low-dose fibrinolytic therapy in hand ischemia. Semin Intervent Radiol 1985;2:367–79.
26. McNamara TO, Bomberger RA. Factors affecting initial and 6 month patency rates after intraarterial thrombolysis with high dose urokinase. Am J Surg 1986;152:709–12.
27. Kremer P, Fiebic R, Tilsner V, et al. Lysis of left ventricular thrombi with urokinase. Circulation 1985;72:112–8.
28. Graor RA, Risius B, Young JR, et al. Thrombolysis of peripheral arterial bypass grafts: surgical thrombectomy com-

pared with thrombolysis. A preliminary report. J Vasc Surg 1988;7:347–55.
29. Durham JD, Geller SC, Abbott WM, et al. Regional infusion of urokinase into occluded lower-extremity bypass grafts: long-term clinical results. Radiology 1989;172:83–7.
30. Gardiner GA, Harrington DP, Koltun W, et al. Salvage of occluded arterial bypass grafts by means of thrombolysis. J Vasc Surg 1989;9:426–31.
31. Belkin M, Donaldson MC, Whittemore AD, et al. Observations on the use of thrombolytic agents for thrombotic occlusion of infrainguinal vein grafts. J Vasc Surg 1990;11:289–96.
32. Risius B, Graor RA, Geisinger MA, et al. Recombinant human tissue-type plasminogen activator for thrombolysis in peripheral arteries and bypass grafts. Radiology 1986;160:183–8.
33. Nevelsteen A, Suy R, Daenen W, et al. Aortofemoral grafting: factors influencing late results. Surgery 1980;88:642–53.
34. Brewster DC, LaSalle AJ, Robinson JG, et al. Clinical consequences and success of secondary reconstruction. Arch Surg 1983;118:1043–7.
35. Whittemore AD, Clowes AW, Couch NP, Mannick JA. Secondary femoropopliteal reconstruction. Ann Surg 1981;193:35–42.

15 Pulsed-Spray Pharmacomechanical Thrombolysis

Karim Valji, M.D., Joseph J. Bookstein, M.D.

Most widely practiced thrombolytic methods for treating peripheral vascular occlusions involve infusion of urokinase (UK) at the site of thrombosis, often with progressive catheter advancement through a channel created with a guide wire.[1–3] This technique has increased the consistency of fibrinolysis and reduced complications compared with early experience with intravenous streptokinase (SK).[1] However, conventional thrombolytic therapy remains incompletely effective, costly, and time-consuming.

For several years, we have conducted both laboratory and clinical experiments designed to increase the consistency and speed of thrombolysis. Laboratory experience has suggested that the rate of diffusion of exogenous activators into a clot is an important limiting factor in clinical thrombolysis.[4,5] We developed new methodology, combining physical disruption of the clot matrix with mechanical dispersal of fibrinolytic agent throughout the clot, to increase the surface area for plasminogen activation. Direct intrathrombic deposition of the entire dose of UK has proven to increase dramatically the speed and consistency of lysis. The reduced dose required to effect lysis and the sequestration of UK from systemic plasminogen apparently decrease the risk of hemorrhage. Acceleration of thrombolysis has reduced procedure time, decreased hospital costs, and improved patient and physician acceptance of the procedure.

EXPERIMENTAL MODELS

The process of diffusion of plasminogen, plasminogen activators, and plasmin inhibitors into thrombus is poorly understood. In vitro studies have demonstrated that incorporation of plasminogen[4] and UK[5] into deep layers of preformed clot occurs slowly. We studied the acceleration of thrombolysis from direct admixture of clot and fibrinolytic agents in an in vitro system.[6] A significant increase in the amount and speed of clot lysis was observed after exposing macerated ^{125}I-labeled thrombus to UK or SK compared with simple soaking of clots. By also increasing the concentration of UK from 2200 to 96,000 U/ml, we obtained 90% clot lysis in 45 minutes. No significant difference in lysis rates was noted among the plasminogen activators tested (SK, UK, and tissue-type plasminogen activator [t-PA]).

Based on these experiments, we postulated that clinical thrombolysis could be accelerated via dispersal of small volumes of highly concentrated agent throughout the clot. We tested a prototype apparatus in a canine model of subacute venous thrombosis.[7] Intrathrombic injection was achieved by placing a tip-occluded 19 gauge stainless steel catheter with multiple side holes directly into a 2-day-old clot. Brisk taps to the plunger of the attached syringe caused a fine, high-pressure spray to permeate the thrombus. Clots treated by intrathrombic injection of UK or t-PA with intermittent infusion lysed significantly more rapidly and completely than clots treated by constant infusion at equivalent doses. Kandarpa and colleagues[8] noted similar results using SK in a pulsatile infusion system in rabbit inferior vena cava thrombosis. Based on our experimental observations, we developed and refined a clinical pulsed-spray technique that has become our standard transcatheter approach to peripheral vascular occlusions, including clotted hemodialysis grafts, native arteries, and arterial bypass grafts.[9,10,11]

TECHNIQUE OF PULSED-SPRAY THROMBOLYSIS

Catheter Construction and Placement

The pulsed-spray method requires access to the entire length of thrombus. For native arteries and bypass grafts, a single catheter is generally sufficient, usually placed through an ipsilateral femoral approach. For hemodialysis grafts, two catheters are placed in a criss-cross fashion via punctures near the center of the graft.[9,10]

The occlusion is crossed with a guide wire. A glide wire (Terumo, Medi-tech, Watertown, MA) may facilitate passage through fresh thrombus in dialysis grafts. Chronic arterial occlusions may require a stiffer wire; judicious use of a beaded tip-occluding wire (Cook, Bloomington, IN) is occasionally helpful. If a wire will not pass through the entire occlusion, subsequent fibrinolysis is unlikely to be clinically successful, even though the thrombus proximal to an atherosclerotic plaque may be lysed.[3,10] Injection of contrast material through a diagnostic catheter placed beyond the occlusion defines the distal extent of thrombus and permits proper evaluation of runoff vessels.

Therapeutic catheters for pulsed-spray therapy are commercially available or can be custom-made for each case. Side holes are punched into a tapered 5 F catheter at 8 mm intervals in a spiral pattern, using a 27 gauge needle. The number of holes is determined by the length of clot the catheter will span. Perforated catheter segments longer than 25 cm create an uneven spray; therefore long thrombi should be lysed in stages. The diagnostic catheter is exchanged for the therapeutic one; a tip-occluding wire is inserted until it fits snugly at the catheter tip, and a hemostatic Y adapter is fitted onto the catheter and flushed with heparinized saline. Care is taken to keep the entire perforated catheter segment within the lumen during injection to prevent extravasation of UK.

Heparin Administration

The importance of adequate anticoagulation during thrombolysis cannot be overemphasized. We have observed in canine models[7] and in patients[10] that lack of adequate heparinization during pulsed-spray thrombolysis prevents or retards complete clot lysis. In addition, some investigators have shown that heparin promotes plasminogen activation by UK in vitro.[12,13]

Therefore once the thrombus has been crossed, the patient is given 5000 to 7000 U of heparin intravenously and continued at 1000 to 2000 U per hour during the procedure. Recently, we have begun injecting most of the initial heparin dose directly into the clot along with UK. We have not found it necessary or useful to monitor coagulation parameters when fibrinolysis is completed within 1 to 3 hours.

Urokinase Delivery

A 250,000 U vial of UK (Abbokinase) is diluted in 10 ml sterile water to a concentration of 25,000 U/ml. About 150,000 U are spray-injected over 20 minutes in 0.2 ml increments with a tuberculin syringe. With some practice, a rapid, limited thrust of the syringe plunger can be performed, which will cause a high-pressure spray to permeate the clot. We are currently testing a mechanical pulse injector to replace manual injection. The catheter is turned 90° periodically to improve UK distribution. Additional UK is injected at a reduced rate or reduced concentration (5000 to 10,000 U/ml).

Our method, using small volumes of highly concentrated UK, allows rapid intrathrombic injection without high risk of downstream embolization. However, we advise against trying more rapid intrathrombic injection than just outlined. In thrombosed canine arteries, UK pulses given every 10 seconds frequently led to downstream emboli that failed to lyse spontaneously (unpublished data).

Our delivery protocol has proven very safe with hemodialysis grafts, and any small emboli that may be produced seem to be well tolerated. We are, however, more concerned about the possibility of downstream embolization in arterial or bypass graft occlusions. For that reason, the distal 1 to 2 cm of these occlusions are often not pulse-sprayed during the first 30 minutes of thrombolysis, in order to retain UK proximally and prevent immediate embolization of large thrombi. This distal plug is then pulse-sprayed after some proximal lysis is noted. To reduce further the chances of embolization, we delay transluminal angioplasty (TLA) of underlying arterial or bypass graft stenoses until near-complete clot dissolution is documented.

Angiograms are obtained frequently through the therapeutic catheter or an indwelling arterial sheath to monitor progress. Pulses of UK are given until satisfactory lysis has been achieved, or up to 1,000,000 U have been given in about 4 hours. The average total dose required in our first reported series was 368,000 ± 132,000 U.[10] Following successful thrombolysis, an underlying stenosis responsible for thrombosis is sought, usually found, and treated with TLA to prevent recurrent occlusion. Occasionally, no abnormality is found and graft thrombosis may be attributed to prolonged hypotension, sepsis, trauma, or mechanical pressure (such as overzealous compression of dialysis graft puncture sites). Heparin is generally not continued after recanalization unless significant clot remains or results of transluminal angioplasty are suboptimal. Patients are given aspirin (325 mg/day) on the day of and for 4 to 6 months after the procedure.

Delayed thrombolysis, or thrombosis progressing during the procedure, should suggest one of the following problems:

1. Presence of old, organized thrombus or large volume of atherosclerotic material
2. Ineffective anticoagulation
3. Lack of adequate inflow or outflow
4. Inadequate delivery of UK to part of the clot
5. Graft infection

Known or suspected graft infection is a relative contraindication to thrombolysis. We have found infected clot to be less responsive to exogenous fibrinolytic agents, and partial thrombolysis may precipitate sepsis.

SPECIFIC APPLICATIONS AND RESULTS

Hemodialysis Vascular Access

Transcatheter techniques for salvaging thrombosed hemodialysis grafts have recently been advocated. Although some investigators have had promising results with both SK and UK in recanalizing grafts,[14–16] others have been less encouraged.[17] Local infusion therapy has been plagued with bleed ing from recent needle puncture sites, arterial and venous embolization, and prolonged infusion times.

Since 1985, almost all clotted hemodialysis grafts at our institution have been treated with pharmacomechanical methods, followed by immediate TLA when indicated. Our initial approach, in which lacing of the clot with UK was combined with mechanical disruption using a hockey-stick-shaped catheter, was applied to 41 grafts, with successful recanalization in 90% in a mean time of 86 minutes. With repeat treatments after recurrent obstruction, about two thirds of these grafts remained functional for 6 to 18 months.

The pulse-spray technique described herein has been applied to 99 dialysis grafts. Our mean lysis time was 42 ± 97 minutes. Thrombolysis was initially successful in all cases, and 94% were patent at 24 hours. In the few instances of early rethrombosis, underlying abnormalities were uncovered, thus directing surgical revision (i.e., pseudoaneurysm repair, arterial steal, and subclavian vein stenosis necessitating graft replacement). No major complications, hemorrhagic or otherwise, occurred.

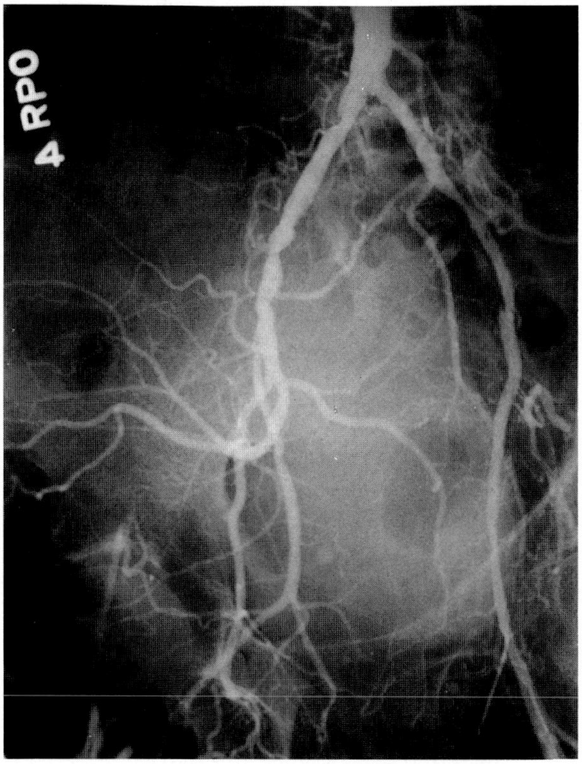

A

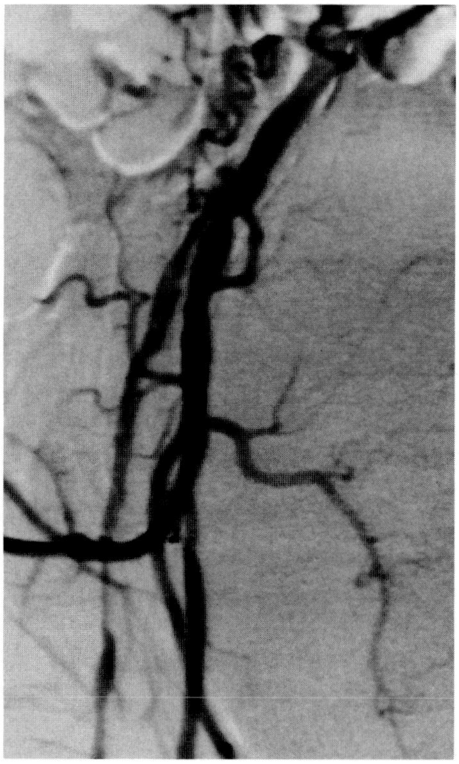

B

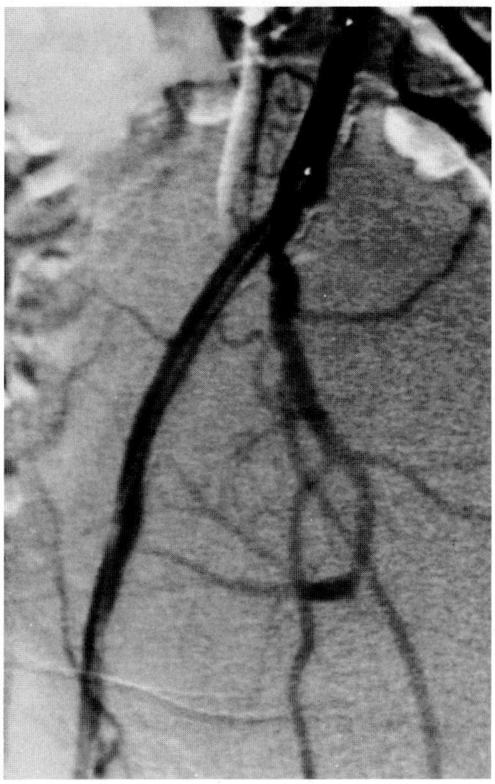

C

Figure 15–1. Pulsed-spray thrombolysis of iliac artery occlusion in a 59-year-old man with 1 year of bilateral thigh claudication. **A:** Initial pelvic arteriogram in right posterior oblique projection demonstrates complete occlusion of the right external iliac artery from its origin with partial reconstitution of the common femoral artery. **B:** After 20 minutes of pulsed-spray injection of 150,000 U of urokinase (UK), partial clot lysis is noted. **C:** Complete recanalization of the right iliac artery is observed after 1 hour of thrombolysis with 250,000 units of UK, followed by transluminal angioplasty. The patient noted a marked improvement in right-sided symptoms, which remain improved at 1-year follow-up.

Peripheral Arteries

Conventional techniques using UK infusion and angioplasty restore patency to occluded arteries in 60 to 80% of cases, but have generally required 18 to 26 hours for complete thrombolysis.[3,18–20] We treated 25 arterial occlusions with pulsed-spray injection (Fig. 15-1). Twenty-two lysed fully in 75 ± 29 minutes. Pulsed-spray injection recanalized vessels with thrombi older than 4 days as frequently as those with relatively fresh clot, although lysis times were slightly longer.[10]

Our experience indicates that inability to cross the entire occlusion with a guide wire or lack of significant clot dissolution after an hour of therapy predicts an unsuccessful clinical result. Our immediate failures involved arteries with extremely poor and untreatable runoff or severe underlying atherosclerotic disease unresponsive to angioplasty.

Arterial Bypass Grafts

These vessels may be well-suited for thrombolytic therapy.[21,22] The patients are often poor operative candidates and the results of surgical revision are mixed.[23,24] In our series of 37 synthetic and saphenous vein bypass grafts treated with pulsed-spray thrombolysis, all but one were successfully recanalized in 104 ± 73 minutes. Lysis was usually performed in stages because of the length of the thrombus.

COMPLICATIONS

Our complication rate was comparable to or better than most reported series using more conventional urokinase therapy.[3,16,21,22] Of 166 cases that we treated with pulsed-spray thrombolysis, only one patient, who developed bilateral groin hematomas, required treatment for bleeding. A second patient had self-limited gastrointestinal hemorrhage from excessive anticoagulation. Four episodes of minor bleeding at puncture sites were observed.

Accelerated thrombolysis and more vigorous catheter manipulation within the thrombus may produce clinically significant distal emboli.[9,11,19] These emboli are aggressively pursued by infusing UK locally with the therapeutic catheter or a smaller catheter placed coaxially. Seven patients in our series of 29 arterial and bypass graft occlusions developed downstream embolization during the procedure. In three cases, emboli were successfully lysed with local UK infusions; four patients required surgical correction.

GUIDING PRINCIPLES

The technical details of pulsed-spray thrombolysis will vary from case to case. Nonetheless, a successful result requires a thorough understanding of the general principles underlying the technique. A number of basic concepts guide every case:

1. UK is preferred over SK because of its greater safety and more predictable dose-response pattern. In addition, UK is not antigenic and therefore allows repeat thrombolysis whenever necessary.
2. Intrathrombic spray-injection of UK increases the speed and consistency of fibrinolysis over conventional parathrombic infusion.
3. Inability to initially cross the entire occlusion with a guide wire or sluggish clot dissolution within the first hour of therapy predicts a poor clinical outcome.
4. The risk of embolization increases as the UK delivery rate is accelerated; the delivery protocol described herein has proven safe for native artery and graft occlusions.
5. A plug of distal thrombus is initially left untreated to prevent embolization; however, the entire occlusion must eventually be spray-injected to achieve a successful result.
6. Continuous heparin administration and pre-treatment with aspirin is critical to prevent rethrombosis, and possibly to enhance the activity of UK.
7. Successful treatment of underlying stenoses is necessary to maintain vessel patency.

REFERENCES

1. Collen D, Stump DC, Gold HK. Thrombolytic therapy. Ann Rev Med 1988;39:405–23.
2. van Breda A, Katzen BT, Deutsch AS. Urokinase versus streptokinase in local thrombolysis. Radiology 1987;165:109–11.
3. McNamara TO, Fischer JR. Thrombolysis of peripheral arterial and graft occlusions: improved results using high-dose urokinase. AJR 1985;144:769–75.
4. Iga Y, Greenwald SR, Bleakley-Chandler A. Uptake of I-125-lys-plasminogen by in vitro thrombi. Hemostasis 1983;13:25–35.
5. Hisano S. Immunofluorescence study on thrombolysis with special reference to the patterns of distribution and the contents of fibrin, plasminogen, alpha-2-macroglobulin and urokinase in artificial thrombi. Thromb Haemost 1978;39:53–60.
6. Bookstein JJ, Saldinger E. Accelerated thrombolysis: in vitro evaluation of agents and methods of administration. Invest Radiol 1985;20:731–5.
7. Valji K, Bookstein JJ. Fibrinolysis with intrathrombic injection of urokinase and tissue-type plasminogen activator: results in a new model of subacute venous thrombosis. Invest Radiol 1987;22:23–7.
8. Kandarpa K, Drinker PA, Singer SJ, et al. Forceful pulsatile local infusion of enzyme accelerates thrombolysis: in vivo evaluation of a new delivery system. Radiology 1988; 168:739–44.
9. Bookstein JJ, Fellmeth B, Roberts A, Valji K, et al. Pulsed-spray pharmacomechanical thrombolysis: preliminary clinical results. AJR 1989;152:1097–110.
10. Valsi K, Bookstein JJ, Roberts AC, Davis GB. Pharmacomechanical thrombolysis and angioplasty in the management of clotted hemodialysis grafts: early and late clinical results. Radiology 1991;178:243–7.
11. Valsi K, Roberts AC, Davis GB, Bookstein JJ. Pulsed-spray thrombolysis of arterial and bypass graft occlusions. AJR 1991;156:617–21.
12. Fears R. Kinetic studies on the effect of heparin and fibrin on plasminogen activators. Biochem J 1988;249:77–81.
13. Andrade-Gordon P, Strickland S. Interaction of heparin with

plasminogen activators and plasminogen. Effects on the activation of plasminogen. Biochemistry 1986;25:4033–40.
14. Rodkin RS, Bookstein JJ, Heeney DJ, et al. Streptokinase and transluminal angioplasty in the treatment of acutely thrombosed hemodialysis access fistulas. Radiology 1983;149: 425–8.
15. Zeit RM, Cope C: Failed hemodialysis shunts: one year of experience with aggressive treatment. Radiology 1985;154: 353–6.
16. Schilling JJ, Eiser AR, Slifkin RF, et al. The role of thrombolysis in hemodialysis access occlusion. Am J Kidney Dis 1987;10:92–7.
17. Young AT, Hunter DW, Castañeda-Zúñiga WR, et al. Thrombosed synthetic hemodialysis access fistulas: failure of fibrinolytic therapy. Radiology 1985;154:639–42.
18. Pilger E, Lammer J, Bertuch H, et al. Intraarterial fibrinolysis: in vitro and prospective clinical evaluation of three thrombolytic agents. Radiology 1986;161:597–9.
19. Katzen BT. Technique and results of "low-dose" infusion. Cardiovasc Intervent Radiol 1988;11:S41–7.
20. Motarjeme A: Thrombolytic therapy in arterial occlusion and graft thrombosis. Semin Vasc Surg 1989;2:155–78.
21. Gardiner GA, Harrington DP, Koltun W, et al. Salvage of occluded arterial bypass grafts by means of thrombolysis. J Vasc Surg 1989;9:426–31.
22. Durham JD, Geller SC, Abbott WM, et al. Regional infusion of urokinase into occluded lower-extremity bypass grafts. Radiology 1989;172:83–7.
23. Whittemore AD. Failure of peripheral arterial reconstruction. Acta Chir Scand Suppl 1988;550:74–80.
24. Bandyk DF, Kaebnick HW, Steward GW, et al. Durability of the in situ saphenous vein arterial bypass graft: a comparison of primary and secondary patency. J Vasc Surg 1987;5:256–67.

16 Thrombolysis

M. Maynar-Moliner, M.D., R. Reyes, M.D., J. M. Pulido-Duque, M.D., J. M. Felices, M.D., E. Gorriz, M.D., W. R. Castañeda-Zúñiga, M.D.

The use of thrombolytic agents in the treatment of peripheral arterial occlusive disease has been widely discussed.[1–3] There are still controversies regarding the fibrinolytic agent of choice, the protocols for drug administration, and the efficacy and durability of this therapy. The cost-effectiveness of this treatment has also been questioned, since subsequent surgery is often required.[2]

Most of the authors agree that urokinase is nowadays the thrombolytic agent of choice. Recent reports advocate the use of new thrombolytic agents such as recombinant tissue-type plasminogen activator (rt-PA), since they cause less systemic effects, and make thrombolysis safer.[4] Although fibrinolytic therapy has been used mainly in acute thrombosis, some authors have used thrombolytic agents in chronic obstructions with high success rates.[5–7]

We report our experience using urokinase in either chronic or acute peripheral arterial occlusions in native arteries and bypass grafts.

MATERIALS AND METHODS

Fifty patients with 50 occlusions of peripheral arteries or grafts were treated with local urokinase infusion from June 1988 to September 1989. The series included 47 men and 3 women, ranging in age from 30 to 88 years (mean, 57 years). Diabetes was present in 39% of the patients, 82% were currently smokers, and 8% were hypertensive. Forty-nine patients presented with ischemia of the lower limbs, 24 acute and 25 chronic, and one patient presented with acute ischemia of the right upper extremity. Forty-three patients had native vessel arterial occlusion and seven were occluded grafts. The segmental distribution of the occluded native arteries was as follows: 14 in the iliac artery (Fig. 16-1), ten in the superficial femoral artery, 17 involving the distal superficial femoral-popliteal artery area, one in the anterior tibial artery, and one in the axillary artery. There were also seven occluded grafts (Figs. 16-2, 16-3).

The axillary approach was used to treat all the occlusions of the common iliac artery and also in some patients with occlusion of femoropopliteal bypass grafts.

Patients presenting with clinical evidence of severe claudication or acute ischemia were considered candidates for fibrinolytic therapy. The patients were examined by a vascular surgeon and an interventional radiologist. On admission, all patients had a full physical examination with measurement of the ankle-arm indexes.

Baseline hematologic evaluation included platelet count, hemoglobin and hematocrit levels, thrombin time, plasma fibrinogen, and fibrinogen degradation products (FDP).

If embolic occlusion was suggested by the patient's history, echocardiography was performed to exclude the presence of intracardiac thrombus.

Internal bleeding and active intracranial processes were considered the only absolute contraindications. After diagnostic angiography, a 5 or 7 F angiographic catheter was introduced to the level of the occlusion (Fig. 16-4). A 0.035 inch open-ended guide wire was passed coaxially through the angiographic catheter and advanced through the occlusion. Connecting the segment above the occlusion with the distal blood flow was considered an important factor in the success of fibrinolytic therapy. As the open-ended guide wire was withdrawn through the thrombus, 250,000 IU of urokinase was infused over 30 minutes. After this initial bolus, a continuous infusion of urokinase was started at a rate of 100,000 U/hour. The patients were returned to the ward where the thrombolytic agent was infused using a pump.

Hematologic tests were performed before the treatment started and 4 hours after. Additional control was obtained every 12 hours with urokinase infusions longer than 24 hours. Angiographic follow-up was obtained every 12 hours. If complete lysis of the clot was not achieved after 24 hours, the infusion was continued for 24 hours more, up to a maximum of 48 hours (Fig. 16-5). Angioplasty or atherectomy was performed if an underlying stenosis was discovered. Clinical follow-up with measurement of ankle-arm index was made every 3 months.

RESULTS

The initial success rate was 88% (44 patients). The fibrinolytic treatment was unsuccessful in six patients, five chronic and one acute occlusion. Two treatments were considered unsuccessful because of reocclusion within the first week after the infusion of urokinase. These two patients were diabetic with poor distal runoff vessels. Another patient had a reocclusion after 2 months and a new attempt was unsuccessful. The infusion of urokinase was discontinued in one patient due to a neurologic complication of an axillary approach. The sixth patient considered unsuccessful developed an intracranial hemorrhage and died.

Adjunctive therapy included angioplasty in 33 patients (Fig. 16-6), atherectomy in three, and in five patients,

A 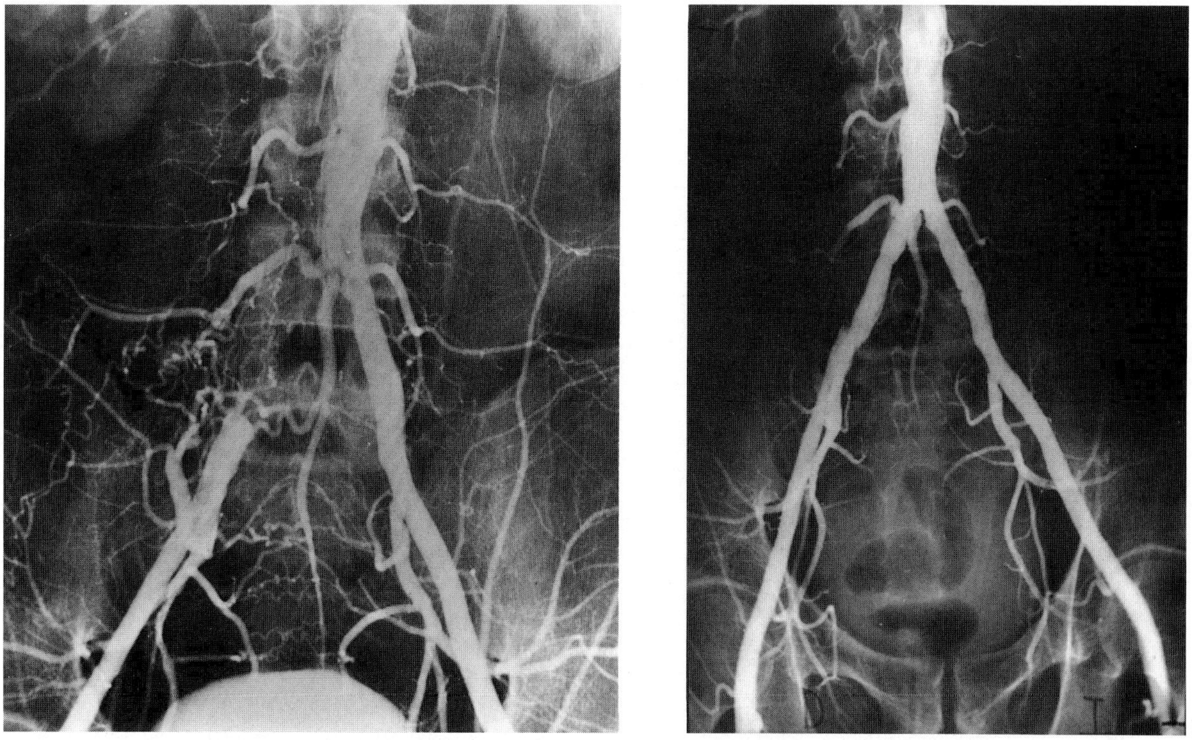 B

Figure 16–1. **A:** Arteriogram shows chronic occlusion of the right iliac artery. **B:** Follow-up angiography after urokinase infusion and angioplasty shows a widely patent lumen.

A 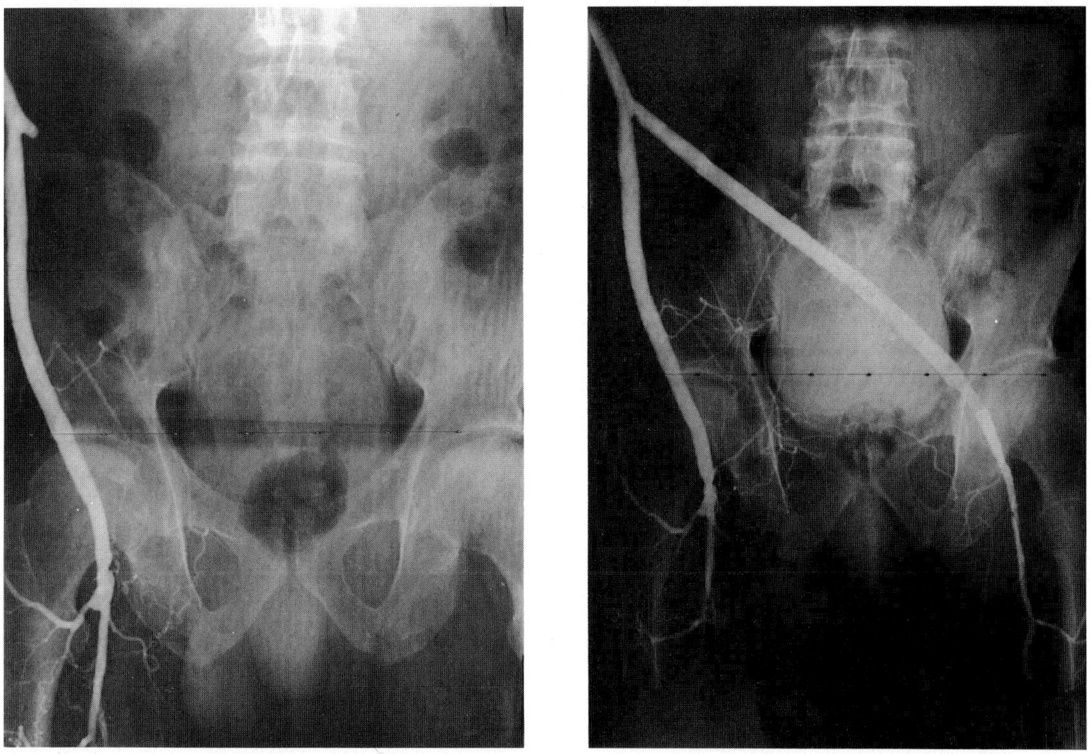 B

Figure 16–2. **A:** Angiography shows occlusion of the left branch of axillobifemoral graft. **B:** Follow-up angiography shows patency of the occluded segment.

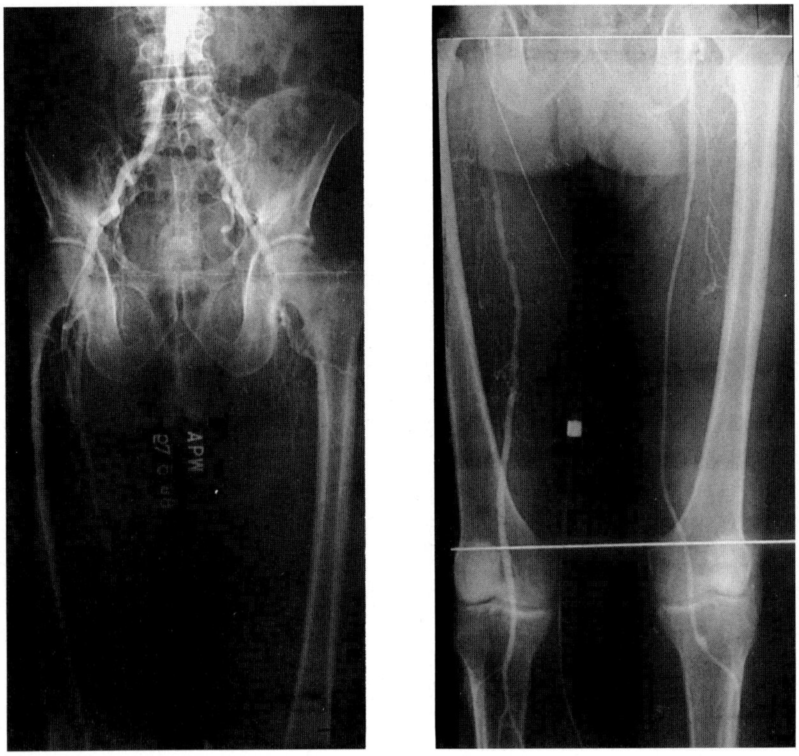

A B

Figure 16–3. **A:** Angiography shows occlusion of left femoropopliteal bypass graft. **B:** Follow-up angiography after urokinase infusion and angioplasty at the anastomotic site shows patency of the graft.

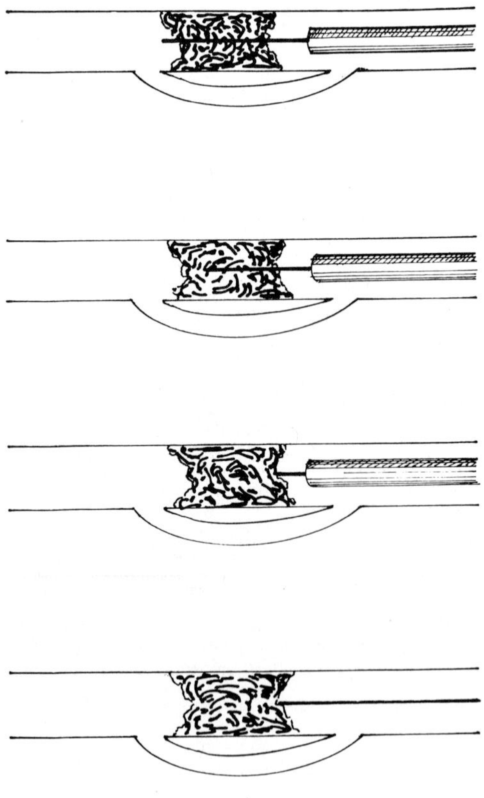

Figure 16–4. Technique for delivery of urokinase bolus. The open-ended guide wire is advanced through the entire length of the occlusion. As the open-ended guide wire is withdrawn the urokinase bolus is delivered.

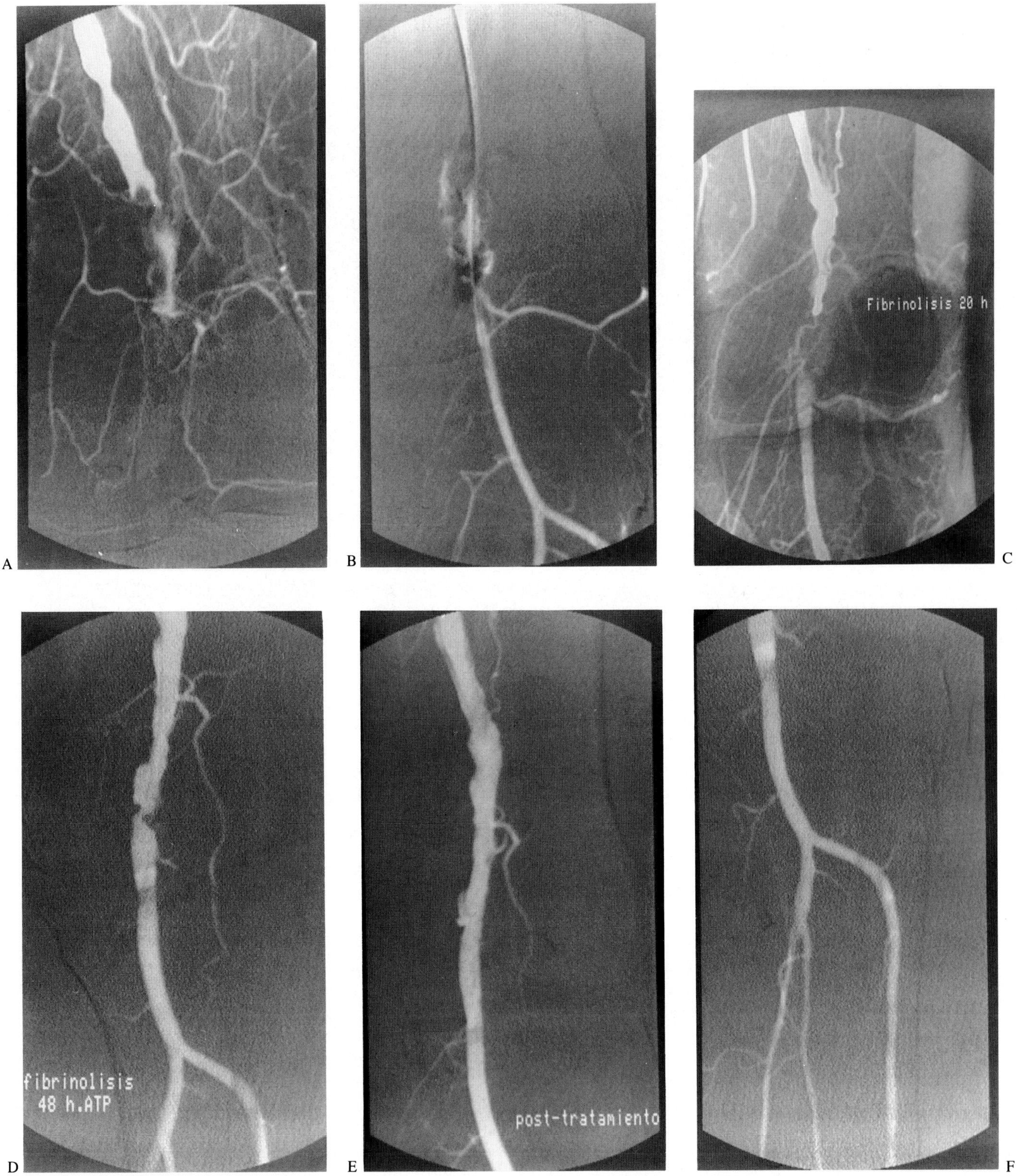

Figure 16–5. **A:** Femoral angiography shows 100% occlusion at the femoropopliteal segment. **B:** Angiography shows patent distal vessels. **C:** Follow-up angiography after 20 hours' infusion of urokinase shows a short occlusion of the popliteal artery. **D:** Follow-up angiography after 48 hours of urokinase infusion shows patent lumen at the previously occluded segment. **E:** Angiography after atherectomy shows patent lumen. **F:** Angiography shows patent runoff vessels.

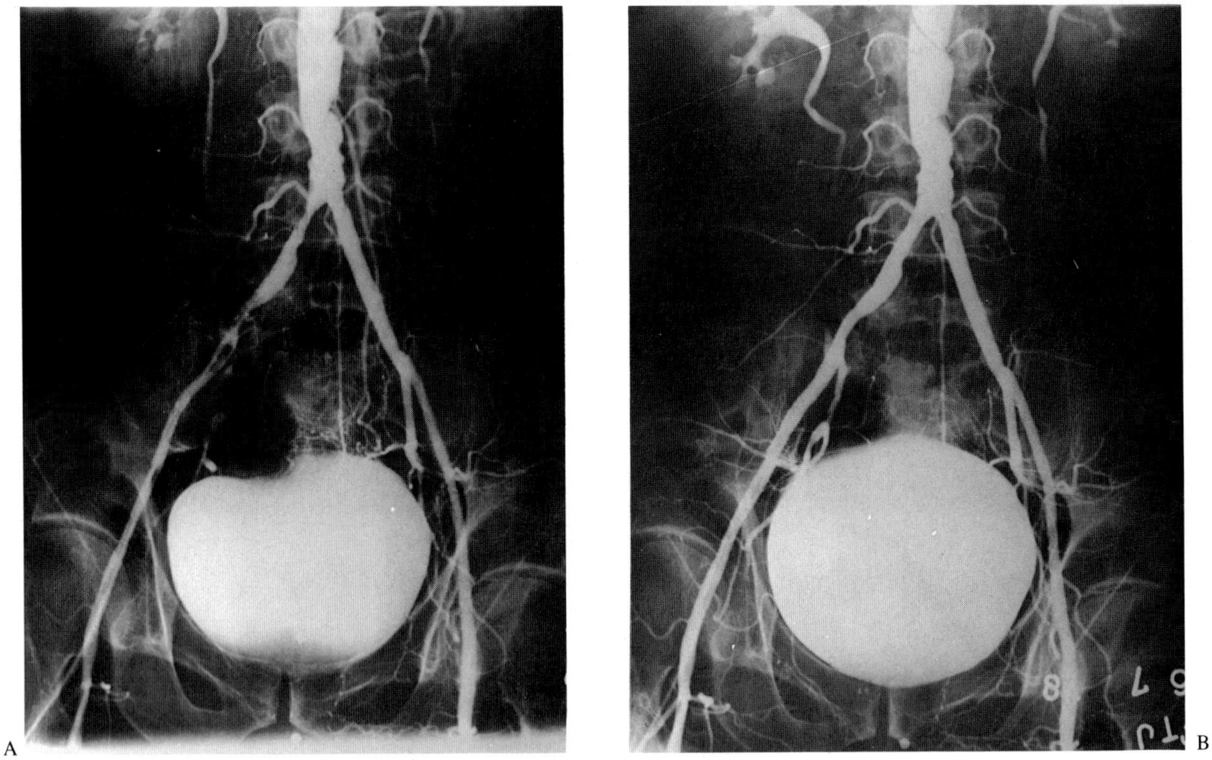

Figure 16–6. A: Angiogram shows acute occlusion of both right internal and external iliac arteries. **B:** Follow-up angiogram after urokinase and angioplasty shows a patent lumen.

angioplasty plus atherectomy; surgery in one patient; and medical treatment (anticoagulation) in two patients.

Clinical follow-up ranged from 3 to 26 months, with a mean of 16 months. Thirty-three of the native arteries or bypass grafts remained patent (66%), seven patients had reocclusion (14%), and four were lost to follow-up.

Major hemorrhage requiring blood transfusion occurred in one patient. This patient developed a large retroperitoneal hematoma (Fig. 16-7). One patient died due to an intracranial hemorrhage (Fig. 16-8). One patient had a transient cerebral ischemic event during an axillary approach. Three hematomas occurred at the puncture site. Pericatheter thrombosis occurred in two cases and resolved successfully by prolonging the infusion time. Distal embolism occurred in one case and it was solved by advancing the guide wire into the embolized segment and prolonging the infusion time (Fig. 16-9).

DISCUSSION

Local infusion of thrombolytic agents for the treatment of peripheral arterial occlusion has become the treatment of choice following the first report of patients treated with intra-arterial fibrinolysis by Dotter et al.[8] Although some authors have limited the use of thrombolytic therapy to acute occlusions,[1,9–11] this therapy has also been used successfully in chronic occlusions.[5–7]

The initial success rate in chronic occlusions is lower.[5–7] However, fibrinolysis of chronic occlusions is justified in patients who are poor surgical candidates or whose only surgical alternative is amputation.

Urokinase remains the thrombolytic agent of choice. This is based on its higher success rate and lower complications compared with streptokinase. New thrombolytic agents such as acylated plasminogen activated complex (APSAC) and rt-PA have the advantage of inducing fibrinolysis while protecting the plasma fibrinogen from degradation. These agents have a high affinity for fibrin-bound plasminogen and little activity against circulating plasminogen.[4] However, an increase in the incidence of intracranial hemorrhage with t-PA compared to urokinase has been reported.[12]

The technique used to deliver the fibrinolytic agent is very important. Connecting the segment above the occlusion with the distal vessels is essential to the success of the therapy, especially in chronic occlusions. Chronic occlusions have on their proximal end a thin layer of thrombus that is more organized than that of the remaining thrombus. This barrier needs to be broken so that the thrombolytic agent can have access to the remainder of the thrombus. Once a channel has been created through the thrombus with antegrade blood flow, the thrombolytic agent will be in close contact with the thrombus, facilitating its lysis. In those patients in whom connection with the distal vessels is not achieved, the treatment is frequently unsuccessful.

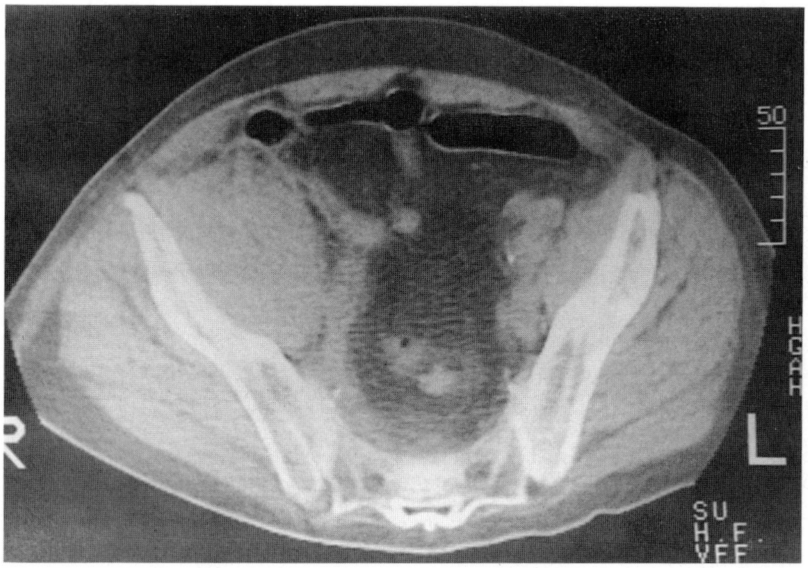

Figure 16–7. Abdominal computed tomography shows a large retroperitoneal hematoma on the right side.

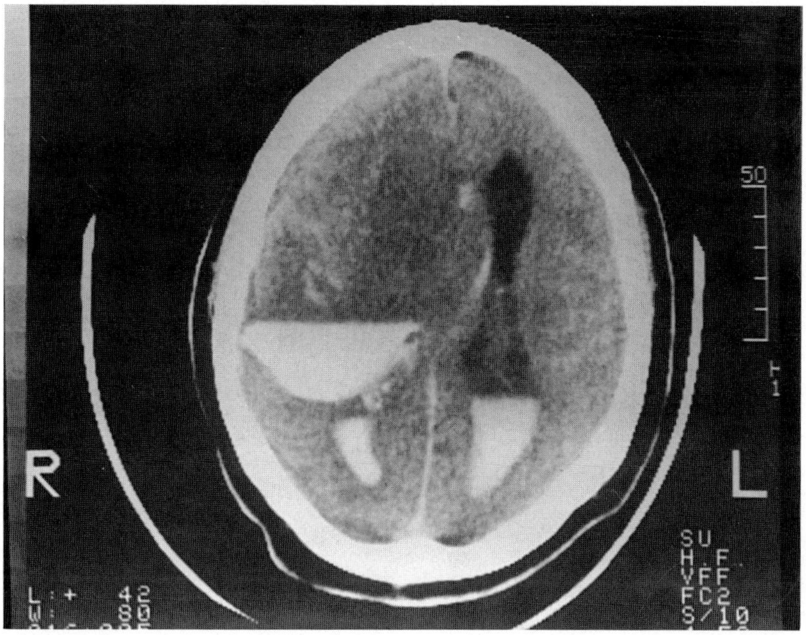

Figure 16–8. Computed tomography shows parenquimatous and intraventricular hemorrhage.

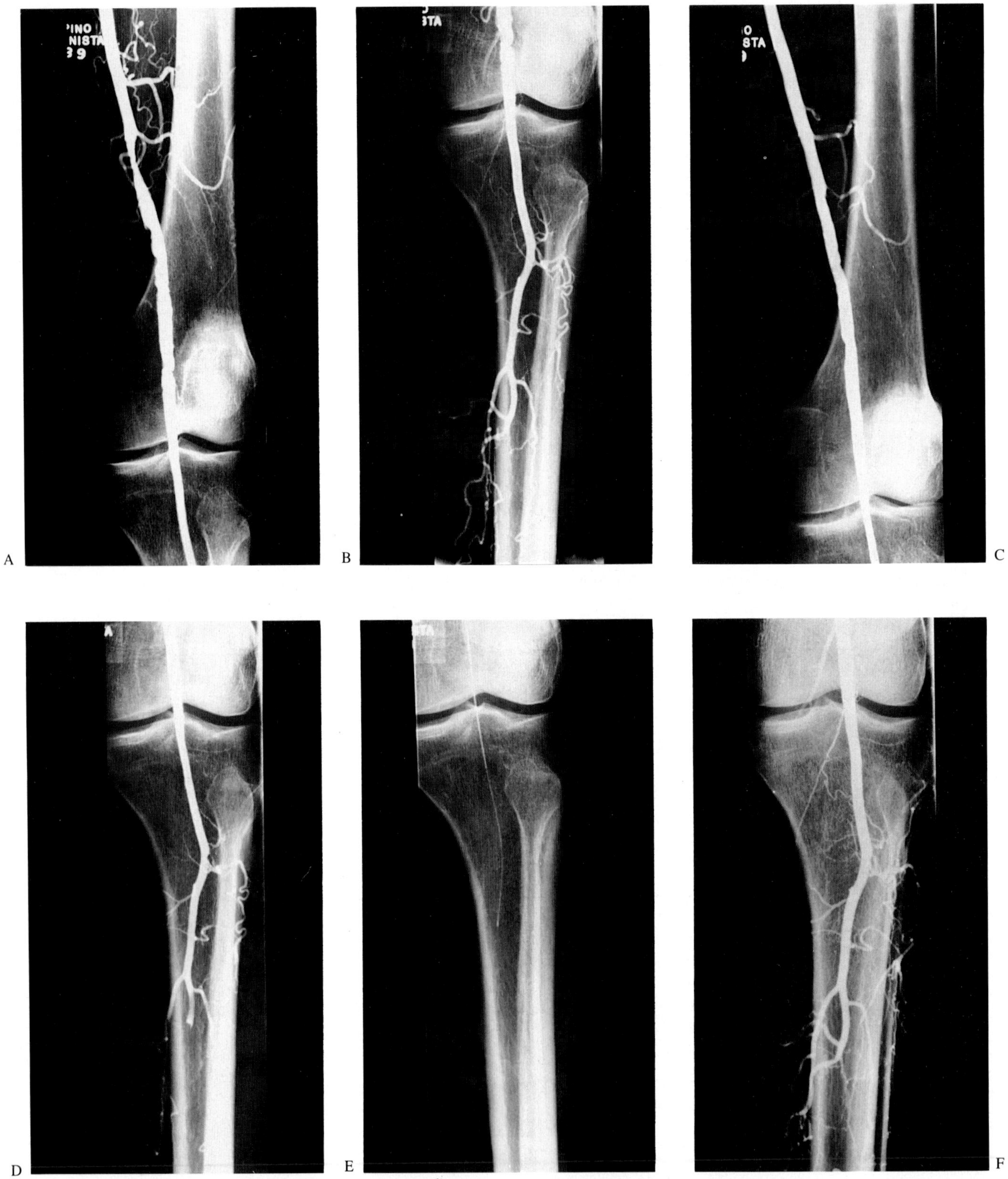

Figure 16–9. Distal embolism after fibrinolysis and angioplasty. **A:** Angiography shows residual stenosis at the occluded segment after urokinase infusion. **B:** Angiography shows patent runoff vessels. **C:** Follow-up angiography after angioplasty shows patent lumen at the stenotic site. **D:** Follow-up angiography shows embolism to distal vessels. **E:** The open-ended guide wire is advanced into the embolized segment. **F:** Follow-up angiogram after 30-minute infusion of urokinase shows total lysis of embolus.

The infusion of a bolus dose (250,000 U of urokinase), as the tip of the recanalizing catheter is withdrawn toward the proximal end of the occlusion, seems to decrease the thrombolysis time and lower the complication rates.[13] The mechanism by which the direct injection of thrombolytic agents within the thrombus accelerates its lysis is not clear. It is known that urokinase can convert plasminogen within the thrombus to plasmin.[14] The plasmin is less susceptible to inhibition within the thrombus by its most important inhibitor, $alpha_2$-antiplasmin, due to the presence of fibrin. On the other hand, $alpha_2$-antiplasmin is inactivated when it binds to and inhibits plasmin.[15] The part of the plasmin formed within the thrombus is inactivated by the $alpha_2$-antiplasmin, but the rest of plasmin can freely act over fibrin, since the circulating $alpha_2$-antiplasmin has little effect on plasmin activity within the thrombus.

The dose of thrombolytic agent continues being controversial. High-dose therapy has been used to treat patients who present with acute ischemic limb, since more rapid lysis is accomplished with these higher doses.[12] However, most of the authors use doses ranging from 40,000 to 100,000 U/hour regardless of the patient's symptoms.[3,9,16] Low-dose therapy seems to diminish the systemic effects of lytic therapy.

The fibrinolytic parameters monitored during the infusion are used more to confirm the lytic state than to control the clinical events. These parameters are not useful in predicting either clinical response or bleeding complications.[16]

The primary success rates of thrombolytic treatment varies from 30 to 100%.[2,3,16] Most series do not show differences between graft and native artery thrombolysis in the initial success rate.[3,4]

There is disagreement concerning the use of thrombolysis in bypass grafts, since the occlusion is commonly due to progression of disease and surgery is often required.[11–18] Nevertheless, there are some important arguments that justify the use of fibrinolytic agents in the treatment of bypass graft occlusions. The fibrinolytic treatment produces lysis of thrombus in small outflow vessels that may be inaccessible to thrombectomy techniques. Thus, thrombolysis decreases runoff vessel resistance, creating a better situation for long-term graft patency. In addition, by lysing the thrombus within the bypass graft, the cause of graft occlusion is uncovered and it can be treated either percutaneously (angioplasty or atherectomy) or surgically.

Complication rates range from 4 to 35%.[2,3,10,19] Because of the potential complications of thrombolytic therapy, the benefit for the patient must be weighed against the risks. The complications can be divided into two groups: management errors and complications in which no underlying error could be identified. These errors are mainly related to the inadequate management of bleeding, wrong selection of patients, and deviation from thrombolytic administration protocol. These avoidable sources of complications can be minimized, making thrombolytic therapy safer and more suitable for many patients.

CONCLUSION

Fibrinolysis as an efficient method of recanalization for either native peripheral artery or graft occlusions is still controversial. Some reports consider thrombolysis less safe, less effective, and more expensive compared with surgery.[3,16] Other authors consider that thrombolysis continues to be an important tool in arterial occlusion treatment.[1,9,12,20] However, a proper patient selection and a close follow-up during infusion time must be carried out to make thrombolytic therapy safe and more useful.

New fibrinolytic agents and improvements in infusion techniques will probably make thrombolysis safer and faster.

REFERENCES

1. McNamara T. Role of thrombolysis in peripheral arterial occlusion. Am J Med 1987;83(suppl 2A):6–10.
2. Dacey LJ, Dow RW, McDaniel MD, et al. Cost-effectiveness of intra-arterial thrombolytic therapy. Arch Surg 1988;123:1218–23.
3. van Breda A, Katzen B. Thrombolytic therapy of peripheral vascular disease. Semin Intervent Radiol 1985;42:354–66.
4. Graor RA, Risius B, Lucas FV, et al. Thrombolysis with recombinant tissue-type plasminogen activator in patients with peripheral artery and bypass graft occlusions. Circulation 1986;74(suppl I)I-15–20.
5. Motarjeme A. Thrombolytic therapy in arterial occlusion and graft thrombosis. Semin Vasc Surg 1989;2:155–78.
6. Hartman J, McKeever L, Teran J, et al. Prolonged infusion of urokinase for recanalization of chronically occluded aortocoronary bypass grafts. Am J Cardiol 1988;61:189–91.
7. Risuis B, Zelch M, Graci R, et al. Catheter-directed low dose streptokinase infusion: a preliminary experience. Radiology 1984;150:349–55.
8. Dotter CT, Rosch J, Seaman AJ. Selective clot lysis with low-dose streptokinase. Radiology 1988;11:541–7.
9. Katzen BT. Technique and results of "low-dose" infusion. Cardiovasc Intervent Radiol 1988;11:541–7.
10. Earnshaw JJ, Gregson RH, McKim GS, Hopkinson BR. Acute peripheral arterial ischemia: a prospective evaluation of differential management with surgery or thrombolysis. Ann Vasc Surg 1989;3:374–9.
11. Gardiner GA, Harrington DP, Koltun W, et al. Salvage of occluded arterial bypass grafts by means of thrombolysis. J Vasc Surg 1989;9:426–31.
12. McNamara TO. The use of lytic therapy with endovascular "repair" for the failed infrainguinal graft. Semin Vasc Surg 1990;3:59–65.
13. Sullivan KL, Gardiner GA, Shapiro MJ, et al. Acceleration of thrombolysis with a high-dose transthrombus bolus technique. Radiology 1989;173:805–8.
14. Hisano S. Immunofluorescence study on thrombolysis with special reference to the patterns of distribution and the contents of fibrin, plasminogen, $alpha_2$-macroglobulin and Urokinase in artificial thrombi. Thromb Haemost 1978;39:53–60.
15. Sakata Y, Aoki N. Significance of cross-linking of $alpha_2$-plasmin inhibitor to fibrin in inhibition of fibrinolysis and in hemostasis. J Clin Invest 1982;69:536–42.
16. Durham JD, Geller SC, Abbot WM, et al. Regional infusion of urokinase into occluded lower-extremity by-pass grafts: Long-term clinical results. Radiology 1989;172:83–7.

17. Marder VJ. Relevance of changes in blood fibrinolytic and coagulation parameters during thrombolytic therapy. Am J Med 1987;83:15–9.
18. Perler BA, White RI, Ernst CB, Williams GM. Low-dose thrombolytic therapy for infrainguinal graft occlusions: an idea whose time has passed? J Vasc Surg 1985;2:799–805.
19. Hirshberg A, Schneiderman J, Garnick A, et al. Errors and pitfalls in intraarterial thrombolytic therapy. J Vasc Surg 1989;10:612–6.
20. Graor RA, Risius B, Young JS, et al. Thrombolysis of peripheral arterial bypass grafts: surgical thrombectomy compared with thrombolysis. J Vasc Surg 1988;7:347–55.

17 Percutaneous Aspiration Thromboembolectomy

E. Starck, M.D., H.-J. Wagner, M.D.

"Dotter defined transluminal angioplasty as a fluoroscopically guided catheter treatment of vascular stenosis or obstructions."[1] Now more and more we perform percutaneous transluminal plastic microoperations to restore artery patency and flow by multiple means. At this time, the angioplastic methods we routinely use in our department are: Dotter technique, balloon dilation, local thrombolysis by urokinase infusion, percutaneous aspiration thromboembolectomy (PAT), rotating aspiration thromboembolectomy (RAT), percutaneous transluminal atherectomy, and stent implantation. Occasionally for the same purposes, we have used a laser, the Fogarty catheter, a biopsy forceps, or a stone basket. New angioplastic techniques developed dramatically and the spectrum for tomorrow will be different. Since 1981, we used the aspiration tool, first to remove thrombotic occlusive material in insufficient and endless local thrombolysis, later also for embolic material related to balloon dilation or local lysis and unrelated to percutaneous transluminal angioplasty (PTA), mainly from cardiogenic origin. In 1985 we published the procedure as "Percutaneous Aspiration Thromboembolectomy (PAT)."[2] The idea of removing embolic material by aspiration was presented in 1960 by Greenfield et al[3] for transvenous aspiration of pulmonary emboli through a femoral venotomy. In 1974 Buxton and Müller[4] reported the successful removal of an iatrogenic clot from a renal artery by catheter aspiration. In 1978 Horvath[5] suggested that emboli caused by balloon angioplasty might be removed by aspiration without citation of clinical experience. In 1984 Sniderman et al[6] reported on five successful removals of such post-PTA emboli in six patients.

Today PAT is our third main angioplastic tool besides balloon dilation and local lysis. We used PAT alone and more often in combination with some of the techniques just mentioned. The application is tailored to the specific situation to achieve luminal patency and flow, thus improving the results of the previous angioplastic procedures.

For the future, there is a strong tendency that aspiration will also be a major component of modern rotating angioplastic techniques as it is in the RAT[7] or in the transluminal endartherectomy catheter system.[8,9]

MATERIAL

Besides regular angiographic equipment, digital subtraction angiography (DSA) with roadmap facilities is very useful for steering aspiration while decreasing mechanical trauma to the vessel wall at the site of disease.[10]

Our regular regimen of drugs is listed in Table 17-1.

The material required for PAT is a sheath, the aspiration catheter, a large syringe, and guide wires. Now, we always use a regular 8 F sheath (Cordis). Its hemostasis valve must be removable, to facilitate removal of entrapped clot material, and big enough to fit the width of the aspiration catheter and a small wire to maintain continuous access. The sideport of the valve serves for flushing and angiographic contrast injections.

The sheath and its components are obligatory because large fragments of occlusive material would not fit through the sheath valve. Clot aspiration may be performed with any catheter without sideholes, but effectiveness for aspiration increases significantly with luminal width. Our aspiration catheters from 5 to 9 F (Angiomed) are thin walled and minimally tapered. Most often, 8 and 7 F sizes are used, according to vessel size, with 5 F in the distal tibial region. To steer the Terumo wire or the Amplatz wires for exchange into the tibial vessels, we use a 5 (or 7) F Berenstein catheter.

TECHNIQUE

The application of PAT is flexible, depending on the individual situation with respect to site, length, volume, consis-

Table 17–1. Drugs in Transluminal Angioplasty

Antiplatelet therapy before and after the procedure
- Aspirin 325 mg/day

Antispasmodics before and during the procedure in case of renal, mesenterial, distal popliteal, and tibial lesions
- Nifedipine 10 mg (capsule sublingually with punched holes)
- Nitroglycerin 100–200 μg in a glass syringe in case of severe spasm
- (Lidocaine 20 cc at least for extensive local anesthesia)

Anticoagulant
- Heparin during the procedure at least 2000 U
  - Normally 5000 U
  - Seldom 100 U/kg
  - Maximum individually
  - After local lysis or below the knee:
    - About 1000 U/hour/3 days for only slight thrombin time prolongation

Thrombolysis
- Urokinase 100,000 U bolus/15 minutes, diffusely into the occlusion, same dose/hour to a maximum of 4 (6) hours into the proximal site of occlusion

tency, and age of the occlusion. The basic technique is shown in Figure 17-1. If an embolus is lodged at a bifurcation of the vessel, the aspiration catheter is advanced over a wire to the site of occlusion. After removal of the wire, the catheter is advanced to get contact with the embolus. DSA roadmapping is useful. Negative pressure for aspiration is applied with a 50 cc syringe and steered by hand. Firmer material will be engaged at the tip and has to be extracted with the catheter through the sheath. We therefore disconnect the hemostasis valve and occlude the sheath with the finger tip to prevent major bleeding.

If blood readily enters the syringe during catheter extraction, the occlusive material either has cleared the catheter or dropped distally. The syringe is removed and its contents are expressed over a gauze-draped basin. Firmer particles remaining on the gauze serve the diagnostic purpose of determining how to proceed. Blood filtering into the basin is an indicator of blood loss. Contrast material is then injected through the aspiration catheter to reassess the situation. Multiple aspirations can be performed if necessary.

In case of a thrombotic occlusion the application of PAT does not differ principally. The most decisive factor for the applicability of PAT is the consistency of the occlusive material. Soft material is better because it has to pass a small catheter lumen (Fig. 17-2). The firmer the material, the more passes that are required to remove the blockage stepwise. In case of firm material, pretreatment is necessary to loosen, break, and increase flexibility by local thrombolysis or balloon dilation or other rotating mechanical devices. How do we get the information about the required type of pretreatment? We get it from the patient's history and by the resistance during initial wire and catheter passage. So, at first, we pass an occlusion in the regular fashion, as in normal balloon angioplasty.

PERCUTANEOUS ASPIRATION THROMBOEMBOLECTOMY BEFORE BALLOON DILATION IN FRESH OCCLUSIONS

Finally, a high-grade atherosclerotic stenosis will result in total occlusion by thrombosis (Fig. 17-3). The length will be determined by the major collaterals, which carry sufficient flow within the residual mainstream vessel. In such a fresh occlusion, the patient's history is short and the resistance during catheter passage is very low except at the stenotic site. Here, PAT before balloon dilation has two functions: The aspiration of soft clot material minimizes the chance for embolization and reduces the workup time significantly. We can finish the procedure with balloon dilation to remove the stenosis that caused the thrombotic occlusion. In this situation PAT also excludes the need for time-consuming local lysis.

BALLOON DILATION BEFORE PERCUTANEOUS ASPIRATION THROMBOEMBOLECTOMY

In case of firmer embolic material, we predilate the occlusion first. Fragmentation of the material reduces consistency, improving the ability to pass the aspiration catheter. This also decreases the need for local urokinase lysis, which we limit in embolic patients to a total of 100,000 U (maximum 200,000) to prevent systemic effects and minimize the chance for reembolization.[11] The same effects result in better aspiration conditions when we predilate a thrombotic occlusion, which has to be done to remove the stenosis, as mentioned before. If we dilate the most distal part of an

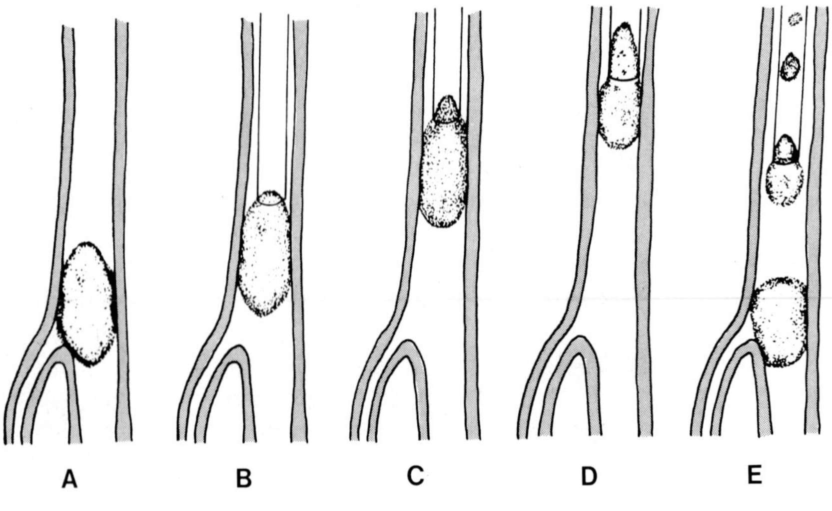

Figure 17–1. Basic technique of percutaneous aspiration thromboembolectomy. **A:** Embolus lodged in a vessel bifurcation. **B:** Aspiration catheter in contact moves the embolus. **C:** Catheter is withdrawn. **D:** Embolus remodels to the distal catheter lumen. **E:** The material becomes fragmented, small particles pass, firmer particles are entrapped at the catheter tip and have to be extracted.

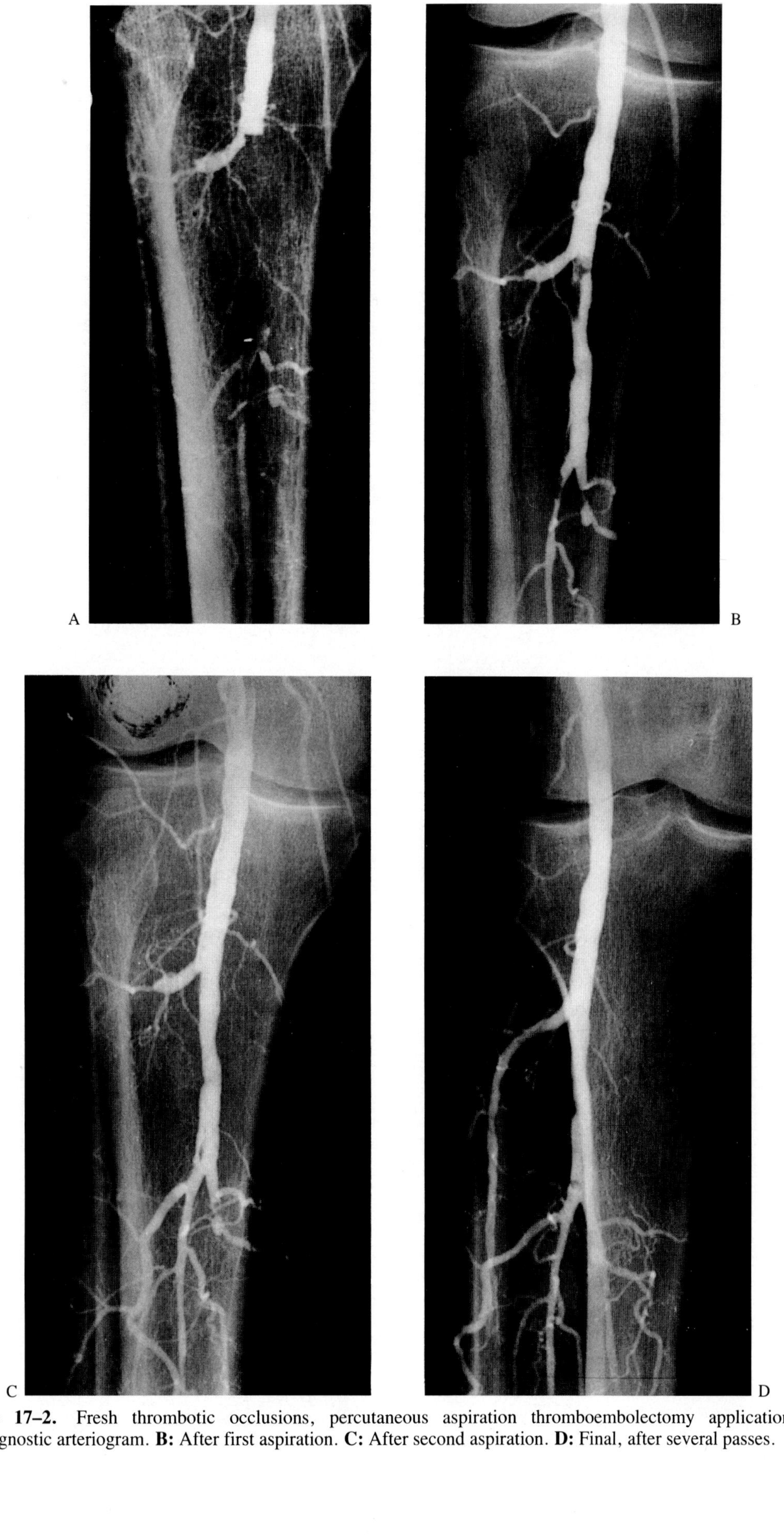

Figure 17–2. Fresh thrombotic occlusions, percutaneous aspiration thromboembolectomy application only. A: Diagnostic arteriogram. B: After first aspiration. C: After second aspiration. D: Final, after several passes.

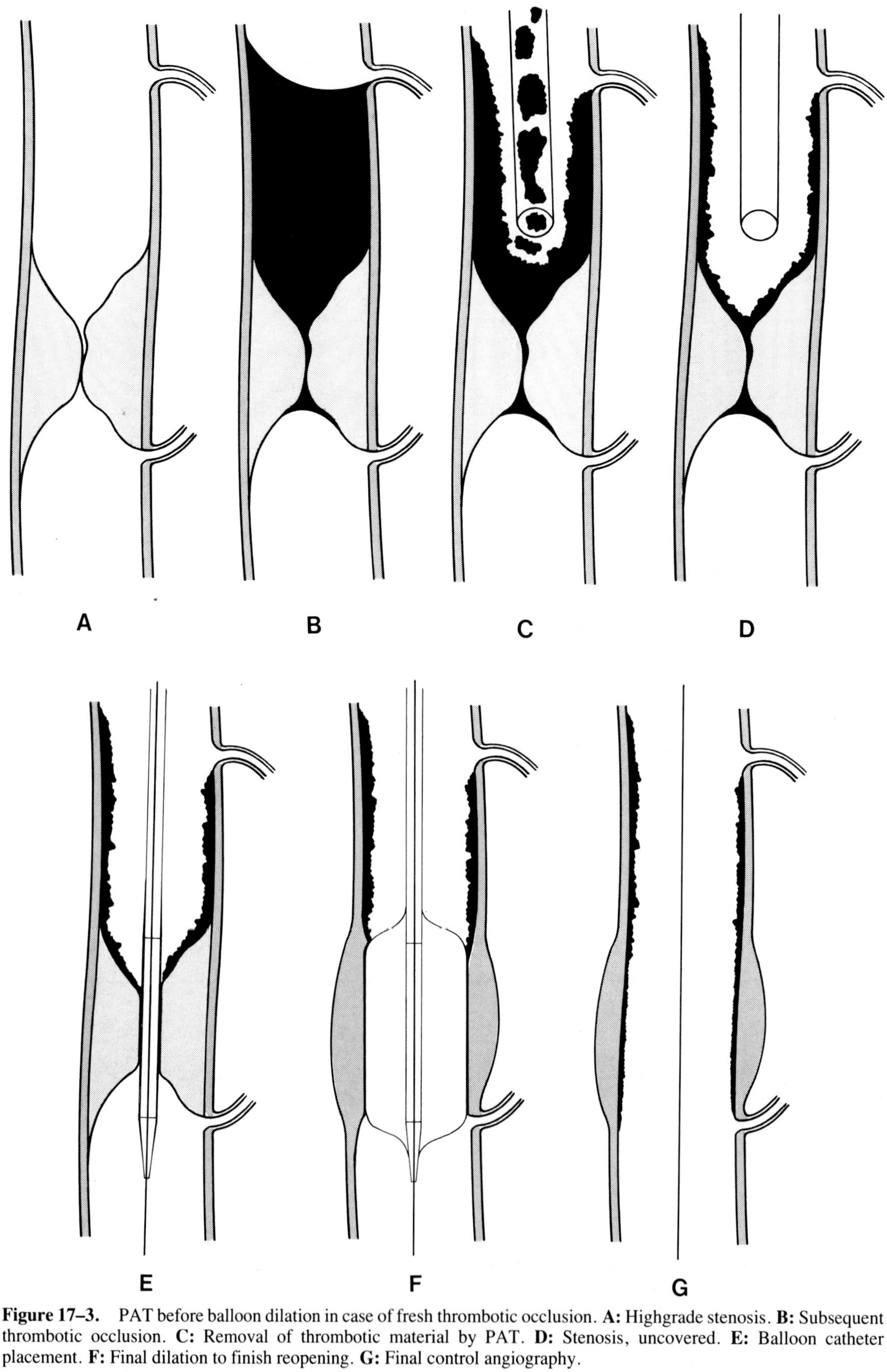

Figure 17–3. PAT before balloon dilation in case of fresh thrombotic occlusion. **A:** Highgrade stenosis. **B:** Subsequent thrombotic occlusion. **C:** Removal of thrombotic material by PAT. **D:** Stenosis, uncovered. **E:** Balloon catheter placement. **F:** Final dilation to finish reopening. **G:** Final control angiography.

occlusion before PAT, we have to anticipate problems by distal embolization. This can be solved by further aspiration, but we might have additional trauma by mechanical manipulations.

PERCUTANEOUS ASPIRATION THROMBOEMBOLECTOMY AND LOCAL LYSIS

Local thrombolytic infusion of urokinase reduces the volume of occlusive material, and it fragments, loosens and increases softness and flexibility. Aspiration of the material is easier than with any other modality. On the other side, the disadvantages that come with the lytic infusion therapy are nearly excluded. These are time consumption and increased bleeding complications by time and dose as well as high embolization rates up to 11 to 16%.[12,13] So PAT and local lysis do very well in combination. By removal of old, bad or nondissolvable thrombus and atherosclerotic debris, we are more often successful than with a single angioplastic tool, especially if we treat old and very long occlusions.

PAT and local thrombolysis act in many ways like a balance scale: the more lysis, the less PAT that is necessary, and vice versa. So with PAT we improve not only success, but also decrease the procedure time. This prompted us to shorten our lysis time and lysis overnight became very exceptional. Our regular schedule (Table 17-1) limits the time of intra-arterial thrombolytic infusion to a maximum of 6 hours. Most often, we finish the procedure within 2 to 4 hours by aspiration in between. With more PAT, we are able to limit the dose of urokinase to 100,000 U. In 65% we do not use any lysis and in 11% we use our minidose regimen, as mentioned before. Only in 24% do we use the regular dose, up to 700,000 U urokinase.

Significant shortening of procedure time is a result of accelerated thrombolysis. This means balloon dilation before thrombolytic medication, as shown in Figure 17-4 to fragment the occlusive material. The increased contact surface for the lytic agent by mechanical alteration enormously speeds reopening.[14–16] Initially, we do not touch the most distal occlusion segment because of the higher embolization risk.

SPECIAL PERCUTANEOUS ASPIRATION THROMBOEMBOLECTOMY PROCEDURES

Aspiration over a wire can be useful to eliminate the risk of subintimal passage. The risk increases at curved vessel sites, for instance, in the popliteal artery and when we move the catheter against resistance, especially with aspiration. A wire in the aspiration channel requires a Touhy-Borst adapter and reduces effectiveness by its size. It also prevents extraction of larger components. We have seldom used this setting after transpopliteal recanalization.

In small vessels we apply PAT during extraction. First a

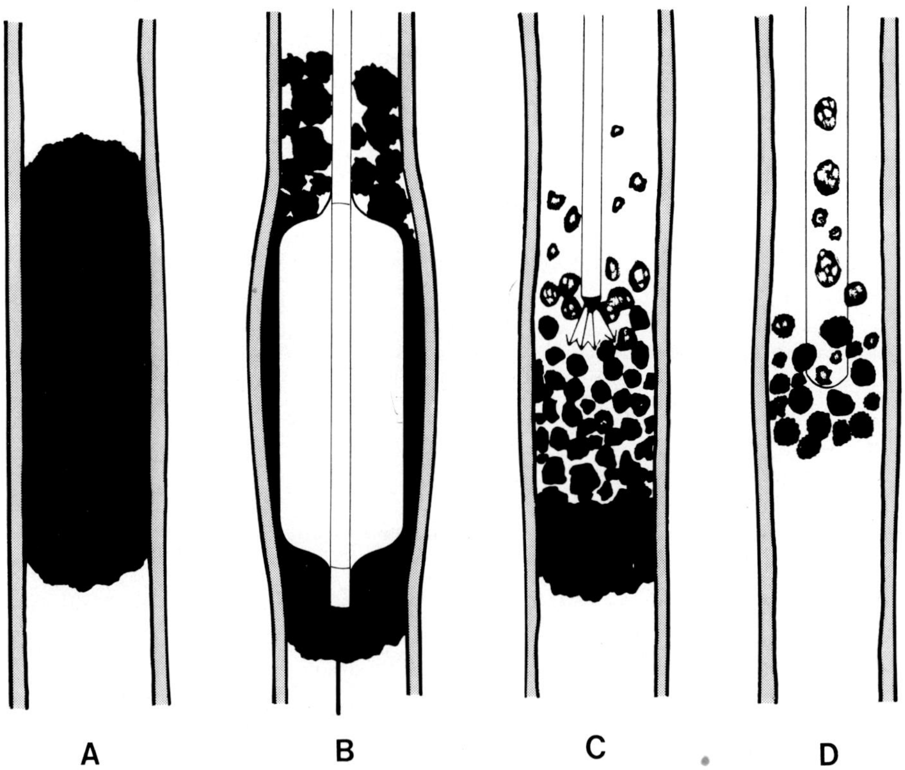

Figure 17–4. Accelerated thrombolysis with percutaneous aspiration thromboembolectomy (PAT). **A:** Thromboembolic occlusion. **B:** Fragmentation by balloon dilation increasing the contact surface for the lytic agent. **C:** Local lytic infusion. **D:** PAT removes badly or unlysable components, thus speeding the reopening significantly.

wire is passed distally, before the catheter (5 to 7 F). After removal of the wire, negative pressure is created and the catheter is withdrawn. If we advance the nontapered aspiration catheter under aspiration in small vessels distally, the risk for subintimal passage is much higher. Aspiration during catheter extraction excludes subintimal passage. Unfortunately, we remove the most distal occlusive part first. So we have to work up the occlusion from distal to proximal. This takes more time and proximal embolic particles sometimes move stepwise distally.

Crossover PAT includes the risk for embolization into the unaffected leg, which no patient will understand. In this situation we have to be very sure that the embolic material fits perfectly to the size of the aspiration catheter, so it can be withdrawn through the sheath without a chance of getting lost.

The "big fish" problem occurs once in about 25 procedures and can be vexing. This means we catch a large, hard thrombus that cannot pass through the small catheter lumen and is extracted into the distal portion of the sheath. This situation is signaled by lack of back-bleeding if we remove the hemostasis valve. Then, for better fixation of the material, we directly apply aspiration to the sheath by a 50 cc syringe. A Terumo wire is then passed while continuous suction is transmitted through the sideport of the repositioned hemostasis valve. When the wire pushes the large thrombus back into the artery, blood will enter the syringe immediately. If it does not, we remove the sheath under suction, avoiding kinks and external pressure to the puncture site. The sheath is cleaned and repositioned over the wire. If the thrombus has been pushed back, usually into the same position as before, a second wire is inserted through the sheath. This is then removed and reintroduced over one wire alone. The second wire remains outside the sheath, functioning as a safety wire. If the thrombus is caught during the next aspiration pass within the sheath, we then perform PAT directly after removal of the hemostasis valve. PAT with the sheath material is more effective because of greater luminal width. We have to avoid kinks and external manual pressure at the puncture site again. The second wire serves for reintroduction of the cleaned sheath to reassess the situation angiographically. We always solve the problem by several attempts, which results in a major step toward final success. Our "big fish" record up to now is 7.2 cm in length.

Intimal flap-atherectomy is a rare but sometimes extremely difficult problem. The reason is that the intimal flap or plaque material is less elastic and does not fit easily into the catheter lumen like clot material. This means we cannot fix this sufficiently for extraction. We also face this problem if such material embolizes. Occasionally, in former times, distal deposition into the peroneal vessels was the only way to minimize the perfusion deficit. Now, we catch and mobilize these flaps or emboli with our specially developed spherical tipped spiral. The RAT instrument (Fig. 17-5) (Angiomed) is rotated by hand or with a motor and pulled out under continuous aspiration.[7]

GENERAL INDICATIONS

With respect to the individual situation, we apply PAT below the inguinal ligament in thrombotic as well as embolic occlusions, causing clinical symptoms according to Fontaine classification IIb, III, and IV. The indications for PAT embolectomy were mainly severe or emergency situations (Table 17-2), representing a negative selection in comparison to the regular balloon angioplasty group. Most of the embolizations not related to angioplasty were cardiogenic (Fig. 17-6) or from abdominal aneurysms. Rare opportunities for PAT are renal or mesenteric embolizations. Those patients have to be attended to as fast as possible so as not to exceed the ischemic tolerance time of the organs. PAT in mesenteric vessels depends on vital bowel tissue, which we believe is signaled by perfusion distal to the embolic occlusion in DSA. For PAT in these regions, we need a transaxillary approach.

We do not recommend PAT for thromboembolic occlusions of the pulmonary, the abdominal aorta, and iliac

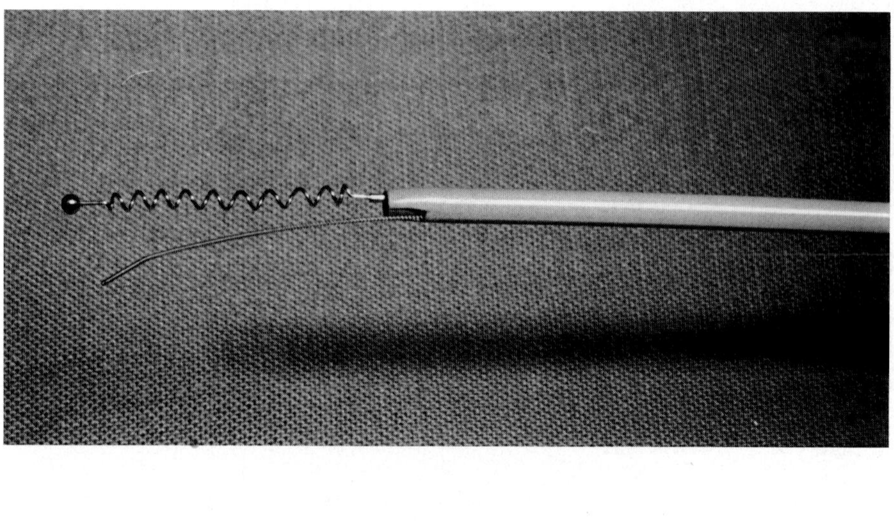

Figure 17–5. Spherical tipped spiral for rotating aspiration thromboembolectomy together with the double-lumen aspiration catheter for simultaneous thrombolytic contrast injection. The spiral also catches intimal flap material or emboli for extraction under aspiration.

Table 17–2. Material and Clinical Success of Percutaneous Aspiration Thromboembolectomy (PAT) in 1989

	PATIENTS		CLINICAL SUCCESS	
	No.	*%*	*No.*	*%*
Thrombotic occlusion	45	55%	41	91%
Embolic occlusion related to PTA	24	29%	24	100%
Embolic occlusion unrelated to PTA	13	16%	11	84%
	82		76	(93%)

arteries because of the large amount of material that has to be withdrawn by a relatively small catheter lumen. We also have to mention that it is nearly impossible to aspirate embolized material distal to the central end of the sheath in retrograde femoral punctures. Most of these patients went directly to the operating room. Sometimes PAT improves patency and flow after iliac balloon dilation or local lysis when a small amount of occlusive material reoccluded the lumen, acting like a valve. So by far the main indications are below the inguinal ligament after antegrade puncture. Crossover PAT is very exceptional, as mentioned before.

RESULTS

Since the first application in 1981, we have treated more than 400 patients with PAT, mainly in combination with other angioplastic methods. The inclusion of the aspiration angioplastic tool improved our former clinical balloon dilation results[17] in the leg region from 59–75% to 91% of the first 156 treatments in which PAT was applied.[18] In 50% of these, local lysis was combined as well. Since PAT, we have not had significant embolization after angioplasty requiring surgical embolectomy.

As mentioned initially, today angioplastic treatment requires a multitechnique approach until we achieve sufficient perfusion. So it is important to know the results of PAT. We have analyzed this throughout 1989. In this period we had 489 angioplasties of the lower extremities. Among these were 82 (17%) PAT procedures. Of these patients, 43 (52%) were in stage IIb, seven (9%), in stage III, and 32 (39%), in stage IV, according to Fontaine, before any angioplastic treatment, not including the emergency situations because of distal embolization after balloon dilation or local lysis.

In 55% of the cases we performed PAT for thrombotic occlusions, in 29% for embolisms related to PTA, and in 16% from cardiogenic origin. The overall clinical primary success was 92% up to discharge (Table 17-2). The angiographic success rate was higher. Angioplasty includes many

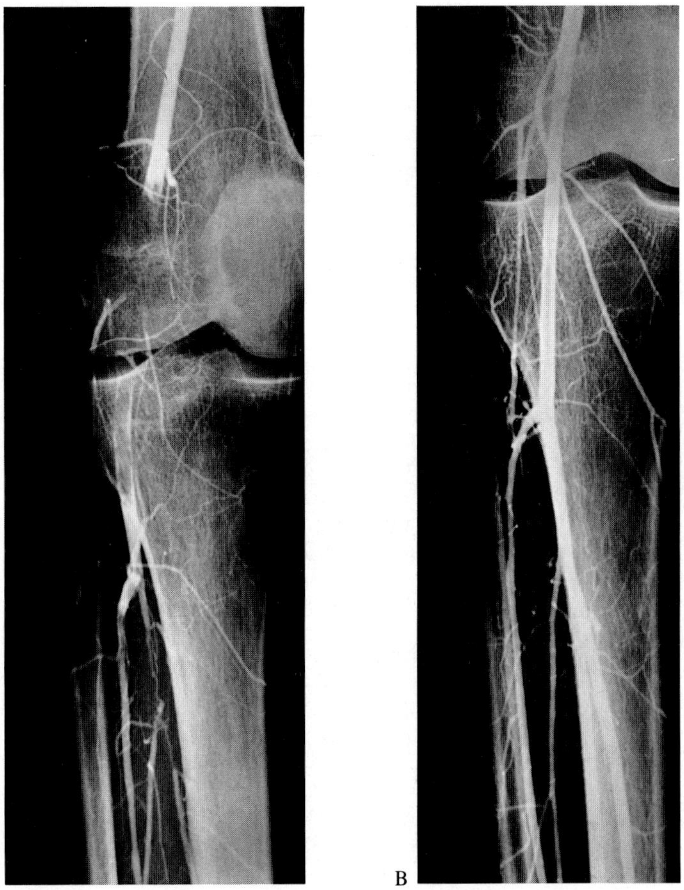

A B

Figure 17–6. Acute cardiogenic embolization, percutaneous aspiration thromboembolectomy application only. **A:** Diagnostic arteriogram. **B:** Final after few aspirations.

Table 17–3. Additional Angioplastic Techniques in 82 Percutaneous Aspiration Thromboembolectomy Patients*

Balloon dilation	162 (61 tibial)
Local thrombolysis	29 (35%)
RAT†	7 (9%)
Endartherectomy (TEC†)	2
Stent implantation	3

*Of a total of 489 leg angioplasties in 1989.

†RAT: rotating aspiration thromboembolectomy; TEC: transluminal endartherectomy catheter.

techniques to optimize flow. Only in very fresh thrombotic occlusions is PAT used first (Fig. 17-2). We add other techniques stepwise, with escalation depending on the individual situation. So the PAT group has more severe and difficult situations, including embolizations not represented in the preangiographic Fontaine stages. Most often, balloon dilation is used with it at different sites (Table 17-3). The figures where we apply local thrombolysis for recanalization decreased from 50 to 35%. Not included are those patients we routinely give 100,000 U urokinase to improve distal perfusion, as in diabetic small vessel disease. This patient group is relatively large with respect to the fact that 38% of the additional balloon dilations within the PAT group were carried out in the tibial region. In three patients of the thrombosis group we had to stabilize perfusion finally by stent implantation (Strecker). The best clinical success (100%) was achieved after PTA embolizations. Less clinical success (84%) with the most complications resulted in the group of cardiogenic emboli. Despite this, our results are superior to the published data for the Fogarty embolectomy.[19,20] In our department all patients with acute embolic occlusions below the inguinal ligament are primarily treated by PAT embolectomy. Until now, we also had a chance to treat successfully seven of seven mesenteric and three of four renal cardiogenic embolizations. Two of the mesenteric arteries were operated on later because the surgeons felt uncomfortable about believing in sufficient reperfusion. There was no bowel resection, and one mycotic aneurysm after embolization caused by endocarditis had to be removed.

A major advantage of PAT embolectomy is the simplicity of the technique. Combining the diagnostic with the therapeutic procedure saves time, reduces tissue loss, and thereby reduces the release of toxic substances. This, together with the reduced invasiveness, results in less mortality. Most of the patients had older emboli with firm organization or atherosclerotic stenosis resulting in occlusions that the Fogarty catheter could not pass. We do not have problems of recanalizing these with multiple angioplastic devices, including treatment of tibial and pedal vessels under regular angiographic equipment and control.

COMPLICATIONS

There is only one PAT-specific complication, the antegrade dissection. The risk increases if we advance the catheter against resistance under aspiration and at sites of a previous balloon dilation. Until now, we have had four antegrade dissections in over 400 procedures in the femoral-popliteal region, which we could handle by balloon dilation. Subintimal passage and dissection is excluded if we guide the catheter over a wire distally. After removal of the wire, we aspirate during catheter extraction.

PAT is a method of escalation for severe and difficult situations, often when others have failed. This also is expressed in the type and number of complications, which are much higher than in the regular angioplastic group. Many of those are related to the underlying life-threatening disease. In the 82 patients, two hematomas at the puncture site required operative treatment. There was one rupture of the artery after balloon dilation without further treatment and one pseudoaneurysm had to be resected. Two compartment syndromes due to severe ischemia before successful angioplasty required fasciotomy and had a good clinical outcome. Two below-knee amputations were unavoidable. One patient from the cardiogenic embolic group of 13 (7.7%) died 24 hours after successful aspiration embolectomy because of severe heart disease.

The figure for mortality in the embolic group nonrelated to PTA is higher than we experienced in over 100 treatments. However, it is still far less than rates published following surgery, from 14 to 22% in the femoral and popliteal region.[19–21]

REFERENCES

1. Castañeda-Zúñiga W (ed). Transluminal Angioplasty. New York: Thieme-Stratton, 1983:1.
2. Starck E, McDermott JC, Crummy AB, et al. Percutaneous aspiration thrombolectomy (PAT). Radiology 1985:156:61–6.
3. Greenfield LJ, Kimmell GO, McCurdy WC. Transvenous removal of pulmonary emboli by vacuum-cup catheter technic. J Surg Res 1960;9:347.
4. Buxton DR Jr, Müller CF. Removal of iatrogenic clot by transcatheter embolectomy. Radiology 1974;111:39–41.
5. Horvath L, Illes I, Varo J. Complications of the transluminal angioplasty excluding the puncture site complications. In Zeitler E, Grüntzig A, Schoop W (eds): Percutaneous Vascular Recanalization. Berlin: Springer, 1978:126–140.
6. Sniderman KW, Bodner L, Saddekni S, et al. Percutaneous embolectomy by transcatheter aspiration. Radiology 1984; 150:357–61.
7. Starck EE, McDermott JC. Rotating aspiration thromboembolectomy. Radiology 1988;169:366.
8. Greenfield JC. An explosion of technology. Am J Cardiol 1988;62:1F–24F.
9. Wholey HM, Jarmolewski CR. New reperfusion devices. Radiology 1989;172:947–52.
10. Crummy AB, Starck EE, McDermott JC, et al. Digital subtraction arteriography (DSA) "road map." Semin Intervent Radiol 1984;1:247–50.

11. Paulson EK, Miller FJ. Embolization of cardiac mural thrombus: complication of intraarterial fibrinolysis. Radiology 1988;168:95–6.
12. Hess H. Clot lysis in peripheral arteries. In: Dotter CT, Grüntzig AR, Schoop W, Zeitler E. eds. Percutaneous Transluminal Angioplasty. Berlin: Springer, 1983:145–53.
13. Roth FJ, Capius G, Schmitdke I. Early experience of catheter lysis. In Dotter CT, Grüntzig AR, Schoop W, Zeitler E (eds): Percutaneous Transluminal Angioplasty. Berlin: Springer, 1983:154–60.
14. Bookstein JJ, Saldinger E. Accelerated thrombolysis: in vitro evaluation of agents and methods of administration. Invest Radiol 1985;20:731–5.
15. Davis GB, Dowd CF, Bookstein JJ, et al. Thrombosed dialysis grafts: efficacy of intrathrombic deposition of concentrated urokinase, clot maceration, and angioplasty. AJR; 1987; 149:177–81.
16. Bildsoe MC, Moradian GP, Hunter DW, et al. Mechanical clot dissolution: new concept. Radiology 1989;171:231–3.
17. von Heydwolff A. Percutane Transluminale Angioplastie. Dissertation, University of Frankfurt, Frankfurt, 1986.
18. Starck E, McDermott JC. Advantages of percutaneous aspiration thromboembolectomy. In Zeitler E. Seyferth W (eds). Pros and cons in PTA and auxiliary methods. Berlin: Springer, 1989:241–7.
19. Abbott WM, Maloney RD, McCabe CC, et al. Arterial embolism: a 44 year perspective. Am J Surg 1982;143:460–74.
20. Connett MC, Murray DH Jr, Wenneker WW. Peripheral arterial emboli. Am J Surg 1984;148:14–9.
21. Elliott JR, Hageman JH, Szilagyi E, et al. Arterial embolization: problems of source, multiplicity, recurrence and delayed treatment. Surgery 1980;88:833.

18 Percutaneous Thrombectomy

Wilfrido R. Castañeda-Zúñiga, M.D., Eugenio Ponomar-Sulepov, M.D., Ph.D., D. W. Hunter, M.D., Joseph Yedlicka, M.D., John Carlson, M.D., Ph.D., Kurt Amplatz, M.D.

Mechanical removal of clot from acutely occluded vessels or grafts using balloon catheters has been shown to be a reliable method for prompt restoration of perfusion.[1,2] However, restoration of flow may be incomplete, due to distal location of thrombi or emboli, thrombus propagation beyond the reach of the catheter, and atherosclerotic obstruction that prevents passage of the catheter into occluded distal arteries.[1] Repeated futile attempts to remove thrombus under these circumstances may cause significant intimal damage and, on occasion, perforate the vessel wall.[1] Failure to restore distal circulation, rethrombosis, or hemorrhage into the soft tissues may ensue.[1]

Chemical fibrinolysis has recently become an effective treatment for vascular thrombosis, but potential drawbacks exist. Chemical thrombolysis often requires prolonged infusion times and may be contraindicated when an immediate need to restore perfusion precludes a 24- to 48-hour trial of lytic therapy.[1] In addition, prolonged infusion of these agents eventually produces a systemic lytic state with increased risk of bleeding.[1] Also, it is often difficult for the patient to maintain a supine position for up to 48 hours (when a femoral approach is used). Furthermore, thrombolytic therapy may fail to achieve recanalization of the occluded vessel. Finally, currently used thrombolytic agents are expensive, as is the required stay in the intensive care unit during infusion.

Because of these limitations, several investigators have directed their attention to percutaneous mechanical rotational thrombectomy devices for clot removal or dissolution.[3-6]

Theoretically, such devices can reduce or even completely remove thrombus from grafts or vessels, thereby obviating the need for or reducing thrombolytic infusion time. This approach may also be useful for thrombus that is refractory to fibrinolytic therapy and should reduce overall patient morbidity as well as the cost of chemical thrombolysis.

Among the mechanical thrombectomy devices are included:

- Transluminal extraction catheter
- Amplatz mechanical thrombolysis catheter
- Ponomar transjugular clot-trapper device
- Rheolytic thrombectomy catheter

TRANSLUMINAL EXTRACTION CATHETER

The transluminal extraction catheter (TEC) was originally designed for the percutaneous removal of atherosclerotic plaque (Fig. 18-1). The catheter has, however, been successfully used by Yedlicka et al[7] for the removal of fresh and chronic thrombus in laboratory animals and in humans.

The TEC device has been used to remove 1-week-old thrombus from Gore-Tex interpositional grafts placed for bypassing surgically created occlusions of the right superficial femoral artery and from the isolated contralateral femoral artery, whose branches were ligated in a canine model (Fig. 18-2). The disrupted thrombus is simultaneously aspirated through the torque tube into a vacuum bottle. The torque tube or cutter is advanced into the thrombus by means of a sliding control. Following the TEC mechanical thrombectomy, angiography is performed to check patency of the treated arteries and the thrombectomy is repeated if necessary. At the conclusion of the procedure, a final angiogram is obtained to check for vascular patency and to evaluate for possible distal embolization. The superficial femoral arteries were removed and sent to Pathology for microscopic evaluation.

The TEC device was successful at removing 1-week-old thrombus in all animals. The thrombectomy was performed quickly and without complications in all dogs. No significant distal embolization was noted in any of the dogs on postprocedure arteriograms. Microscopic examination of the superficial femoral arteries demonstrated mild intimal disruption and no evidence of perforation.

This device has also been used in humans with superior vena cava (SVC) obstruction (Fig. 18-3) and with obstructed hemodialysis grafts.

In conclusion, the TEC endarterectomy system is a safe, convenient, and effective means of removing thrombus from grafts and arteries in experimental animals as well as from central veins in human subjects. We believe that this system will prove to be useful in treating thrombus refractory to thrombolytic therapy as well as in reducing overall fibrinolytic infusion time by debulking thrombus.

AMPLATZ MECHANICAL THROMBOLYSIS CATHETER

The prototype catheter is 100 cm long, 8 F in size and made of polyurethane. At its distal tip is a 1 cm long, open-ended metal capsule with two sideholes (Fig. 18-4). The capsule serves as the housing for a tiny propeller similar to the blade of a household mixer. The propeller is connected to a drive shaft that can be connected either to a high-speed electric or air-driven motor. Rotational speeds of 100,000 rpm can be

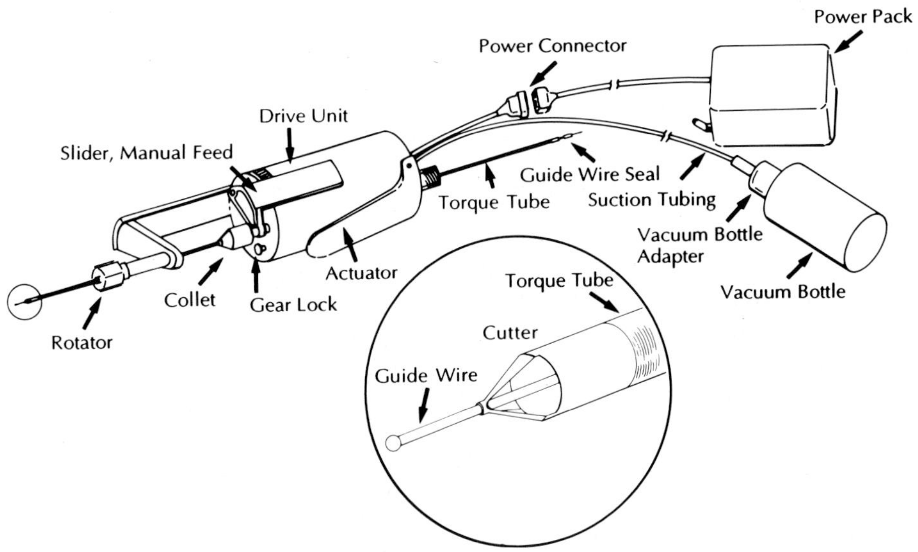

Figure 18–1. Diagrammatic representation of the transluminal extraction catheter system.

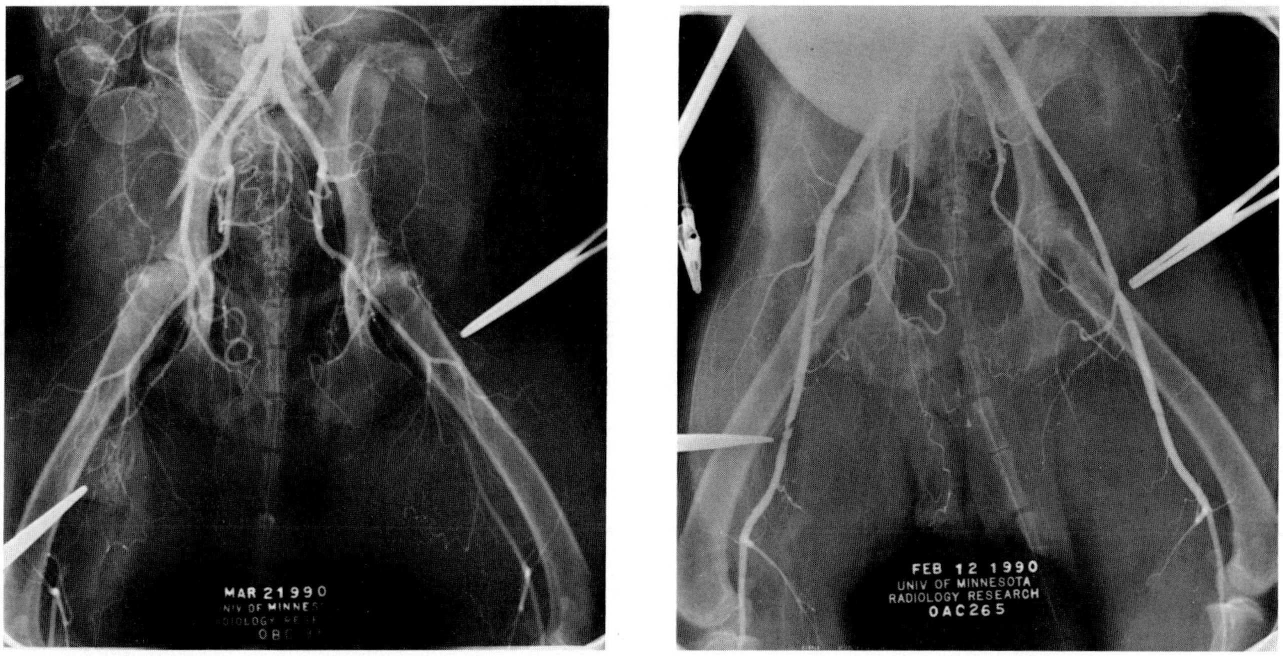

A B

Figure 18–2. **A:** An abdominal aortogram in a dog with occlusion of the left bypass graft and right native femoral artery prior to transluminal extraction catheter (TEC) procedure. **B:** Following the TEC procedure of occluded bypass graft and native right femoral artery, note widely open lumen. Residual narrowing is noted at the site of a stenosis of the bypass graft and the right femoral artery. Note distal patent arteries.

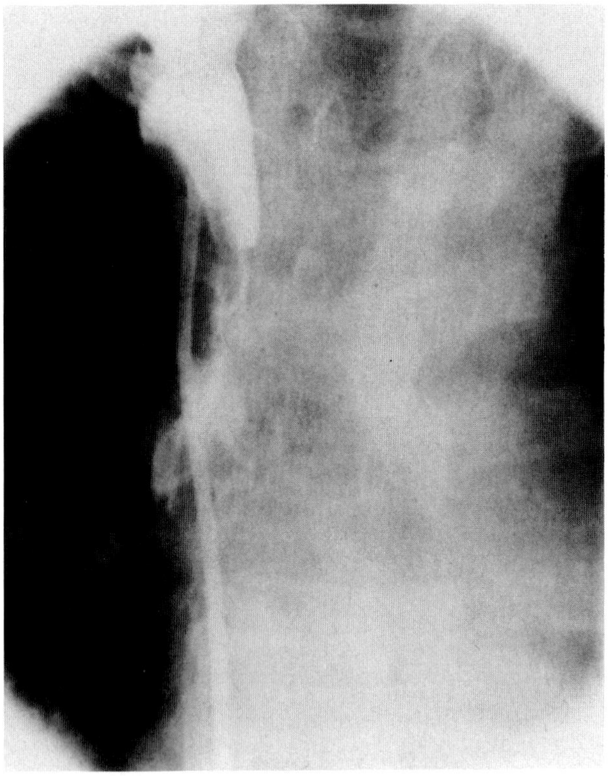

A

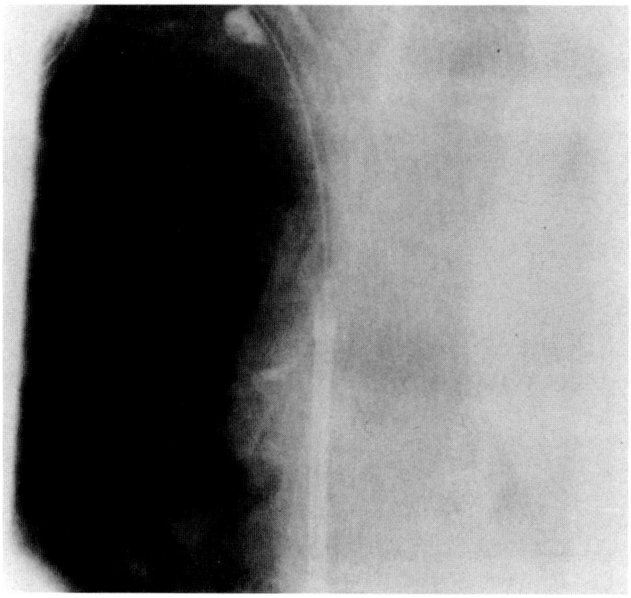

B

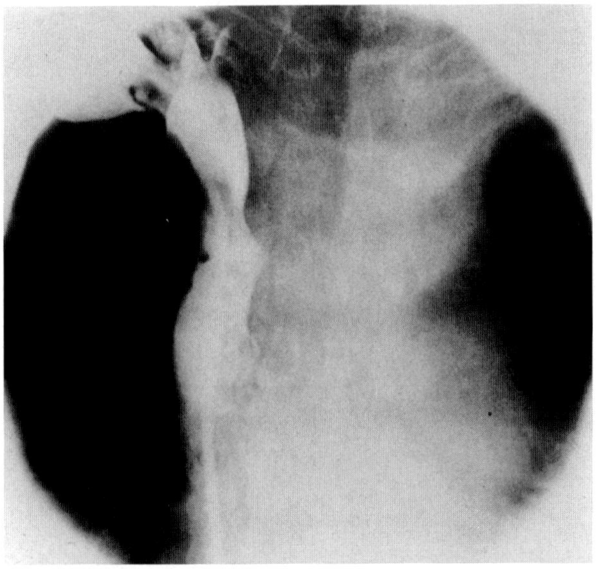

C

Figure 18–3. **A:** Superior vena cavagram in patient with a superior vena cava syndrome caused by thrombosis of the superior vena cava. **B:** Spot film taken during introduction of the transluminal extraction catheter (TEC) device. **C:** Superior vena cavagram following the TEC procedure shows almost complete removal of thrombus in superior vena cava with excellent flow.

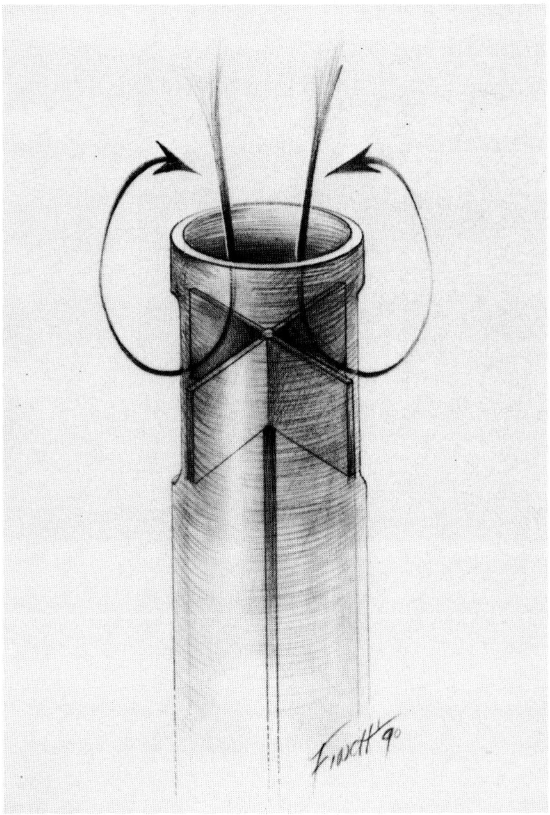

Figure 18–4. Diagram of tip of Amplatz thrombectomy device showing the position of the window in relationship to the propeller blades.

achieved. The drive shaft extends through a "Y" connector at the proximal end of the catheter, which allows the infusion of saline, contrast medium, or fibrinolytic solutions, any of which also serve to lubricate and cool the drive shaft.

Mechanism of Action

The mechanism of this device is identical to that of a blender. A blender contains a cutting blade at the bottom of a vessel. The blade has a cutting edge and is slightly tilted (pitched). This allows for both the cutting of particles and for their recirculation. By recycling cut particles over and over again, particle size is progressively reduced. The effectiveness of a blender depends also on revolutions per minute and duration of application. The miniature version of a blender blade used in this design rotates in a small, metallic housing with two large sideholes made to allow for material recycling. The use of a nonencased rapidly rotating turning blade would be dangerous if used in the vascular system. Consequently, the blade is recessed in the metal housing, preventing contact with the vessel wall.

Results

The completeness of clot dissolution is directly related to both the duration and the speed of rotation of the propeller. It should be noted that simply moving the catheter back and forth within the clot without rotation of the propeller, 50% clot disruption was achieved after 2 minutes. However, at 10,000 rpm, 2 minutes of application resulted in 95% dissolution. A similar degree of clot dissolution occurred after only 27 seconds at 60,000 rpm. Finally, at 80,000 rpm, 97% dissolution was achieved after just 10 seconds.

The vast majority of the residue after fragmentation was normal-appearing red blood cells. In addition, there was a sparse scattering of inhomogeneous aggregates of amorphous, nonstaining material that contained basophilic clumps of material resembling disrupted white cell nuclei. The largest of these measured 208 μm in greatest diameter. No fibrin fragments or other potentially embolic debris was seen.[3,8]

Plasma hemoglobin prior to clot formation was 159 mg/dl (for our laboratory, normal is less than 15 mg/dl). Following clot formation and mechanical lysis, plasma hemoglobin was 228 mg/dl.[3,8]

Discussion

Clinical application of this technique may be possible in both the venous and arterial systems (Fig. 18-5).[9–13]

Probably the most promising application of this new technique is the mechanical dissolution of clotted arterial bypass grafts. These thromboses are usually recent because they are immediately clinically evident. Therefore clot dissolution can be expected to be similar to the in vitro experiments. Occlusion of the distal anastomosis or outflow vessels should not be necessary in order to prevent embolization. The extremely forceful, retrograde flow produced by the device should allow the clot to be dissolved from its proximal extent to its distal extent without any tendency to push or expel debris of any significant size distally. Mechanical dissolution may be accomplished in a few minutes compared to hours or days for enzymatic thrombolysis. Advantages of mechanical dissolution over enzymatic thrombolysis are ones of time and expense, since current thrombolytic regimens require intensive care unit monitoring, often for several days, multiple angiographic procedures to monitor the progress of thrombolysis, and repeated laboratory tests such as the prothrombin time, partial thromboplastin time, thrombin time, and fibrinogen level.[14] In addition, the complications of enzymatic thrombolysis such as hematoma at the puncture site, internal bleeding, distal embolization of large particles (including remote mural thrombi sources), pericatheter thrombosis, graft extravasation, fever, and allergic reactions are eliminated.

Whether the mechanical catheter thrombolysis can become even more effective and faster when combined with the simultaneous administration of low-dose thrombolytic agents infused through the sideport of the catheter currently remains to be demonstrated. One might expect that this would reduce the embolic potential of mechanical clot lysis. However, our present early results would indicate that

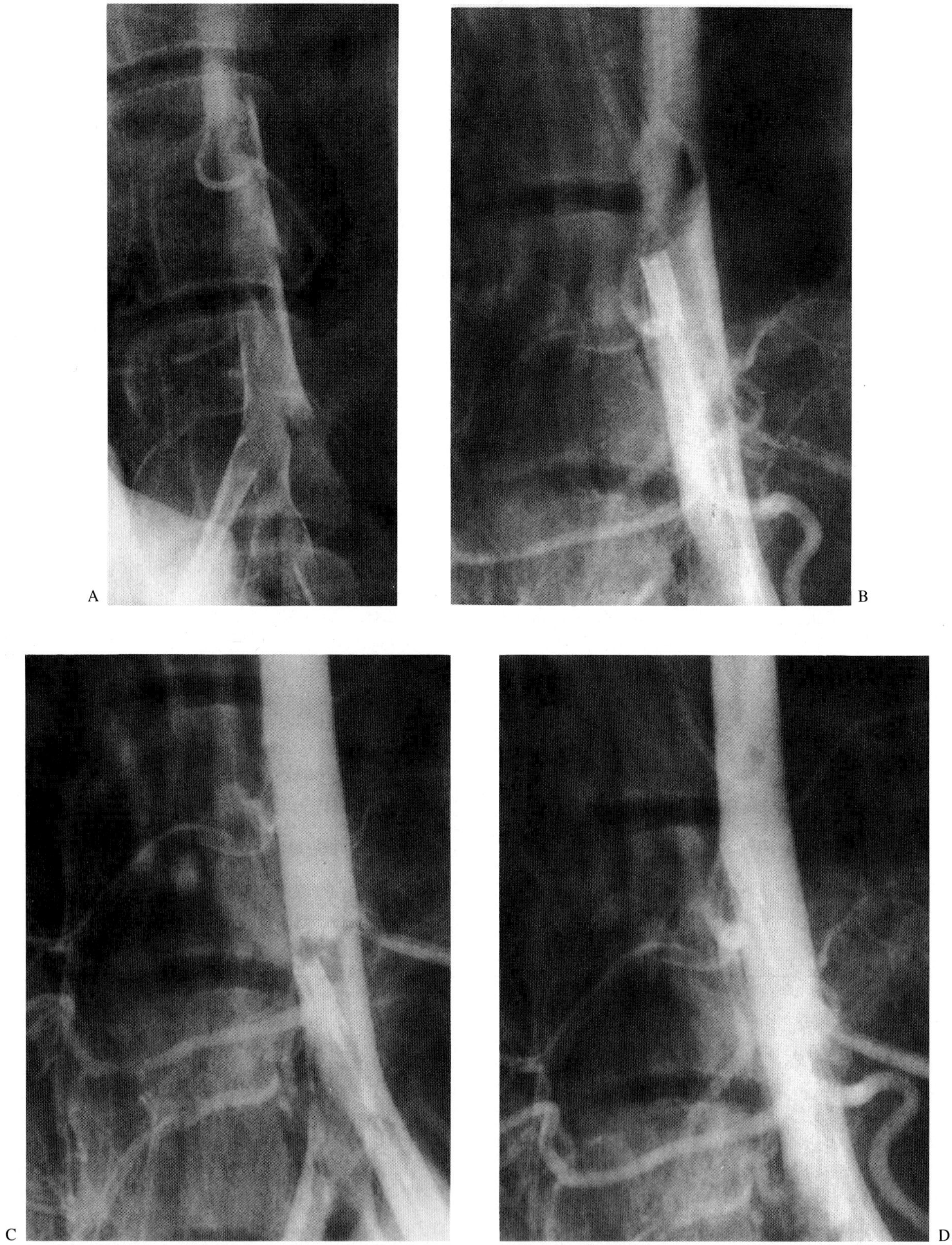

Figure 18–5. **A:** Aortogram in a dog after thrombosis of the abdominal aorta. Note extensive thrombus. **B:** Film taken during the thrombectomy procedure. Note the position on the catheter tip in relationship to the large thrombus in the abdominal aorta. **C:** Toward the end of the thrombectomy procedure. Note that most of the thrombus in the abdominal aorta has been removed. The thrombectomy device is removing the most distal fragments. **D:** Near completion of the procedure, note small fragments in the proximal abdominal aorta and a residual fragment in the right common iliac artery.

simultaneous thrombolytic agent infusion may not appreciably diminish the number and size of particles, since tiny particles most likely represent combinations of cytoplasmic and nuclear cell fragments rather than fibrin.

PONOMAR TRANSJUGULAR CLOT-TRAPPER DEVICE

Pulmonary embolism is a known complication of lower extremity and iliac vein thrombosis, with an estimated nonfatal pulmonary embolism incidence in the United States of 600,000/year, and a mortality rate of 140,000/year.[15]

Most pulmonary emboli originate in the iliocaval (63.8%) and femoral-popliteal segments (36.2%).[16] The presence of free-floating thrombus within the iliac veins or the inferior vena cava (IVC) is a common indication for the placement of an IVC filter, but if the thrombus load is too large, patency of the IVC cannot be guaranteed after filter placement.

Recently, several devices have been described for the percutaneous removal of thrombus, predominantly in the arterial side, but with obvious applications on the venous side, including the thrombus aspiration catheters[13] and mechanical clot dissolution devices.[3–8,18] A mechanical device has also been used for thromboembolectomy in patients with pulmonary emboli.[13] All of these devices need to reach the level where the thrombus is lodged, in order to either aspirate it or mechanically fragment it in situ. The risk with these methods is that a fragment of the thrombus might be dislodged and embolize into the pulmonary arteries. This is particularly risky in the presence of a large free-floating thrombus in the IVC or iliac veins. The clot-trapper device (CTD) was developed for the removal of large amounts of thrombus from the iliac veins and from the IVC. The device can be used in conjunction with a mechanical thrombectomy device[3,8,9,17] to fragment the thrombus once this has been caught within the bag.

The prototype CTD consists of a 12 F double lumen catheter (Fig. 18-6). The smaller lumen of the catheter is 15 cm long in the distal end of the device and houses a stainless steel wire whose distal end emerges as a spring loop at a 90° angle to the shaft. The loop is attached to the distal end of a 15 cm long funnel-shaped polyvinyl bag. The proximal end of the bag is connected to the second lumen. The distal end of the bag can be opened or closed by advancing or retracting the wire. Adjustments on the size of the spring loop allows adaptation to different IVC diameters.

In the proximal end of the large lumen there is a coaxial introducer with a check-flow valve and a sidearm flushing

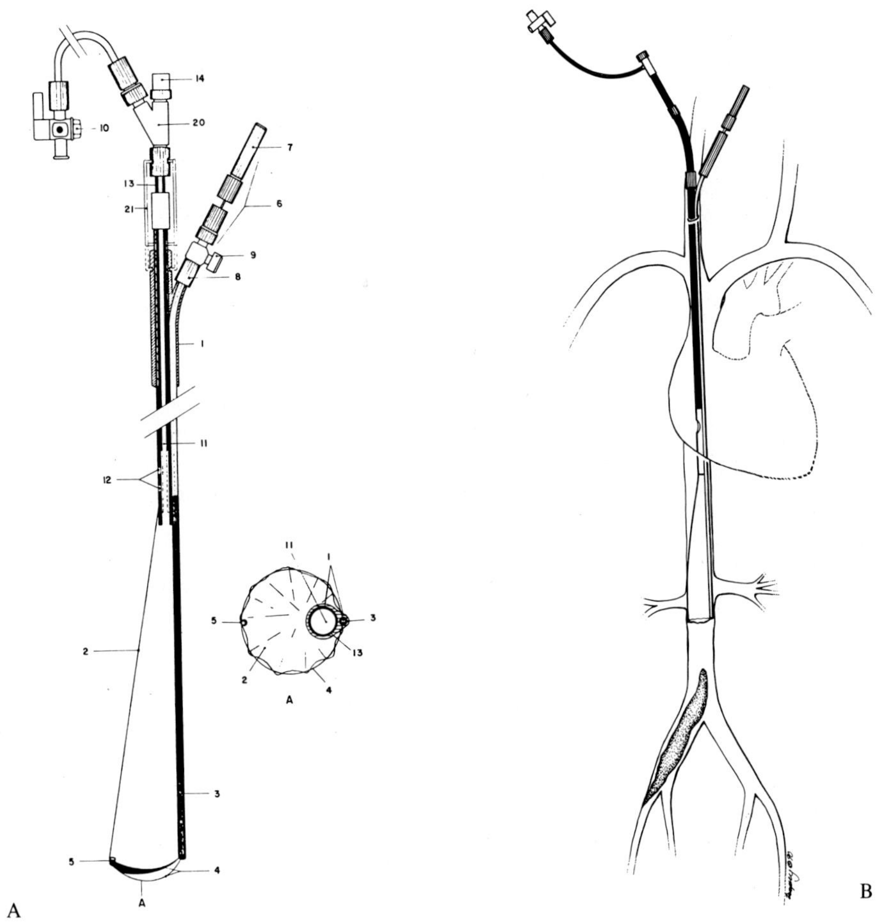

Figure 18–6. **A:** Diagrammatic representation of the Ponomar device. **B:** Diagram illustrating the position of the Ponomar retrieval device below the level of the renal veins. Large thrombus is seen in the right common iliac.

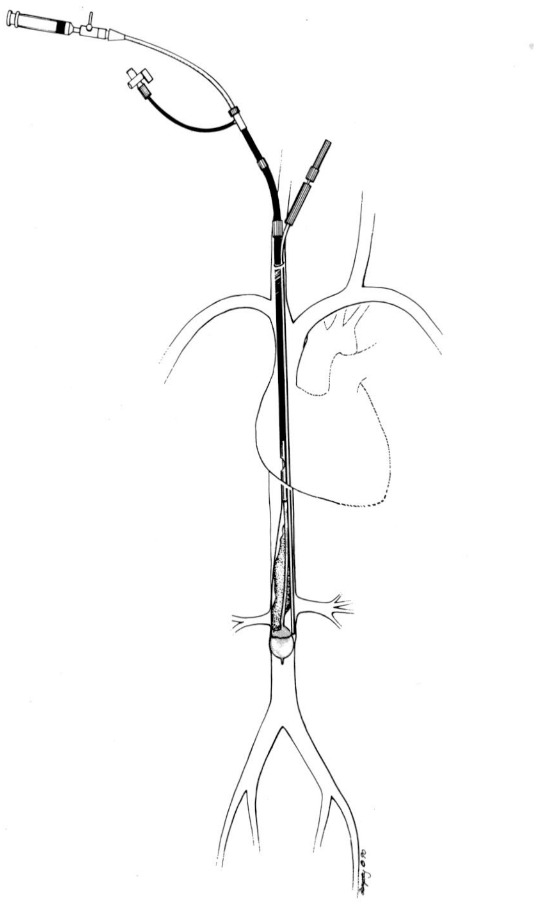

Figure 18–7. A balloon has been used to pull the thrombus into the bag.

port. The forward movement of the introducer closes the sideholes, made in the midsegment of the large lumen just above the connection of the large lumen with the proximal end of the bag.

The CTD for transjugular thrombectomy is introduced using a venous cutdown in the right internal jugular vein to place a 20 F Teflon sheath. The CTD is then introduced through the sheath over a stiffening wire. Commonly, the distal end of the CTD is placed below the level of the renal veins in the IVC (Fig. 18-6B). The bag is opened to allow the blood flow in the vena cava to pass through the bag and go out through the two sideholes in the lateral wall of the large lumen, thereby preserving vena caval flow. A balloon catheter is introduced through the check-flow valve and is advanced over a guide wire into the iliac vein or IVC where the thrombus is lodged. By injecting contrast medium in the iliac vein through the endhole of the catheter, the thrombus is localized; using the inflated balloon, the thrombus is pulled toward the opening of the bag (Fig. 18-7). Once the thrombus is trapped in the bag, the check-flow introducer set is pushed forward to close the sideholes. The injection of contrast material through the sidearm allows verification of the presence of the thrombus in the bag. The balloon is deflated, withdrawn, and the entrance of the bag closed, effectively trapping the thrombus. The injection of contrast material through the sidearm allows verification of the presence of the thrombus in the bag. Flow through the IVC is not blocked during this maneuver for more than a few seconds. The CTD was first tested in an IVC simulator to determine its ability to trap in vitro-created thrombus. In all experiments, the Amplatz mechanical thrombectomy device (MTD) was used to destroy thrombus trapped in the bag (Fig. 18-8).

Results

In vitro-created thrombus (16 contrast labeled and 16 unlabeled) were introduced into the iliac vein and IVC and trapped successfully by the CTD. All the thrombi were then successfully fragmented by the MTD.

In two dogs, extensive semiacute IVC thrombus produced by clipping the infrarenal IVC was removed using the CTD in combination with the MTD (Fig. 18-9).

Histopathologic examinations of the IVC after the use of the CTD showed endothelial desquamation. No evidence of perforation was found.

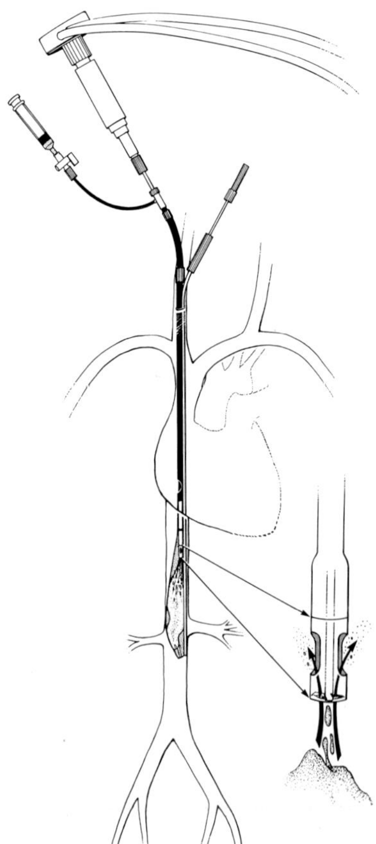

Figure 18–8. After closing the end of the bag, the Amplatz thrombectomy device has been introduced for fragmentation of the captured thrombus.

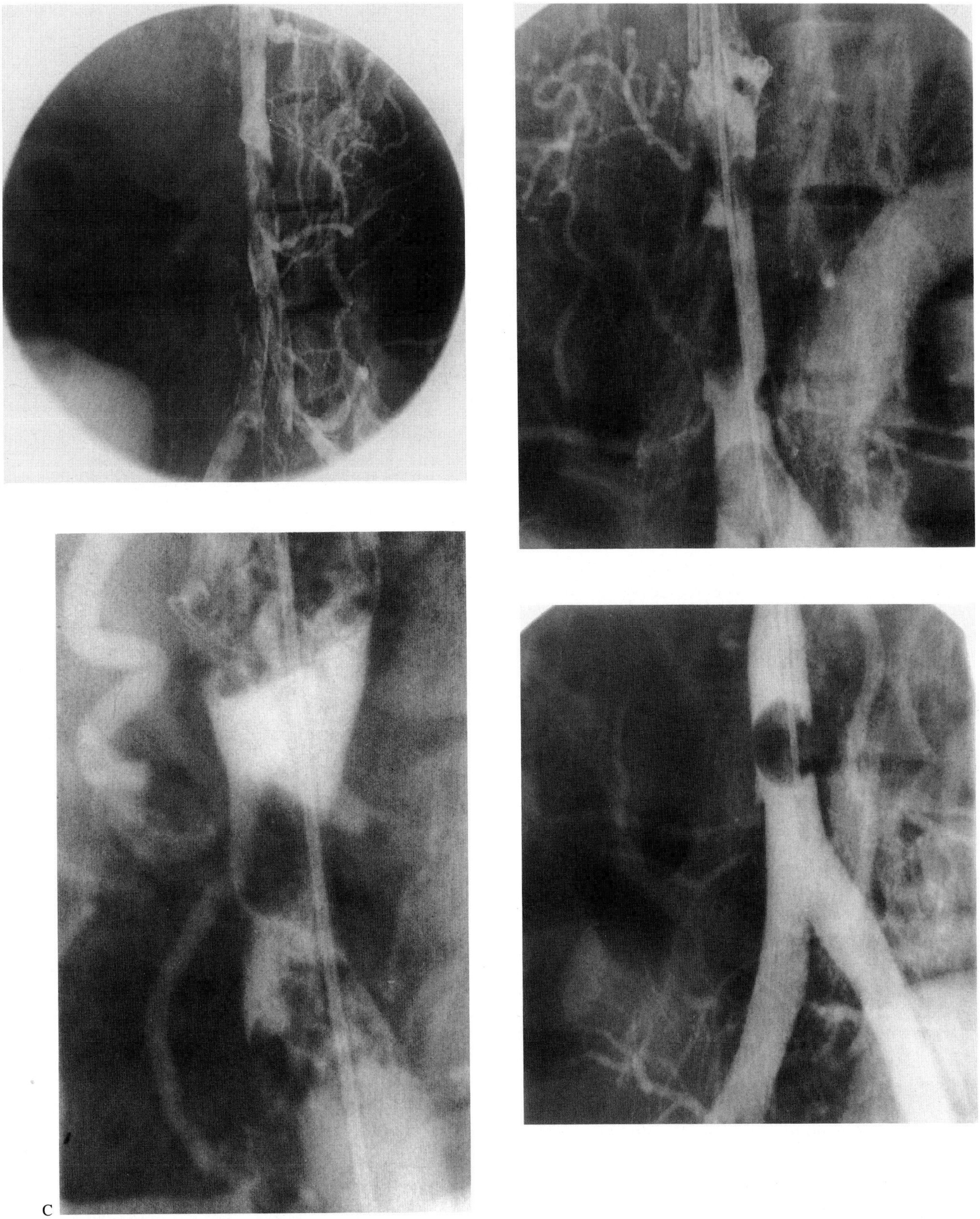

Figure 18–9. **A:** Inferior vena cavagram 7 days after clipping shows extensive thrombosis of the inferior vena cava and proximal iliac veins. **B:** A Ponomar retrieval device has been placed below the level of the renal veins and a balloon is used to pull the thrombus in the inferior vena cava into the bag. **C:** Close-up showing large amount of thrombus being pulled back by the balloon into an almost completely filled bag. **D:** Inferior vena cavagram following thrombectomy shows widely open iliac veins and inferior vena cava.

Discussion

The management of acute iliofemoral venous thrombosis remains a difficult problem, particularly if a large floating thrombus is present in the IVC or iliac veins. Several authors have reported the use of MTDs for the rapid removal of thrombus from arteries or veins.[3–9,18–21] All of these devices have the risk of embolization of the fragmented thrombus. This would be particularly dangerous in the presence of large free-floating thrombus in the IVC or iliac veins. The CTD was developed for the removal of large amounts of thrombus from the iliac veins or IVC.

Mechanical thrombus fragmentation inside the bag of the CTD where the clot is isolated reduces the possibility of embolism. Our preliminary in vitro and in vivo results are encouraging. CTD, used in combination with MTD, will enable the quick and effective removal of large venous thrombi from the IVC and the iliac veins. A large thrombus in the iliac vein or IVC can usually be fragmented and pulled into the bag. Once the bag is filled, its end is closed prior to fragmentation with the MTD. If there is fear of migration of untrapped fragments, the bag can be left open, since the IVC blood flow will keep the trapped thrombus within the bag during fragmentation with the MTD. The suction produced by the MTD further attracts the thrombus against the end of the device. Contrast medium can be injected through the lumen of the MTD to facilitate visualization of the trapped thrombus in the bag.

Further improvements in the technology will allow an easier introduction, since, in its present prototype stage, the device requires a 20 F size introducer sheath. The use of a 30 mm universal diameter bag will allow, in most cases, a good match with the IVC diameter. The diameter of the IVC will be determined by inferior vena cavography. Oversized bags can be made available for large IVCs.

RHEOLYTIC THROMBECTOMY CATHETER

Methods

DEVICE CONSTRUCTION

The rheolytic thrombectomy catheters were fabricated from 4 to 6 F dual-lumen tubing. The smaller lumen contains a high-pressure stainless steel tubing used to supply the saline jets; this lumen also is used as the inflation lumen for a latex balloon, which serves to center the catheter tip in the vessel lumen. A second larger lumen provided for the evacuation of debris can also be used to inject drugs or contrast medium or to pass a guide wire. The stainless steel tubing at the catheter tip has 4 to 8 jet orifices 25 to 50 μm (0.001 to 0.002 inch) in diameter. One jet is directed against the catheter's large lumen to promote the evacuation of debris; the remaining jets are oriented at a retrograde angle to avoid direct impact on the vessel wall, while providing, at the same time, the necessary mixing and recirculation for effective clot lysis (Fig. 18-10). A positive displacement pump supplies pressurized saline to the catheter and is activated by a foot switch by the catheter operator.

Results

IN VITRO TESTING

The rheolytic thrombectomy catheter (RTC) lysed the thrombus in all cases.[21] Thrombi ten centimeters long were lysed by the catheter at 10,000 to 13,000 psi in 1 minute. The RTC left very little remaining thrombus, less than that from the Fogarty procedure. The RTC jets infused saline typically at a rate of 50 ml/min, removing debris at the same rate through the evacuation lumen.

IN VIVO TESTING

The RTC was used to lyse and evacuate thrombi from eight vessels.[21] The average age of the thrombus was 4 days (range, 3 to 7 days); the average pressure used was 12,000 psi. The RTC successfully lysed thrombus and restored patency in all cases. Balloon thrombectomy procedures were used to declot four vessels. There appeared to be more residual thrombus seen on postprocedure radiographs using the balloon procedure than following the use of the RTC.

Excised vessels after thrombectomy using the RTC showed little damage; the excised graft and native vessels from the animals sacrificed in 2 weeks following the thrombectomy procedure showed lack of an endothelialized surface on the expanded polytetrafluoroethylene (ePTFE) graft; the native femoral artery was free of thrombus and showed little wall trauma. Histologic examination demonstrated no damage to the elastica in the vessels in which the RTC was used. The rheolytic catheter was capable of removing 1-week-old thrombus from both the ePTFE graft and the native vessel. In contrast, the vessels after balloon thrombectomy showed a pattern of damage consistent with the radial stress pattern expected using a balloon.

For most of the procedures, the RTC was introduced through a guiding catheter, which helped to position the device and allowed for contrast medium delivery; however, the flexibility of the RTC enabled it to follow a 0.014 inch guide wire when that was desired. No vessel dissection or perforations were evident in any of the experiments.

Debris collected from the evacuation lumen of the catheter consisted of clumps of platelets and red blood cells; effluent blood that was collected downstream of the thrombus during RTC thrombectomy consisted primarily of individual red blood cells with occasional clumping.

Discussion

The ability of the rheolytic thrombectomy catheter to lyse clots at least 1 week old in vivo points to its potential usefulness in a variety of cases.

The RTC advantages over the Fogarty-type balloon embolectomy procedures include reduced vessel wall trauma and

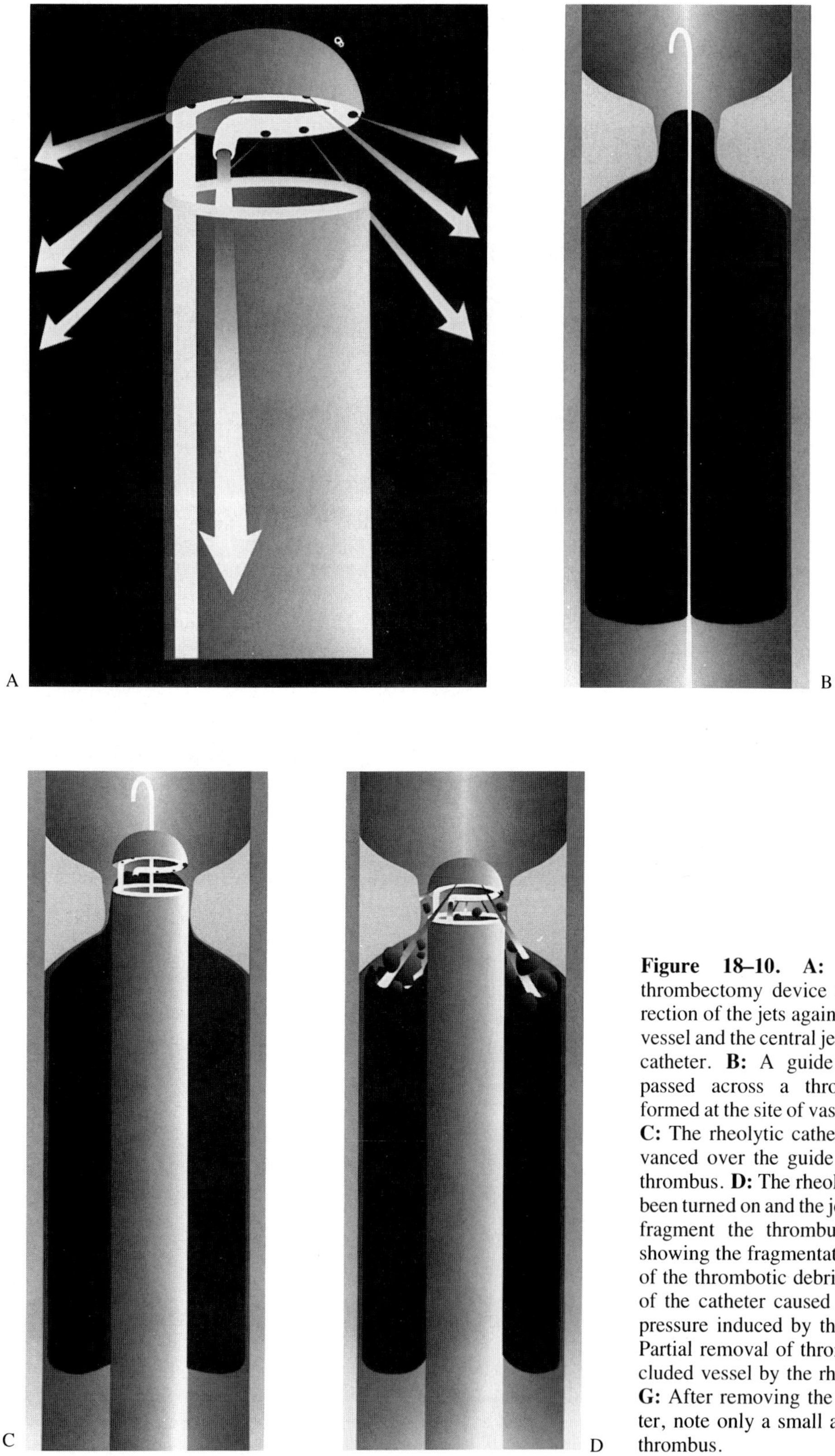

Figure 18–10. **A:** The rheolytic thrombectomy device showing the direction of the jets against the wall of the vessel and the central jet into the luminal catheter. **B:** A guide wire has been passed across a thrombus that has formed at the site of vascular narrowing. **C:** The rheolytic catheter has been advanced over the guide wire across the thrombus. **D:** The rheolytic catheter has been turned on and the jets have began to fragment the thrombus. **E:** Close-up showing the fragmentation and removal of the thrombotic debris into the lumen of the catheter caused by the negative pressure induced by the central jet. **F:** Partial removal of thrombus on the occluded vessel by the rheolytic catheter. **G:** After removing the rheolytic catheter, note only a small amount of mural thrombus.

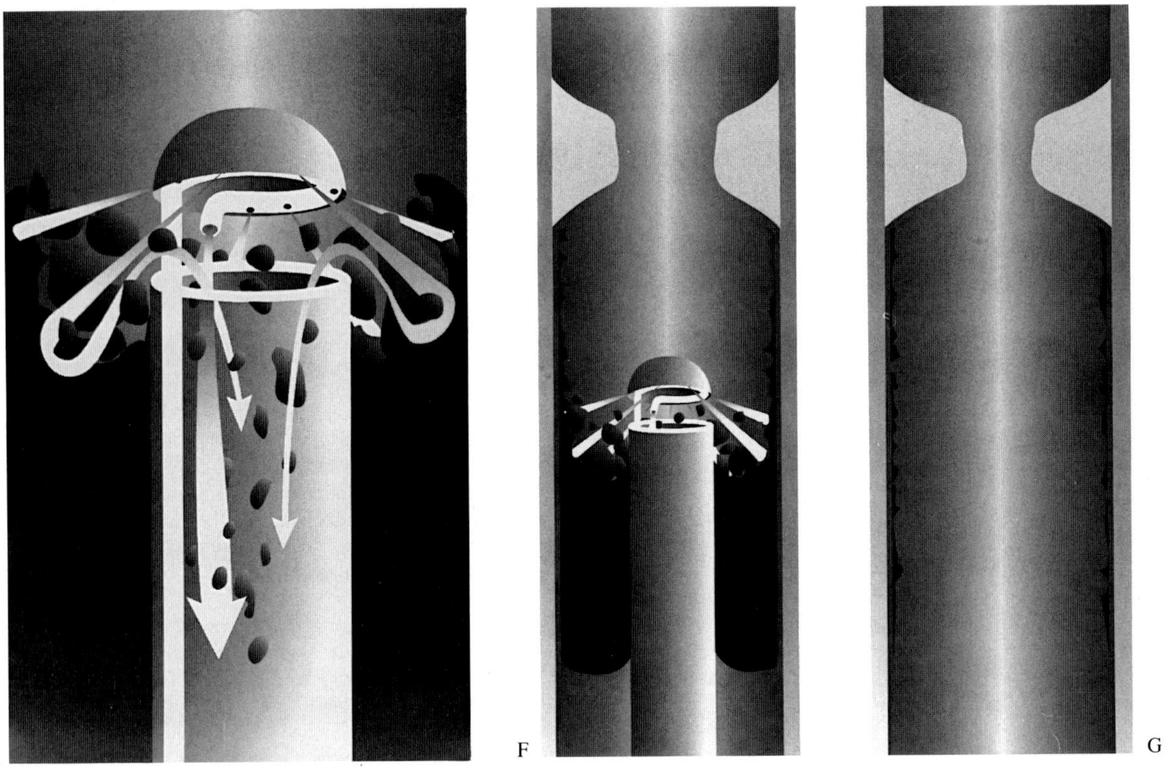

E F G

Figure 18–10 (continued)

the treatment of thrombi not easily treatable by balloon embolectomy because of the percutaneous access combined with fluoroscopic guidance. The removal of the thrombotic debris seems desirable, rather than the mere fragmentation of thrombus achieved by other devices,[3,7–9,17,20] although controlled studies of distal embolization have not been done using the RTC to verify the benefit of debris evacuation. Debris removal, combined with the jet action breaking the thrombus into small fragments, seems preferable to balloon embolectomy procedures or other mechanical thrombectomy devices.

Although heparin anticoagulation would likely be used perioperatively, the local action of the RTC may significantly reduce the incidence of bleeding complications compared with thrombolytic agents. In addition, thrombolytic drugs often require many hours for complete clot lysis, whereas treatment using the RTC may provide rapid symptomatic relief in a matter of minutes.

The main shortcoming of other mechanical thrombectomy devices appears to have been addressed by the RTC system, that is, the ability of the RTC to clear vessels much larger than the catheter diameter. In addition, the RTC may be able to lyse an entire lesion on a single pass of the device, thus avoiding the repeated withdrawal and reinsertion required with other devices.

By infusing radiologic contrast material via the evacuation lumen of the RTC, direct assessment of the vessel lumen may be obtained without the need to use a separate catheter.

Acute pulmonary emboli requiring treatment faces a variety of undesirable choices. Open vessel surgical embolectomy is associated with great operative risk; thrombolytic drug therapy is time-consuming and may be ineffective despite the risk of bleeding complications. The rapid treatment of large pulmonary emboli by a percutaneous device has been advocated; the RTC may offer fast, effective treatment and thus significantly reduce mortality and morbidity. In addition, it may be desirable to lyse any large thrombi found in the deep veins, using the RTC immediately, to reduce the likelihood of recurrent pulmonary emboli.

The ability of the RTC to follow a guide wire and access coronary vessels suggests its possible use in acute myocardial infarction, after sufficient preclinical and clinical testing.

CONCLUSIONS

An effective system for the percutaneous lysing and removal of thrombus utilizing high-velocity saline jets has been presented. The ability of this rheolytic thrombectomy catheter system to lyse thrombus up to 1 week old has been demonstrated both in vitro and in vivo in canine arteries and in vascular grafts. Initial vessel examinations from short-term in vivo studies were favorable, and follow-up in one animal demonstrated patent vessels and ePTFE vascular graft 2 weeks following thrombectomy using the RTC. The size and flexibility of the catheter, and its ability to follow a guide wire, suggest possible application to the treatment of acute coronary thrombosis.

REFERENCES

1. Cohen LH, Kaplan M, Bernhard VM. Intraoperative streptokinase: an adjunct to mechanical thrombectomy in the management of acute ischemia. Arch Surg 1986;12:708–15.
2. Fogarty TJ, Chin AK, Ollott C, et al. Combined thrombectomy and dilation for the treatment of acute lower extremity arterial thrombosis. J Vasc Surg 1989;10:530–4.
3. Bildsoe MC, Moradian GP, Hunter DW, et al. Mechanical clot dissolution: new concept. Radiology 1989;171:231–3.
4. Hansen DD, Auth DC, Vracko R, Ritchie JL. Rotational thrombectomy in acute canine coronary thrombosis. Int J Cardiol 1989;22:13–19.
5. Hansen DD, Auth DC, Vracko R, Ritchie JL. Mechanical thrombectomy: a comparison of two rotational devices and balloon angioplasty in subacute canine femoral thrombosis. Am Heart J 1987;114:1223–31.
6. Kensey KR, Nash JE, Abrahams C, Zarins CK. Recanalization of obstructed arteries with a flexible, rotating tip catheter. Radiology 1987;165:387–9.
7. Yedlicka J, Carlson J, Hunter DW, et al. Thrombectomy with the TEC endarterectomy system: an experimental study. Radiology (in press).
8. Moradian GP, Bildsoe M, Hunter DW, et al. In-vivo mechanical clot dissolution. Experimental work in progress. Radiology 1988;169(suppl):366.
9. Carlson JE, Sunram SE, Kurisu Y, et al. New mechanical thrombectomy device. Radiology 1990;177(suppl):125.
10. Fluid and hemodynamic derangements. In Robbin SL, Cotran RS (eds): Pathologic Basis of Disease, 2nd ed. Philadelphia: WB Saunders, 1979:123.
11. Moser KM, LeMoine JR. Is embolic risk conditioned by location of deep vein thrombosis? Ann Intern Med 1981; 94:439–44.
12. Bomalaski JS, Martin GJ, Hughes RL, Yao JST. Inferior vena cava interruption in the management of pulmonary embolism. Chest 1982;82:767–72.
13. Greenfield LJ, Kimmell GO, McMurdy WC III. Transvenous removal of pulmonary emboli by vacuum-cup catheter technic. J Surg Res 1969;9:347–52.
14. Klatte EC, Becker GJ, Holden RE, Yune HY. Fibrinolytic therapy. Radiology 1986;159:619–24.
15. Dalen JE, Alpert JS. Natural history of pulmonary emboli. Prog Cardiovasc Dis 1975;17:259–70.
16. Savelyev VS, Yablokov EG, Kirienko AI. Surgical prevention of pulmonary embolism. World J Surg 1980;4:709–16.
17. Ponomar E, Carlson JE, Kindlund A, et al. Clot trapper device for transjugular thrombectomy from the inferior vena cava. Radiology (in press).
18. Günther RW, Vorwerk D. A new aspiration thromboembolectomy catheter with propeller-tipped rotating wire. An in-vitro study. J Intervent Radiol 1990;1:17–20.
19. Günther RW, Vorwerk D. Aspiration catheter for percutaneous thrombectomy: clinical results. Radiology 1990;175:271–3.
20. Hawkins IF, Helms R, Spencer C, Hawkins MC. Mechanical spiral embolectomy catheter. Semin Intervent Radiol 1985; 2:414–8.
21. Drassler WJ, Jenson ML, Thielen JM, et al. A rheolytic catheter for percutaneous removal of thrombus. Circulation (in press).

19 Simpson's Atherectomy Catheter: Technical Description, Operating Mechanism

Manuel Maynar-Moliner, M.D., Ricardo Reyes, M.D., J. M. Pulido-Duque, M.D., E. Gorriz, M.D., J. M. Felices, M.D.

The Simpson's Atherocath (Redwood City, CA) allows the percutaneous transluminal removal of atheromatous material from the vessel lumen.[1]

It consists of a double lumen catheter (Fig. 19-1), which is described in three sections for better understanding:

1. The main part of its operating mechanism is located in the distal section. This consists of a cylindrical metal capsule with a longitudinal window on one side measuring 1.5 cm. Opposite the window is a low-pressure (30 psi) balloon that is used to force the window against the atheromatous plaque.

A cylindrical cutting blade is located at the end of a metal cable extending along the catheter. This cutter is used to resect the plaque storing it in the distal part of the capsule. A floppy guide wire is attached to the distal end of the capsule. This steerable guide wire allows manipulation of the Atherocath through the narrowed segments of vessel.

At the proximal end of the catheter, there is one port that is used to inflate and deflate the balloon. A side port allows flushing of either saline or contrast medium through the catheter.

A battery-powered motor drive is used to power the cutter's cable at the base of the catheter. The cutting device rotates at 2000 rpm.

2. Since its invention, the Simpson catheter has undergone a series of improvements in its construction (Fig. 19-2).

A tank made of flexible material has been fitted to the distal end of the metal capsule between the capsule and the floppy guide wire. This permits storage of a greater amount of atheromatous material, thus reducing the number of passes to be made. This new design must be used carefully when dealing with lesions in the distal part of the popliteal artery, since the capsule and storage chamber length together may occlude blood flow to distal arteries (Fig. 19-3).

The floppy guide wire, attached to the distal part, is joined to the storage tank by a screw system (Fig. 19-4). This system enables the guide wire to be replaced if it is damaged, either when passing through the introducer sheath or along the vessel.

The new Atherocath is provided with a sheath at its distal end that protects the floppy guide wire when passing it through the introducer sheath. Another improvement in the Atherocath design is the capability of advancing it over a guide wire. This improvement facilitates the use of the Atherocath in total arterial occlusions after recanalization.

3. Finally, the diameters of the balloon in the capsule have been made larger, as well as the length of the window (20 cm). The Atherocaths available now are 7, 8, 9, 10, and 11 F, which correspond to working diameters of 4.8, 5.7, 6.0, and 7.7 mm.

OPERATING MECHANISM

The most important changes of the atherosclerotic process take place in the intimal layer of the vessel, although minor changes in the internal elastic lamina and media are also common.

The two phenomena that affect the intima, causing a reduction in arterial lumen and producing symptoms of vascular obstruction, are proliferation of modified smooth muscle cells and the deposition of lipid material.

The purpose of the atherectomy procedure is to remove the atherosclerotic material that protrudes into the vessel lumen. Once the Atherocath has been placed at the level of the stenosis, the balloon is inflated, forcing the atheromatous plaque into the window of the capsule. It is essential to match the working diameter of the Atherocath (inflated balloon plus capsule) to the diameter of the vascular lumen at the stenotic site so that the material protruding from the arterial wall can be resected. When the motor is switched on and the cutter is moved toward the distal end of the capsule, the material removed is stored in the tank (Fig. 19-5).

Obviously, if the diameter of the catheter is smaller than the artery, it will be more difficult (if not impossible) for the atheromatous plaque protruding from the wall to enter the capsule.

In our experience with 43 lesions correlated in terms of diameter, we have observed that in 100% of cases in which no material was removed, the arterial diameter was larger than that of the atherectomy device, and in 72% of cases in which the number of pieces removed was greater than 7, the arterial diameter was the same or smaller than that of the Atherocath.

The operating mechanism of angioplasty cannot be explained by the remodeling of atheromatous material alone,[2] since the plaques are not compressible, as opposed to the theory of Dotter and Judkins,[3] which explains the underlying mechanism of the angioplasty as one of compression and remodeling of the atheromatous material. The greatest advantage of atherectomy compared with angioplasty is with

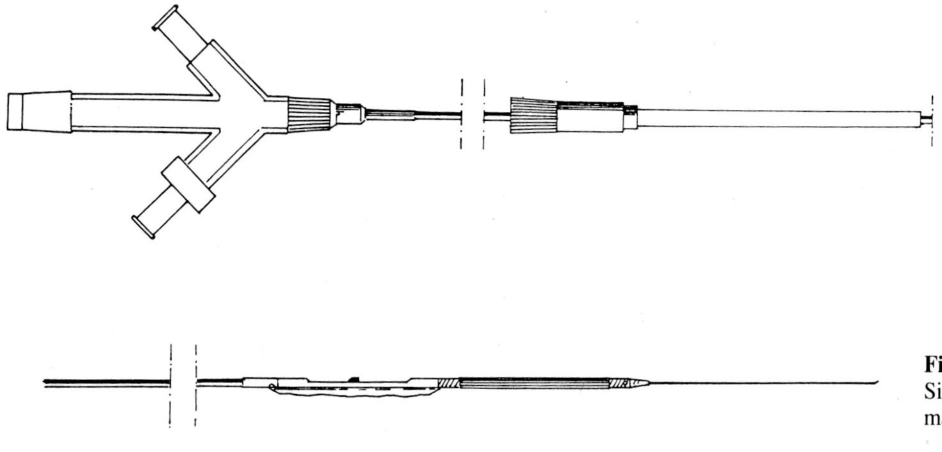

Figure 19–1. Schematic diagram of Simpson's Atherocath shows the proximal and distal parts of the catheter.

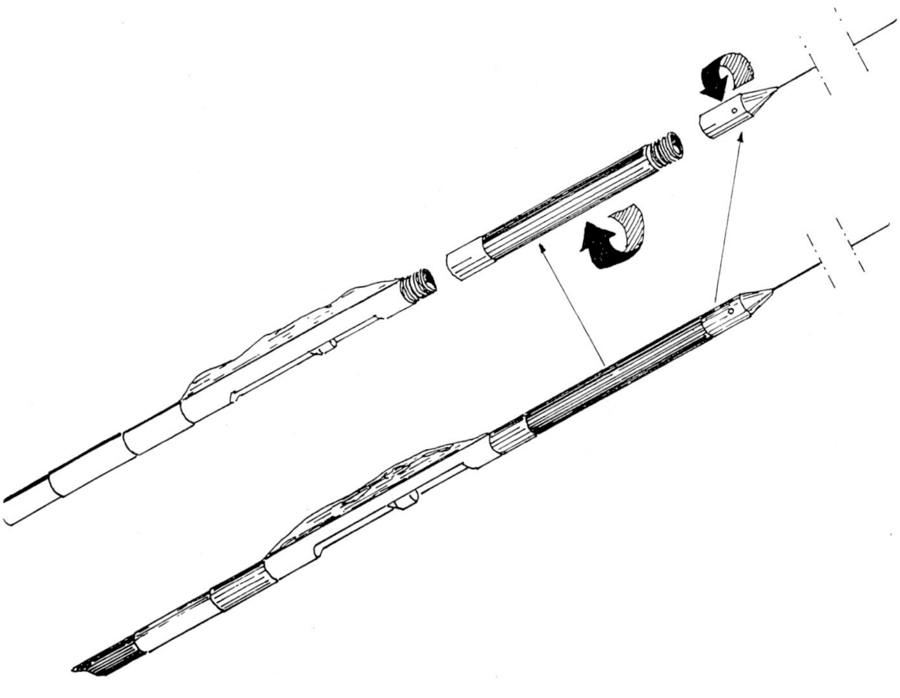

Figure 19–2. New Simpson's Atherocath has a storage tank between the capsule and the floppy guide wire.

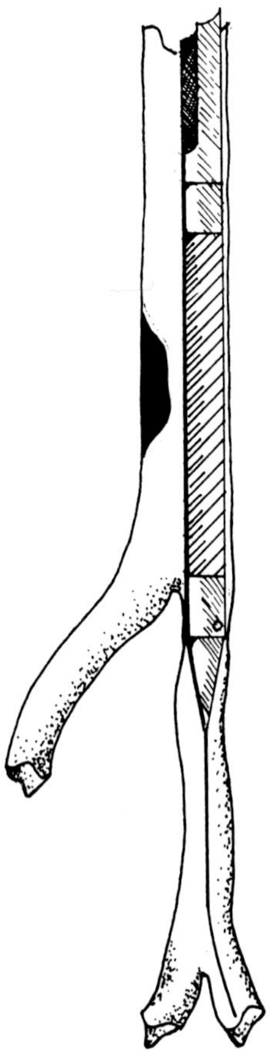

Figure 19–3. This new model must be used carefully in distal vessels because it may occlude the flow.

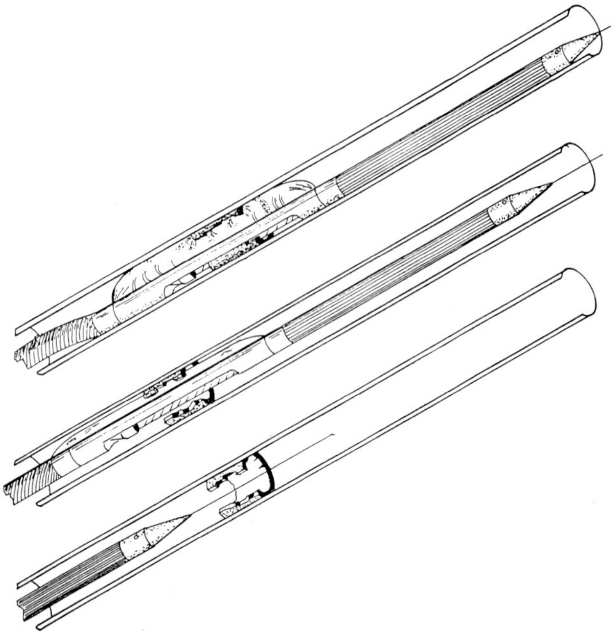

Figure 19–5. It is important to match the working diameter of the Atherocath to the diameter of the vascular lumen at the stenotic site.

regard to the differences in the operating mechanisms of both. The main difference between both procedures is that angioplasty pushes the plaque against the arterial wall after fracturing the intima, while atherectomy removes the plaque that protrudes into the arterial lumen without damaging the wall (Fig. 19-6A-E). In histologic studies of vessels subjected to angioplasty, the most characteristic findings are dehiscences between the intima and media, which may give rise to intimal flaps and, on the other hand, the corkscrew deformity of the smooth muscle cell nuclei.

Unlike in angioplasty, the mechanism of the atherectomy ensures the removal of the plaque without damaging the arterial wall. The potential advantage of this technique compared with angioplasty is that it acts by means of various mechanisms.

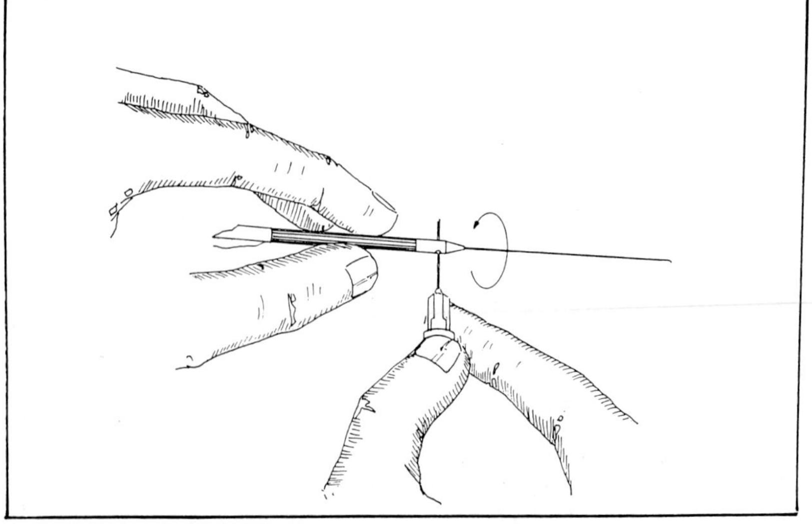

Figure 19–4. The guide wire is removable in this new model. It is joined to the storage tank by a screw system.

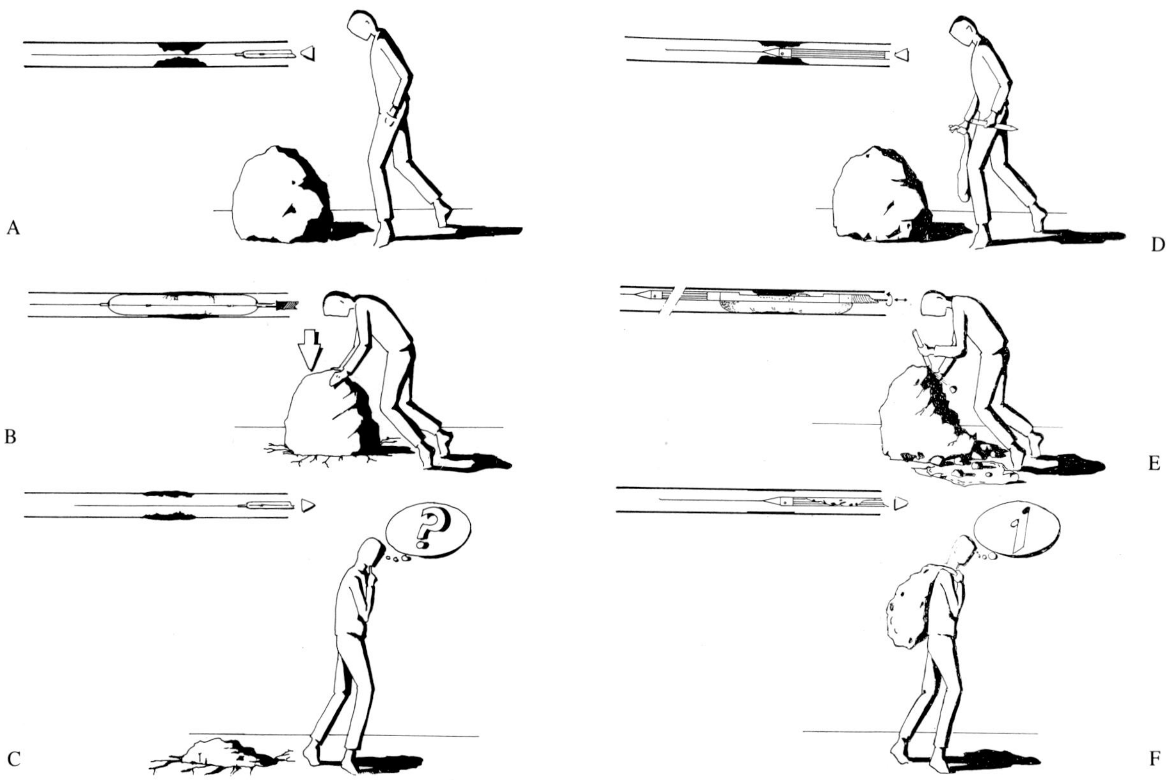

Figure 19–6. Diagrammatic portrayal of the angioplasty balloon compared with the atherectomy catheter. **A, B, C:** When the balloon is inflated, plaque is pushed against the wall. The obstacle is removed by pushing it against the wall. **D, E, F:** Positioning the balloon forces the Atherocath capsule against plaque, which is then cut by the device. The obstacle is then carried away.

In the first place, the most important mechanism is the cutting and removing of atheromatous material. On the other hand, it acts by increasing the lumen by a Dotter coaxial mechanism and a balloon dilation effect caused by the positioning balloon inflation. This dilation phenomenon has been clearly observed in some of our cases in which, despite the removal of a small amount of material, the angiographic result obtained was excellent.

Histologic examination revealed the presence of atheromatous material in all cases. In one case, components of the media layer were found. This finding is explained by the fact that the Atherocath will only cut material protruding into the capsule. The position of the capsule parallel to the arterial wall prevents tissues, other than those protruding into the vascular lumen, to enter the capsule's window.

Using the atherectomy technique, the plaque is removed and turbulence in the vessel reduced following the procedure, which thus improves long-term patency.

MANEUVERING OF THE ATHEROCATH

The Atherocath is introduced through the sheath introducer. This posed a problem in the first generation, since the floppy guide could not cross the diaphragm of the introducer sheath. To overcome this difficulty, a method was designed using a 16 G Teflon catheter.

Using a scalpel, the catheter is cut along its length. The modified catheter is placed over the guide wire (Fig. 19-7). The distal section of the catheter moves forward through the introducer sheath valve, with one hand of the operator holding the proximal part of it and the other inserting the Atherocath. Once the guide has passed through the diaphragm of the introducer sheath, the catheter is removed and used in successive reinsertions of the Atherocath.

Currently, the new catheter model has a Teflon sheath (Fig. 19-8) that opens the valve of the introducer sheath allowing the guide wire to pass through it without being damaged. Once the catheter is in the arterial lumen, it is advanced under fluoroscopic control, ensuring that the guide does not enter a side branch and bend (Fig. 19-9), which would require a repetition of the process after replacing the guide.

Roadmapping is a good aid in positioning the catheter in place, ensuring its position at the stenotic lesion.

Sometimes in tortuous vessels (especially iliac arteries), it is difficult to advance the metal capsule toward the desired area. To overcome this problem, the use of a long introducer sheath is useful, advancing the distal end beyond the lesion. Next, the capsule is positioned within the introducer sheath

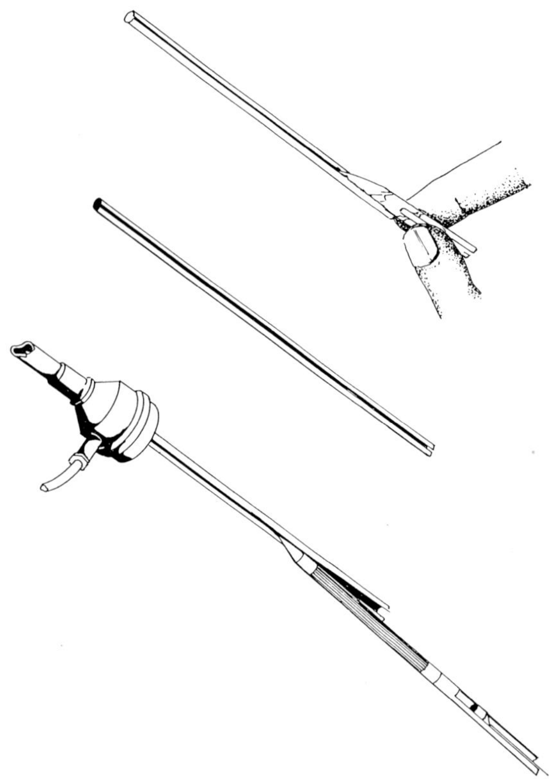

Figure 19–7. This was the method used in old models to introduce the Atherocath without damaging the distal guide wire. Using a scalpel, a catheter is cut along its length. This modified catheter is placed over the guide wire and both are advanced through the introducer sheath.

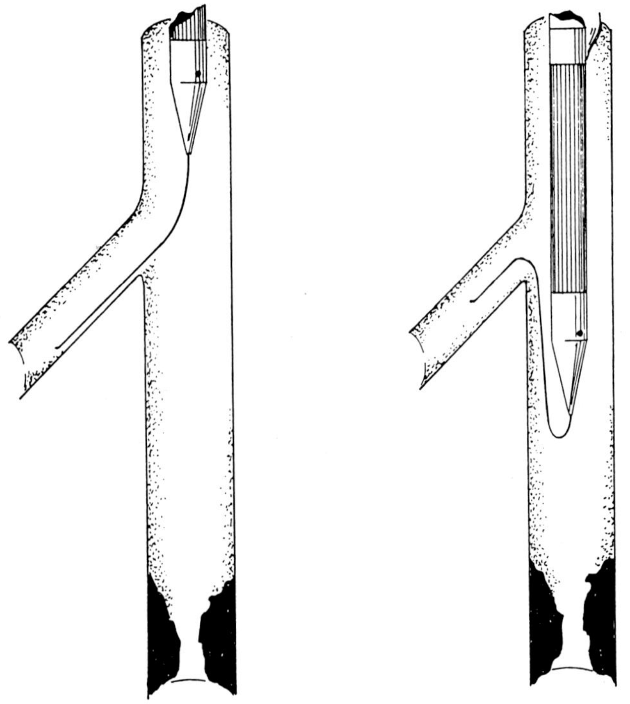

Figure 19–9. The catheter must be advanced through the artery under fluoroscopic control, ensuring that the guide wire does not enter a side branch and bend.

beyond the area to be treated. At this point, the introducer sheath is pulled back distal to the lesion, leaving the capsule at the desired level (Fig. 19-10).

After placing the capsule against the stenosis, the balloon is inflated, the motor drive is activated, and the cutter blade advanced. After deflation of the balloon, the capsule is rotated and the procedure repeated. The capsule window must be in contact with the whole internal surface of the vessel, rotating always in the same direction (from 45° to 45°) until the path is completed (Fig. 19-11).

When the storage compartment is full, the Atherocath is withdrawn. During withdrawal, it is important that the cutter is in the distal part of the capsule to prevent the loss of

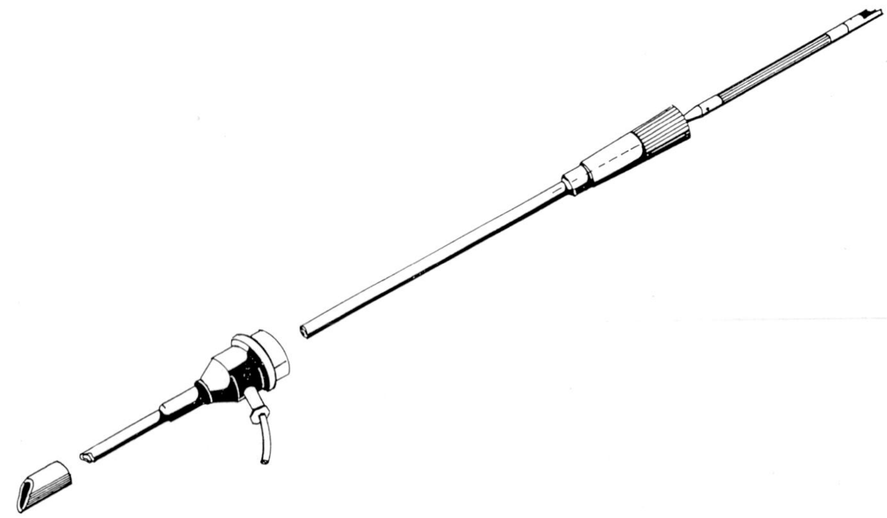

Figure 19–8. New catheter model has a Teflon sheath that allows it to pass through the guide wire without being damaged.

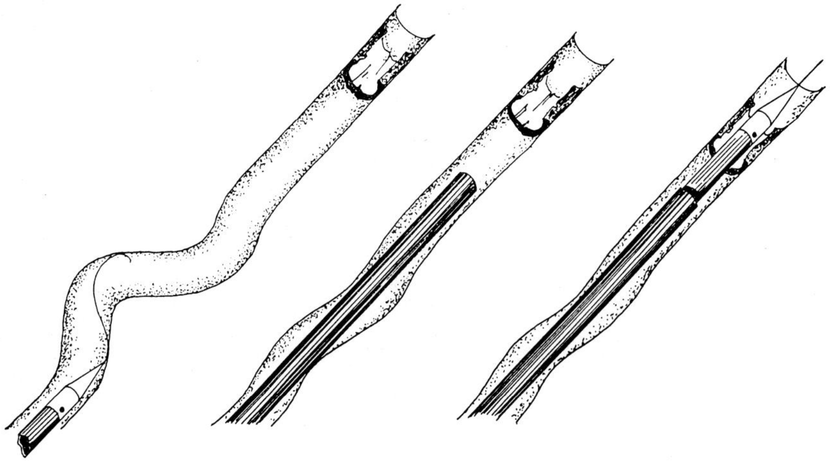

Figure 19–10. Long introducer sheath to advance the metal capsule is useful in tortuous vessels.

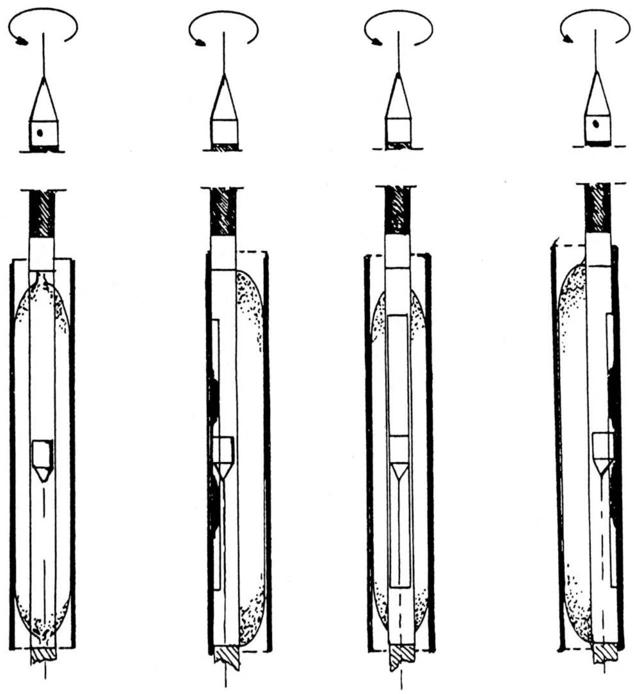

Figure 19–11. The capsule window must be in contact with the whole internal surface of the vessel, rotating always in the same direction.

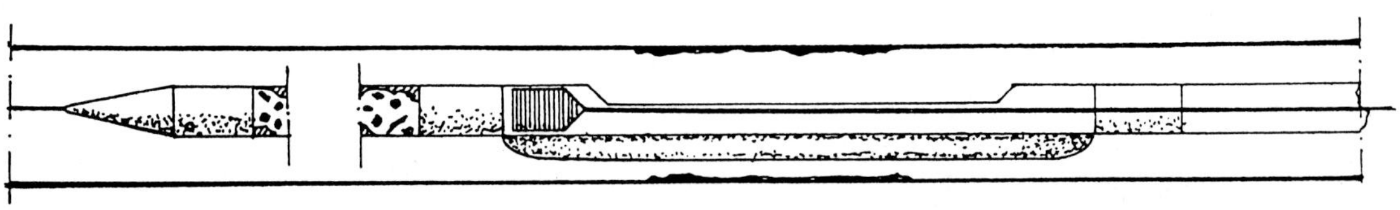

Figure 19–12. The cutter must be maintained in the distal part of the capsule when the Atherocath is withdrawn.

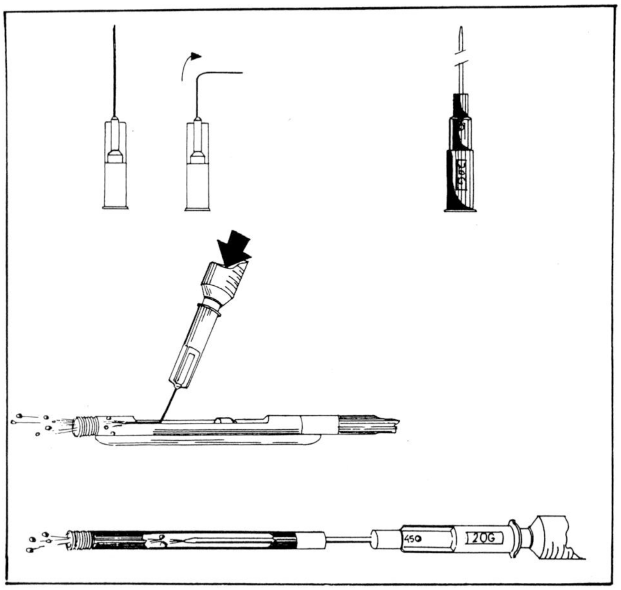

Figure 19–13. A bent insulin needle is used to flush the capsule and the storage tank.

atheromatous material through the window of the capsule, thus leading to possible embolization (Fig. 19-12).

With the capsule above the auxiliary table, the atheromatous material deposited inside is removed. A bent insulin needle can be used to flush the different compartments. In the same way, the tank is flushed once dismantled, using a thin needle (Fig. 19-13).

The samples obtained are sent for histopathologic study and weighing.

A follow-up angiography is performed and the procedure repeated until the best morphologic result for the affected vessel has been obtained. Pressure gradient, angioscopy, and intravascular ultrasound can also be useful to evaluate the results of the procedure. The latter allows a review of the whole inner surface of the artery, showing the amount of atheromatous plaque retrieved with the atherectomy catheter.

REFERENCES

1. Schwarten DE, Katzen BT, Simpson JB, Cutcliff WB. Simpson catheter for percutaneous transluminal removal of atheroma. AJR 1988;150:799–801.
2. Castañeda-Zúñiga WR, Formanek A, Tadavarthy M, et al. The mechanism of balloon angioplasty. Radiology 1980;135:565.
3. Dotter CT, Judkins MP. Transluminal treatment of atherosclerotic obstruction. Circulation 1964;30:654–7.
4. Maynar M, Reyes R, Cabera V, et al. Percutaneous atherectomy as an alternative treatment for postangioplasty obstructive intimal flaps. Radiology 1989;170:1029–31.

20 Percutaneous Atherectomy of the Iliac Arteries

Manuel Maynar-Moliner, M.D., Ricardo Reyes, M.D., J. M. Pulido-Duque, M.D., M. DeBlas, M.D., J. M. Felices, M.D., E. Gorriz, M.D., M. Casal, M.D., Wilfrido R. Castañeda-Zúñiga, M.D.

It is difficult to improve on the results obtained in the iliac arteries by percutaneous transluminal angioplasty, with patency rates between 85 and 90% at 7 years.[1–3] Simpson's Atherocath was developed for the treatment of arterial stenosis and allows the percutaneous removal of atheromatous material without injuring the arterial wall.[4]

The 9 or 11 F Simpson Atherocath was used, depending on the size of the iliac artery to be treated. In total, we have performed 36 atherectomies of the iliac arteries in 31 patients: 29 males and two females, aged between 37 and 80 years (average age, 59.4 years). All had incapacitating claudication, and one had rest pain. Twenty-seven were smokers and 17 were diabetics. All patients were evaluated clinically, hemodynamically (Doppler, ankle and arm levels), and angiographically before the procedure. In total, 27 lesions of the common iliac artery were treated (23 stenoses and four obstructions), and nine stenoses of the external iliac artery. All patients were anticoagulated during the procedure. The material removed was sent for histopathologic examination.

TECHNIQUE

The Simpson Atherocath can be used only through a unilateral retrograde femoral approach. Because of the lack of over-the-wire capability and mostly because of the rigidity of the metal capsule, the Atherocath cannot be advanced from the axillary or contralateral femoral approach. Because of these characteristics, there is a need to use an introducer sheath with hemostatic valve to advance the catheter into the lumen of the vessel. The Atherocath is then advanced under fluoroscopic control to the level of the lesion. Roadmapping is useful to place the capsule with the window opposite to the atheromatous plaque. The accumulation of atheromatous material inside the capsule can be observed under fluoroscopy by observing the cutter stopping short of the capsule's end. When the storage compartment is full, the Atherocath is withdrawn and the atheromatous material is evacuated. During withdrawal of the Atherocath, it is important to maintain the cutter in the distal end of the capsule, in order to prevent the loss of resected atheromatous material through the window of the capsule, thus leading to possible embolization. Follow-up angiograms in various projections are performed after Atherocath withdrawal in order to evaluate the result. The procedure is repeated until a good morphologic result is obtained, although it can be considered terminated when, after various cuts, it is impossible to extract more atheromatous material. However if significant residual atheromatous obstruction (over 30%) is present, and the Atherocath does not resect more material, a larger Atherocath should be used in order to complete the atherectomy procedure.[5] Alternatively, as is the case in the iliac arteries, when the largest Atherocath available is smaller than the arterial diameter, angioplasty is used to achieve a complete reconstitution of the vessel lumen. It is necessary to ensure that the residual stenosis is less than 20%.

In the four cases of total obstruction of the common iliac artery, the obstructions varied in length from 1 to 3 cm. In two of these patients, recanalization was followed by percutaneous atherectomy; in one, a transluminal angioplasty was performed before the insertion of the atherectomy catheter, and in the fourth, thrombolytic treatment was performed initially followed by atherectomy (Fig. 20-1).

In cases with tortuous iliac arteries, it is difficult to advance the Atherocath to the level of the lesion. In these cases, a long introducer sheath can be used, placing the distal end beyond the obstruction (Fig. 20-2). The Atherocath is inserted through the sheath, placing the metal capsule at the desired level. When dealing with complete obstructions, a 0.012 to 0.014 inch guide wire should be passed beyond the obstructing lesion to avoid the risk of losing the access across the recanalized segment[6] (Fig. 20-3).

RESULTS

The primary success of atherectomy alone or in combination with angioplasty was 97.22%. In four cases, no atheromatous material was removed and in 16 others the amount removed was minimal. In all these cases, a significant residual stenotic lesion remained, which made it necessary to use angioplasty afterward to maximize lumen reconstitution. Isolated atherectomy was used in 15 procedures (41.67%) (Figs. 20-4, 20-5); on 19 occasions (52.78%), it was combined with angioplasty balloon. In one case, fibrinolysis was performed prior to atherectomy, and in another, fibrinolysis and angioplasty were combined with atherectomy. Thirty patients showed clear clinical and hemodynamic improvement following treatment, with increase of the ankle to arm indices (average improvement, 0.23). Complications included one arterial thrombosis that required surgery and a dissection that was successfully treated with angioplasty.

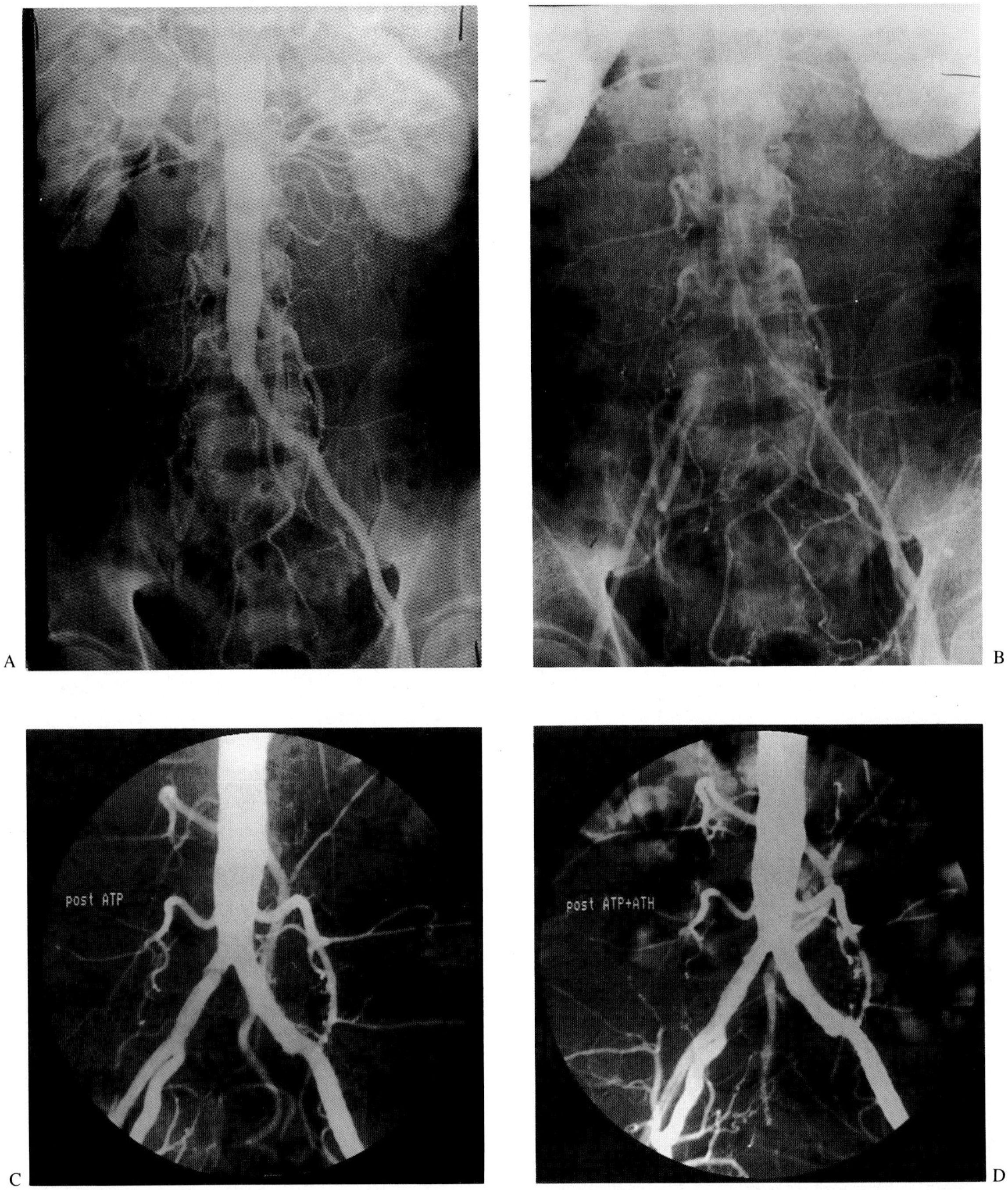

Figure 20–1. **A:** Angiography shows 100% occlusion of the right common iliac artery. **B:** Reconstitution of the external iliac artery by collaterals is demonstrated. **C:** Follow-up angiography after fibrinolysis and angioplasty. Note intimal flap at site of dilation. **D:** Angiography after atherectomy shows a widely patent artery at the site of revascularization. Note disappearance of intimal flap.

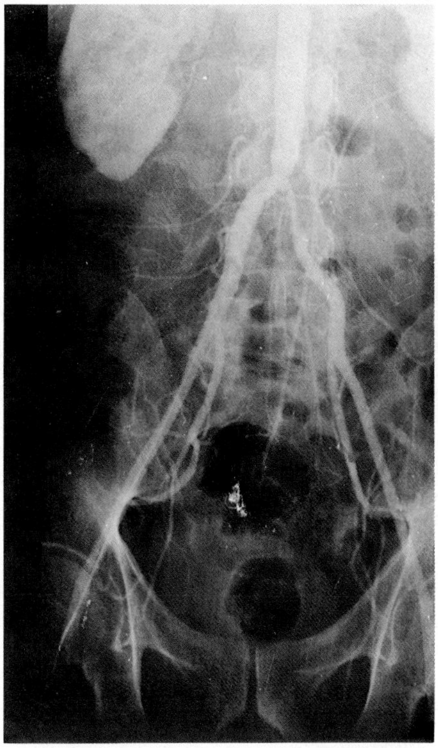

A

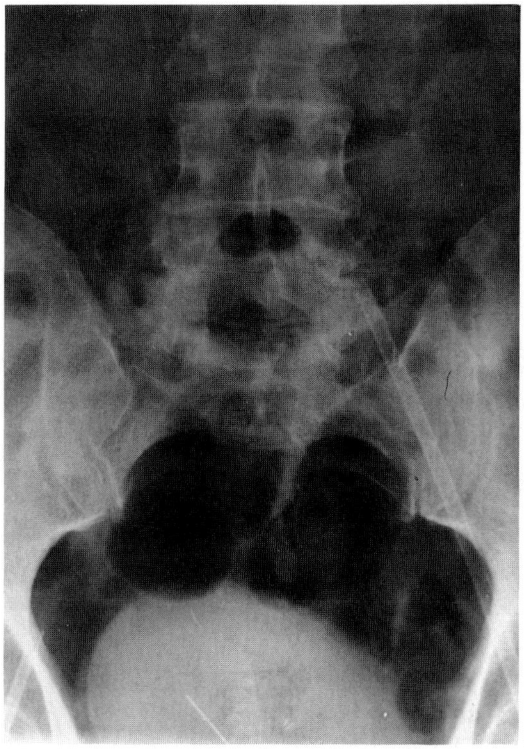

B

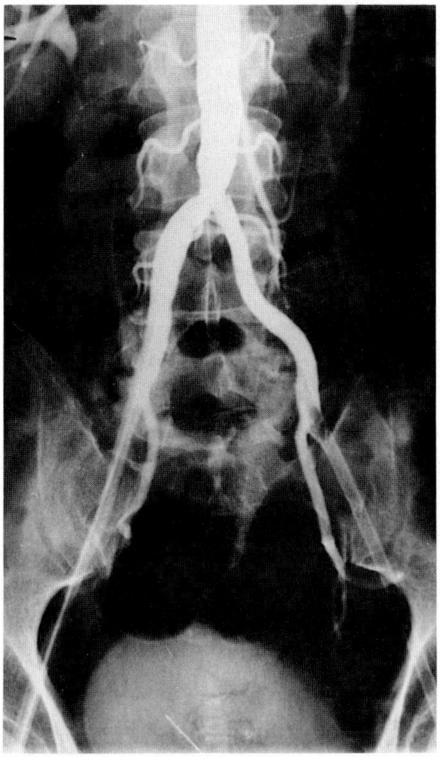

C

Figure 20–2. **A:** Angiography shows a severe stenosis of the left common iliac artery. **B:** Plain film of the abdomen shows the 11 F introducer sheath used for the advancement of the Simpson atherectomy catheter through the tortuous iliac artery. **C:** Follow-up angiography after atherectomy shows a widely open lumen. Note occlusion of flow by introducer sheath at the external iliac artery level.

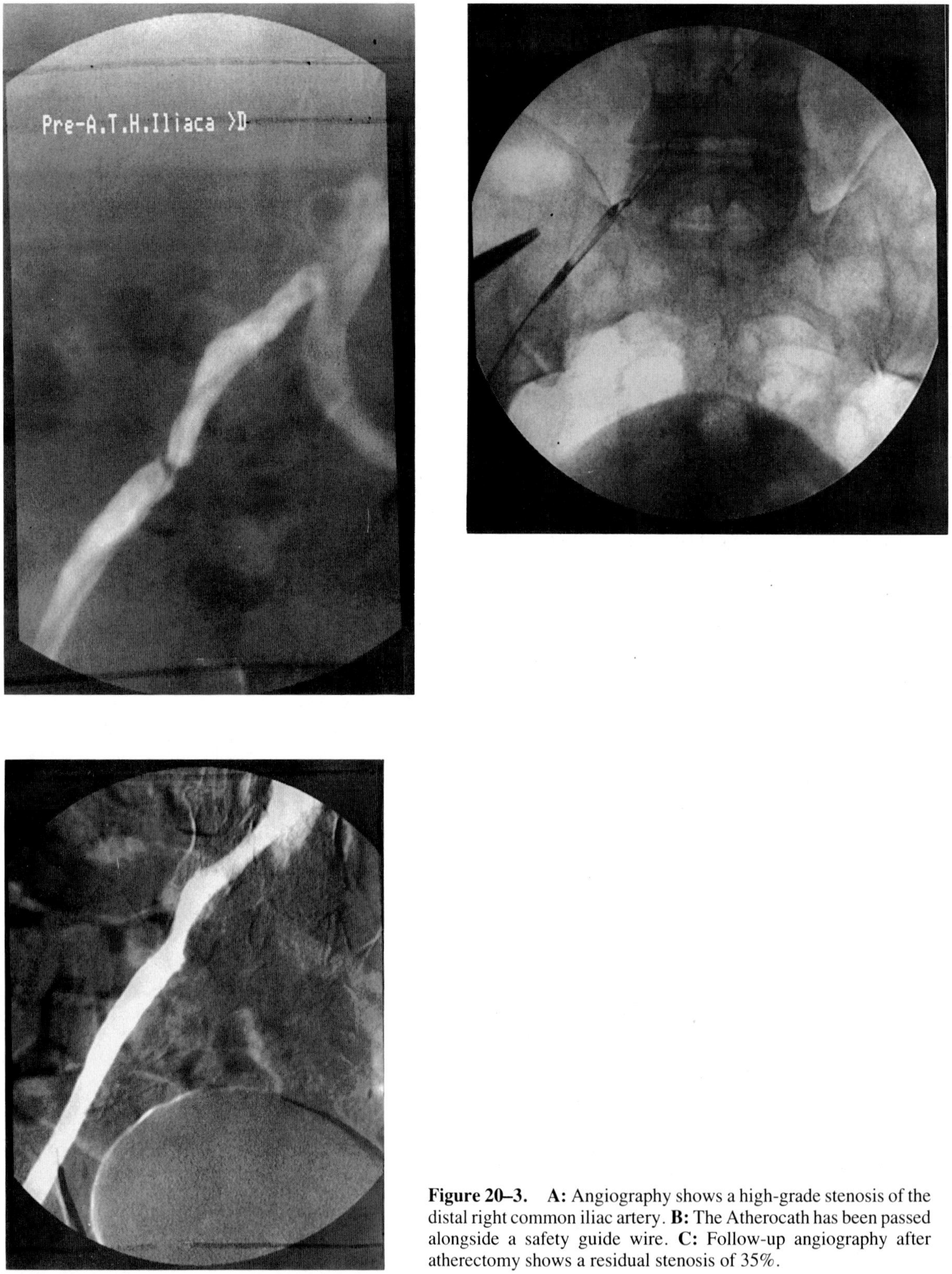

A

B

C

Figure 20–3. **A:** Angiography shows a high-grade stenosis of the distal right common iliac artery. **B:** The Atherocath has been passed alongside a safety guide wire. **C:** Follow-up angiography after atherectomy shows a residual stenosis of 35%.

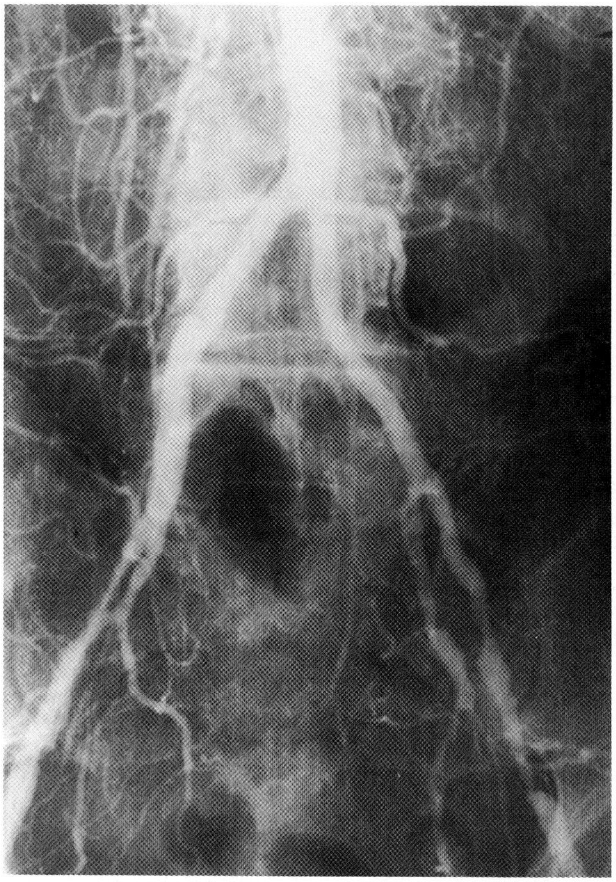

A

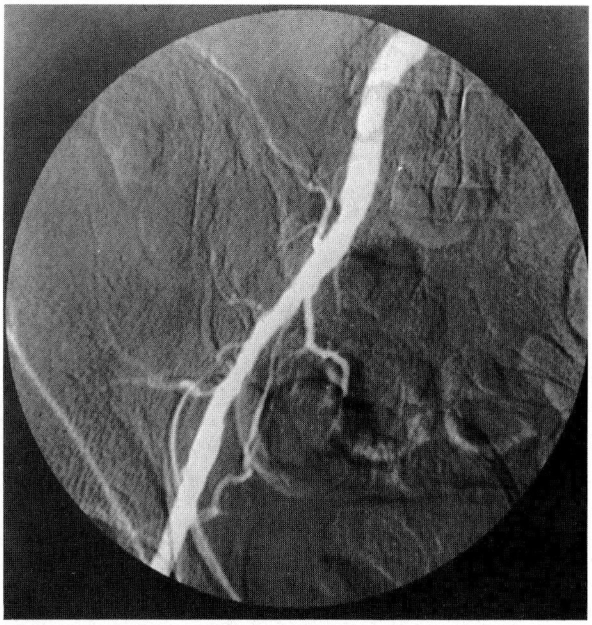

B

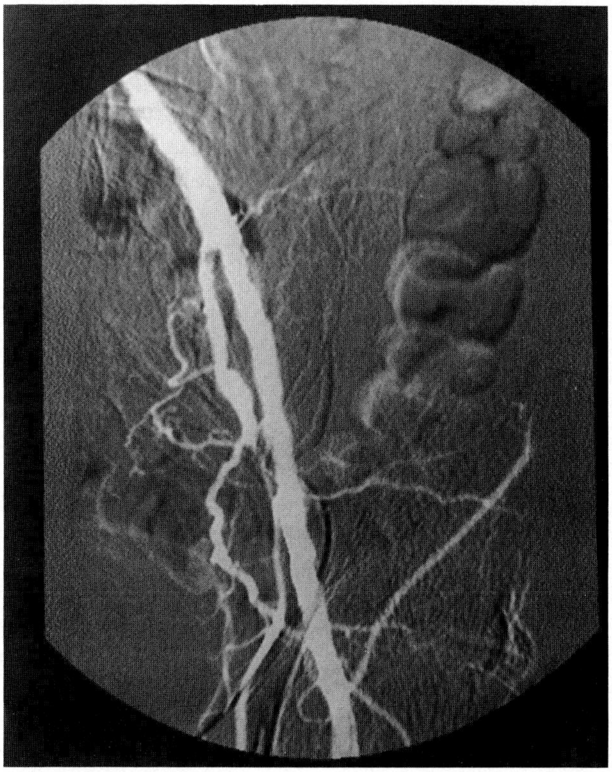

C

Figure 20–4. Bilateral iliac stenotic lesions treated with the Simpson Atherocath. **A:** Angiography shows severe stenotic lesions of both external iliac arteries. **B:** Right iliac arteriogram after atherectomy shows a widely patent lumen with a residual 20 to 30% stenosis. **C:** Left iliac arteriography shows an almost complete reconstitution of the arterial lumen.

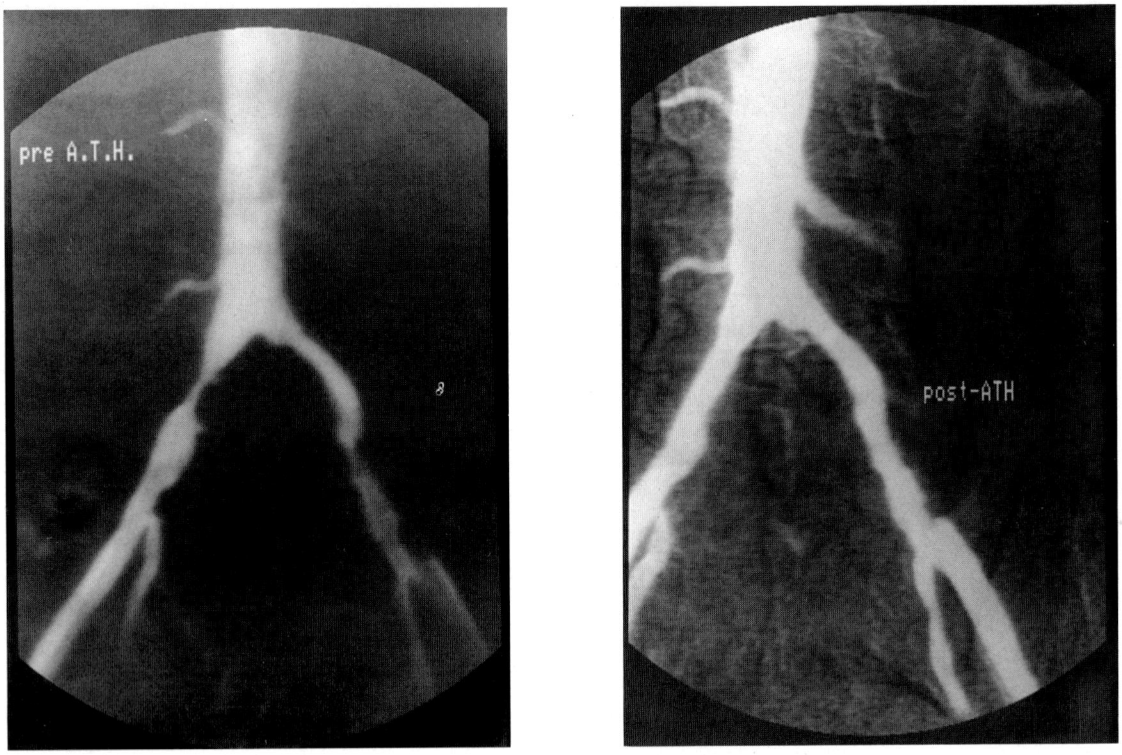

A B

Figure 20–5. **A:** Angiography shows severe stenotic lesions of both common iliac arteries. **B:** Right iliac arteriography after atherectomy shows a widely lumen at the atherectomy sites, but residual 30% stenosis.

DISCUSSION

The small amount of atheromatous material removed in several patients reflects the poor match between the arterial diameter and the diameter of the Atherocath.[7] In these cases, angioplasty had to be performed in order to complete lumen reconstitution. One disadvantage of the Atherocath in the iliac area is the discrepancy between the arterial diameter and the working diameter of the Atherocath (diameter of the capsule plus diameter of the inflated balloon), which makes it impossible to remove all the atheromatous material present. In these cases, an angioplasty must be performed to complete lumen reconstitution, therefore avoiding a significant residual stenosis.

The main argument here is why to use an expensive device like the Atherocath in the iliac arteries, since commonly there is a poor match of the device diameter with the iliac artery diameter. In addition, angioplasty results in the iliac artery are quite satisfactory, in the order of 80 to 90%. The rationale to use atherectomy in the iliac artery, particularly in cases with severe stenosis, is to remove as much atheromatous material as possible in order to improve the results of angioplasty by leaving a smoother lumen after dilation. By debulking the plaque with the Atherocath, fewer intimal flaps will be present following angioplasty and, it is hoped, a better long-term patency rate will be obtained (Fig. 20-6).

Obviously, when a good match between the Atherocath diameter and the arterial diameter is obtained, the post-atherectomy result is angiographically and hemodynamically better than after angioplasty of the iliac artery. Following angioplasty, the atheromatous fractured intima remains in situ, causing turbulent flow, and becoming the potential cause of reobstruction. The atherectomy mechanism is more physiologic and produces less damage to the arterial wall. In addition, atherectomy enables a histopathologic study of the material removed, provides important findings for the evaluation of restenosis, and allows the mechanism of action of drugs on intimal hyperplasia or on the atheromatous plaques to be studied.

Recent improvements in catheter design, namely, the increase in the working diameter of the capsule by using larger balloons, the increase in the size of the storage compartment and window, and the added over-the-wire capability, make it possible to eliminate part of the disadvantages described herein.[8] These improvements also reduce procedure time, since it is possible to remove the atheromatous material with fewer passes of the Atherocath. All the factors just discussed lead us to think optimistically in terms of the future role of atherectomy in the percutaneous treatment of atherosclerotic lesions of the iliac region.

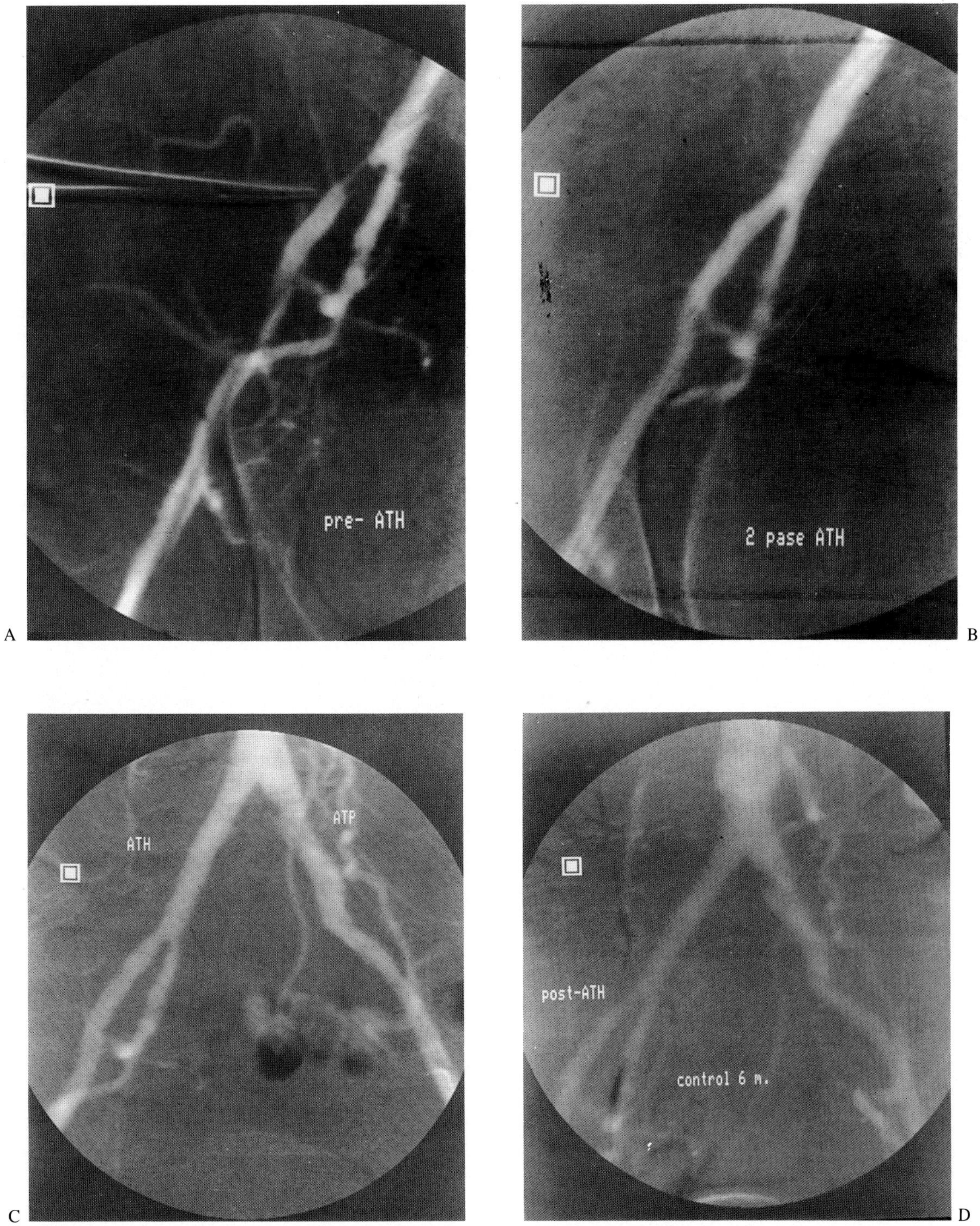

Figure 20–6. Bilateral stenotic lesion of the iliac arteries. **A:** Right iliac angiography shows a severe stenosis of the external iliac artery. **B:** Follow-up angiography after atherectomy shows a widely patent lumen. **C:** Follow-up pelvic angiography shows a widely patent lumen at the atherectomy site and a large intimal defect due to arterial dissection in the left iliac artery where percutaneous transluminal angiography was performed. **D:** Follow-up venous digital subtraction angiography after 6 months of the procedure. Note persistent irregular lumen at the site of the angioplasty.

REFERENCES

1. Waltman AC, Greenfield AJ, Novelline RA, et al. Transluminal angioplasty of iliac and femoropopliteal arteries. Arch Surg 1982;117:1218–21.
2. Schwarten DE. Aortic, iliac, and peripheral arterial angioplasty. In Castañeda-Zúñiga WR, Tadavarthy SM (eds): Interventional Radiology. Baltimore: Wiliams & Wilkins, 1988:268.
3. Spence RK, Freiman DB, Gatenby R, et al. Long-term results of transluminal angioplasty of the iliac and femoral arteries. Arch Surg 1981;116:1377–84.
4. Schwarten DE, Katzen BT, Simpson JB, Cutcliff WB. Simpson catheter for percutaneous transluminal removal of atheroma. AJR 1988;150:799–801.
5. Maynar M, Reyes R, Cabrera V, et al. Percutaneous atherectomy of iliac arteries. Semin Intervent Radiol 1988;5:253–5.
6. Maynar M, Reyes R, Cabrera V, et al. Use of safety wire in atherectomy procedures for recanalization of complete arterial obstructions. Technical note. Semin Intervent Radiol 1988; 5:256–9.
7. Maynar M, Reyes R, Cabrera V, et al. Percutaneous atherectomy with Simpson atherectomy device in the management of arterial stenosis. Semin Intervent Radiol 1988;5:247–52.
8. Katzen BT, Dake MD, Kaplan JO, Dolmatch BL. Percutaneous atherectomy in peripheral vascular disease. International Symposium on Peripheral Vascular Intervention. Florida, January 1989:156–8.

21 Femoral Artery Atherectomy

Donald E. Schwarten, M.D.

Prior to 1988, the generally accepted methods for the treatment of superficial femoral atherosclerotic occlusive disease included bypass surgery using autologous vein grafts,[1,2] synthetic grafts,[3,4] or percutaneous balloon angioplasty.[5,6] Percutaneous balloon angioplasty offers a number of advantages over conventional surgical procedures. It is less expensive, it is easily repeatable, and its morbidity and mortality rates are lower. Productive time lost as a result of the procedure is significantly better with balloon angioplasty than surgery. Balloon angioplasty of lesions longer than 2 to 4 cm suffers from what many believe to be an unacceptably high recurrence rate, and even if recurrence does not occur, there may be progression of disease in the native vessel. Progression has the same impact on the patient as recurrence. To address the issue of recurrent disease that develops after a primary technical success in the superficial femoral artery and the threat of abrupt occlusion related to the development of a large intimal-medial cleft, Simpson and colleagues[7] designed a catheter system that, in essence, is a biopsy tool that removes atheromatous occlusive material from the superficial femoral artery. Simpson coined the term "atherectomy" (ather = atheroma, ectomy = removal) to describe the procedure. For the purposes of this discussion, atherectomy will refer to the Simpson-designed catheter procedure. The Simpson Atherocath (DVI, Redwood City, CA) is a directional atherectomy catheter. There are other atherectomy devices that operate on a rotational principle, one of which has, at the time of this writing, received Food and Drug Administration approval.[8]

PATIENT SELECTION

The clinical indications for percutaneous atherectomy in the superficial artery include lifestyle-limiting intermittent claudication and more advanced stages of ischemia, rest pain, ulceration, or ischemic gangrene. The clinical contraindications to percutaneous atherectomy of the superficial femoral artery include morbid obesity, acute ischemia (unless thrombolysis can be used to reestablish flow and reveal *anatomically suitable* lesion for atherectomy), and evidence of an active, ongoing "trash foot" syndrome.

The angiographic anatomy of the superficial femoral artery occlusive disease determines whether atherectomy is feasible. First, the common femoral and proximal superficial femoral arteries must be of sufficient caliber to permit the placement of a sheath into the proximal superficial femoral artery without creating an extremely low flow or no flow state. Stenotic lesions must be short enough so that the cutting chamber of the catheter can bridge the lesion or at least that the cutting chamber can be positioned at the margins of the lesion and effectively remove the atheroma in a series of passes with the catheter. The catheter is not designed to cross total obstructions in the superficial femoral artery. To perform atherectomy on an occluded segment, a preliminary recanalization must be performed. Dense calcification within a lesion will make for a difficult atherectomy. Recurrent lesions that develop after an initially successful procedure are ideally suited for atherectomy, as are retained valve cusps in in situ bypass grafts that develop myointimal hyperplasia and become hemodynamically significant (Fig. 21-1).

ATHERECTOMY CATHETER

The atherectomy catheter (Simpson's Peripheral Atherocath) consists of a torque-responsive catheter shaft and a cylindrical metal housing that is attached to the end of a braided double lumen catheter and is available in sizes from 7 to 11 F. The cylindrical housing has a longitudinal window. Opposite the window is a balloon similar to those used for angioplasty (Fig. 21-2). The balloon is used to position the window snugly against the occlusive atheromatous material. The balloon is inflated to a pressure less than 35 psi to avoid dilation during the procedure (Fig. 21-3). A separate handheld battery-powered motor drives the cable that is attached to a cutter blade that spins at approximately 2000 rpm. The cable and cutter blade are advanced by a small lever at the cable attachment to the motor drive. Also at the proximal end of the catheter is the balloon inflation port and a flushing port. The distal end of the catheter has a fixed 0.018 inch guide wire that aids safe negotiation to and through the atheromatous segment of vessel. The catheter is also available with a fixed 0.035 inch guide wire at its tip, and soon to be released is an over-the-wire atherectomy catheter. The Simpson Atherocath is designed with an extended, flexible housing that serves as a collection chamber and to which relatively large volumes of atheromatous material can be deposited (Fig. 21-4). At the joint between the rigid metal housing and cutting chamber and the flexible extended collection chamber, there is a slightly greater than 10% stenosis. When advancing the cutter blade past the edge of the window and into the distal portion of the metal housing, a moderate amount of forward pressure on the lever that controls the cable is necessary to force the atheromatous material through the stenosis and into the extended collection chamber, otherwise the atheromatous material will remain in the rigid segment of the catheter and the catheter will need to be removed and emptied of the atheromatous material. The

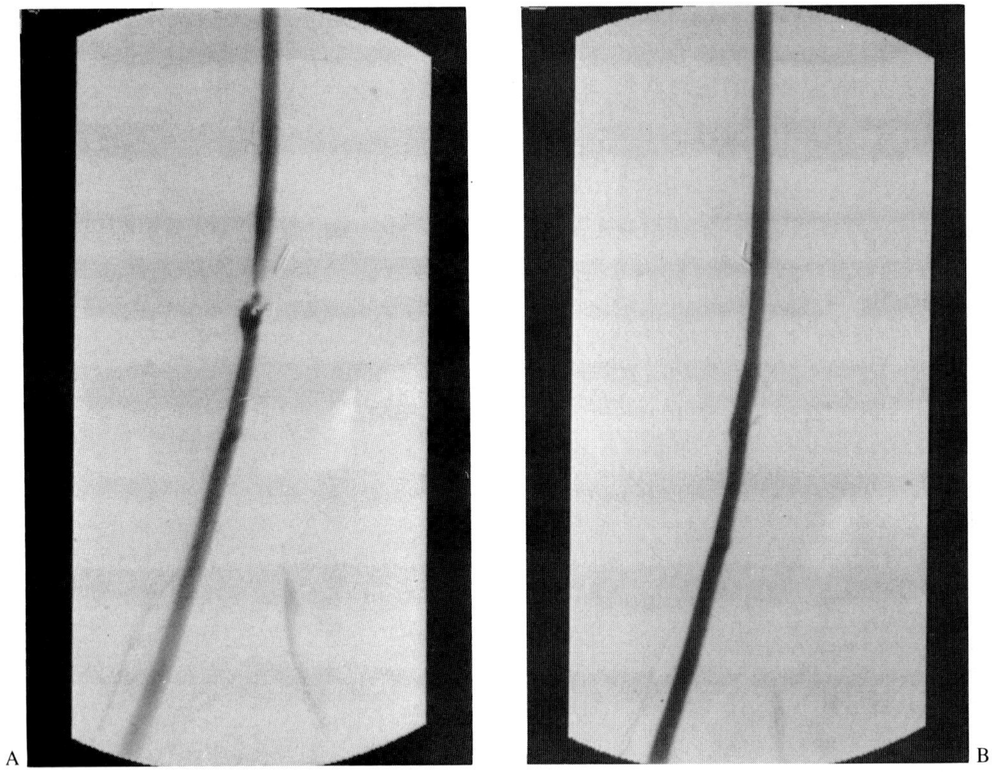

Figure 21–1. **A:** In situ vein bypass with retained valve cusp tissue. **B:** Postatherectomy: tissue removed.

flexible extended collection chamber and nose cone of the catheter are available as separate parts, so that one may purchase a catheter with an additional flexible collection chamber and nose cone and if an extensive area of atheromatous material is to be removed in a timely fashion, once one of the extended chambers if filled and removed, it may be

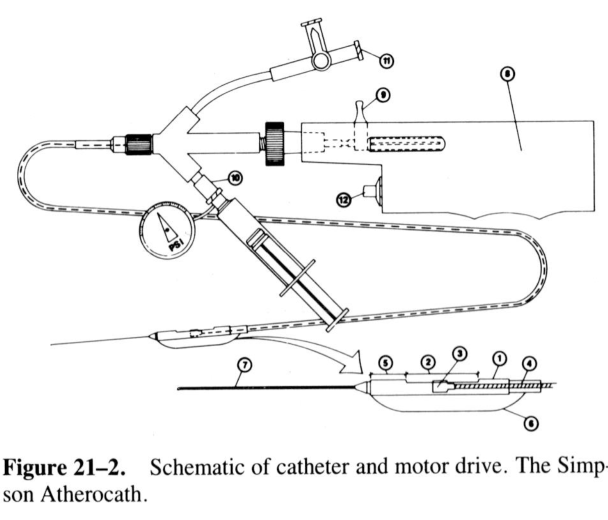

Figure 21–2. Schematic of catheter and motor drive. The Simpson Atherocath.

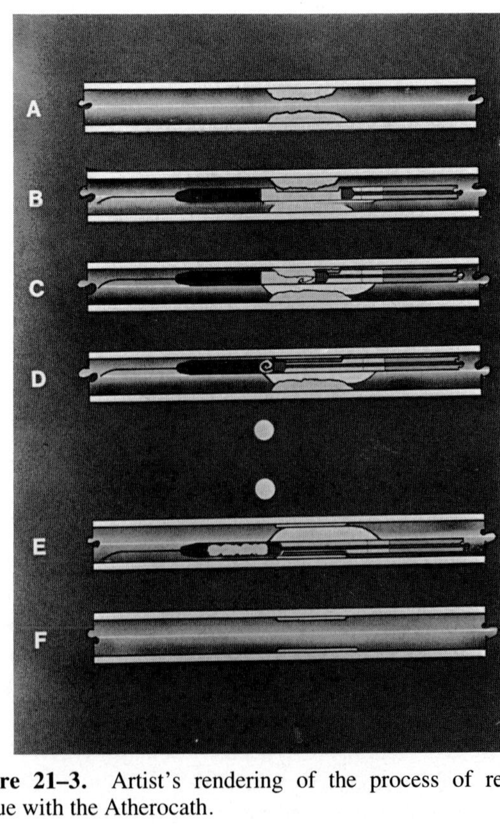

Figure 21–3. Artist's rendering of the process of removing plaque with the Atherocath.

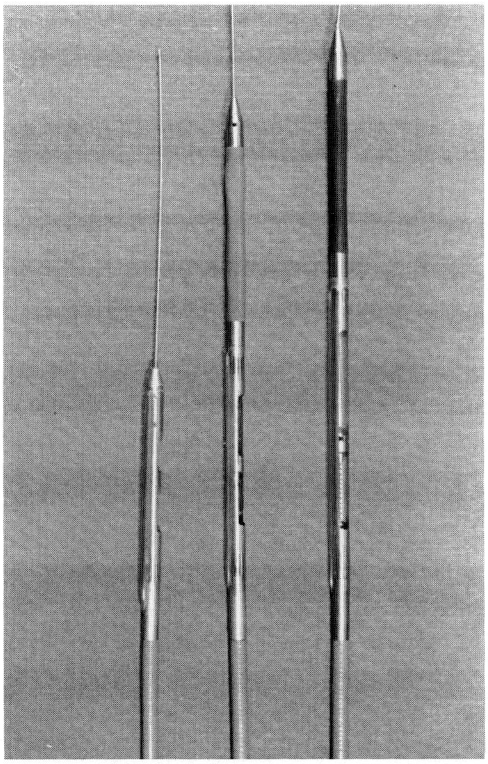

Figure 21–4. The Simpson Atherocath: The original design (left). The first extended housing collection chamber (middle). Current design with 2 cm window (right).

taken off the catheter and replaced by the second one; thus, the procedure can be continued with only a brief interruption.

TECHNIQUE OF DIRECTIONAL ATHERECTOMY OF THE SUPERFICIAL FEMORAL ARTERY

Atherectomy with the Simpson Atherocath must be performed through a sheath; therefore an antegrade ipsilateral puncture is mandatory. It is essential that the antegrade puncture be made as horizontal as possible to prevent kinking of the sheath. A sheath that is kinked makes it extremely difficult to pass the catheter through the sheath without severely damaging the guide wire. It is for this reason that we exclude extremely obese patients. It is almost impossible to obtain a sufficiently horizontal puncture in extremely obese patients. The sheath size selected is based on the catheter size selected, and the catheter size depends on the size of the superficial femoral artery. The 7 F Atherocath and its balloon will have a working diameter of 4.8 mm; the 8 F catheter with its 3 mm balloon gives a total working diameter of 5.7 mm, which is sufficient for most superficial femoral arteries. We most commonly use an 8 F sheath with the 8 F catheter. Measurement of the superficial femoral artery is based on analog films with the nearest "normal" segment of vessel measured without correction for magnification.

PHARMACOLOGIC ADJUNCTS TO ATHERECTOMY

All patients undergoing atherectomy receive antiplatelet therapy (aspirin, 80 to 325 mg orally daily). Patients undergoing atherectomy are also systemically heparinized for the duration of the procedure. Postprocedural heparinization is rarely necessary. Calcium antagonist and nitroglycerin to combat vasospasm are rarely necessary during atherectomy. For whatever reason, the vasospasm that is sometimes seen in balloon angioplasty of the superficial femoral artery is rarely, if ever, encountered during directional atherectomy.

Once vascular access has been achieved and the sheath is in the superficial femoral artery, the patient is heparinized with 2500 to 7000 U administered via the flush port of the sheath. Multiplaner angiography of the occlusive lesion is obtained prior to introducing the atherectomy catheter. It is important to view the superficial femoral artery stenosis with multiplaner angiography prior to the procedure. At the completion of the procedure, it is equally, if not more, important to observe the treated area in multiple projections to ensure that no angiographically visible atheroma remains. After acquisition of the (usually digital) preliminary arteriogram to assess the plaque morphology and to ensure that no fresh thrombus has developed since the original diagnostic study, the atherectomy catheter is introduced through the hemostatic valve of the sheath with "the cheater" that is provided with the catheter. Once the collection chamber has passed the edge of the hemostatic valve, the cheater is retracted back along the catheter shaft to the attachment with the motor drive. The catheter is advanced under fluoroscopic guidance into the superficial femoral artery. The field of view is positioned so that the guide wire and the occlusive lesion are both visible and a roadmap image is required. With the roadmap image superimposed on live fluoroscopy, the catheter is advanced carefully through the occlusive lesion. The 0.018 inch guide wire is very delicate and is unlikely to pass into the subintimal plane. The catheter is very torque responsive, and with a gentle curve placed on the tip of the guide wire, it is possible to negotiate it through even the tightest, most irregular, stenoses (Fig. 21-5). With a very tight stenosis, a moderate amount of forward pressure is necessary to get the flexible housing and metal chamber to pass the stenosis (Fig. 21-6). We have never failed to cross a stenosis (Fig. 21-7). When advancing a catheter, the cutter blade should be positioned at the distal end of the rigid metal housing. Once across the stenosis, the window is positioned under fluoroscopic guidance. Within the occlusive lesion, the balloon is inflated to 10 to 20 psi and the cutter blade is retracted, the balloon is then inflated to 35 psi, the motor is activated, and the cutter blade is advanced and shaves off a piece of atheroma, which is deposited firmly into the flexible distal housing. The balloon is then deflated, the cutter blade is maintained at the distal end of the chamber while the catheter is repositioned, and the procedure is repeated. We find that it is best to rotate the catheter either clockwise or

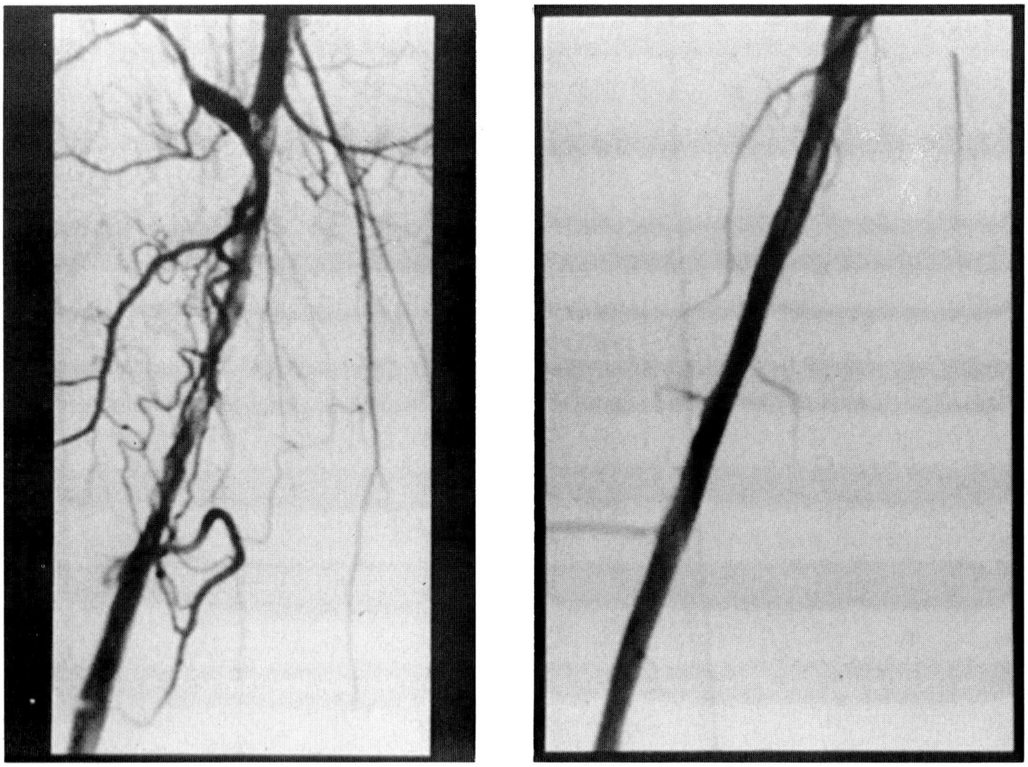

A B

Figure 21–5. **A:** Long irregular lesion of the superficial femoral artery. **B:** Postatherectomy.

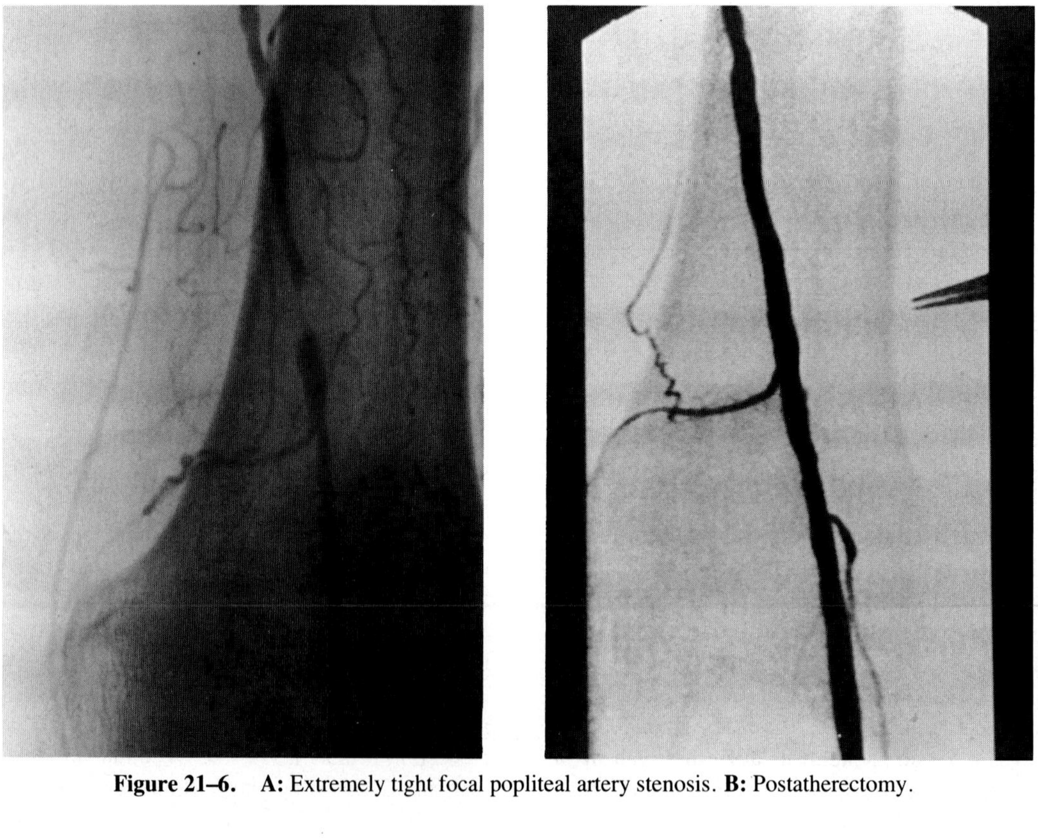

A B

Figure 21–6. **A:** Extremely tight focal popliteal artery stenosis. **B:** Postatherectomy.

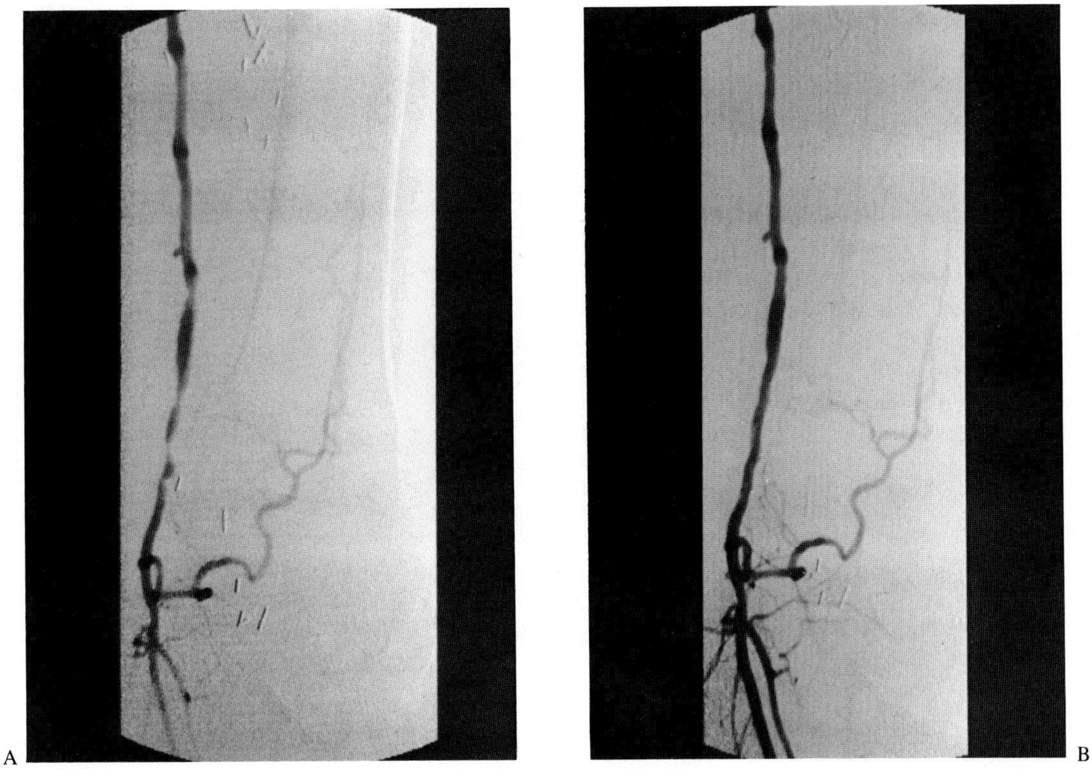

Figure 21–7. **A:** Multiple stenoses in a distal vein bypass to posterior tibial artery. Successful balloon angioplasty 6 months prior. **B:** Postatherectomy. Note: procedure done with investigational over-the-wire device.

counterclockwise in approximately 10° to 20° increments until the 360° circumference has been treated. The catheter has some tendency to follow the path of least resistance. Once the initial cut has been made and a piece of atheroma removed, if the operator does not maintain control of the torque of the catheter, the next time the balloon is inflated, the catheter will tend to return to the initial "groove." Therefore it is our habit, once the procedure has begun, never to let go of the shaft of the catheter at the groin. This greatly reduces the likelihood that the catheter will be malpositioned when the balloon is inflated, or that anterior-posterior directionality will be lost to the operator. It also ensures that the operator will probably develop a muscle cramp in his or her thenar eminence, which tends to speed the procedure along. In most instances if only one pass with the catheter is necessary to complete atherectomy of a superficial femoral artery stenosis, the atherectomy procedure will take no more than 5 to 10 minutes longer than the balloon angioplasty procedure of a comparable lesion. As noted before, a completion digital angiography is performed in multiple projections and should be performed with dilute contrast material so that no angiographically visible residual atheroma will be left. Primary anatomic success is not considered to have been achieved until, at worst, a residual 30% stenosis is left.

Roadmapping capabilities are not necessary for directional atherectomy. It is quite adequate to localize the window of the catheter within the stenosis to be treated using small volumes of contrast material injected via the flush port of the sheath. If fact, after initial localization with roadmapping, we frequently remove the roadmap image and avail ourselves of the very helpful feedback that the inflated balloon gives about the character of the lesion that it is up against. It becomes quite obvious that, when the balloon is indented by a stenosis on the wall of a vessel opposite the open window, we must rotate the catheter and position the window in that region, and only when the balloon inflates with its silhouette parallel to the long access of the vessel with no indentation is it evident that there is no residual atheroma that can be removed from that segment of the artery.

Percutaneous directional atherectomy for total occlusions is possible and, we believe, desirable. We begin the procedure the same way we would atherectomy for stenoses, and after a horizontal antegrade puncture has been made, the sheath is placed into the superficial femoral artery. The patient is heparinized and then a 5 or 6 F catheter is advanced to just proximal to the occlusion and the occlusion is recanalized with the catheter and a guide wire. Once a true intraluminal position has been confirmed with a contrast injection, is has been our habit to perform a preliminary balloon angioplasty. The balloon angioplasty is performed with a balloon equal to the diameter of the nearest normal segment of the vessel, measured on analog films, without correction of magnification. Once the angioplasty has been completed, the angioplasty catheter is removed, the guide wire is removed, and the atherectomy catheter is introduced, and as much as possible of the fractured intima, media, and atheroma are removed. The atherectomy procedure continues until no additional material is retrieved (Fig. 21-8).

Preliminary angioplasty of the recanalized occluded segment of vessel may or may not enhance the outcome of the procedure. Casteñada-Zúñiga[9] has described simply passing an 8 F catheter through the occluded segment to establish a lumen large enough to permit passage of the atherectomy catheter and then perform an atherectomy to optimize the anatomic result. In our own experience we have employed Casteñada-Zúñiga's method on several occasions and have found that we retrieve more material and spend somewhat more time because of the volume of clot, intima, media, and atheroma that were removed. His method certainly is more cost-effective.

RESULTS

Since October 1986 we have performed more than 250 superficial femoral artery atherectomy procedures. Between October 1986 and October 1987, we performed atherectomy in 41 patients. These 41 patients had a total of 80 lesions; 67 (84%) were in the superficial femoral artery. Nineteen (24%) of the lesions were eccentric, and nearly two thirds were tandem lesions. Primary anatomic success was, as defined in the preceding text, achieved in 92% of the patients without supplemental balloon angioplasty. During the year that this series was accumulated, 8 F catheters were not available and we confined ourselves to using 7 F devices. Patients who did not have a satisfactory anatomic result from atherectomy alone received a supplemental balloon angioplasty so that nearly 99% of the patients had satisfactory lumen at the conclusion of the procedure.

COMPLICATIONS

The original group of patients enrolled in 1986 to 1987 experienced no complications. There were no instances of distal embolization, acute occlusion, or groin hematoma resulting in prolongation of hospital stay, transfusion, or surgical intervention. In the more than 200 superficial femoral artery atherectomy procedures performed since 1987, there still have been no distal embolizations or acute occlusions. Three groin complications requiring operative intervention have occurred.

LATE RESULTS

All of the patients enrolled in the original series have passed the 2-year anniversary of their original procedure. We have defined recurrence at the atherectomy site as follows: (1) recurrent claudication to the pretreatment level (no patients in the original series had signs of resting ischemia); (2) loss of 50% of the initial gain by Doppler examination; and (3) angiographic documentation of a greater than 50% stenosis at the site of the atherectomy. At 6 months, 32 superficial femoral artery atherectomy sites were available for follow-up, and two restenoses had occurred, for a 6-month follow-up restenosis rate of 6%. At 1 year, 30 superficial femoral artery atherectomy sites were available for follow-up and five restenoses had redeveloped, for a 1-year restenosis rate of 17%. At 2 years, 27 superficial femoral atherectomy sites were available for follow-up. There were six restenoses for a recurrence rate of 22%.[10] This 78% 2-year patency rate compares favorably with comparable series of percutaneous balloon angioplasty of the superficial femoral artery. We have observed on follow-up angiograms of patients with recurrent symptoms and diminished noninvasive indices that

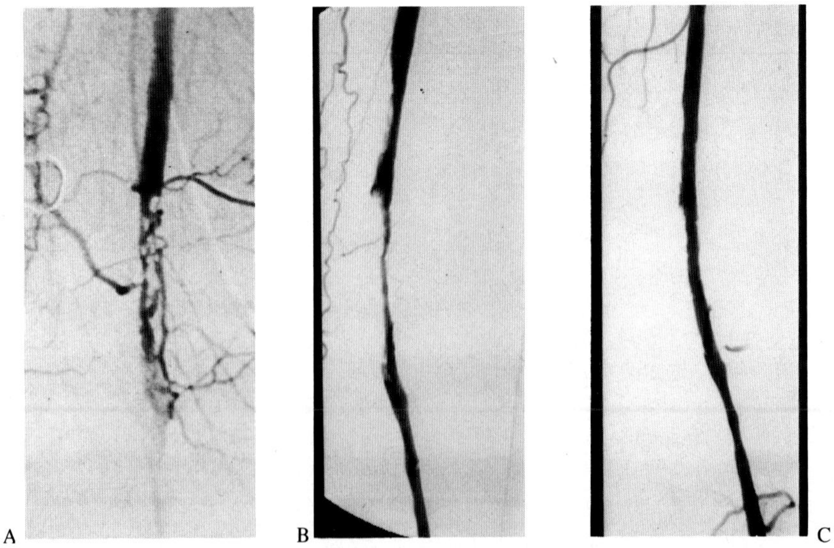

Figure 21–8. **A:** Irregular total occlusion of SFA. **B:** After preliminary recanalization. **C:** Appearance after directional atherectomy.

many of the patients not only have recurrence at the atherectomy site, but have evidence of significant progression in more proximal areas of the superficial femoral artery. We have noted the development of the stenoses at or near the site of the tip of the sheath as well as other sections of the proximal and midsuperficial femoral artery. Most of the recurrent lesions were near the distal end of the adductor canal. It appears that when recurrences occur and are associated with new disease developing within a year of the atherectomy procedure, the frequency of the new disease increases when larger caliber catheters and sheaths were employed. It was less common to see extensive new disease proximal to the atherectomy site when we used 7 F catheters.

Histologic examination of material removed from the superficial femoral arteries in the course of an atherectomy procedure has revealed in native lesions that atherosclerotic plaque was present and consisted of densely fibrous, libid-laden tissue. Lesions tended to be complex, and many exhibited surface thrombus even though no patients appeared to be actively embolizing distally. In our initial series of patients, atherectomy was performed with catheters without the extended flexible housing and collection chamber, so no more than three to five cuts could be made before the chamber was filled and the catheter had to be removed and emptied of the material in the chamber. Each pass with the catheter was considered as an individual entity. On the first pass, the material retrieved was placed in a bottle of buffered formalin labeled 1. The second pass was placed in a bottle and labeled 2, and so on, until no additional material could be removed. Histologic examination revealed in many cases that as the procedure came to a conclusion, the last one or two bottles of formalin contained small amounts of media. Unlike reports in coronary atherectomy, no adventitial tissue was removed.

We have had some experience using endovascular ultrasound in conjunction with atherectomy. The ultrasound catheter that we used is a 6 F device with a 20 MHz transducer in the distal tip of the catheter (Diasonics, Milpitas, CA). The transducer is mechanically rotated and a scan of 360° enabled us to view not only the lumen of the superficial femoral artery, but also the wall of the artery. We were able to characterize an inner (closest to the catheter) bright layer that is believed to represent the intima and the internal elastic membrane. We were able to identify media, and less clearly, adventitia. It was possible to characterize thrombus, plaque, and calcified plaque and to see where atherectomy cuts had been made.

At the time of this writing, no changes in the course of an atherectomy procedure were made as the result of information provided by the ultrasound images and as yet no therapeutic decisions have been made based on endovascular ultrasound information (Fig. 21-9). We have noted, as have others, that occasionally an atherectomy catheter will be passed through a high-grade stenosis and multiple cuts will be made, resulting in markedly improved angiographic appearance, yet in some occasions very little, if any, material was retrieved from the atherectomy chamber and no evidence of distal embolization was present. Clearly, the passage of a 7 or 8 F catheter through a high-grade stenosis will have some "Dotter effect," and we have documented that both with ultrasound and angiography by passing the catheter through the stenosis, making no cuts, removing the catheter, and repeating the angiography and the ultrasound.

Truly effective atherectomy does remove atheroma. Simpson has shown that aggressive atherectomy resulting in restoration of the caliber of the lumen to near normal results in patency rates at 6 months that are clearly superior to those achieved if there is a 50% residual stenosis at the conclusion of the atherectomy procedure.[11] It may be, however, that being extremely aggressive with the atherectomy catheter may result in removal of not only plaque, intima, internal elastic membrane, and small amounts of media, but large amounts of media and perhaps adventitia may be removed, and this setting may actually have a negative impact on long-term patency. There may be, in fact, so much media exposed to circulating and tissue mitogens that a myointimal hyperplasia is inevitable, resulting in a "restenosis lesion."

Rousseau reported a 10% restenosis rate in patients initially treated successfully with percutaneous atherectomy of the superficial femoral artery. The mean follow-up time was 11 months in his series.[12] He and his colleagues concluded that atherectomy restores a large and smooth lumen without vessel wall stretching, which they believed may be responsible for decreasing the restenosis rate compared with plain old balloon angioplasty.

We are confronted with widely divergent data on restenosis rates in percutaneous directional atherectomy of the superficial femoral artery. Different endpoints for restenosis further cloud the issue. Clearly, the 6- to 9-month follow-up time that has been widely accepted for predicting when recurrences will occur in superficial femoral artery following balloon angioplasty are not appropriate for percutaneous atherectomy. The timing of recurrent disease following atherectomy is not as well defined as it appears to be for percutaneous balloon angioplasty of the superficial femoral artery. Atherectomy may not only have a different recurrence rate than balloon angioplasty, but it may occur in a different time frame. Answers to these and other questions await the results of prospective randomized trials that are currently underway at several centers.

CONCLUSION

Percutaneous transluminal atherectomy using the Simpson Atherocath is an effective way to manage atherosclerotic occlusive disease at the superficial femoral artery. Within certain clinical and angiographic guidelines, the procedure is technically simple to perform and, with current catheter design, requires only several minutes more to complete than percutaneous balloon angioplasty of a comparable lesion. Percutaneous atherectomy does not appear to subject the

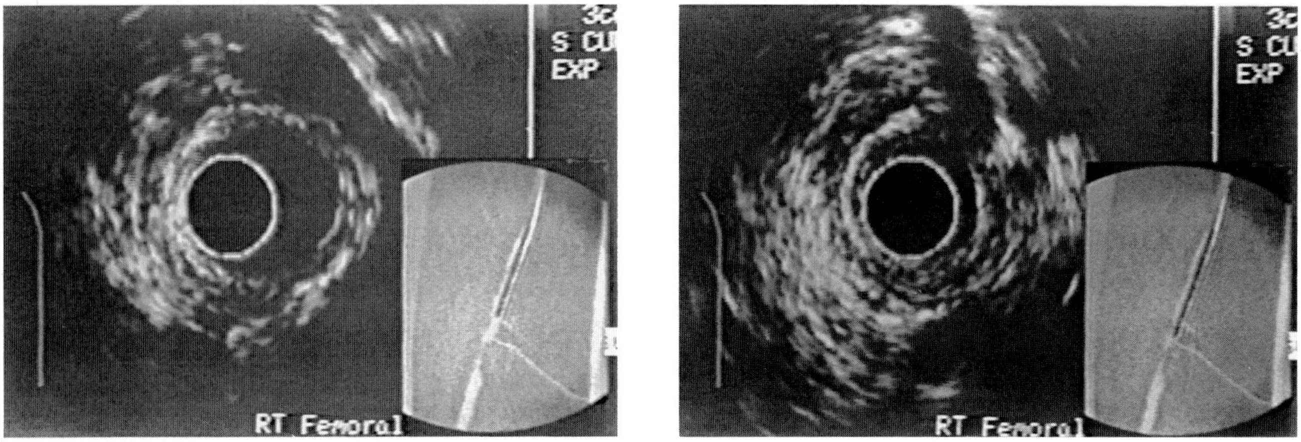

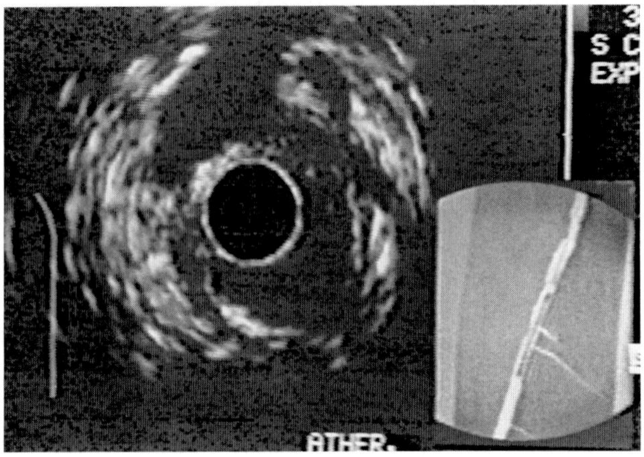

Figure 21–9. Ultrasound and roadmap (insert) images of **A:** Minimally diseased vessel proximal to collateral. **B:** Entrance into high-grade stenosis at collateral branch. **C:** Postatherectomy images with ultrasound catheter in treated segment.

patient to any risk not associated with percutaneous balloon angioplasty. In fact, the creation of large intimal-medial clefts and the possibility of acute thrombosis are not seen with atherectomy. When properly performed, atherectomy results in a relatively smooth lumen that may be more favorable to laminar flow than the lumen resulting from balloon angioplasty. This, in turn, may not only reduce the risk of acute occlusion, but may have important implications for long-term patency.

REFERENCES

1. Taylor LM Jr, Phinney ES, Porter JM. Present status of reversed vein bypass for lower extremity revascularization. J Vasc Surg 1986;3:28–97.
2. Buchbinder D, Rolins DL, Verta MJ, et al. Early experience with in situ saphenous vein bypass for distal arterial reconstruction. Surgery 1986;99:350–6.
3. Veith FJ, Gupta SK, Ascer E, et al. Six-year prospective multicenter randomized comparison of autologous saphenous vein and expanded polytetrafluoroethylene grafts in infrainguinal arterial reconstructions. J Vasc Surg 1986;3:104–14.
4. Szilagyi DE, Elliott JP Jr, Smith RF, et al. A thirty-year survey of the reconstructive surgical treatment of aorto iliac occlusive disease. J Vasc Surg 1986;3:421–36.
5. Krepel VM, Van Andel GJ, Van Erp WFM, Breslace PJ. Percutaneous transluminal angioplasty of the femoropopliteal artery: initial and long-term results. Radiology 1985;156: 325–8.
6. Katzen BT. Percutaneous transluminal angioplasty for arterial disease of the lower extremities. AJR 1984;142:23–5.
7. Simpson JB, Johnson DE, Thapllyal HV, et al. Transluminal atherectomy: a new approach to the treatment of atherosclerotic vascular disease. Circulation 1985;72(suppl 2):111–46.
8. Wholey MH. "TEC" endarterectomy catheter; an analysis of 132 patients with 204 lesions in the peripheral circulation. Presented at RIPCV 2, Toulouse, France, March 1990.
9. Casteñada-Zúñiga WR. Response to question at SCVIR. Workshop on New Devices, San Diego, 1989.
10. Schwarten DE, Cutcliff WB, Krol KL. The late results of femoral directional atherectomy. Presented at RIPCV-2, Toulouse, France, March 1990.
11. Simpson JB, Selmon MR, Robertson GC, et al. Transluminal atherectomy for occlusive peripheral vascular disease. Am J Cardiol 1988;61(suppl G):96G–101G.
12. Rousseau, H, Joffre, F. Results of directional atherectomy. Presented at RIPCV-2, Toulouse, France, March 1992.

22 Use of Simpson's Atherocath in the Treatment of Arterial Obstruction

Manuel Maynar-Moliner, M.D., Ricardo Reyes, M.D., J. M. Pulido-Duque, M.D., E. Gorriz, M.D., J. M. Felices, M.D.

Simpson's Atherocath was designed for the treatment of vascular stenosis.[1–4] Because of the lack of over-the-wire capability and the presence of a soft steerable guide wire attached to the tip of the capsule, the device cannot be advanced through a complete vascular obstruction. We have, however, used the Atherocath alone or in combination with angioplasty in the management of 29 patients with complete vascular obstruction.

The use of atherectomy in these cases is based on the principle that the irregular channel produced by recanalization can be enlarged by the Atherocath, leaving a smoother vascular lumen by removing the plaque than would be produced by compressing the plaque against the arterial wall, as in angioplasty.

MATERIALS AND METHODS

After a decision is reached following the clinical evaluation and diagnostic angiographic examination to recanalize an obstructed vascular segment, the approach is selected. Normally, when the obstructed segment to be treated is in the iliac artery, the method of choice is the retrograde femoral artery. This is also the case in patients in whom fibrinolysis of the obstructed segment has been carried out using the axillary approach. It is necessary to puncture the ipsilateral femoral artery in order to approach the iliac lesion with the Atherocath, since the device cannot be advanced from the contralateral approach. In obstructions of the femoropopliteal area, an anterograde femoral approach is used.

In those patients in whom fibrinolysis is not used, the obstructed segment is recanalized using the conventional guide wire and catheter system. A moveable core 0.035 inch J guide wire and a straight 6.5 F catheter with a distal and lateral sidehole are used during the recanalization. This catheter allows the injection of contrast medium while advancing the guide wire until the area distal to the obstruction is reached.

Once continuity with the distal end is obtained, the subsequent therapeutic method to be used might include:

1. Fibrinolysis followed by atherectomy
2. Angioplasty
3. Angioplasty plus atherectomy
4. Atherectomy alone

Fibrinolysis Followed by Atherectomy

In the event that the area proximal to the obstruction is recanalized easily, which will favor the predominance of the thrombotic vascular occlusive component over the fibrous atheromatous component, particularly if this is corroborated by the typical angiographic image, an infusion with urokinase at 100,000 IU/hour is initiated.

Following angiographic follow-up 12 or 24 hours afterward, the site of atheromatous obstruction is localized and the Atherocath is used to treat the lesion.

In those cases in whom the axillary approach was used for the fibrinolytic treatment, a subsequent retrograde femoral approach will allow use of the Atherocath for the treatment of the subjacent vascular lesion (Fig. 22-1).

Angioplasty and Atherectomy

In cases in which the Atherocath cannot be advanced distally following recanalization, an angioplasty is performed. If the result of the angioplasty is acceptable, that is, less than 20% residual stenosis, the treatment is concluded.

More commonly, after performing recanalization of occluded vascular segments followed by angioplasty, extensive irregularities of the arterial wall occur (Fig. 22-2). Because these wall irregularities make manipulations difficult, a technique was designed to avoid the risk of losing the recanalized channel while trying to advance the Atherocath. A 0.012 or 0.14 inch guide wire is passed through the 6.5 F catheter after the recanalization, beyond the obstructed vascular segment, removing the catheter afterward. This guide wire will allow the passage of the 7 F Atherocath through an introducer of the same bore, while at the same time ensuring access to the area distal to the recanalization. This is of great help in the event of serious complications, such as arterial perforation, distal embolization of an atherotomatous plaque, or subintimal dissection.[5]

The main advantage of using the Atherocath in these cases is that it permits removal of all the irregularities of the vessel wall, leaving a smoother vascular lumen (Fig. 22-3).

Another useful application of atherectomy is in the management of intimal flaps following angioplasty, which may cause partial or complete obstruction of the vascular lumen.[6] These flaps are produced by the rupture of the atherotomatous intima with proximal dehiscence of the atheromatous

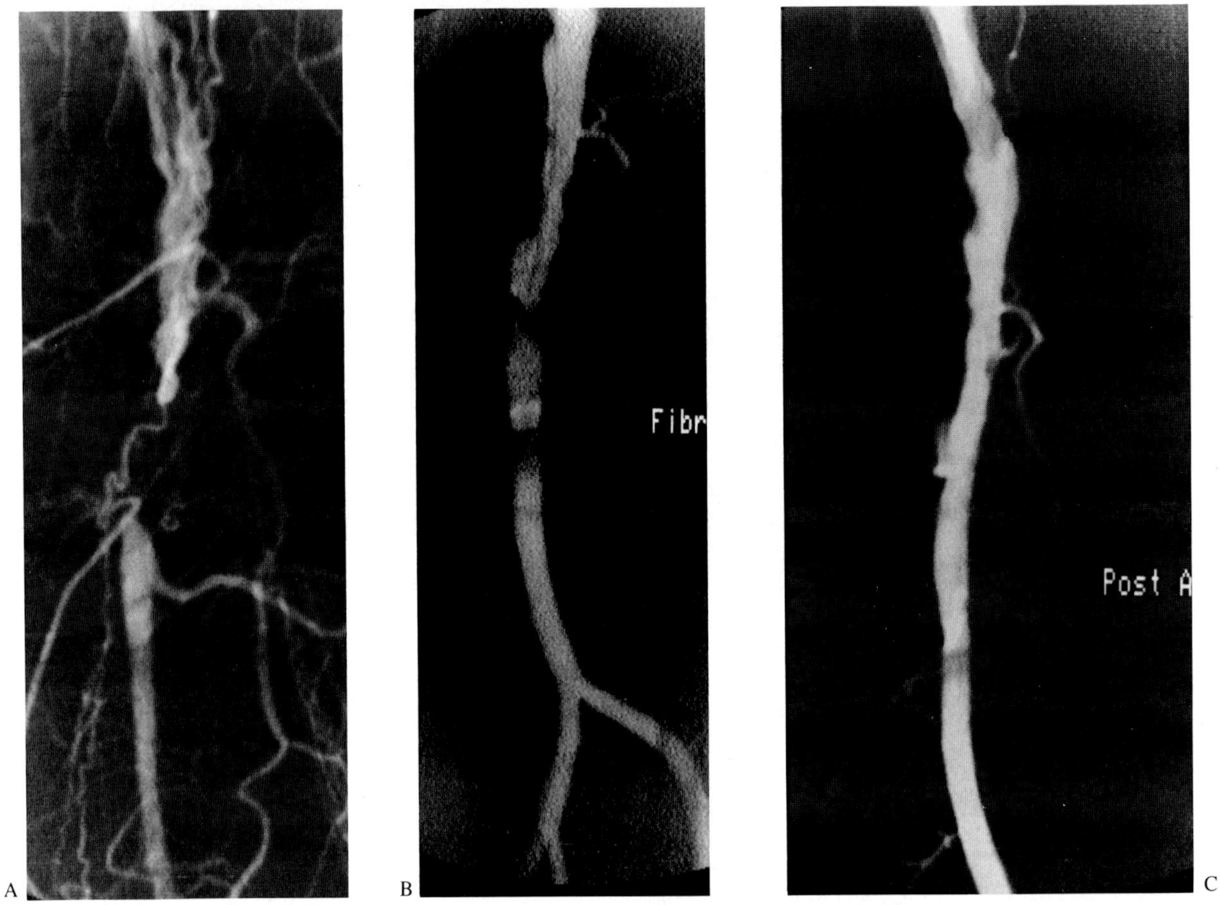

Figure 22–1. A: Angiography shows occlusion of a 3 cm segment in the popliteal artery. **B:** Follow-up angiography after 40 hours of fibrinolytic infusion shows the presence of a severe stenosis. **C:** Follow-up angiography after atherectomy with 7 F Atherocath shows a widely open lumen.

plaque from the vascular wall, following balloon angioplasty. When this complication occurs, the site can be redilated trying to remodel the plaque against the vascular wall; this maneuver is, however, not generally effective. Intimal flaps may lead to acute obstruction of the vessel or, more commonly, to an early recurrence of the obstruction. In the event that an acute thrombosis occurs, the only treatment available in the past was surgical repair. However, it has been shown that the Atherocath can be used effectively in resolving these complications, thus preventing surgery.[6]

Atherectomy

In those cases in which the Atherocath can be passed across the recanalized segment, atherectomy can be used as the only therapeutic method. In these cases, a safety guide wire is initially placed across the recanalized segment. The Atherocath is then passed alongside this guide wire, ensuring access at all times to the area distal to the obstruction. The diameter of the Atherocath must be selected carefully, in direct correlation to the arterial diameter proximal or distal to the obstructed segment, taking into account that the diameter of the Atherocath is given by the sum of the diameter of the capsule plus the inflated balloon diameter.

Once the atherectomy has been performed, an angiographic control study is obtained in several projections for a better evaluation of the results of the procedure (Fig. 22-4).

Atheromatous material removal should be as complete as possible, as assessed by angiographic control or by intravascular ultrasound. It is necessary to ensure that the residual stenosis is always less than 20%, since, as has been shown by Simpson's experience, the rate of reobstruction may reach 27% at 6 months when a residual stenosis of more than 30% remains.[2] This is one of the disadvantages of the Simpson Atherocath, since it forces us to make as many cuts with the Atherocath as necessary until the maximal arterial diameter is achieved. This problem has been partly solved by a new Atherocath design with a longer storage capsule that allows a larger amount of atheromatous material in one pass.

RESULTS

Atherectomy with Simpson's Atherocath has been used in 29 patients with arterial obstruction either by itself or in combi-

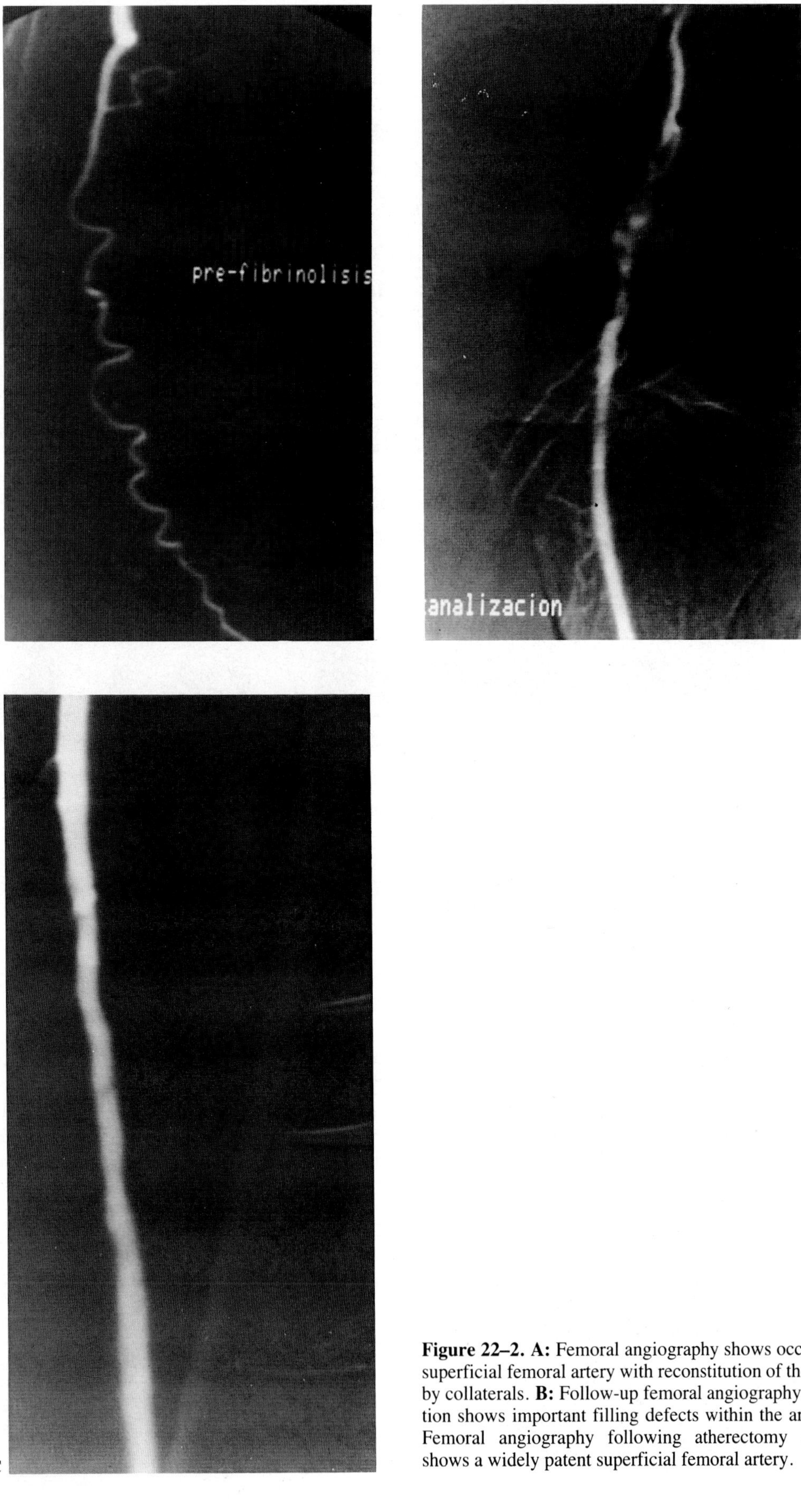

A B C

Figure 22–2. A: Femoral angiography shows occlusion of the left superficial femoral artery with reconstitution of the popliteal artery by collaterals. **B:** Follow-up femoral angiography after recanalization shows important filling defects within the arterial lumen. **C:** Femoral angiography following atherectomy and angioplasty shows a widely patent superficial femoral artery.

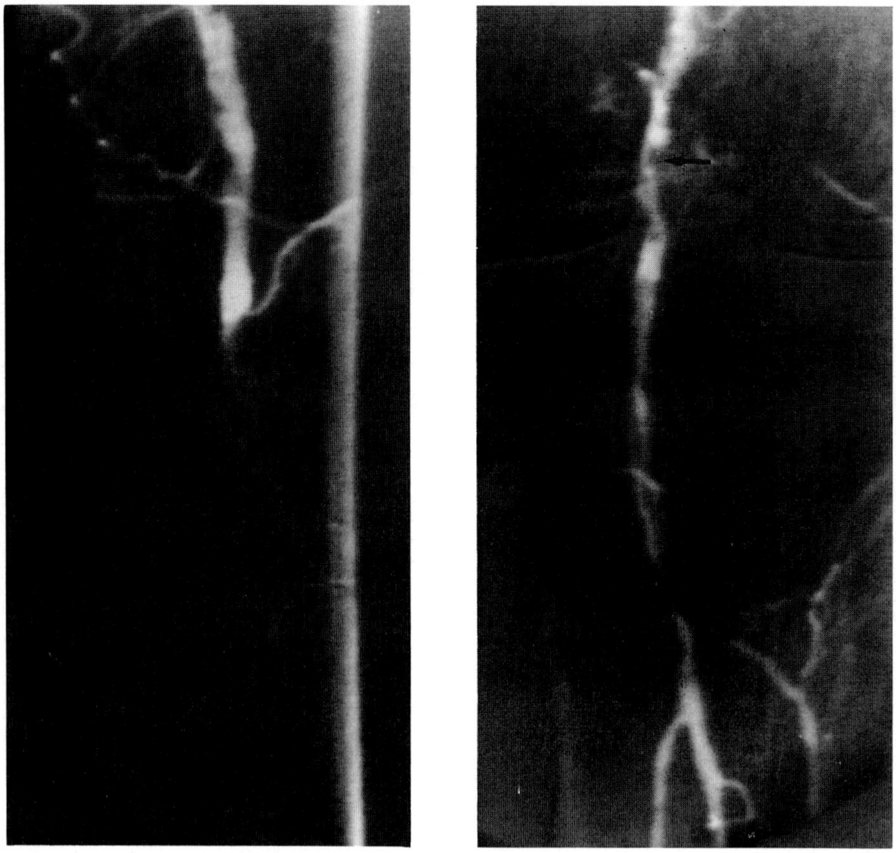

A B

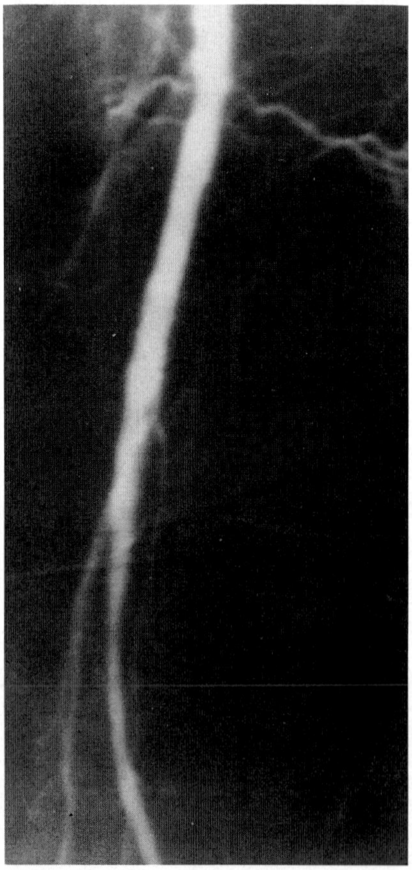

C

Figure 22–3. A: Femoral angiography shows occlusion of superficial femoral artery. **B:** Follow-up angiography after 18 hours of urokinase infusion shows the presence of severe stenosis (arrows). **C:** Femoral angiography after atherectomy and angioplasty shows a patent lumen.

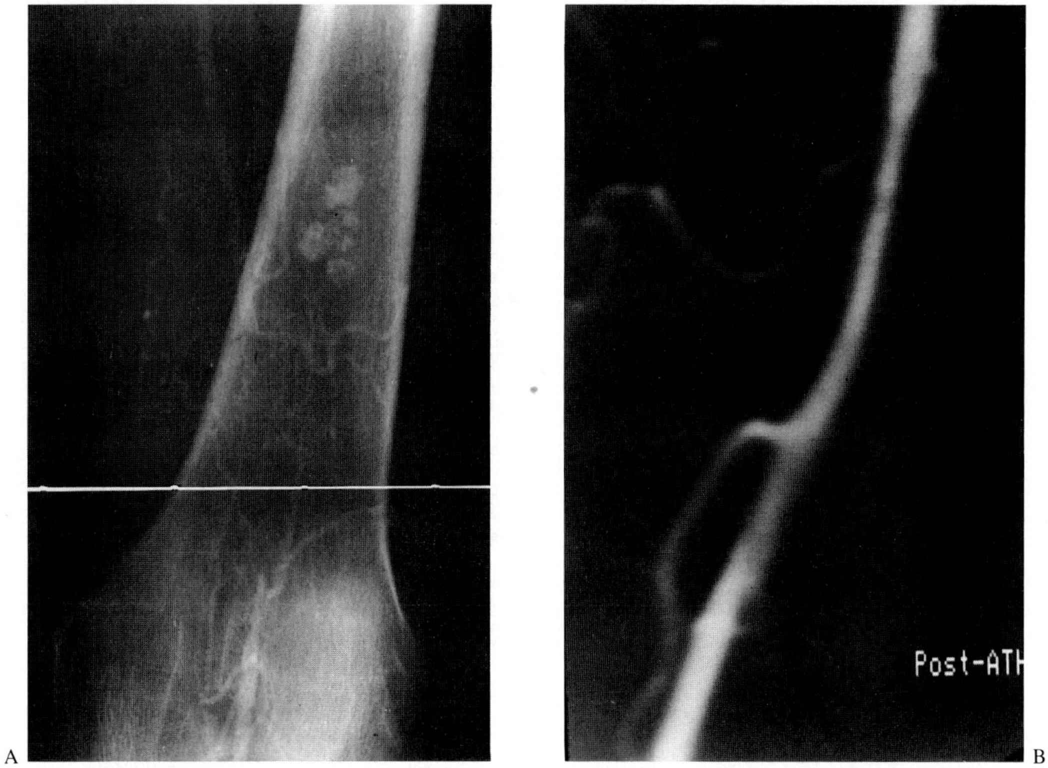

Figure 22–4. A: Angiography shows 100% occlusion of the left superficial femoral artery with reconstitution of the popliteal artery by collaterals. **B:** Follow-up angiography after atherectomy with a 7 F catheter shows patent lumen.

nation with fibrinolysis or angioplasty. Of these, 27 were males and two were females. With regard to anatomic distribution, four were performed in the iliac artery, seven in the superficial femoral artery, 12 in the popliteal artery, and eight in vascular occlusions involving the superficial femoral and popliteal arteries. The average length of the obstructed segment was 8.2 cm, with a maximum length of 19 cm and a minimum of 2.5 cm.

Periodic follow-up examinations were performed after 3 and 6 months, and 1 and 2 years, with patency rates at 2 years of 75%, obstructions of 25%; five patients were lost to follow-up.

In three of the patients, atherectomy alone was performed; in two, atherectomy was combined with fibrinolysis; in 19, atherectomy was performed in combination with angioplasty; and in five cases, fibrinolysis, angioplasty, and atherectomy were used in combination.

A total of four complications occurred: two arterial perforations, one early thrombosis, and one intimal dissection. The two cases of arterial perforation occurred during the recanalization maneuvers using a guide wire and catheter and were satisfactorily resolved after successfully recanalizing the obstructed segment. In these patients, however, the angiographic study after angioplasty showed the existence of partially obstructing intimal flaps. The Atherocath was used in the same setting to remove the obstructing flap.

Thrombosis occurred 7 days following atherectomy in a patient who had had a saphenous vein patch of the popliteal artery 12 months prior. Seven days after atherectomy, the patient presented with acute thrombosis of the treated segment. This was successfully treated with urokinase, with complete lysis after 24 hours.

A distal intimal dissection was observed in a patient on whom an Atherocath slightly larger than the arterial diameter had been used. The anatomic-pathologic study revealed the existence of a fragment of medial layer. The patient, however, did not have any clinical symptoms and no further therapeutic interventions were necessary.

DISCUSSION

Percutaneous transluminal angioplasty in the management of arterial occlusion has a 5-year patency rate of 50 to 60%.[7–10] These patency rates become even worse when the arterial occlusions are longer than 7 cm.[9] These poor results in the treatment of vascular occlusion, especially in the femoropopliteal territory, has led to the development of new devices. Simpson's atherectomy catheter is one of these new devices, although it was not designed for the treatment of vascular occlusion. After recanalization of complete occlusions, the arterial lumen obtained has extensive irregularities. The purpose of the use of the Atherocath in these areas is to obtain a smoother lumen by removing the atheromatous plaque instead of fracturing and compressing it against the arterial wall. The long-term patency of an artery following angioplasty or atherectomy is closely related to the residual stenosis following the revascularization procedure. As has been shown in the series published by Simpson,[2] the recurrence rate may reach 27% at 6 months when the residual stenosis is more than 30%. In total vascular occlusion in whom the amount of atheromatous plaque present is large, it is difficult to widen the lumen by pushing the plaque into the arterial wall. For this reason, it is hoped that the atherectomy will improve postprocedural patency rates over and beyond those seen in angioplasty. The initial results and follow-up obtained are encouraging, although the role of the atherectomy technique is not well defined at the present time. Long-term follow-up is needed to know the exact role of the Simpson Atherocath in the treatment of total vascular occlusion.

REFERENCES

1. Simpson JB, Johnson DE, Thapliyal HV, et al. Transluminal atherectomy: a new approach to the treatment of atherosclerotic vascular disease. Circulation 1985; 72(suppl 3): III–146.
2. Simpson JB, Zimmerman JJ, Selmon MR, et al. Transluminal atherectomy: initial clinical results in 27 patients. Circulation 1986; 74(suppl 2):II-203.
3. Schwarten DE, Katzen BT, Simpson JB, Cutcliff WB. Simpson catheter for percutaneous transluminal removal of a theroma. AJR 1988;150:799–801.
4. Maynar M, Cabrera V, Reyes R, et al. Percutaneous atherectomy with the Simpson atherectomy device in the management of arterial stenosis. Semin Intervent Radiol 1988;5:247–52.
5. Maynar M, Reyes R, Cabrera V, et al. Use of safety wire in atherectomy procedures for recanalization of complete arterial obstructions. Semin Intervent Radiol 1988;5:256–9.
6. Maynar M, Reyes R, Cabrera V, et al. Percutaneous atherectomy as an alternative treatment for postangioplasty obstructive intimal flaps. Radiology 1989;170:1029–31.
7. Hewes RC, White RI, Murray RR, et al. Long-term results of superficial femoral artery angioplasty. AJR 1986;146:1025–9.
8. Krepel VM, van Ardel GJ, van Erp WF. Percutaneous transluminal angioplasty of the femoropopliteal artery: initial and long-term results. Radiology 1985;156:325–8.
9. Murray RR, Hewes RC, White RI, et al. Long segment femoropopliteal stenosis: is angioplasty a boom or a bust? Radiology 1987;162:473–6.
10. Becker GJ, Katzen BT, Dake MD. Non-coronary angioplasty. Radiology 1989;170:921–40.

23 Percutaneous Atherectomy of the Obstructive Postangioplasty Intimal Flaps

Manuel Maynar-Moliner, M.D., Ricardo Reyes, M.D., J. M. Pulido-Duque, M.D., E. Gorriz, M.D., J. M. Felices, M.D.

Until the studies of Castañeda-Zúñiga et al[1] in 1979, it was considered that the mechanism of angioplasty was by compression and remodeling of the atheromatous plaque against the arterial wall to increase the arterial lumen.[2] Based on microscopic and physiologic studies, Castañeda-Zúñiga et al[1] concluded that the arterial wall does not react in the same manner as a rigid tube, but that its external diameter increases. Angioplasty effectiveness is based on its ability to rupture the arterial wall layers, thus causing an increase in the vessel diameter.[1,3]

Anatomic-pathologic studies in autopsy specimens following balloon angioplasty showed a partial or complete separation of the atheromatous plaque from the media, with or without associated rupture of the media. These arterial wall changes appear in angiography as linear filling defects in the arterial lumen.

The intima, partially separated from the media, is commonly joined to the artery wall at its proximal and distal ends. Fortunately, total separation from the media with distal embolization is uncommon.[4] Intimal flaps usually do not cause any clinical effects, since they are not obstructive. In some cases, they are partly separated from the media and can become obstructive flaps, blocking the blood flow.

Simpson's Atherocath can be used to manage intimal flaps.[5,6] The Atherocath was used to treat five obstructive intimal flaps following angioplasty.

CASE REPORTS

Case 1

An 80-year-old patient presented with severe claudication and rest pain. Distal pulses were not palpable. Angiography showed complete occlusion of the distal femoral artery. The artery diameter proximal to the occlusion was 4 mm. Initial recanalization of the artery was carried out with an angiographic catheter and guide wire. Dilation was achieved with a 4 mm diameter balloon. Follow-up angiography after angioplasty showed a large intimal flap at the junction of the superficial femoral and popliteal arteries, which was almost completely obstructing blood flow. An attempt to relocate the flap against the arterial wall with an angioplasty balloon was unsuccessful. Using a 7 F Simpson Atherocath, the flap was removed and the arterial flow restored. The follow-up angiogram showed a widely patent lumen at the site of angioplasty-atherectomy. Heparin was administered for the next 48 hours. Rest pain disappeared and the ankle-arm index increased from 0.24 to 0.66. On long-term follow-up at 2 years, the patient remains asymptomatic with an ankle-arm index equal to the one after the atherectomy.

Case 2

A 39-year-old patient, smoker, with no other known risk factors presented with right lower extremity claudication. Two years prior to admittance, the patient underwent angioplasty and atherectomy of the right common iliac artery. Six months prior to admittance, the patient presented with intermittent claudication of the right leg of 100 m. Arteriography showed obstruction of the right common iliac artery of approximately 3 cm in length.

After recanalization of the occluded segment, urokinase was infused for 24 hours. Follow-up angiography showed a 50% stenosis. The stenosis was dilated with a 7 mm diameter angioplasty balloon. Follow-up angiography after angioplasty showed the presence of an intimal flap that partially obstructed the arterial lumen. An atherectomy was then performed with a 9 F Atherocath. Follow-up angiography showed complete restoration of the arterial lumen. The patient recovered the distal pulses and the ankle-arm index rose from 0.5 to 1. At 6 months follow-up, the patient remained asymptomatic and with an ankle-arm index still equal to 1 (Fig. 23-1).

Case 3

A 58-year-old patient with diabetes presented with rest pain in the left leg and necrotic lesions. Distal pulses were not palpable and ankle-arm index was 0.57. Arteriography showed total obstruction in the middle third of the superficial femoral artery, 6 cm long, and a poor distal vessel runoff. The caliber of the artery proximal to the stenosis was 3.5 mm.

After recanalization with a guide wire and catheter, an angioplasty was performed with a 4 mm balloon. Follow-up angiography showed an intimal flap obstructing intermittently the distal flow. After several passes with a 9 F Atherocath, a normal luminal caliber was reestablished. Heparin was administered for the next 48 hours. Ankle-arm index rose to 0.71 and the rest pain disappeared.

One month after atherectomy, the patient underwent a below-knee amputation. On angiography prior to amputation, the segment treated was permeable (Fig. 23-2).

Case 4

A 51-year-old patient presented with left leg claudication. Distal pulses were not palpable. Arteriography showed a 1.5

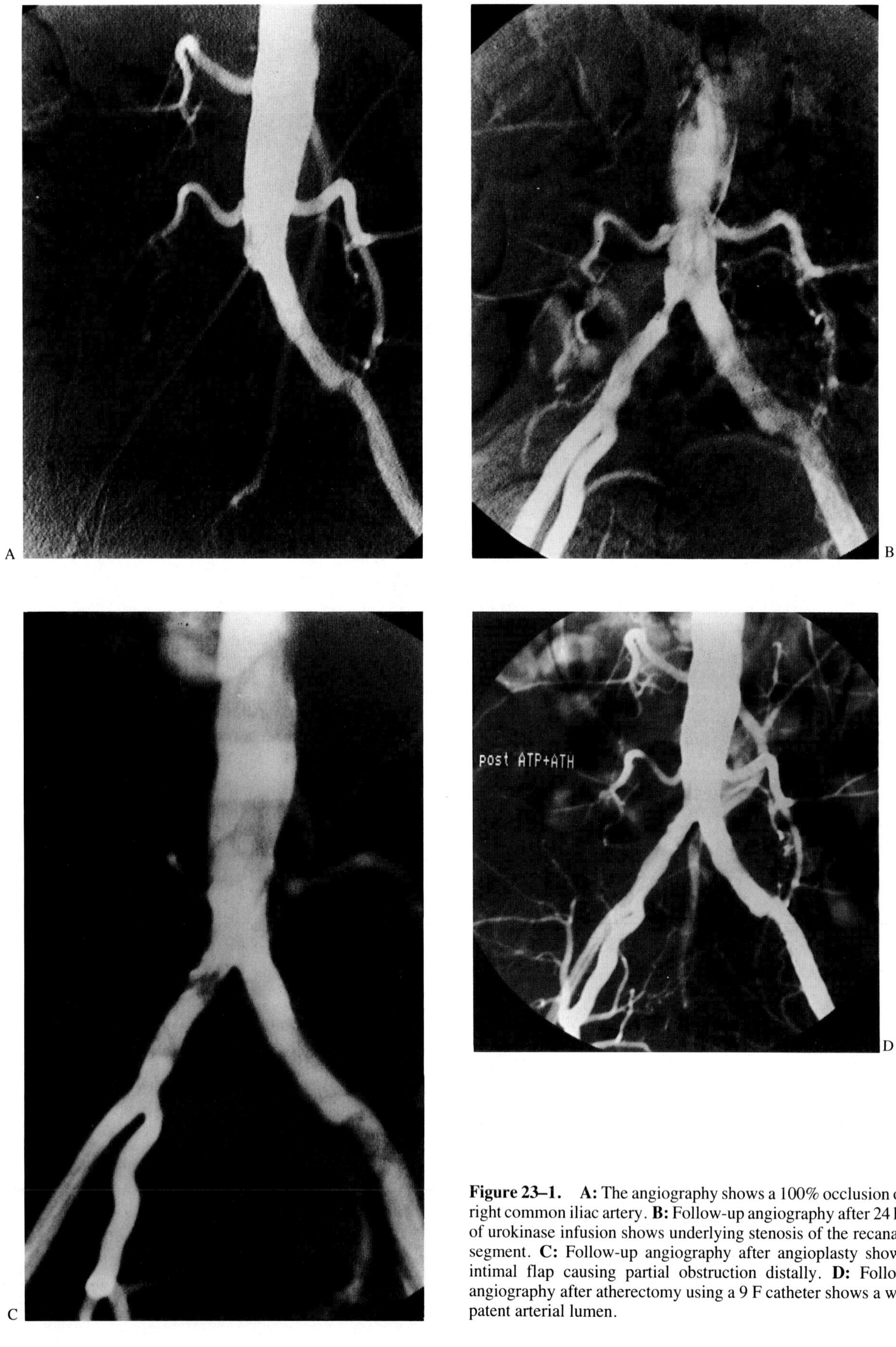

Figure 23–1. **A:** The angiography shows a 100% occlusion of the right common iliac artery. **B:** Follow-up angiography after 24 hours of urokinase infusion shows underlying stenosis of the recanalized segment. **C:** Follow-up angiography after angioplasty shows an intimal flap causing partial obstruction distally. **D:** Follow-up angiography after atherectomy using a 9 F catheter shows a widely patent arterial lumen.

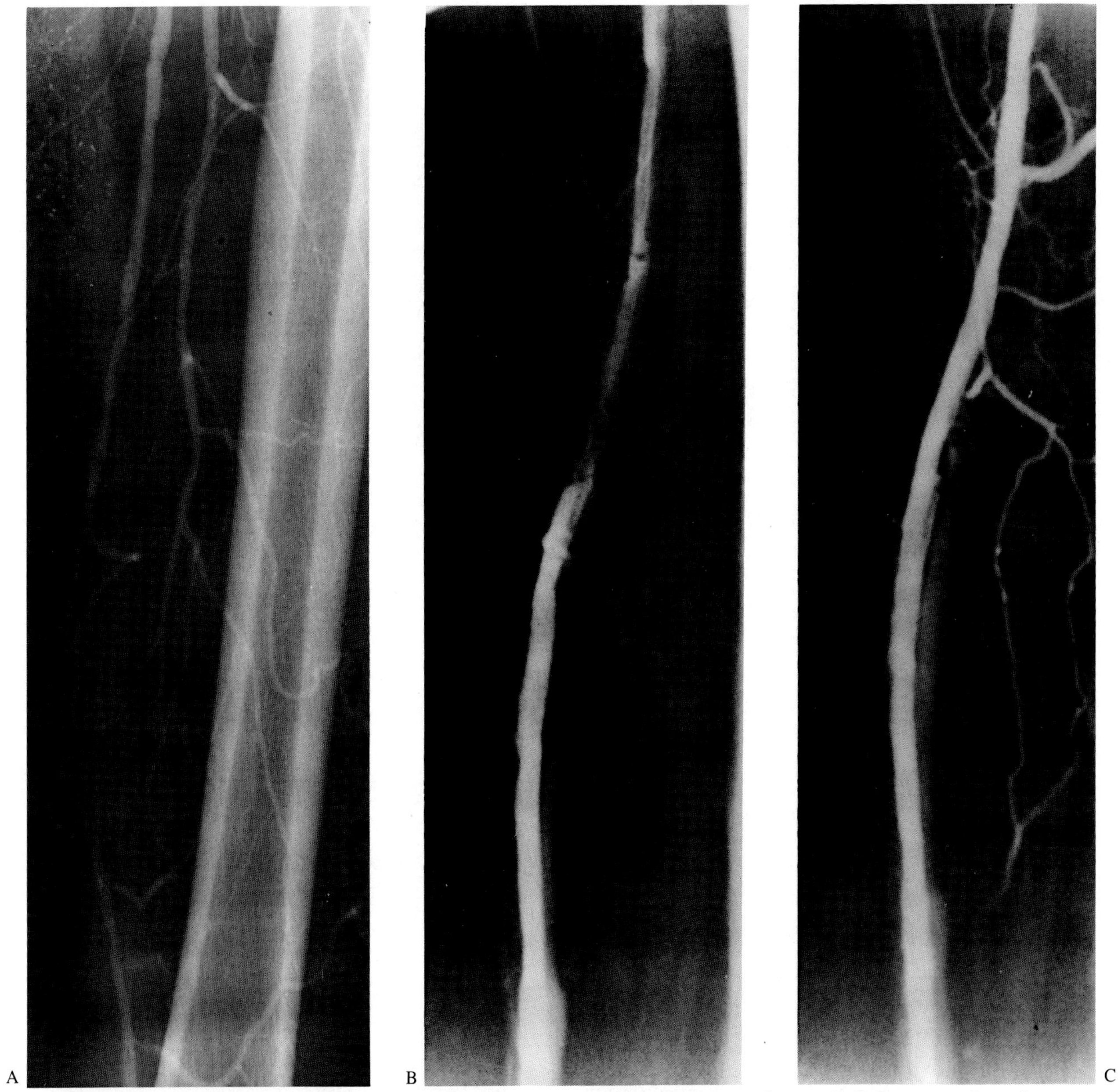

Figure 23–2. **A:** The femoral angiography shows occlusion at the superficial femoral artery. **B:** Follow-up angiography after angioplasty shows intimal flap partially obstructing the arterial lumen. **C:** Follow-up angiography after 9 F atherectomy catheter shows patent lumen.

cm long occlusion in the distal third of the left superficial femoral artery.

After recanalization with a guide wire and angiographic catheter, angioplasty was performed with a 4 mm diameter, 4 cm long balloon catheter. Follow-up angiography showed an intimal flap partly obstructing the arterial lumen. An attempt was made to resect the flap with a 7 F Atherocath, but due to the poor match with the arterial diameter, plaque removal was inadequate. A 9 F Atherocath was subsequently used. The lumen of the femoral artery was reconstituted to 100% of its normal caliber. Ankle-arm index rose from 0.47 to 0.7, and the patient recovered distal pulses.

At 1-year follow-up, the patient presented with recurrent claudication of the left leg, and the ankle-arm index dropped to 0.6. Angiographic follow-up has not been obtained (Fig. 23-3).

Case 5

A 59-year-old patient presented with claudication of the left leg and absent distal pulses. The arteriography showed a 7 cm long occlusion in the distal segment of the left superficial femoral artery. Arterial diameter above the obstruction was 4.5 mm. After recanalization of the obstructed segment,

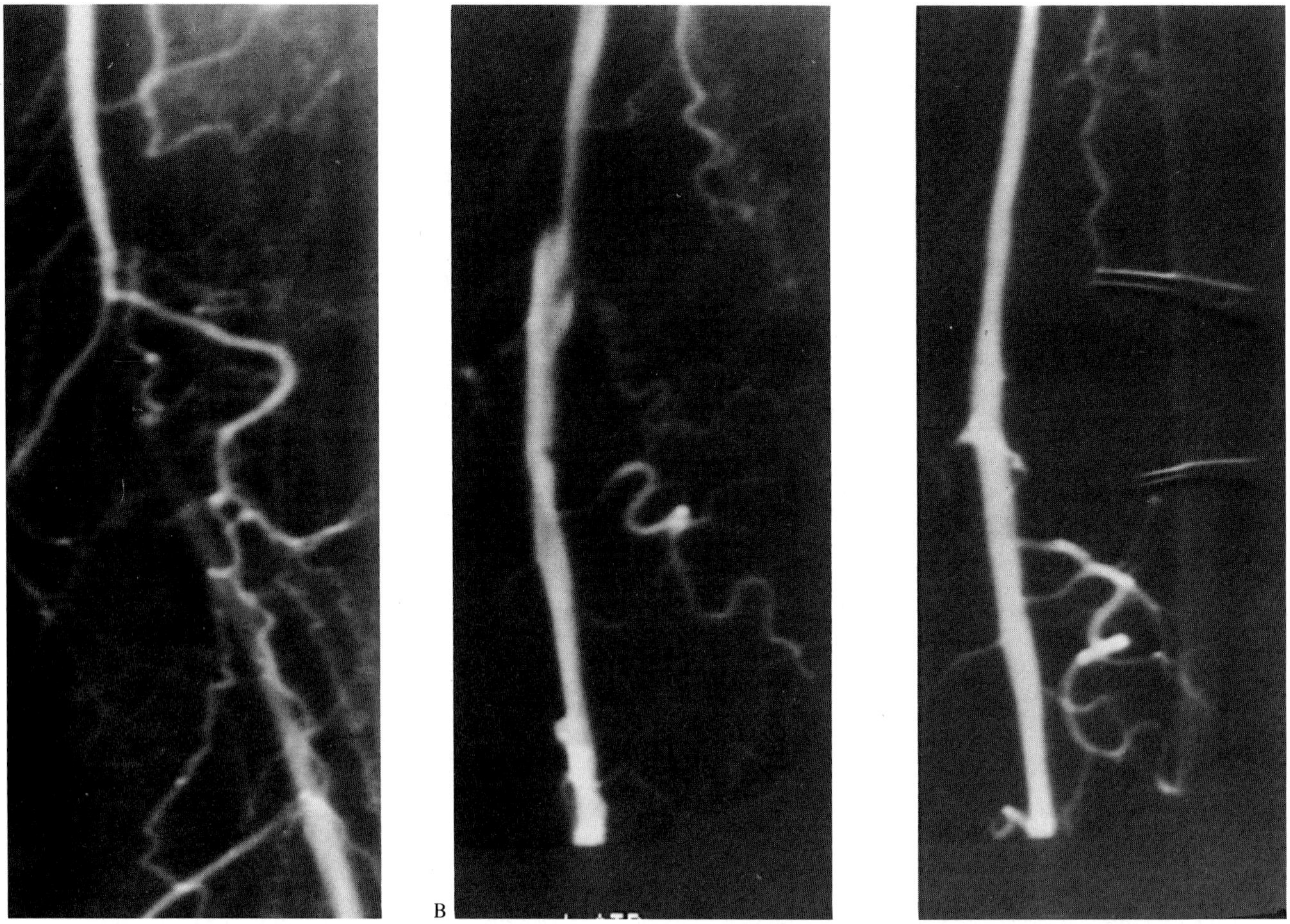

A B C

Figure 23–3. **A:** Femoral angiogram shows occlusion of the superficial femoral artery. **B:** Follow-up angiography after atherectomy and percutaneous transluminal angioplasty shows a large intimal flap causing partial obstruction. **C:** Follow-up angiography after atherectomy shows normal diameter of the artery at the treated segment.

dilation was accomplished with a 5 mm diameter, 4 cm long balloon catheter. Follow-up arteriography showed an intimal flap blocking 50%, of the arterial lumen. After five passes with the 7 F Atherocath and removing a large amount of plaque, normal arterial lumen was established. Heparin was administered for 48 hours. Ankle-arm index rose from 0.40 to 0.95.

Follow-up angiography at 1 year showed occlusion at the origin of the superficial femoral artery (Fig. 23-4).

DISCUSSION

Nonobstructive intimal flaps are commonly observed following angioplasty. These flaps are the result of the fracture and partial dehiscence of the arteriosclerotic intima from the media. The flap remains commonly joined to the artery by the proximal and distal ends. If the proximal end is separated, the flap can produce intermittent obstruction, acting like a valve. This rarely occurs, but can be the cause of acute thrombosis following treatment. What usually occurs is that these flaps produce delayed restenosis or obstruction.

If an intimal flap is observed after angioplasty, the site can be redilated trying to remodel the plaque against the vascular wall. This maneuver is not commonly effective. Until recently, the only therapeutic alternative for obstructive flaps was surgical repair. Currently, atherectomy and intravascular stents are other viable alternatives. The use of atherectomy enables removal of the intimal flaps and restoration of blood flow.[7] The atherectomy catheter must be carefully selected in relation to the diameter of the artery at the lesion site. If an Atherocath of a diameter smaller than the diameter of the vessel is used, it will be impossible to remove the flap in its entirety with the potential risk of causing embolization.

CONCLUSIONS

The use of the Simpson Atherocath for the removal of either obstructive or nonobstructive intimal flaps following angioplasty is extremely useful.

Nonsurgical removal of the flaps was not possible until the development of the Simpson Atherocath. These flaps tended to cause an acute or chronic obstruction of the vessel

24 Recanalization of Chronic Occlusions: Low-Speed Rotational Angioplasty

Christian Vallbracht, M.D., Dieter Liermann, M.D., Ingeborg Prignitz, M.D., Christa Paasch, M.D., Helmut Landgraf, M.D., Wolfgang Beinborn, M.D., Jürgen Kollath, M.D., Franz-Josef Roth, M.D., Werner Schoop, M.D., Martin Kaltenbach, M.D.

Nonoperative dilation of stenosed atherosclerotic vessels, first performed by Charles Dotter in 1964 on peripheral arteries[1] and essentially refined by the introduction of Andreas Grüntzig's technique of balloon angioplasty,[2] has widely become routine in clinical centers worldwide. Favorable experience has been gained specifically with coronary stenoses[3] and renal stenoses in addition to the arteries of the lower extremities. Various technical innovations, particularly in the field of steerable balloon catheters,[4] accounted for a rapid improvement, so that more than 90% of all attempted arterial stenoses can now be dilated successfully.[3,5]

Today, the limits of this technique are total occlusions; occlusions of peripheral arteries more than 10 cm in length and subacute coronary occlusions can be reopened successfully only in about 50 to 60% of all cases.[3,6] The possibility of reopening decreases with the duration of occlusion and the amount of calcification. Chronic occlusions of the iliac artery have not yet become an indication for angioplasty due to unsatisfactory acute treatment results (acute success rate is 30 to 40%) and frequent complications (dissections, emboli) and are consequently referred to surgery.[7]

We have been working on a new technique in Frankfurt since 1984 with which recanalization can be achieved by means of a slowly rotating, flexible, and blunt catheter.[8,9,14] Experimental investigations on postmortem human arteries have demonstrated that even old and calcified occlusions that were not accessible to conventional techniques yielded to the new one.[8] There were no perforations during the investigation and histologic and angioscopic examinations showed relatively smooth channel surfaces.

In this chapter we shall report on our clinical experience obtained with patients with chronic occlusions of the peripheral arteries.

MATERIAL AND METHOD

Patients

From December 1986, when we first applied our new technique,[9] to January 1989 a total of 100 patients, 29 female and 71 male, aged 35 to 90 years (mean age, 68.5 years) were treated with low-speed rotational angioplasty. The superficial femoral artery was chronically occluded in 62 patients, the popliteal artery in 26, and the iliac arteries (communis, 8; externa, 1; both segments, 3) in 12 patients. Occlusion lengths ranged from 4 to 35 cm, with a mean of 12 cm. Calcifications in the occluded area were found in 73 patients.

Patients were allocated to 4 groups:

- Group 1: 18 patients with primary intervention, occluded femoral or popliteal artery and occlusion length less than 10 cm
- Group 2: 46 patients with primary intervention, occluded femoral or popliteal artery and occlusion length more than 10 cm
- Group 3: 24 patients with secondary intervention, after failure of conventional techniques on occluded femoral or popliteal artery
- Group 4: 12 patients with occluded iliac artery, occlusion length from 5 to 20 cm (mean occlusion length, 9.8 cm)

Clinical and Angiographic Findings on Admission

The clinical stage was IIb according to Fontaine in 87 patients, IIa in three patients; the distance to claudication ranged from 30 to 300 m, with a mean of 105 m. In ten patients the clinical stage was IV with necrosis and pain at rest; seven of these had been refused surgical revascularization and were consequently facing amputation. The ankle-brachial index in Doppler pressure measurements before treatment was between 0 and 0.86 (mean, 0.53).

Duration of occlusion was estimated according to the respective case history (patients were asked about present claudication symptoms and their onset) and varied between 5 and 48 months. Earlier angiographic findings from seven patients gave evidence for a minimum occlusion duration of 6 to 36 months.

Technique

The electrically driven rotating catheter (outer diameter, 2.2 mm) consists of 4 V_2A steel coiled wires of 0.2 mm each, with an inner lumen that allows introduction of exchange wires and injection of contrast agents; it is covered with a highly flexible Teflon shrinking tube and has an olive-shaped blunt tip (Fig. 24-1). The motor unit, offering a continuously variable speed ranging between 0 and 500 rpm, formerly ran directly off the mains with speed control via the foot switch of a transformer.[9] It is now battery operated (9 V battery) with potentiometric speed control that guarantees smooth adjustment and a high level of electrical safety (Fig. 24-2).

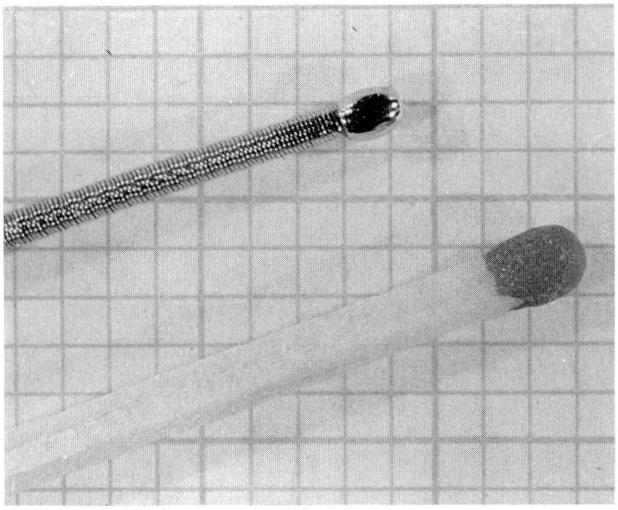

Figure 24–1. Rotating catheter consisting of 4 × 0.2 mm V_2A-steel coiled wires covered with a highly flexible Teflon shrinking tube and an olive-shaped, blunt tip (see difference in size to the match).

(Producer: Dr. Ing. P. Osypka GmbH, Baseler Straße 109, D-7889 Grenzach-Whylen, Germany.)

After antegrade puncture of the femoral artery and subsequent intra-arterial injection of 5000 U of heparin, a conventional 7 or 8 F sheath of appropriate length was introduced and angiography performed of the entire extremity. A frozen picture of the occluded area was obtained via digital subtraction angiography, which was used as a roadmap to mark the obstructed area from behind the live x-ray image.

An initial retrograde puncture of the contralateral femoral artery was performed in 12 patients with occlusion of the iliac artery (group 4) who were first treated when we had used the new technique for 1 year. A 4 F pigtail catheter was then entered into the abdominal aorta and a frozen picture selected that subsequently helped—via roadmapping—with retrograde puncture of the femoral artery at the distal end of the occlusion. This procedure has proven to facilitate both finding the artery with absent pulsation in the groin as well as careful insertion of the valve into a relatively short distal vessel stump.

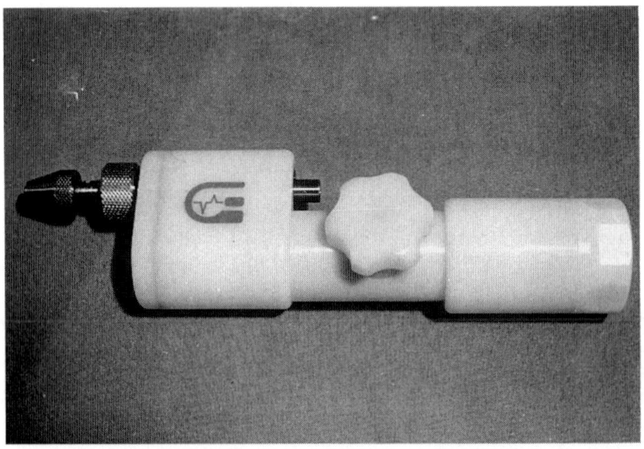

Figure 24–2. Battery-driven electric motor. The 9 V battery is placed in a sterilized compartment with screw fixture.

The rotation catheter was introduced directly through the plastic sealing into the conventional hemostatic valve and advanced carefully, under fluoroscopic control, to the obstructed area. Due to technical modifications, it is no longer necessary to use the more complicated rotating hemostatic valve (see Vallbracht et al[9]) used at the beginning of our clinical examinations. When the occlusion was reached, the small electric motor placed in the right hand of the investigator was started and the obstructed area slowly passed using low rotational speed of 100 to 200 rpm, under slight axial thrust, and continuous fluoroscopical monitoring (Fig. 24-3). Once the occlusion was passed, blood was aspirated and disposed of and contrast material was injected through the rotating catheter to document its intraluminal localization distal to the occlusion. A 0.35 inch exchange wire on standby in the rotating catheter approximately 2 cm behind the tip was then advanced and placed distal of the obstruction. After retraction of the rotating catheter, the new channel was documented by angiography and further dilated using a conventional balloon catheter.

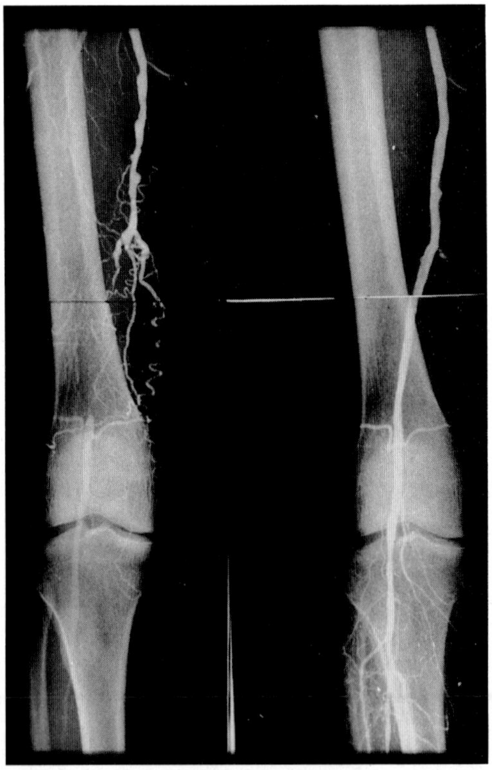

Figure 24–3. Chronic occlusion of the superficial femoral artery (length 11 cm). Left side: before the procedure; right side: after reopening with low-speed rotational angioplasty and balloon dilation.

Medication

All patients received aspirin (0.5 to 1.5 mg/day[10]) from at least 24 hours before the intervention until control angiography, in a mean of 6 months. The valve was continuously perfused during the intervention with 2000 U of heparin per hour.[3]

Immediately after the intervention, 1000 to 1200 U of heparin per hour were administered intravenously and monitored over a period of 48 hours. Only in rare cases (with very long occlusions, intolerance to aspirin) was permanent anticoagulation indicated.

RESULTS

Angiographic Results

Group 1: 18 patients with primary intervention and occluded femoral or popliteal artery, <10 cm, mean length: 5.8 cm. Occlusions were successfully reopened in 17 of the 18 patients.

Group 2: 46 patients with primary intervention and occluded femoral or popliteal artery, more than 10 cm; mean length, 14.8 cm; maximum length, 35 cm. Reopening was successful in 38 of the 46 patients (Fig. 24-3).

Group 3: 24 patients after failure of conventional reopening techniques, including three patients with more than one attempt. Mean occlusion length, 10.5 cm. Twenty of the 24 patients were treated with low-speed rotational angioplasty more than 4 weeks following failure of conventional attempts. Occlusions were successfully reopened in 13 of 20 cases. Four of the 24 patients were treated less than 4 weeks following failure of conventional attempts. Reopening was only achieved in one patient.

Group 4: 12 patients with chronic occlusions of the iliac artery; mean occlusion length, 9.8 cm. Occlusions were successfully reopened in 7 of 12 patients (Fig. 24-4); two patients had subsequent local urokinase lysis of some remaining thrombotic deposits in the formerly obstructed area; a stent was implanted in one patient with elastic stenosis.

Limitations

Vessels with fluoroscopically evident "plaque-shaped" calcifications in the occluded area more or less regularly obstructing the entire vessel lumen along the cross-sectional diameter—the respective resistance can be "felt" by the operator—are not likely to be successfully reopened. In contrast, those calcifications spreading along the vessel wall in longitudinal direction marking the path of the vessel, however, do not restrict the chances of success even in case of substantial stenosis. In a total of four patients with very old occlusions, major proximal collaterals had developed with minimum angular distance that paralleled the native vessel. Since there was no definite proximal vessel stump, both the rotating catheter and the conventional guide wires kept on slipping into the respective collateral, yet without inflicting any damage to the collateral.

Complications

In none of our patients did perforation or other severe complications occur through the rotating catheter. Dissection was observed in seven patients that caused, however, no further problems; in one patient there was a small peripheral embolism without any clinical consequences; hematoma formation at the puncture site, found with five patients, required surgical correction and transfusion in one patient.

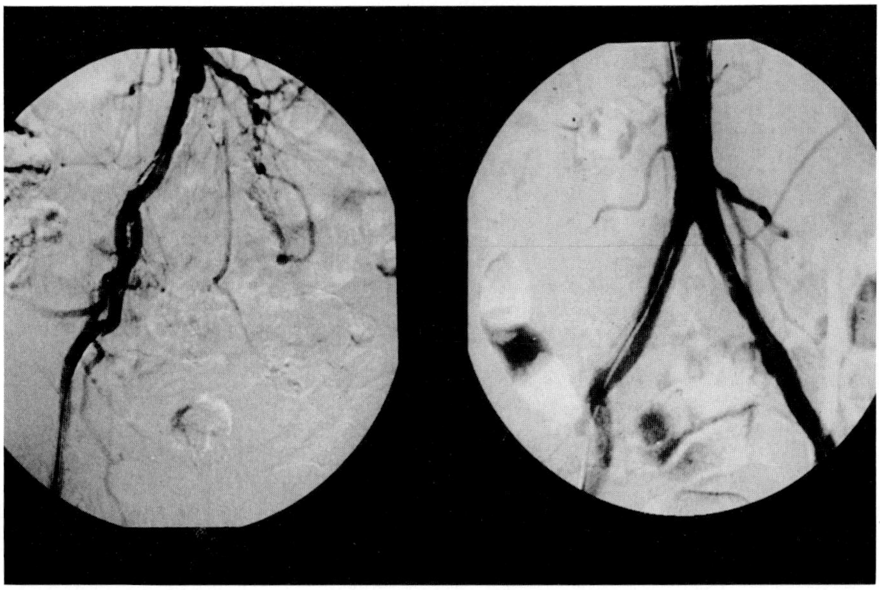

Figure 24-4. Chronic occlusion of the left common iliac artery. Left side: before the procedure; right side: after reopening with low-speed rotational angioplasty and balloon dilatation (guide wires in both sides).

Functional Results

The ankle-brachial index in Doppler measurements, determined on the second day after the intervention, increased from a mean of 0.53 to 0.89 in the 75 successfully treated patients.

In four of the seven patients with clinical stage IV who had been refused surgical revascularization, reopening was successful, the impending amputation consequently averted and, finally, the clinical stage decreased to stage IIb. There was no deterioration in any of the patients.

Preliminary Long-Term Results of Follow-up Angiography

Until March 1989, a total of 31 patients had angiographic control at 2 to 24 weeks (mean time interval, 16.4 weeks). There were favorable long-term results: the absence of hemodynamically significant stenoses, in a total of 15 patients; significant stenosis in the formerly occluded segment was found with five patients; another 11 patients showed reocclusion. The mean length of the initial stenosis in patients with reocclusion or restenosis (mean, 12.9 cm) was clearly higher than that obtained from patients with favorable long-term results (9.9 cm). Eleven of 16 patients were again treated with rotational angioplasty or conventional balloon angioplasty, two patients were treated medically, and another two patients were referred for bypass surgery. In no case, however, was amputation necessary.

DISCUSSION

Chronic arterial vessel occlusions are likely to be caused in most cases by ulcerating atherosclerotic plaques that stenose the vessel lumen subsequently occluded by thrombotic deposition.

Two major consequences may be derived from this type of pathophysiologic process: first, there is a clear risk of dissection and even wall perforation involved in the attempt to reopen mechanically occlusions due to preformed rupturing, a risk that rises with increasing occlusion length; second, there is a "soft point," a point of least resistance among concentrated obstructions in the occluded area that may persist for a yet unknown longer period—the final occluding thrombus that indicates the last real lumen—and that might help in pioneering through the occlusion.

Therefore the relatively thin and straight wires commonly used in conventional recanalization techniques may easily enter into such preformed dissections. Even with successful reentry into the vessel lumen and ensuing neolumen there are unsatisfactory acute and long-term results. The risk of wall perforation is especially high when such a wire is advanced through a vessel bend and approaching a delicate wall portion.

Thin wires therefore seem to be more dangerous than the relatively large and flexible catheter with an ideally blunt tip applied in our new rotational angioplasty technique. Low-speed rotation is associated with minimum adhesive friction, thus facilitating forward movement, passage through the vessel bends, and an especially sensitive transmission of any resistance from distal to proximal.

These properties may be responsible for the definitely low tendency toward dissection observed so far in all of our experimental and clinical studies, as a result of which we may conclude that there is virtually no risk of vessel wall perforation derived from this procedure.

High-speed rotation techniques[11,12] are not comparable with our technique; they differ fundamentally and technically, namely, with regard to the mechanism of recanalization. Abrasive catheters rotating at high speeds of up to 150,000 rpm, some of them with diamond-covered sharp drilling heads, are geared to remove obstructive material by abrading, as opposed to rotational angioplasty, which aims at gently displacing or compressing the vessel-occluding material and consequent volume reduction as a result of fluid expression.[13] The procedure can be compared to exposing without cutting.

Once the olive-shaped, blunt tip has approached the obstructing material by slight axial thrusts, low-speed rotation leads the catheter to "search" the path of least resistance. Since the final occluding thrombus "lags behind" the other obstructive components in its organization and calcification, it represents and remains the softest part of the obstruction, offering easy penetration for a long time, possibly over years.

It can be assumed that the rotating catheter will thus pass the obstruction through the last "real" lumen, as is also indicated by the often astonishing smooth channel surfaces achieved with subsequent balloon dilation, which is always performed.

Our experimental and clinical studies now of more than 5 years standing demonstrated that reopening occluded vessels by means of low-speed rotational angioplasty has proven to be a particularly gentle and safe procedure with a low complication rate and virtually no risk of perforation. Acute success rate with primary intervention exceeds 80%; even the very long occlusions were successfully reopened. These results are clearly more favorable than those obtained with both the conventional and the high-speed techniques.

In case of failing conventional attempts, successful recanalization of formerly nontreatable occlusions can be achieved in more than 60% of cases applying low-speed rotational angioplasty at a minimum time interval of 4 weeks to the primary intervention. This time period seems necessary for the sites of predilection and dissections to close following unsuccessful conventional reopening procedures.

Meanwhile, the indication has been extended for complete occlusions of the iliac artery (Fig. 24-4) and, additionally, for coronary vessel occlusions. The first documented long-term results obtained from angiography are promising, yet require further research owing to small numbers and short time periods.

SUMMARY AND CONCLUSIONS

One hundred patients with chronic occlusions of the peripheral arteries were treated with low-speed rotational angioplasty between December 1986 and January 1989 by means of a reopening technique that comprises the application of a relatively thick and flexible catheter with an olive-shaped head providing an ideally blunt tip. Rotational reopening was performed at very low speeds of 100 to 200 rpm using a small motor unit.

Acute success rate at the initial intervention was 90% in the femoral and popliteal arteries with occlusion lengths of less than 10 cm and 80% in occlusions of more than 10 cm. Following unsuccessful conventional recanalization attempts, 13 of 20 occlusions were reopened by thc rotating catheter at a minimum time interval of 4 weeks; the rate was, however, clearly lower (one of four) with shorter time intervals. Successful reopening of chronic common iliac artery occlusions was achieved with this technique in 7 of 12 patients. There were no perforations and other severe complications.

It is concluded that effective and gentle reopening of chronic arterial occlusions may be obtained by low-speed rotational angioplasty, even in case of obstructions otherwise subject to operation.

The rate of successful recanalization of chronically occluded arteries is significantly higher with this new technique than with conventional techniques, and formerly nontreatable occlusions can be successfully reopened in more than 60% of cases.

Update, May 1992

PERIPHERAL VESSELS

To date more than 350 patients with chronic occlusions of peripheral vessels have been treated in Frankfurt. As in our hospital, the technique has become part of the clinical routine in more than 130 centers in Europe. A questionnaire gathering the experience from learning curves of other centers was started in 1991. The results of 74 centers and 1252 patients are available now. Indications included superficial femoral and popliteal arteries (80.5%), lower limb (11%) and iliac arteries (7.3%), and more recently, subclavian and carotid arteries and the tuba uterina. In 70% of the cases low-speed rotational angioplasty was used as the first attempt in 30% only after failure of conventional techniques. The overall success rate was 979/1252 (78.2%). In patients after failure of conventional techniques the system was successful in 66.5%. Complications: one death (0.08%), dissections or perforations, 31 (2.4%), emergency surgery, 14 (1.1%), peripheral embolization without consequences (mostly in fresh occlusions), 42 (3.3%).

CORONARY ARTERIES

To date more than 200 patients with chronic complete occlusions of coronary arteries, in whom the attempt to pass the obstruction with a conventional wire failed, have been treated with low-speed rotational angioplasty in Frankfurt. The acute success rate is 70%. Three patients (1.2%) underwent emergency surgery; no patient died. Meanwhile, the coronary system is used in some other centers too and randomized studies were started comparing low-speed rotational angioplasty to other new techniques.

REFERENCES

1. Dotter CT, Judkins MP. Transluminal treatment of arteriosclerotic obstruction: description of a new technique and a preliminary report of its application. Circulation 1964;30:654.
2. Grüntzig A, Hopff H. Perkutane Rekanalisation chronischer arterieller Verschlüsse mit einem neuen Dilatationskatheter. Modifikation der Dottertechnik. Dtsch Med Wochenschr 1974;99:2502–10.
3. Kober G, Vallbracht C, Lang H, et al. Transluminale koronare Angioplastik 1977–1985: Erfahrungen bei looo Eingriffen. Radiologe 1985;25:346.
4. Simpson JB, Blaim DS, Robert E, Harrison DC. A new catheter system for coronary angioplasty. Am J Cardiol 1982;49:1216–22.
5. Faxon DP, Kelsey S, Kellet MA, et al. Predictors of a successful angioplasty (PTCA-registry). Circulation 1986; 74(suppl II):768.
6. Zeitler E. Die perkutane transluminale Rekanalisation chronischer Stenosen und Verschlüsse peripherer Arterien. Wien Med Wochenschr 1985;135:384–92.
7. Graziani L. Percutaneous recanalization of total iliac and femoro-popliteal artery occlusions. Eur J Radiol 1987;7:91–3.
8. Vallbracht C, Kress J, Schweitzer M, et al. Rotationsangioplastik-ein neues Verfahren zur Gefäßwiedereröffnung und -erweiterung. Experimentelle Befunde. Z Kardiol 1987; 76:608–11.
9. Vallbracht C, Schweitzer M, Kress J, et al. Rotationsangioplastik-erste klinische Ergebnisse bei peripheren Gefäßverschlüssen. Z Kardiol 1988;77:352–7.
10. Breddin HK. Treatment with platelet function inhibitors. In Kaltenbach M, Grüntzig A, Rentrop K, Bussmann WD (eds): Transluminal Coronary Angioplasty and Intracoronary Thrombolysis. Heidelberg: Springer-Verlag, 1982:41–3.
11. Ritchie JL, Hansen DD, Vracko H, Auth D. In vivo rotational thrombectomy-evaluation by angioscopy. (Abstr.) Circulation 1986;74(suppl II):1822.
12. Kensey RK, Nash JE, Abrahams C, Zarius CHK. Recanalization of obstructed arteries with a flexible, rotating tip catheter. Radiology 1987;165:387–9.
13. Kaltenbach M, Beyer J, Klepzig H, et al. Effect of 5 kg/cm^2 pressure on atherosclerotic wall segments. In Kaltenbach M, Grüntzig A, Rentrop K, Bussmann WD (eds): Transluminal Coronary Angioplasty and Intracoronary Thrombolysis. Heidelberg: Springer-Verlag, 1982:189–93.
14. Kaltenbach M, Vallbracht C. Rotationsangioplastik-ein neues Katheterverfahren. Fortschr Med 1987;105:412–4.

25 Kensey Catheter: Technical Description

Kenneth R. Kensey, M.D.

DEVICE DESCRIPTION AND OPERATING SYSTEM

The Kensey catheter is a flexible high-speed rotating tip catheter used for recanalization of stenotic and occluded vessels (Fig. 25-1). Its primary indication is in treating lesions unable to be passed with a guide wire. The rotating tip is essentially a blunt rotating stainless steel cam. The flexible polyurethane catheter body, available in 5 and 8 F sizes, encloses a motor-driven cable that drives the cam at speeds of 30,000 to 100,000 rpm. The catheter also contains a lumen that carries pressurized fluid to the base of the cam. A combination of nonionic contrast media and saline is injected through the lumen and into the vessel at flow rates of up to 60 ml/min. The ejected contrast medium serves to identify the occluded vessel and map out the recanalization procedure. As the rotating cam selectively ablates diseased tissue, the resulting vortex draws in the ablated particulate for micropulverization while the ejected fluid acts to center and cool the high-speed rotational cam.

As shown in Figure 25-2, the Kensey catheter system is composed of the catheter itself and a drive motor, a control console, and a fluid injector with a supply of injection solution. The rest of this chapter will describe how the Kensey catheter system should be used for recanalization of totally occluded arteries.

OPERATING PRINCIPLES

The safety and efficacy of the Kensey catheter is based on two major assumptions: (1) diseased tissue can be selectively pulverized based on inherent differences in its viscoelasticity, organization, and fibrous make-up; and (2) microembolization of diseased tissue is clinically innocuous to the distal organ, as shown clinically with this and other devices that microembolize tissue. Using these principles, this section will describe how the catheter utilizes the rotating cam and fluid jets to ablate diseased tissue selectively. Understanding the principle of action is very important because this device is highly technique-sensitive.

Rotating Cam

The major component of the Kensey catheter is the spinning cam. The shape of the cam is extremely critical and gives the tip its ability to pulverize selectively nonviscoelastic material. No cutting is involved. There are no sharp edges. The tip acts more like a high-speed rotary hammer to pulverize nonviscoelastic material in much the same way as a cast cutter removes a cast from an injured limb. The vibrating saw that removes the cast selectively destroys the plaster, without damaging normal skin.

In a similar manner, the rotating cam differentiates between normal artery wall and atherosclerotic tissue based on differences in tissue viscoelasticity. This allows the catheter to pulverize atheroma selectively while leaving the arterial wall intact.

Normal arterial walls have a high degree of elasticity that allows the tissue to yield under the stress imparted by the rotating cam, as shown in Figure 25-3A. The amount to which the tissue deforms is proportional to the cam size, the applied rotational energy, and the tissue elasticity. There is an elastic limit, however, which is defined as the amount of stress a material can withstand and still return to its original shape. Normal arterial tissue has a higher elastic limit than material such as calcium, fatty tissue, thrombus, and fibrous tissue. As shown in Figure 25-3B, when the rotating cam imparts a stress surpassing the elastic limit of atheromatous material, the material deforms and is subsequently pulverized. Meanwhile, the healthy elastic tissue remains undamaged (Fig. 25-4).

Pressurized Fluid

The high-speed rotating catheter tip also directs fluid jets laterally against the artery wall. These lateral jets are important in guiding the catheter through a total occlusion, in dilating the artery, and in opening collaterals. The working tip creates a powerful vortex that, in turn, creates a significant negative pressure at the tip of the catheter. The vortex recirculates debris and repeatedly reduces the size of parti-

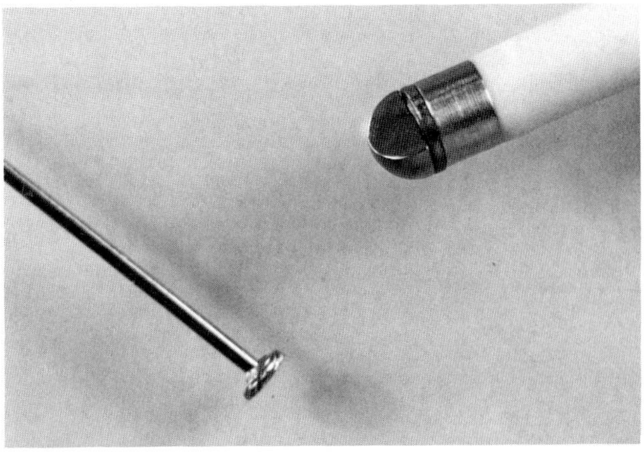

Figure 25–1. The Kensey catheter (8 French).

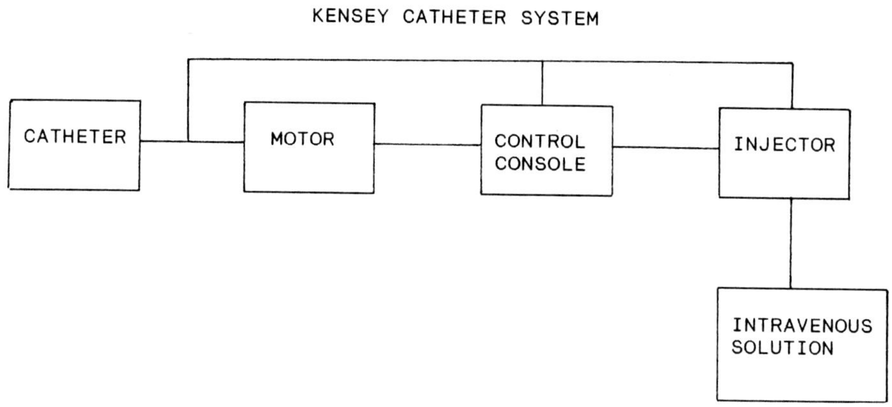

Figure 25–2.

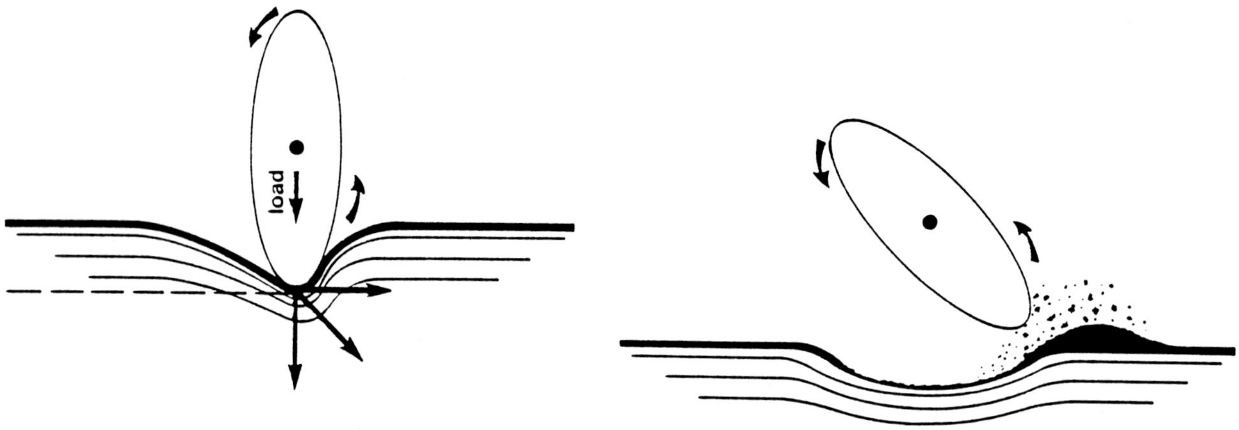

Degree of deformation of the arterial wall is proportional to the cam size and applied energy (rotational speed) of the Kensey catheter.

The difference in elastic limits enables arterial deposits to be pulverized while keeping the arterial wall intact.

Figure 25–3.

WORKING TIP

A) THE WORKING TIP FUNCTIONS LIKE A HIGH SPEED "ROTARY HAMMER" TO PULVERIZE NONVISCOELASTIC MATERIAL.

NO CUTTING INVOLVED

B) THE WORKING TIP DILATES THE ARTERY WITH FLUID JETS PROPELLED LATERALLY AGAINST THE ARTERY WALL.

C) THE WORKING TIP CREATES A VORTEX TO RECIRCULATE DEBRIS AND REPEATEDLY REDUCES THE SIZE OF THE PARTICLES PRODUCED.

D) THE FLUID JETS PRODUCED BY THE WORKING TIP HELP THE TIP "SELF GUIDE" ITSELF. THE TIP REMAINS IN THE LUMEN OF THE ARTERY BY FOLLOWING THE PATH OF LEAST RESISTANCE.

Figure 25–4.

FLUID

A) COOLS SYSTEM

B) LUBRICATES SYSTEM

C) ALLOWS VISUALIZATION OF PROCEDURE (DYE)

D) ALLOWS INTRODUCTION OF MEDICATION

1) ANTICOAGULANTS/ANTIPLATELETS
2) UROKINASE, ETC.
3) ANTISPASMODICS - CALCIUM CHANNEL BLOCKERS, NITRO
4) OXYGEN?
5) ETC.

Figure 25–5.

cles produced. This feature of the working tip will be described in more detail later (Fig. 25-5).

The fluid also acts to cool and lubricate the system, allows visualization of the procedure, and allows addition of any type of medication to the site of treatment. Thrombolytic agents such as urokinase and heparin are generally added to the solution in subclinical doses. Antispasmodics, oxygen, and perhaps other types of medications to produce multiple other effects could also be added. The fluid is injected under pressure by the usual injector system found in a catheterization laboratory at rates of 30 to 60 cc/min. The higher flow rates probably open more collaterals and better control the catheter, but the most efficacious fluid formulation is still unknown. Up to this point, patients have been treated empirically. Note that high viscosity concoctions will result in lower flow per minute through the catheter because of a pressure limit in each catheter. Higher flow rates may be very advantageous and therefore additional studies are necessary to determine the best perfusate mixture.

Path of Least Resistance

The theory of the "path of least resistance" plays an important role in guiding the working tip. Implied in this theory is that total occlusions have an area of least resistance that correlates to that area in the artery that was last patent. Depending on the age of the obstruction, this area of least resistance will be made up of fresh thrombus or organized thrombus. Obviously, as the obstruction becomes older, the area of least resistance becomes more fibrous or more calcified. The Kensey catheter tip finds the area of least resistance through several mechanisms. Fresh thrombus is very nonviscoelastic. Thrombus usually fills the area of least resistance and therefore the catheter tip will remove this area first, since it is most easily pulverized (Figs. 25-6, 25-7). The fluid jets tend to guide the catheter to the area of least resistance (Fig. 25-8). The amount of pressure created by these lateral jets of fluid have been measured and are exponentially related to the revolutions per minute of the tip (Fig. 25-9).

Of unknown significance is the fact that a spinning tipped catheter reduces the amount of forward friction created by the forward movement of the catheter. This phenomenon is seen in daily life when a cork is removed from a wine bottle. If the cork is twisted as a forward force is applied to the cork, there will be less resistance required to remove the cork. A similar effect is seen as the catheter's spinning tip is passed down an artery (Figs. 25-10, 25-11).

Another important component is that the catheter tip tends

EASILY PULVERIZED = AREA OF LEAST RESISTANCE

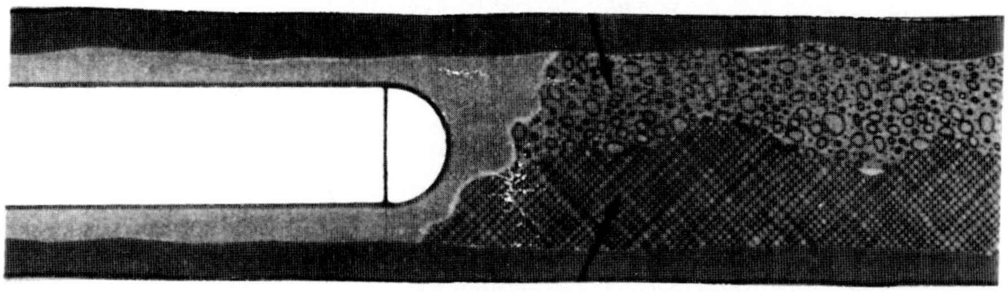

FIBROUS

Figure 25–6. Total occlusion. Recanalization by differences in tissue properties.

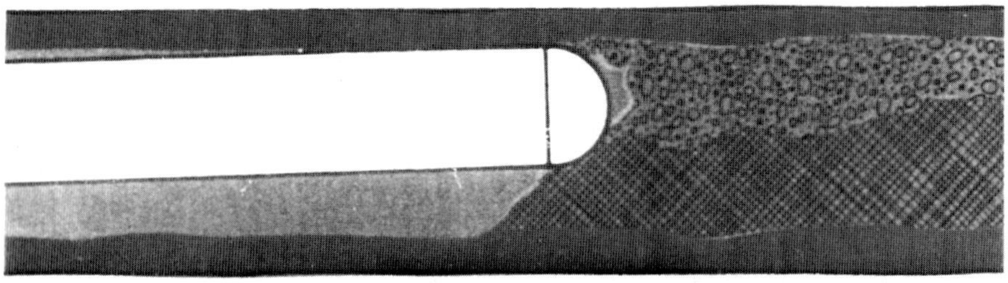

Figure 25–7. Area of least resistance removed first, exposing more easily pulverized material.

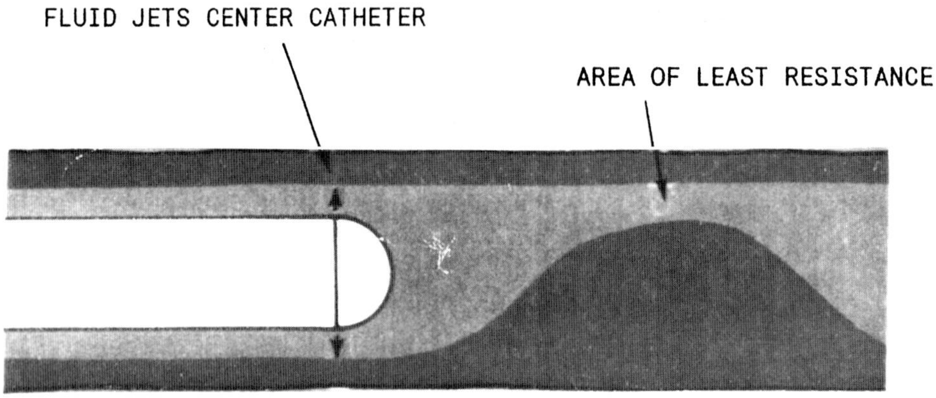

Figure 25–8.

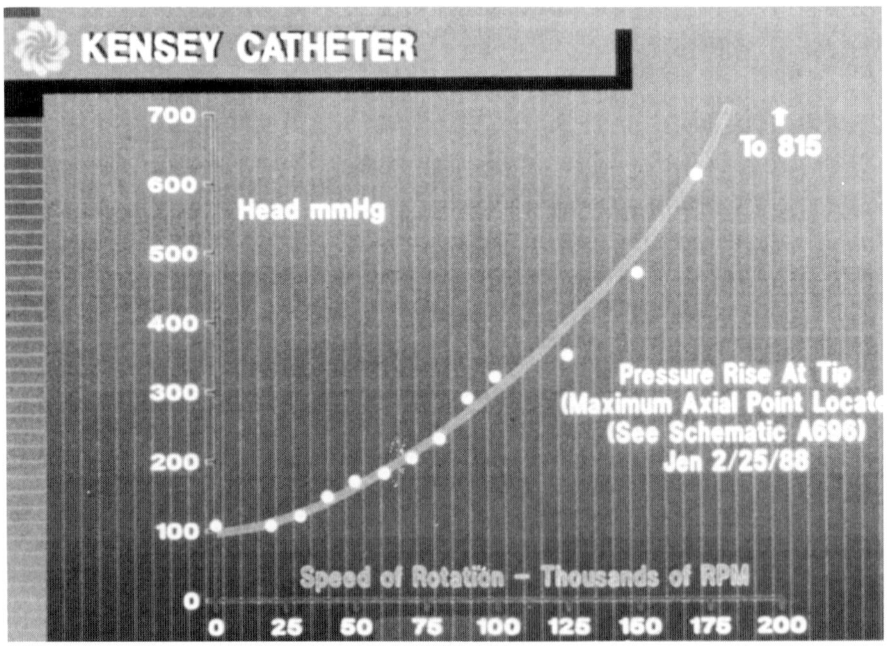

Figure 25–9.

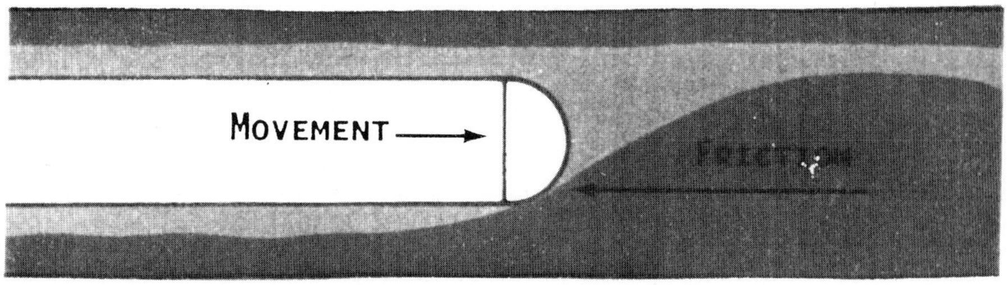

Figure 25–10. Nonrotating friction vector.

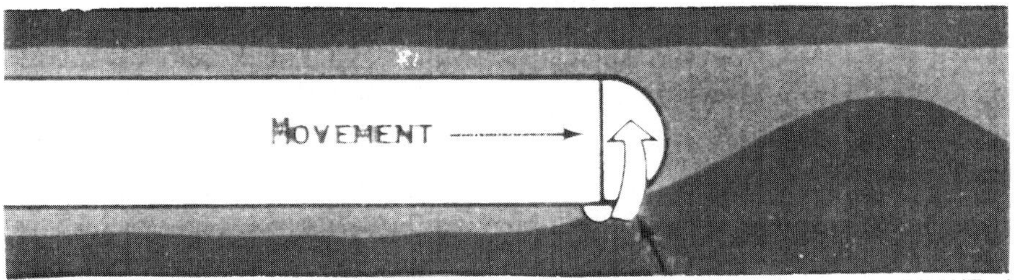

Figure 25–11. Force required to pass catheter down lumen is reduced.

to vibrate when it comes in contact with a less easily pulverized surface. A "bouncing" tip or vibration deflects the tip from the "hard" areas into the area of least resistance (Fig. 25-12).

In addition, the tip itself creates an area of high negative pressure. This negative pressure also tends to pull the catheter tip into the area of least resistance once a small nipple of material has been removed. The catheter tip will always be directed to the nipple where the negative pressure at the tip is magnified by the shape of the occlusion (Fig. 25-13).

These multiple forces combine synergistically to find the area of least resistance of a total occlusion. The relative significance of any one of these forces is unknown, but our in vitro testing of this system in areas such as the destruction of kidney stones has confirmed these basic principles. Future testing is required to identify the roles each mechanical property plays in finding the area of least resistance.

GUIDELINES FOR USING THE DEVICE

As mentioned previously, this device is highly technique-sensitive. The main principle to remember is to go slowly. In the hands of a skilled operator, one can achieve greater than 90% acute success in recanalizing long total occlusions. A few points to remember will perhaps shorten the learning curve. Allow the tip to do its work. Watch for extravasation and deflection of the tip laterally. Remember, it is not a race. Go slowly.

Extravasation of Dye

When using this catheter, extravasation of contrast medium through the artery wall is an important safety parameter that must be watched for. If the operator pushes the catheter too hard, goes too fast through a lesion, or if the catheter is deflected from an obstruction or stenosis, the catheter tip will be jammed into the arterial wall. With continued force on the tip, perforation of the artery may occur. If the operator is alert and observant, he will notice extravasation of dye occurring through the artery wall into the soft tissue surrounding the artery before actual perforation occurs. Extravasation warns of impending perforation before vessel wall puncture, allowing the operator to proceed with caution or withdraw totally and reanalyze the situation (Fig. 25-14). Extravasation of dye is not usually associated with any clinical ill effect. Acutely and in long-term studies, clinical deleterious effects have not been observed from extravasation. If the contrast solution is too concentrated, extravasation will cause opacification of the soft tissue surrounding the artery and obscure visualization for the rest of the procedure. It is for this reason that no greater than a 30% nonionic dye solution is used in the perfusate of this catheter.

Use of Guide Wires

It is also recommended that an occlusion should not be instrumented with a guide wire prior to the use of this catheter. The guide wire does not have a "smart tip" and cannot determine the ideal passage through a total occlusion, and thus a guide wire will create an area of least resistance which may or may not be in the desirable area. If the guide

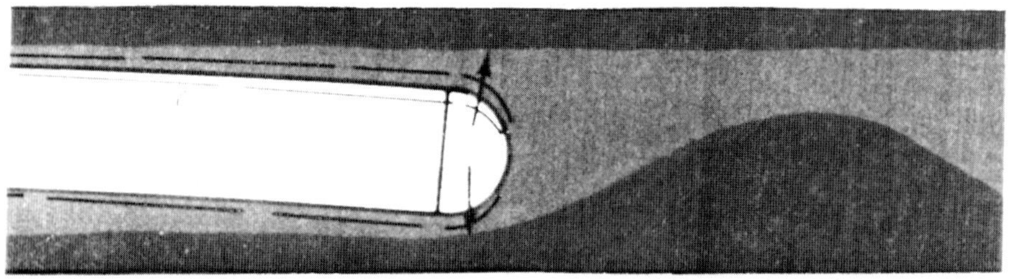

Figure 25–12. Bouncing tip will direct tip away from hard areas into the area of least resistance.

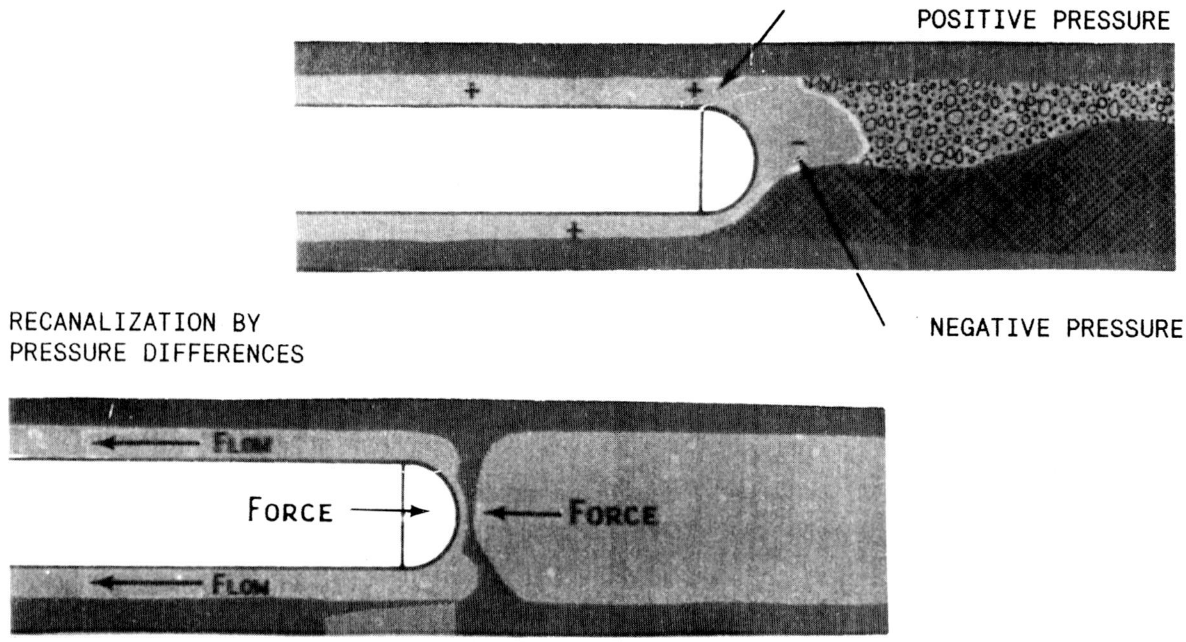

Figure 25–13.

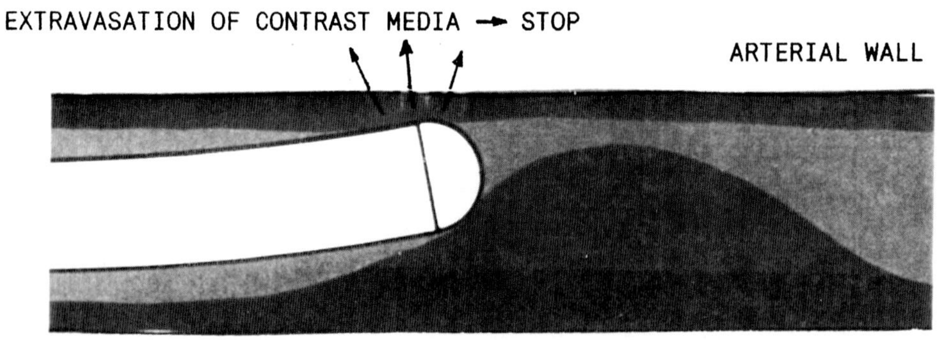

Figure 25–14.

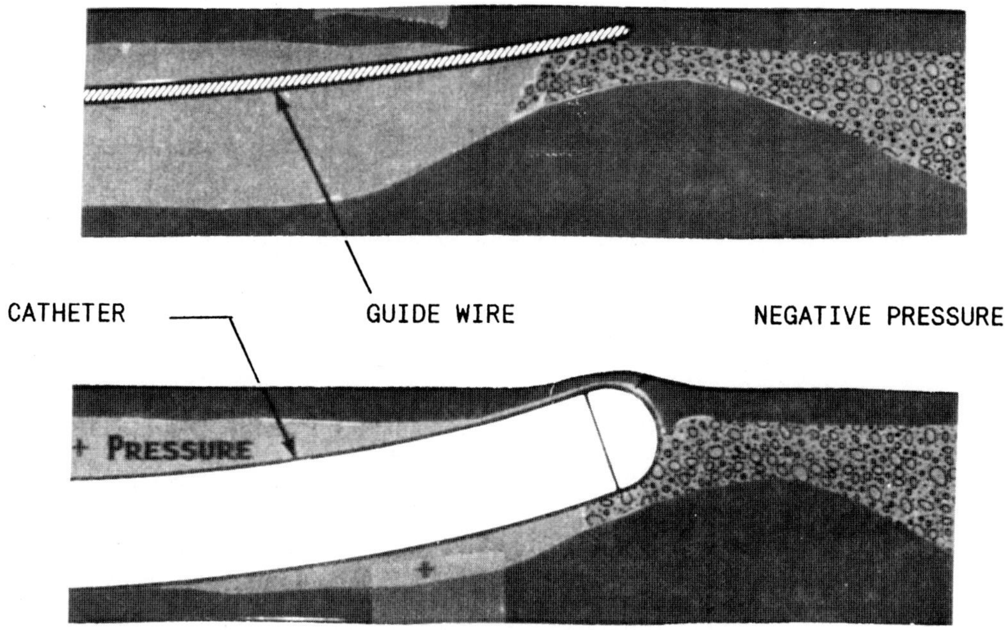

Figure 25–15.

wire begins to perforate the arterial wall, an area of least resistance has been created in the artery wall and therefore the Kensey catheter will follow the previous tract made by the guide wire (Fig. 25-15).

Recommended Speeds and Fluid Pressures

The catheter should be introduced at about 20,000 rpm and at a relatively low flow rate of 20 to 30 cc/min until the lesion has been contacted by the tip. At this point, increasing to 90,000 rpm and increasing the flow to the maximum tolerated by the catheter is recommended. The viscosity of the fluid should be as low as possible to allow the highest flow possible. Passage of the catheters should be extremely slow, with a to-and-fro motion. The operator should watch for defection of the tip caused by a viscoelastic lesion, i.e., the wave sign. The catheter tip will wave at the operator. If this occurs, the catheter should be allowed to sit in the nonwave state allowing the spinning tip to pulverize the deflecting lesion. The operator should be alert and aware of any extravasation and, prior to total recanalization, the fluid flow should be reduced to 10 to 20 cc/min again until the total occlusive distal end lesion has been recanalized. Reducing the flow reduces the risk of breaking off the end of the total occlusion causing a potentially large embolus. Finally, once the total occlusion has been recanalized, increase the flow and the RPM again to its maximum state to allow perfusion and dilation of collaterals of the distal limb or organ. Withdrawal of the catheter should be at the highest revolutions per minute and flow rate possible.

In an artery that is totally occluded with calcified material, it is important that the catheter be near or equal to the size of the internal lumen of the artery. The catheter jacket and catheter itself will guide the tip through the calcific lesion. Calcium requires a great deal of energy to pulverize and therefore much more time is needed to pulverize calcific tissue than a thrombosed vessel. Be patient when recanalizing calcified lesions.

DISCUSSION

Even at this very early stage in the development of the Kensey catheter, significant advances have been made. With the use of this device, greater than 50% of preamputation cases have been salvaged from amputation, and bypass surgery has been obviated in a much higher percentage per patient. When used carefully, clinically significant embolic events occur in less than 1% of patients. The procedure is quick, simple, and safe. The introduction of other treatment modalities can follow unhindered.

In conclusion, the Kensey catheter system has been shown to be useful in limb salvage cases with totally occluded peripheral arteries. Only future studies will determine its usefulness in other applications.

26 Percutaneous Atherectomy: A New Rotary Atherectomy System

Amir Motarjeme, M.D.

In recent years several atherectomy devices for percutaneous removal of atherosclerotic plaques from the arterial system, both peripheral and coronary, have been developed and initial human trials have been reported.[1–10] We are reporting our clinical experience on atherectomy of peripheral arteries using the Bard Rotary Atherectomy System (BRAS).

BARD ROTARY ATHERECTOMY SYSTEM

BRAS is designed for percutaneous extraction of atheroma causing arterial stenoses or occlusions (Fig. 26-1). The system consists of: (1) atherectomy catheter; (2) system's guide wire (retrieving device); (3) motor drive; (4) power pack; (5) arterial sheath; and (6) accessories.

The cutting device is an 8 F catheter, similar to an angiographic catheter, tipped with a 9 F small stainless steel cutter. The cutter has an outside diameter of 0.115 and an inside diameter of 0.105 inch and is 0.180 inch long. The thickness of the cutting tip is 0.010 inch (Fig. 26-2).

The guide wire is auger-shaped, especially designed to collect excised atheromas. The wire is 0.038 cm in diameter with a soft flexible tip. The working length of the wire is 25 cm (Fig. 26-2).

The motor drive is a hand-held battery driven motor with a push-button activator (Fig. 26-1). The power pack allows two modes of speed and torque: a lower speed of 600 and a higher one of 1200 rpm. It also offers normal and high torque selections (Fig. 26-1).

The arterial sheath is a 9 F Teflon check valve, with a sidearm for injection, available in short and long lengths.

Accessories include: (1) a metal introducer, inserted into the exit hole of the motor drive to facilitate passage of the system's guide wire; (2) Tuohy-Burst adapter, tightened around the wire, preventing blood leakage from the exit hole of the motor drive; and (3) wire fixer, tightened on the wire behind the motor drive, to immobilize the wire.

OPERATION AND MECHANISM

The arterial sheath is first inserted into the common femoral artery under local anesthesia with the usual technique. The stenosis is crossed with the system's wire. If the stenosis appears difficult to cross or a total occlusion is to be treated, the lesion is first negotiated with the usual wire and catheter technique. The regular angiographic wire is then exchanged for the system's wire. Once the auger wire is in place, the catheter is first connected to the motor drive, then it is advanced over the system's wire to the sheath. The catheter can be advanced into the artery to the diseased segment manually or with the help of the motor drive. Just before atherectomy, special attention is made to ensure that the wire remains absolutely stationary while the cutting catheter is being activated.

The mechanics of BRAS consists of excising the atheroma from the arterial wall and affixing it around the wire. The system is designed around the joint function of the cutting catheter and retrieving guide wire. The auger wire across the lesion remains stationary while the cutting catheter, activated by the motor drive, revolves around the wire at the speed of 600 to 1200 rpm. During these revolutions, the excised atheromas are wrapped around the wire. When cutting is completed the catheter remains in place while the wire is removed along with atheromas (Figs. 26-3A–E, 26-4).

MATERIALS AND METHODS

Fifty arteries in 40 patients, 27 males and 13 females, from 39 to 78 years of age, were treated. The occlusive lesions ranged from 75 to 100%. Of the 50 arteries, 41 were treated for stenoses, and nine patients had total occlusions. The length of the lesions varied from 0.5 to 45 cm. Two patients had atherectomy of both superficial femoral arteries (SFAs), 38 patients had claudication, and two were treated for gangrene. Thirty-four patients were smokers, and 20 had diabetes. Atherectomy was performed percutaneously in 39 patients and intraoperatively in one patient.

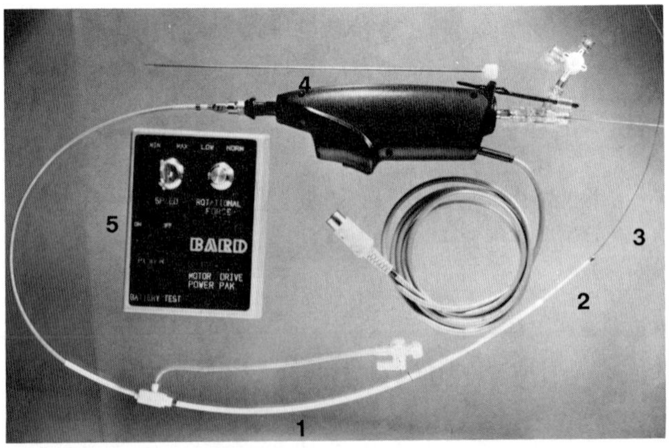

Figure 26–1. Bard Rotary Atherectomy System (BRAS): (1) arterial sheath; (2) atherectomy catheter; (3) system's guide wire; (4) motor drive; and (5) power pack.

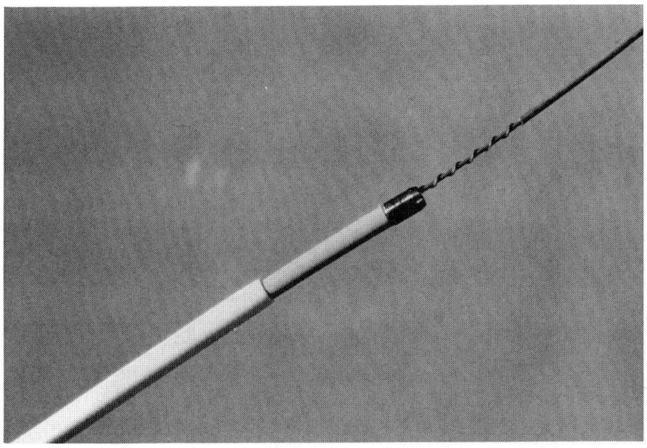

Figure 26–2. Atherectomy catheter, metal cutter, and system's guide wire.

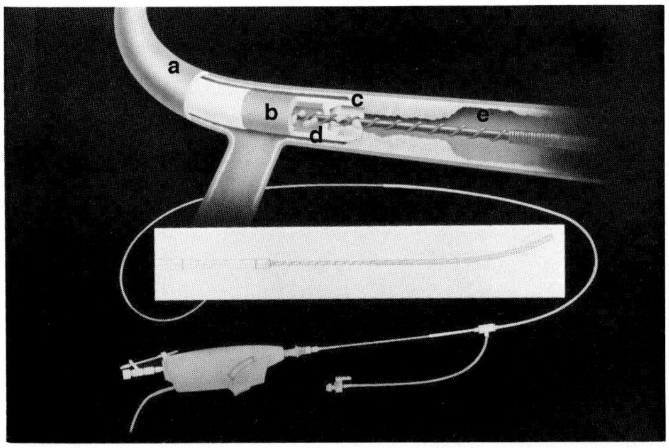

Figure 26–3. Schematic drawing of the Bard Rotary Atherectomy System in cross-section. **A:** Artery; **B:** atherectomy catheter; **C:** cutter tip; **D:** excised atheroma wrapped around the wire; and **E:** system's guide wire.

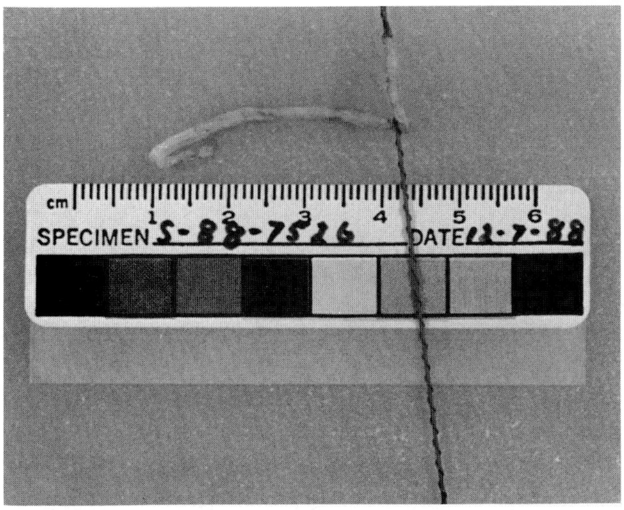

Figure 26–4. A 6 cm long cylindrical atheroma affixed to the wire was removed from a totally occluded superficial femoral artery.

Thirty-eight patients were treated with additional percutaneous transluminal angioplasty (PTA) and two arteries in two patients were treated with atherectomy alone. A pulse volume recording (PVR) was performed on all patients, both before and after the procedures. All patients were anticoagulated with 5000 U of heparin intravenously and/or intra-arterially during the procedure. Heparin was not reversed for removal of the arterial sheath. Patients in whom a long segment occlusion (longer than 10 cm) was recanalized were treated with Warfarin for 6 months with the desired prothrombin time of 18.0 seconds. The remaining patients were treated with dipyridamole (75 mg three times daily) and aspirin (325 mg daily). Arteriograms were performed prior to and after atherectomy and also after additional PTA. The first ten patients had follow-up (clinical examinations and PVR) every month, but the next 30 patients, after the initial 1-month visit, were seen for follow-up every 2 months for a 6-month period. All patients were followed every 3 months thereafter. Six to 18 months follow-up arteriograms were performed on 19 patients.

RESULTS

The results were evaluated in three areas: (1) technical success when atheroma was excised; (2) clinical success when the arterial lumen was improved; and (3) failure when neither technical nor clinical success was seen. Thirty-three patients (82.5%) had both technical and clinical success, and six patients (15%) had only clinical success, presumably due to dotterization with no atheroma removed. Atherectomy failed in one patient (2.5%) following an unsuccessful PTA. The overall success was 97.5%.

An improved ankle-brachial index of 50 to 100% was seen in 39 patients. There were four reocclusions and five restenoses during the first year (22.5%). The cumulative follow-up is 14 months, ranging from 1 to 24 months. An overall 1 year patency rate for total occlusions and stenoses is 74.5%. However, the angiographic examinations of patients with clinical evidence of reocclusions showed progression of the disease, mostly in other areas rather than in the atherectomized segments (Fig. 26-6).

No restenoses or reocclusions were seen after 1 year, and the 2-year patency rate remains at 74.5%.

COMPLICATIONS

Thrombosis of the SFA at the site of insertion of the sheath happened in two arteries, both in the same patient and both treated successfully with intra-arterial infusion of urokinase. No distal emboli, arterial perforation, or thrombosis at the site of the atherectomy was seen. There was one large local hematoma of the groin and scrotum in a patient who had a high antegrade femoral puncture.

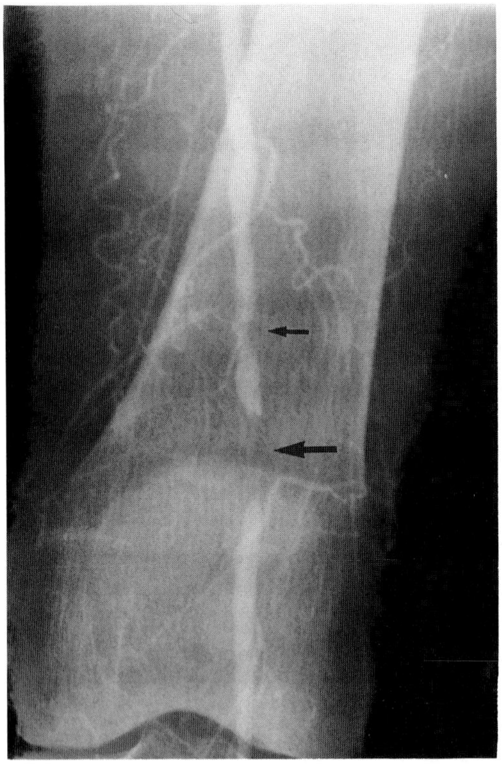

A

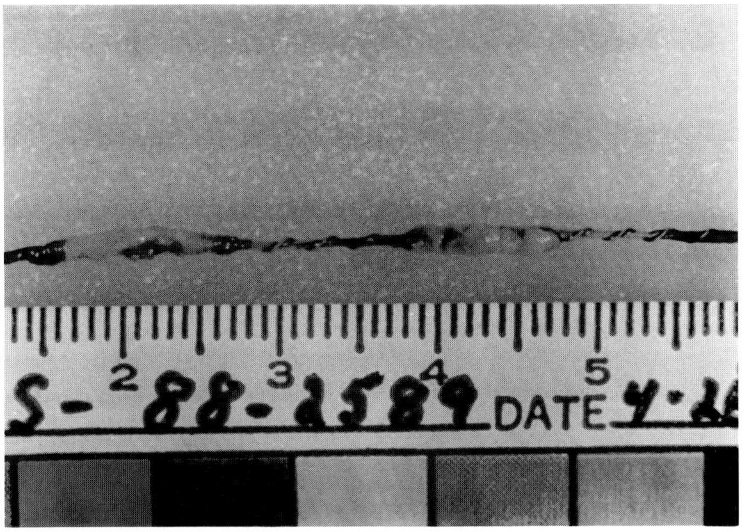

B

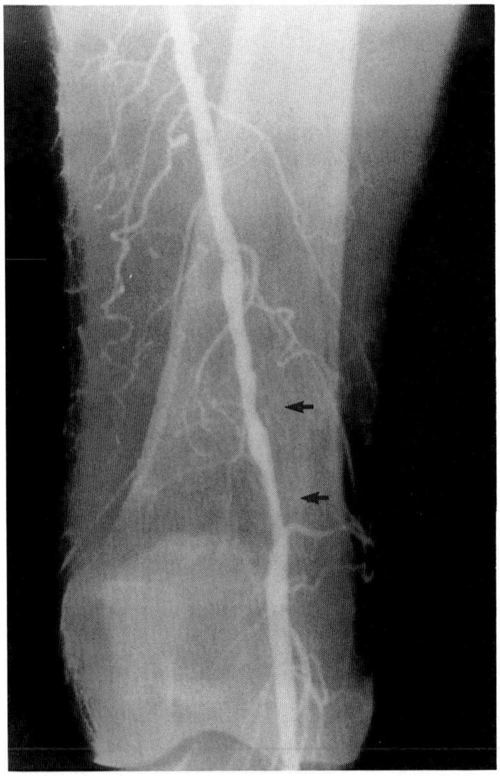

C

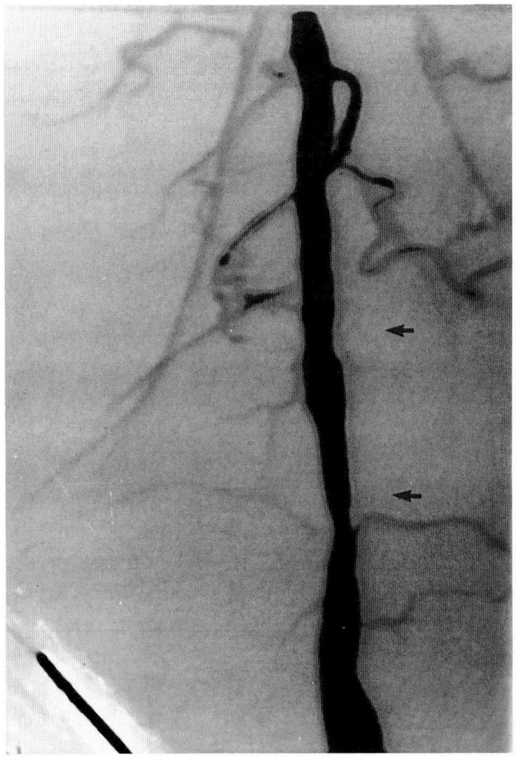

D

Figure 26–5. **A:** A femoral arteriogram of a 72-year-old woman complaining of intermittent claudication shows a focal stenosis (small arrow) and a 2 cm occlusion (large arrow) of the popliteal artery. **B:** Excised atheromas. **C:** Postatherectomy arteriogram showing residual stenosis, not greater than 50% (arrows). **D:** At 18 months follow-up, arteriogram revealed no progression of disease (arrows).

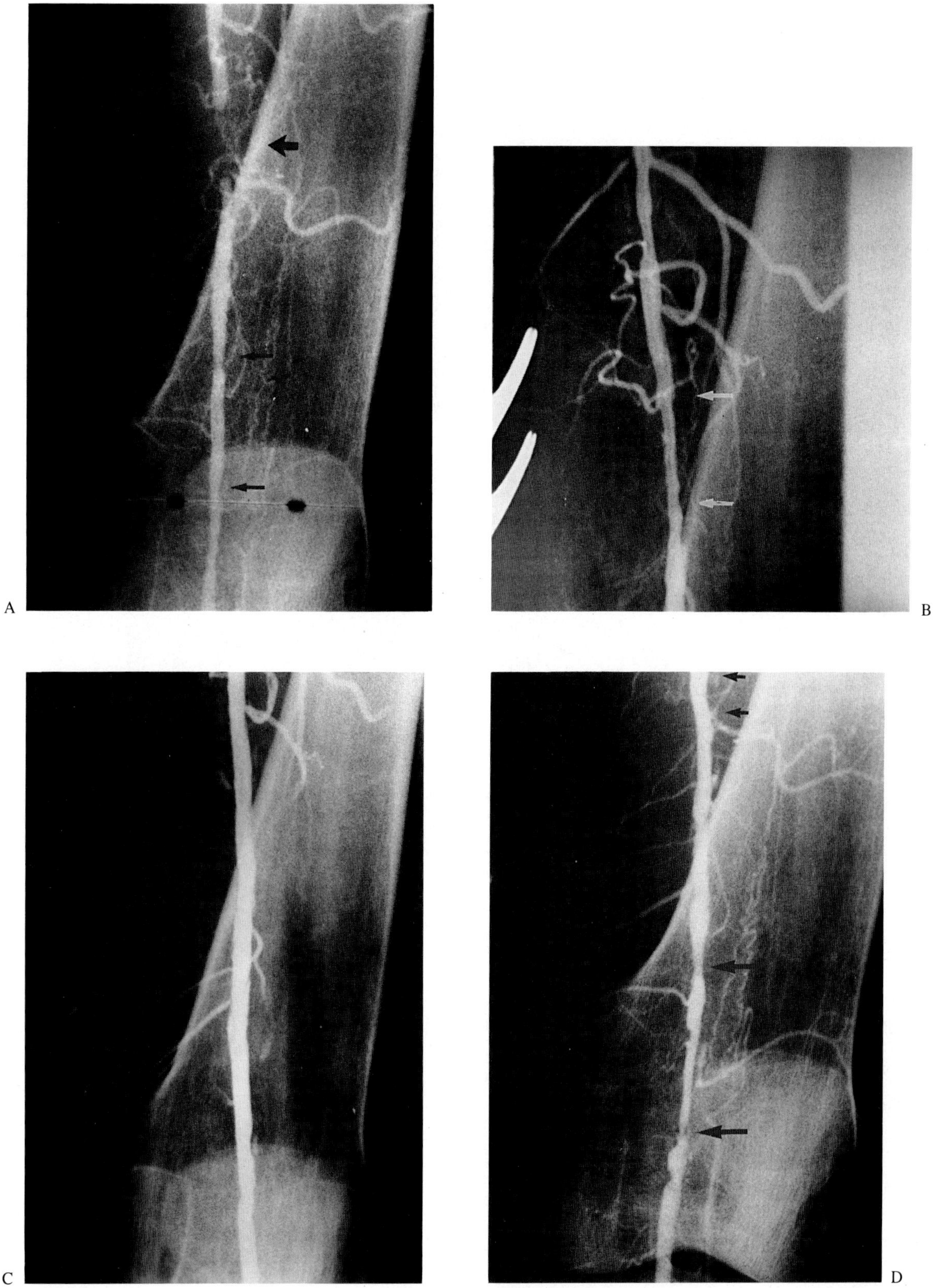

Figure 26–6. **A:** A femoral arteriogram of a 52-year-old man showing a 3 cm total occlusion of the distal superficial femoral artery (large arrow) and two focal stenoses of the popliteal artery (small arrow). **B:** Postatherectomy arteriogram shows recanalization of the totally occluded segment with only minimal residual stenosis (between arrows). **C:** Postatherectomy and percutaneous transluminal angioplasty (PTA) arteriograms showing no residual stenosis of the occluded segment and focal stenosis (treated only with PTA). **D:** A 6-month follow-up arteriogram showed no evidence of progression of disease where atherectomy was performed (between small arrows) whereas restenoses are seen where only PTA was performed (large arrows).

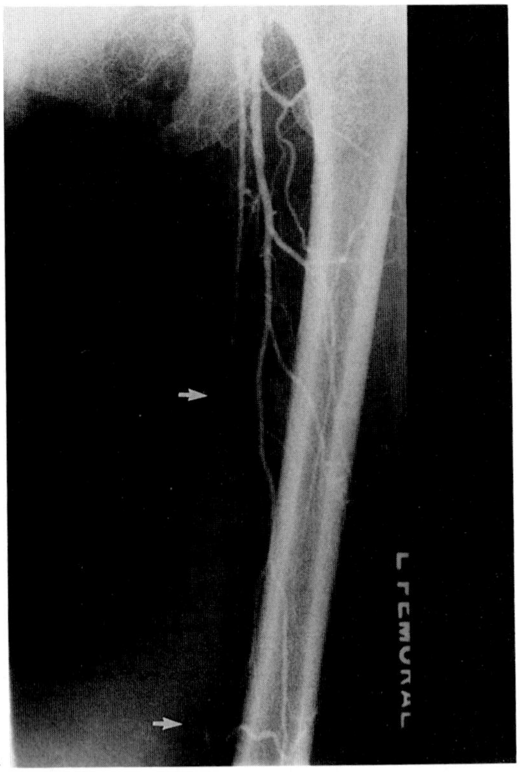

A

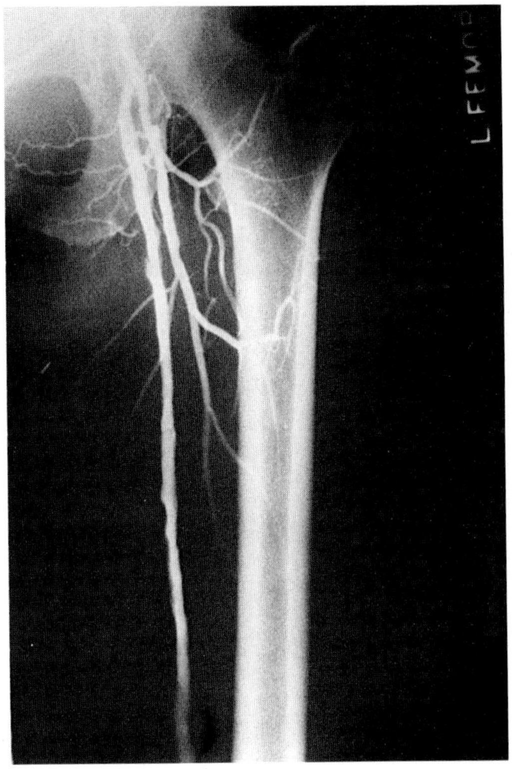

B

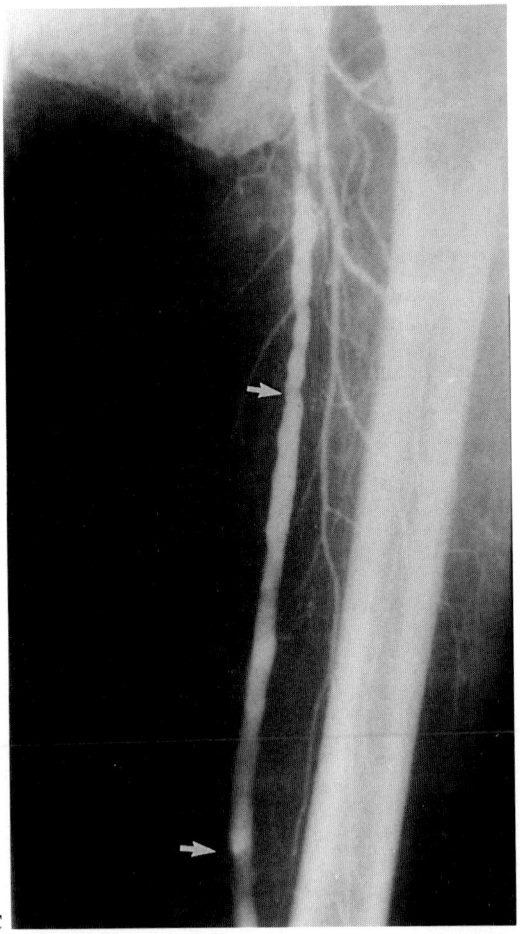

C

Figure 26–7. **A:** A femoral arteriogram showing stenosis of the proximal superficial femoral artery (SFA) and long segment with total occlusion of the distal SFA (between arrows). **B:** Postatherectomy and percutaneous transluminal angioplasty (PTA) arteriogram. Atherectomy was only done on occluded segment. **C:** A 6-month arteriogram shows patent and further dilation of atherectomized segment (between arrows) whereas restenosis is seen in the proximal SFA where no atherectomy was done prior to PTA.

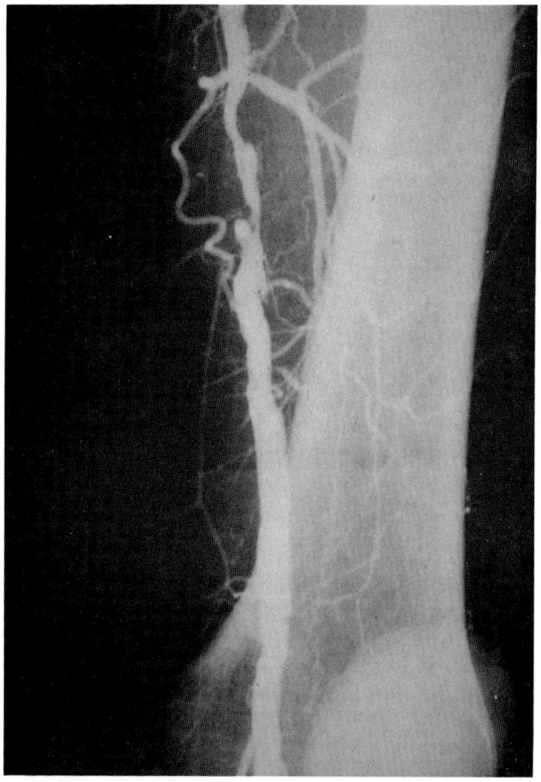

A

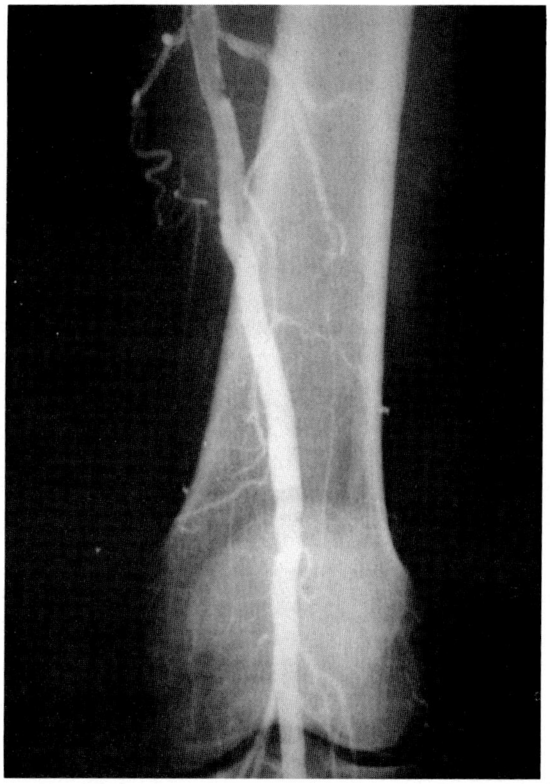

B

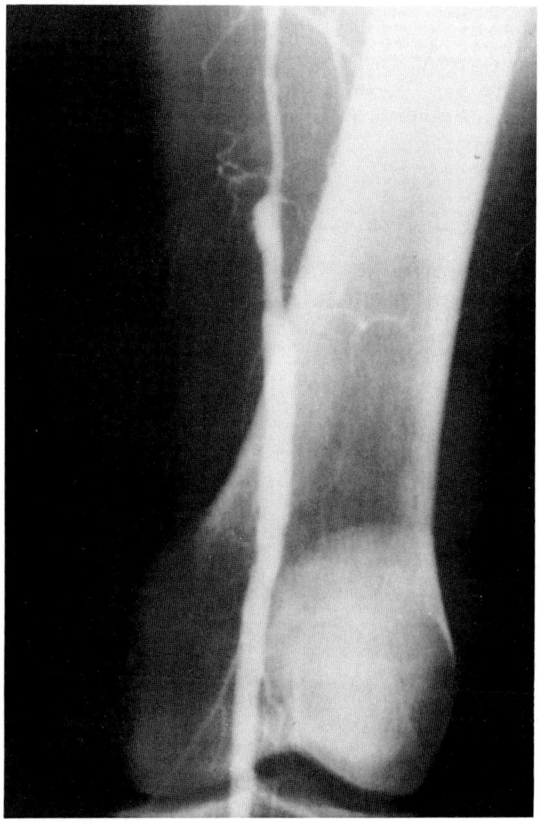

C

Figure 26–8. **A:** Stenosis of the superficial femoral artery in a 62-year-old man complaining of claudication. **B:** Postatherectomy and percutaneous transluminal angioplasty arteriogram show no further stenosis. **C:** A 6-month follow-up arteriogram showing smooth and elongated restenosis suggestive of intimal hyperplasia.

DISCUSSION

PTA, although very effective and successful in the treatment of peripheral vascular occlusive disease, has a restenosis rate of 25 to 60%.[11] Angiographic evidence of dissection is commonly seen in most of the vessels dilated but extensive dissection is complicated by arterial occlusion.[12] We are led to believe that atherectomy catheters could excise atheromas without dissection.[8] On the other hand, debulking the occlusive lesions by removing the atheroma without damaging the media and adventitia might increase the long patency rate of the arteries with and without subsequent PTA.

Among our patients, restenoses were mainly seen where sufficient atheroma was not removed and the residual stenosis, prior to PTA, was greater than 50%. This finding has been also experienced by Simpson et al.[4] These findings support the hypothesis that the patency rate might be directly related to the bulk of atheroma removed during atherectomy. Findings supporting these ideas are seen on follow-up arteriograms.

ANGIOGRAPHIC OBSERVATIONS

1. Patients who were treated with atherectomy without adjunct PTA showed no progression of disease (Fig. 26-5).
2. Most of those arteries treated with atherectomy and PTA showed no evidence of progression of disease at the atherectomized segment, whereas restenoses were frequently seen in areas treated with PTA alone (Fig. 26-6).
3. When all atheromas were removed, follow-up arteriograms showed an overdilated artery (Fig. 26-7).
4. Morphologic appearance of restenoses of the atherectomized arteries varies with PTA, suggesting intimal hyperplasia rather than progression of atherosclerosis[13] (Fig. 26-8).

These findings strongly suggest that the atherectomized lumen might remain patent longer than those treated with PTA only.

The BRAS appears to be safe, rapid, and simple to operate. Because of the over-the-wire system, it has no risk of arterial perforation, as is seen by other atherectomy systems.[4] We have not experienced thrombosis at the atherectomy site, nor have we seen distal emboli, either clinically or angiographically. However, overenthusiasm is guarded until more data have been collected on a larger number of patients.

REFERENCES

1. Ahn SS, Auth D, Marcus DR, et al. Removal of focal atheromatous lesions by angioscopically guided high-speed rotary atherectomy. J Vasc Surg 1988;7:292–300.
2. Zacca NM, Raizner AE, Noon GP, et al. Treatment of symptomatic peripheral atherosclerotic disease with a rotational atherectomy device. Am J Cardiol 1989;63:77–80.
3. Kensey KR, Nash JE, Abrahams C, et al. Recanalization of obstructed arteries with a flexible, rotating tip catheter. Radiology 1987;165:387–9.
4. Simpson JB, Selmon MR, Robertson GC, et al. Transluminal atherectomy for occlusive peripheral vascular disease. Am J Cardiol 1988;61:96G–101G.
5. Hansen DD, Auth DC, Vracko R, et al. Rotational atherectomy in rabbit iliac arteries. Am Heart J 1988;115:160–5.
6. Newman GE, Miner DG, Sussman SK, et al. Peripheral artery atherectomy: description of technique and report of initial results. Radiology 1988;169:677–80.
7. Hofling B, Backa D, Lauterjung L, et al. Percutaneous removal of atheromatous plaques in peripheral arteries. Lancet 1988;1:384–386.
8. Simpson JB, Zimmerman JJ, Selmon MR, et al. Transluminal atherectomy: initial clinical results in 27 patients. Circulation 1986;74(suppl 2):II–203.
9. Hofling B, Simpson JB, Remberger K, et al. Percutaneous atherectomy in iliac, femoral and popliteal arteries. Klin Wochenschr 1987;65:528.
10. Simpson JB, Johnson DE, Thapliyal HV, et al. Transluminal atherectomy: a new approach to the treatment of atherosclerotic vascular disease. Circulation 1985;72(suppl II):III–146.
11. Widlus D, Osterman F Jr. Evaluation and percutaneous management of atherosclerotic peripheral vascular disease. JAMA 1989;261:3148–53.
12. Gardiner GA Jr, Meyerovitz MF, Harrington DP, et al. Dissection complicating angioplasty. AJR 1985;145:627–31.
13. Vom Polnitz A, Backa D, Remberger K, et al. Restenosis after atherectomy shows increased intimal hyperplasia as compared to primary lesions. J Vasc Med Biol 1989;1:283–7.

27 Percutaneous Atherectomy: Transluminal Endarterectomy Catheter and the Atherolytic Reperfusion Wire Device

Mark H. Wholey, M.D., Robert G. Levitt, M.D., Deborah Fein-Millar, M.D.

Over 200,000 patients are currently being treated for inoperable peripheral vascular disease or failed prior surgery. Percutaneous transluminal angioplasty (PTA) is an important alternative to surgery in these patients. Major factors limiting its use include acute occlusion due to uncontrolled injury and a restenosis rate of 15 to 25% at 1 to 2 years, increasing to 30 to 45% at 4 to 5 years.[1,2] Atherectomy was developed with the hypothesis that removal of plaque instead of remodeling of plaque (PTA) would result in a lower acute occlusion rate and restenosis rate than PTA.[3,4] Several atherectomy devices are now under evaluation. In this chapter we discuss our experience with two such devices.

TRANSLUMINAL ENDARTERECTOMY CATHETER

Technical Description

The transluminal endarterectomy catheter (TEC; Interventional Technologies, San Diego, CA) was designed by R.S. Stack and his coworkers at Duke University.[5] This unit is the first atherectomy device for recanalization and reperfusion through total obstructions that continuously removes the debris by the vacuum effect, thereby reducing the incidence of distal embolization.[6]

The TEC system includes a cutter mounted on the distal end of a torque tube that passes freely over a 0.014 inch steerable wire. The cutter consists of three blades that form the sides of a triangle (Fig. 27-1). The torque tube cutter assembly (TEC) is connected to a motorized drive assembly and power source that rotates the torque tube and cutter at 750 rpm to circumferentially pare atheromatous tissue from occluded or stenotic peripheral vessels (Fig. 27-2). The excised tissue is removed through the torque tube by an attached 125 ml vacuum bottle under 1 atm negative pressure. Large amounts of plaque may be removed using this device (Fig. 27-3). The TEC system comes in a 5 F (1.7 mm), 7 F (2.3 mm), and 9 F (3 mm) sizes. In contrast to the Simpson atherectomy catheter, the cutter is exposed on the end of the torque tube, not protected within a catheter housing unit. Also, unlike the Simpson atherectomy catheter, the TEC does not require removal of the device (to remove excised debris) until the recanalization process is completed.

Indications

The TEC is designed for use in short (less than 2 cm) or long (more than 2 cm) stenoses or occlusions of peripheral vessels or grafts. It may also be used for percutaneous thrombectomy. There is no restriction on the number, length, or severity of lesions so long as the Interventional Technologies (IVT) 0.014 inch guide wire may be advanced across the lesion of interest. TEC is contraindicated in peripheral vessels when the IVT 0.014 inch guide wire cannot be positioned across the lesion of interest. The outside diameter of the selected TEC device should never exceed the intraluminal diameter of the native vessel or graft immediately proximal or distal to the lesion or lesions of interest. Atherectomy should be performed with a smaller French size TEC (5 F, 7 F) initially and followed with the larger TEC (9 F) if necessary. TEC may be used in conjunction with other recanalization techniques, including thrombolysis and PTA. Only the IVT 0.014 inch guide wire should be used with the TEC device.

Technique

After angiographic documentation of the lesion of interest, introduce an appropriately sized sheath (5 F, 7 F, 9 F) percutaneously, either retrograde or antegrade, depending upon the vessel involved. Avoid sharp angulation or kinking of the sheath. Administer heparin (5000 U) intra-arterially. Advance the IVT 0.014 inch guide wire across the lesion under fluoroscopic control. Back-feed the proximal end of the guide wire through the appropriately sized TEC drive unit and rear extension tube assembly. Advance the TEC through the hemostasis valve over the guide wire and position the cutter proximal to the lesion. Administer 100 to 200 μg nitroglycerin if the lesion is below the knee. Activate the drive unit and vacuum and advance the TEC *slowly* under fluoroscopic control to excise atheromatous tissue from the lesion. Continuously monitor flow into the vacuum bottle and change the bottle when full. Evaluate the postatherectomy site by removing the TEC while holding the guide wire in position and inject contrast medium through the sheath. If a larger lumen is necessary, replace the TEC with a larger TEC and repeat the atherectomy. Alternatively, consider adjunctive PTA.

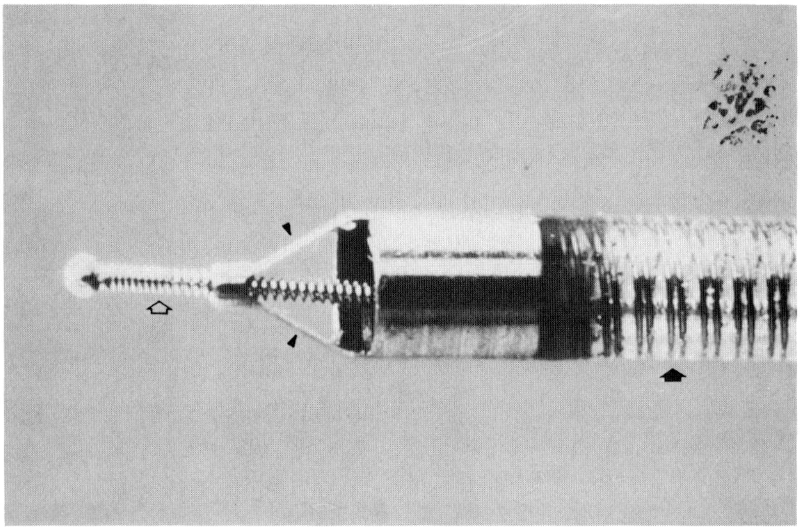

Figure 27–1. The transluminal endarterectomy catheter cutter consists of three triangular blades (arrowheads) mounted on the distal end of the torque tube (closed arrow). The Interventional Technologies 0.014 inch guide wire (open arrow) passes through the cutter and torque tube.

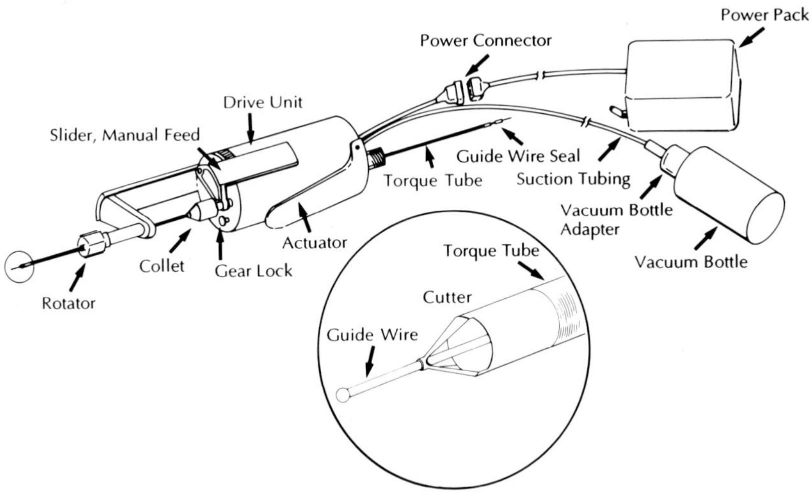

Figure 27–2. Diagram of components of the transluminal endarterectomy catheter peripheral atherectomy device.

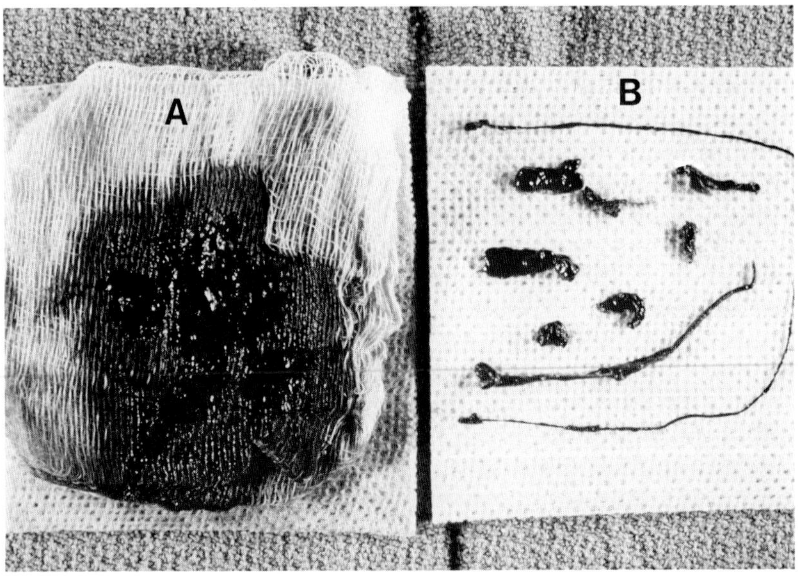

Figure 27–3. Atherosclerotic debris retrieved from transluminal endarterectomy catheter atherectomy of occluded superficial femoral artery. A: Debris from vacuum bottle filtered through gauze. B: Retrieved debris consists of several long cores.

Technical Results

A 16 center trial of the TEC device involving 132 patients has been performed (Table 27-1). A total of 204 lesions in this population were treated by TEC atherectomy. Slightly less than two thirds of the lesions were short segment (less than 2 cm) stenoses, and approximately one quarter of the lesions were long segment (more than 2) stenoses or total occlusions respectively (Table 27-2). The mean stenosis of the nonocclusion lesions was 80%. Greater than 60% of the lesions involved the superficial femoral artery, and 20% of the lesions were located at or below the knee (Table 27-3).

A TEC atherectomy was classified a technical success if a residual stenosis less than 50% was achieved; this was achieved in 88% of TEC procedures (Table 27-4). When the residual stenosis was 30% or greater, PTA was performed. A supplemental PTA was required in 50% of total occlusions, 40% of long segment stenoses and 25% of short segment stenoses (Table 27-4).

Complications

In the multicenter study, 23% of patients had complications related to the TEC procedure (Table 27-5). Hematoma at the puncture site was the most frequent complication (8%). Thrombosis at the atherectomy side, dissection, and intimal flap each occurred in approximately 5% of procedures. Regional intra-arterial urokinase restored patency in thrombotic occlusions at the atherectomy site. Intimal flaps were "tacked up" by adjunctive PTA. No distal embolization occurred in the multicenter study, but this complication has been reported in a smaller study.[7]

Clinical Results

Six-month clinical follow-up has been obtained in nearly 50% of the 132 patients entered in the multicenter study (Table 27-6). This follow-up is comprised of 75% of patients with lesions treated by TEC alone, but only 25% of patients with lesions treated by TEC and supplemental PTA. Clinical improvement was defined by no symptoms or only mild symptoms (7 to 10 block claudication) in the 6-month follow-up period. Restenosis or reocclusion was defined clinically by the development of moderate (three block claudication) to severe (minimal exertion claudication) symptoms of ischemia during the 6-month follow-up period. Patients with total occlusions or short segmental stenoses (Fig. 27-4) had good clinical results; 86% of patients with total occlusions and 77% of patients with short segment stenoses had no symptoms or mild symptoms 6 months post-TEC atherectomy. Patients with long segment stenoses did poorer; 50% of patients had moderate or severe symptoms at 6 months (Table 27-7).

Patients with lesions requiring supplemental PTA following TEC atherectomy (Table 27-8) did not do nearly as well as the TEC only group. Only patients with total occlusions undergoing TEC and supplemental PTA (Figs. 27-5, 27-6) had good clinical results; 71% of these patients had no symptoms or mild symptoms at 6 months. Patients with stenotic lesions had poor results; 50% of patients with short segment stenoses had moderate or severe symptoms at 6 months and 100% of patients with long segment stenoses had moderate or severe symptoms at 6 months. The poorer results of the TEC plus PTA group compared with the TEC only

Table 27–1. Transluminal Endarterectomy Catheter Multicenter Study Population

Patients:	132
Gender:	75 men, 47 women
Mean age:	65 years

Table 27–2. Transluminal Endarterectomy Catheter Multicenter Study Lesions

Total number of lesions: 204	
Occlusions:	48
Stenosis*:	156
≤2 cm	129
≥2 cm	27

*mean diameter reduction = 80%.

Table 27–3. Location of the 204 Lesions

Iliac artery:	10
Superficial femoral artery:	140
Femoral-popliteal artery graft:	10
Popliteal artery:	29
Tibial/peroneal artery:	15

Table 27–4. Transluminal Endarterectomy Catheter (TEC) Technical Success*

	NO. LESIONS	TEC ONLY	TEC + PTA	SUCCESS
Occlusion	48	24	24	41 (85%)
Stenosis ≤ 2 cm	129	94	35	114 (88%)
Stenosis ≥ 2 cm	27	16	11	24 (89%)
Total	**204**	**134**	**70**	**179 (88%)**

*residual stenosis < 50%.

Table 27–5. Transluminal Endarterectomy Catheter (TEC) Complications in 132 Cases

Hematoma:	10
Thrombosis:	6
Dissection:	8
Intimal flap:	7
Embolization:	0
Perforation:	0

Table 27–6. Transluminal Endarterectomy Catheter (TEC) 6-Month Clinical Follow-Up

	NO. PATIENTS	TEC ONLY	TEC + PTA
Occlusion	14	7 (50%)	7 (50%)
Stenosis ≤ 2 cm	41	35 (85%)	6 (15%)
Stenosis ≥ 2 cm	6	4 (67%)	2 (33%)
Total	**61**	**46 (75%)**	**15 (25%)**

Table 27–7. Transluminal Endarterectomy Catheter Only 6-Month Clinical Follow-Up

	MILD/NO SYMPTOMS	MODERATE/SEVERE SYMPTOMS
Occlusion	6 (86%)	1 (14%)
Stenosis ≤ 2 cm	27 (77%)	8 (23%)
Stenosis ≥ 2 cm	2 (50%)	2 (50%)
Total	**35**	**11**

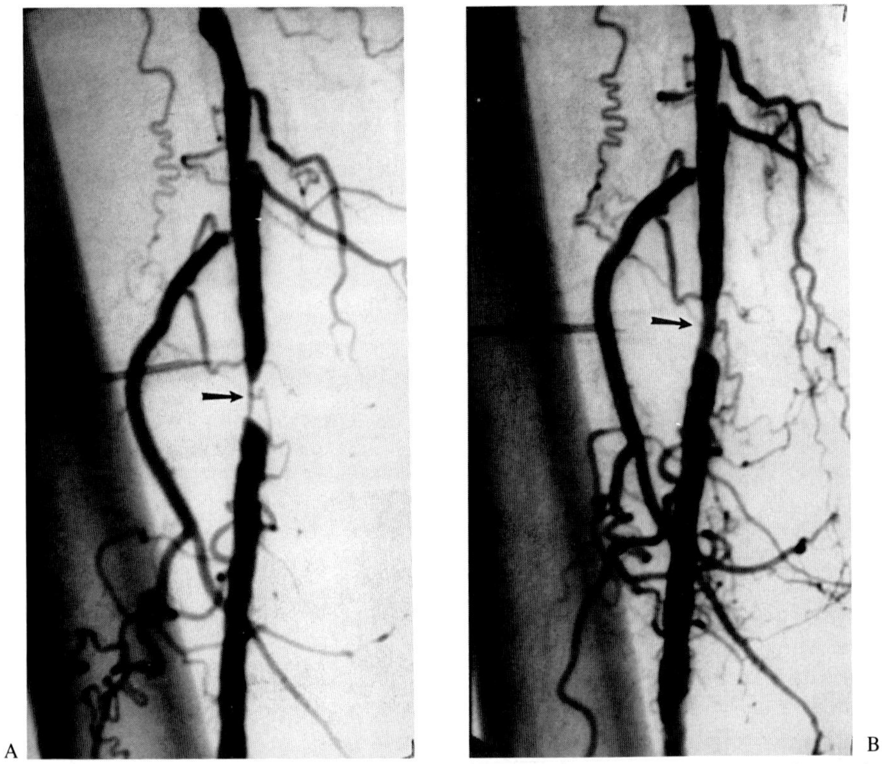

Figure 27–4. Short segment stenosis of superficial femoral artery (SFA). **A:** Digital subtraction angiogram (DSA) reveals high-grade stenosis of SFA (arrow). **B:** DSA shows improved diameter of stenotic segment (arrow) after passage of 7 F transluminal endarterectomy catheter.

Table 27–8. Transluminal Endarterectomy Catheter plus Percutaneous Transluminal Angioplasty 6-Month Clinical Follow-Up

	MILD/NO SYMPTOMS	MODERATE/SEVERE SYMPTOMS
Occlusion	5 (71%)	2 (29%)
Stenosis ≤ 2 cm	3 (50%)	3 (50%)
Stenosis ≥ 2 cm	0	2 (100%)
Total	**8**	**7**

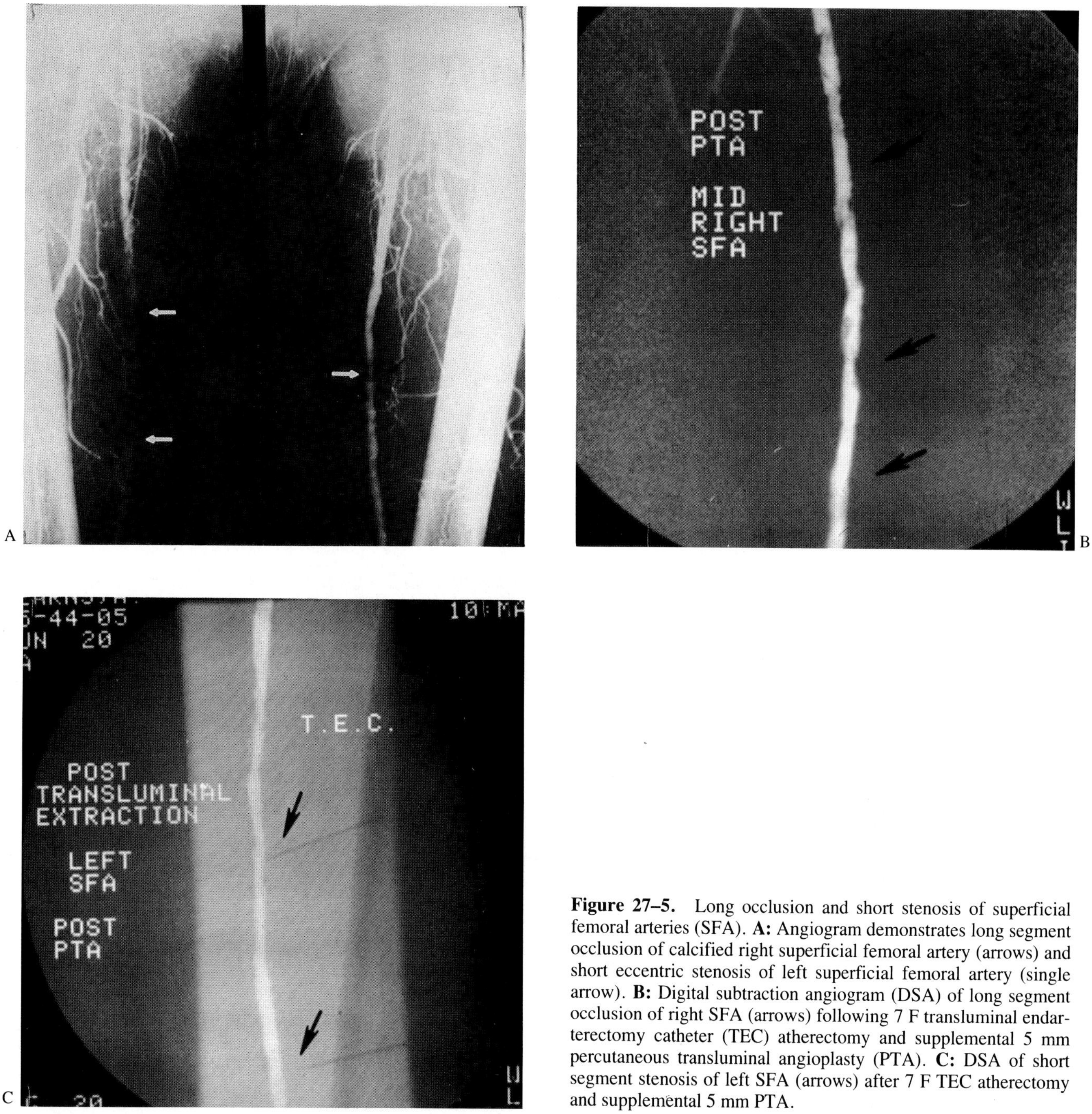

Figure 27–5. Long occlusion and short stenosis of superficial femoral arteries (SFA). **A:** Angiogram demonstrates long segment occlusion of calcified right superficial femoral artery (arrows) and short eccentric stenosis of left superficial femoral artery (single arrow). **B:** Digital subtraction angiogram (DSA) of long segment occlusion of right SFA (arrows) following 7 F transluminal endarterectomy catheter (TEC) atherectomy and supplemental 5 mm percutaneous transluminal angioplasty (PTA). **C:** DSA of short segment stenosis of left SFA (arrows) after 7 F TEC atherectomy and supplemental 5 mm PTA.

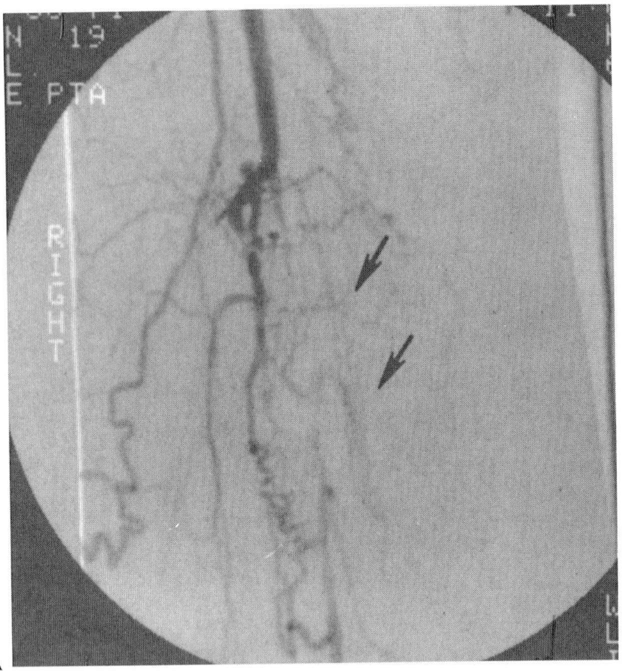

A

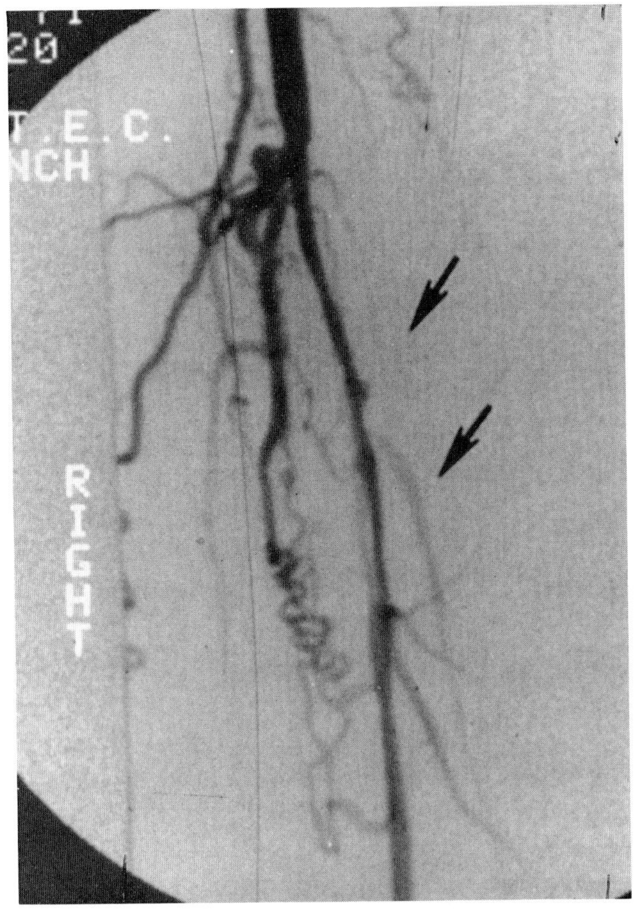

B

Figure 27–6. Occlusion of the right common peroneal trunk (CPT). **A:** Digital subtraction angiogram (DSA) of right CPT occlusion (arrows). **B:** DSA of recanalized CPT (arrows) after passage of 5 F transluminal endarterectomy catheter. A supplemental percutaneous transluminal angioplasty of the residual stenosis in the mid-CPT was performed.

group are to be expected. As noted earlier, restenosis of peripheral vessels after balloon angioplasty continues to be a major problem. We have recently started using the Simpson atherectomy device to remove residual eccentric plaque following TEC atherectomy of critical stenoses in an effort to reduce the restenosis rate (Fig. 27-7).

CURRENT STATUS OF TRANSLUMINAL ENDARTERECTOMY CATHETER ATHERECTOMY

The results of the multicenter study show that TEC atherectomy is a safe and efficacious therapy for occluded peripheral vessels and short segment stenoses if no residual stenosis greater than 30% remains postatherectomy. In the TEC only patient follow-up, the patency rate for total occlusions was 85% and the clinical improvement (no symptoms/mild symptoms) for short segment stenoses was 77%. TEC atherectomy is not effective in long segment stenoses; the clinical restenosis rate (moderate/severe symptoms) was 50% at 6 months. IVT redesigned the cutter in 1990 so that the blades are of microtome-like sharpness. Early reports show a decrease in the restenosis rate at 6 months.[9] When TEC atherectomy of a total occlusion left a residual stenosis greater than 30% requiring supplemental PTA, the combined procedure was effective; 71% of the total occlusions were patent at 6 months. TEC atherectomy of stenoses that required supplemental PTA was not effective; clinical restenosis developed in 50 to 100% by 6 months.

The major problem with the TEC atherectomy device is its small working diameter. The largest 9 F device has a working diameter of only 3 mm. In contrast, the Simpson 9 F atherectomy catheter has a working diameter of 6 mm. The small working diameter of the TEC device explains the frequent requirement for supplemental PTA. For example, a 9 F (3 mm) TEC atherectomy successfully performed on a critical stenosis or a normal-sized superficial femoral artery (6 to 8 mm) leaves a residual stenosis of 50 to 60%, requiring supplemental PTA. Conversely, the small size of the TEC device allows recanalization of occluded or highly stenotic vessels below the knee. These cases have been our most rewarding because threatened limb loss has been reversed (Fig. 27-8).

We currently recommend TEC atherectomy for total occlusions above and below the knee with supplemental PTA or Simpson atherectomy if a residual stenosis greater than 30% exists after TEC atherectomy.

A
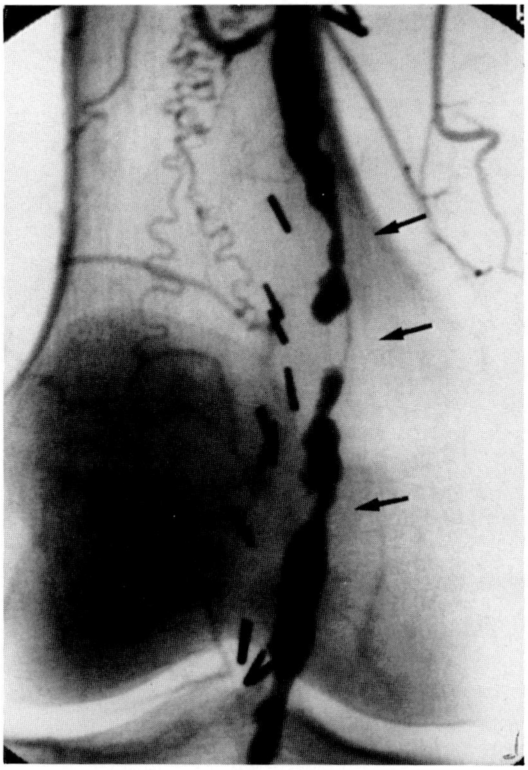

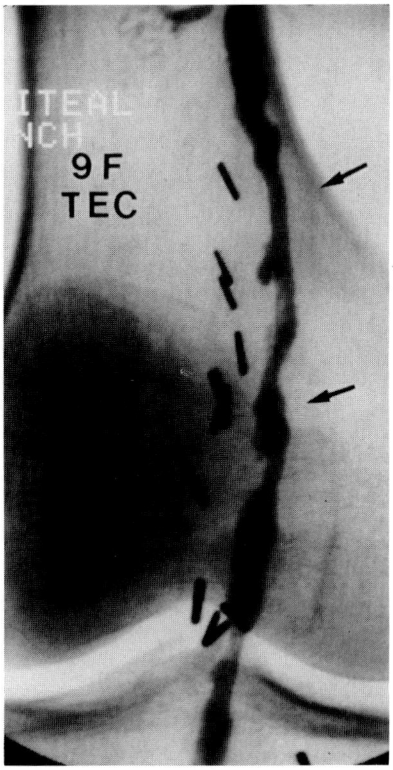

B

C
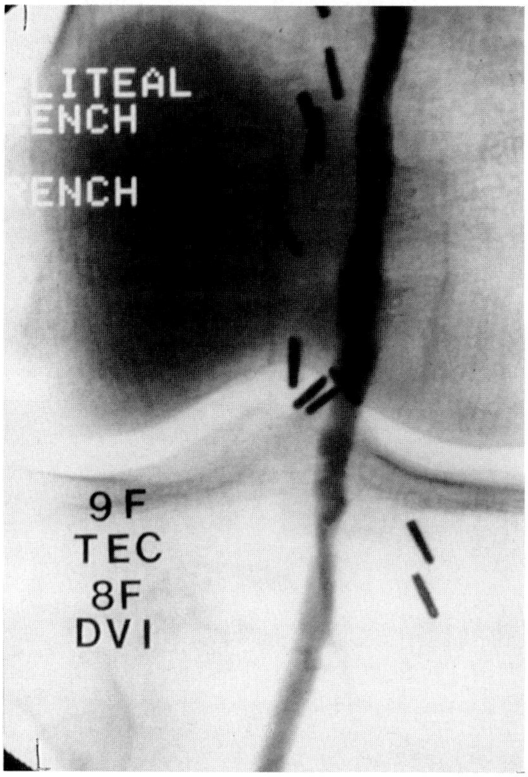

Figure 27–7. Multiple stenoses of vein interposition graft placed after popliteal artery aneurysm resection 7 years earlier. **A:** Digital subtraction angiogram shows multiple high-grade stenoses and one critical stenosis of proximal vein interposition graft (arrows) and moderate stenoses of distal graft. **B:** Following a 9 F transluminal endarterectomy catheter atherectomy, the high-grade and critical stenoses are relieved (arrows) but moderate stenoses are still present distally. **C:** After an 8 F Simpson atherectomy, the distal moderate stenoses are no longer present.

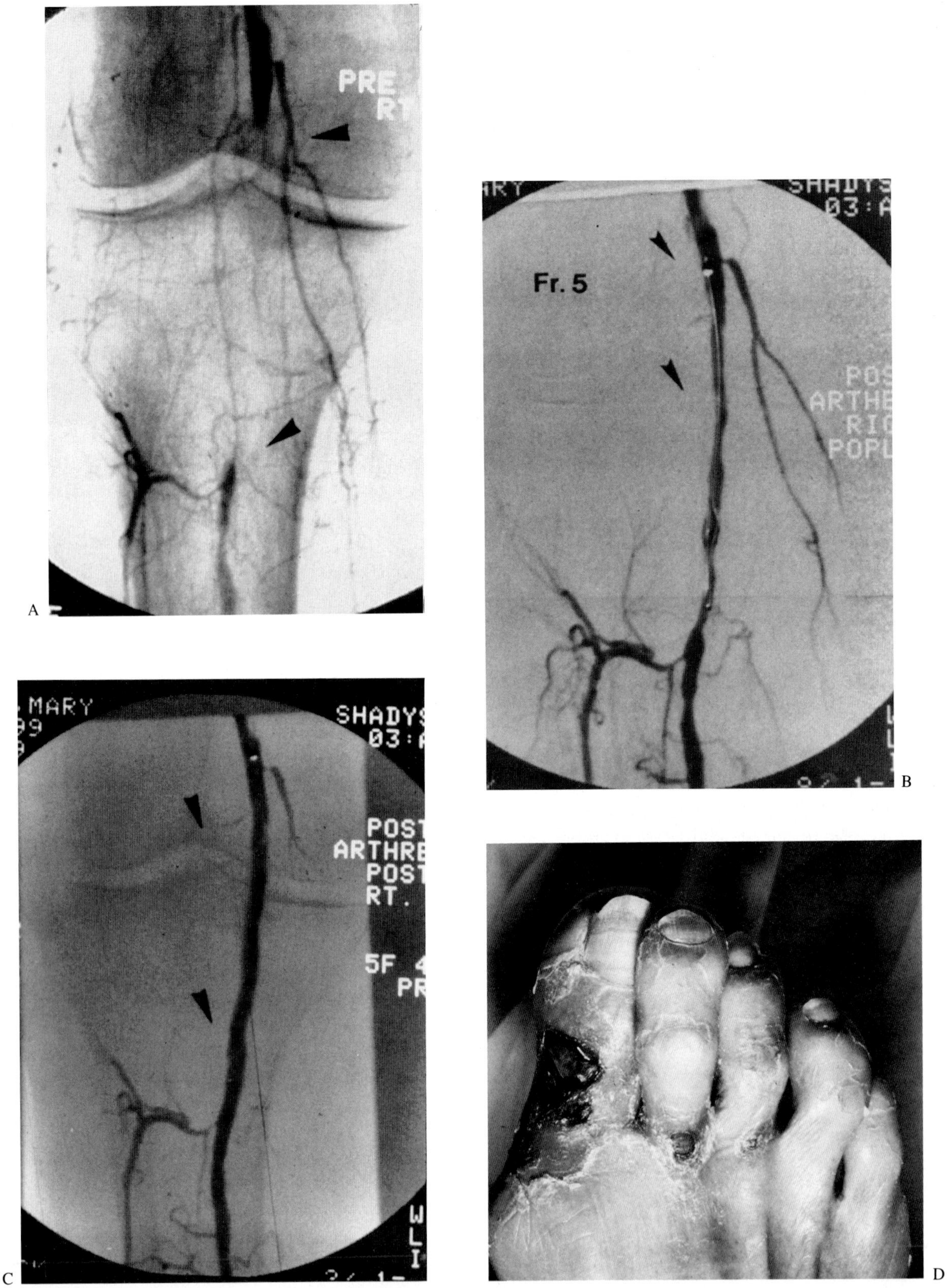

Figure 27–8. Occluded popliteal artery in a woman with pregangrenous changes of her great toe. **A:** Digital subtraction angiography (DSA) shows occluded popliteal artery (arrowheads). **B:** DSA showing recanalization of popliteal artery (arrowheads) after passage of a 5 F transluminal endarterectomy catheter (TEC). The 0.014 inch wire remains across the lesion. **C:** After supplemental percutaneous transluminal angioplasty, the previously occluded popliteal artery (arrowheads) has normal lumen diameter. **D:** Gangrenous changes of great toe prior to TEC atherectomy.

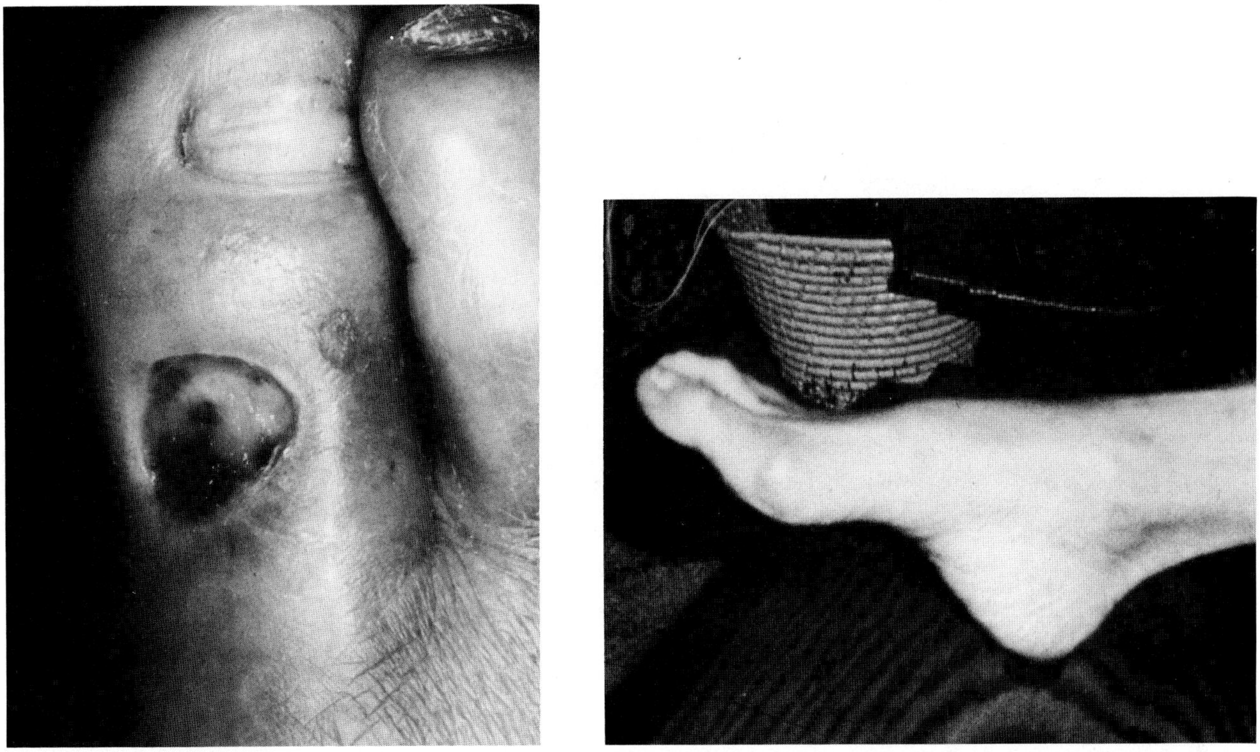

E F

Figure 27–8 *(continued)*. **E:** Healing ulcer 4 weeks postatherectomy. **F:** Great toe was completely healed at 6 months.

ATHEROLYTIC REPERFUSION WIRE DEVICE

Technical Description

Although the TEC endarterectomy device was designed for use in total occlusions and stenoses, the atherolytic wire device (Medrad, Pittsburgh, PA) was designed for recanalization of total occlusions only. The device consists of a 0.035 inch coil spring wire with ellipsoid-shaped distal tip. The distal tip may be notched or un-notched (Fig. 27-9). The proximal segment of the wire device is connected to a hand-held, battery operated motor drive unit which rotates the wire at 600 rpm (Fig. 27-10). The wire passes through a conventional 5 F catheter or any angioplasty catheter with a 0.035 inch end hole. The wire device is used to create a "pilot-hole" through a short or long segment occlusion.[6]

Indications

The first step in recanalization of an occluded vessel is to create a lumen through the obstruction. Most occlusions are composed of organized thrombus with single or multiple short segment of atheromatous occlusion.[10] Often, the lumen may be recanalized by a steerable 0.035 inch torque-controlled Wholey Wire (Advanced Cardiovascular Systems, Santa Clara, CA) beyond a soft-tipped 5 F polyethylene catheter.[11] When excessive resistance to this system is encountered, the atherolytic wire device allows additional force through the rigid segment of obstruction. The device is best applied in relatively straight vessels: iliac, superficial femoral, or popliteal arteries. The wire may serve as a guide for leading other recanalization devices, including atherectomy devices and conventional angioplasty balloon catheters.

Technical Results

Clinical experience with the atherolytic wire device is limited. We have attempted recanalization in 12 patients. Eight patients had total occlusions of the superficial femoral artery, varying in length from 8 to 15 cm. Two patients had more than 3 cm in length external iliac artery occlusions; two patients had common iliac artery occlusions, both of which were close to the aortic bifurcation and measured 2 cm in length (Table 27-9). Eight of the 12 patients were successfully recanalized and subsequently had conventional angioplasty (Figs. 27-11, 27-12). Four patients had rigid (calcified) occlusive disease which could not be crossed with the atherolytic wire device (Table 27-10).

COMPLICATIONS

Vessel dissection occurred in all four patients with rigid occlusive disease that could not be recanalized (Table 27-11). In three patients the dissections were limited, but one patient with a common iliac occlusion had an extensive dissection. Other potential complications, including vessel

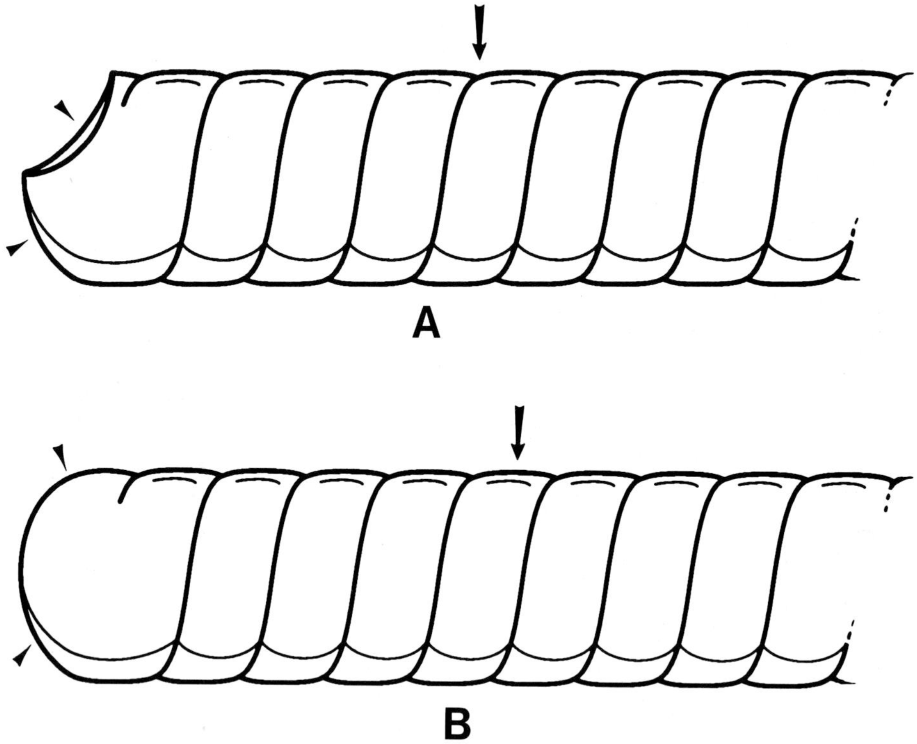

Figure 27–9. Atherolytic wire device consists of a 0.035 inch coil spring wire (arrow) with an ellipsoid-shaped distal tip (arrowheads). This tip may be notched **(A)** or un-notched **(B).**

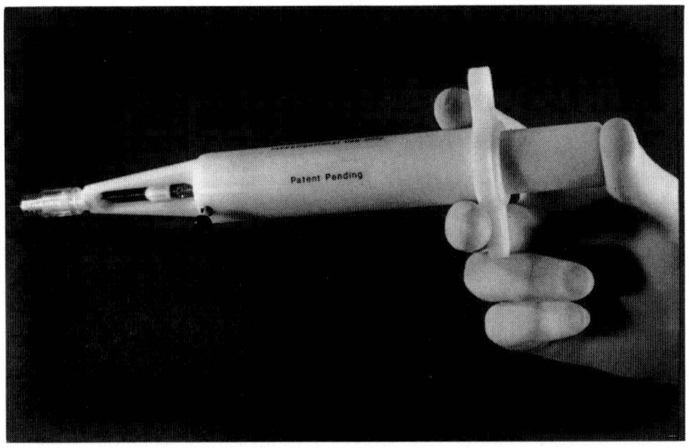

Figure 27–10. Self-contained battery pack for atherolytic wire. Power is activated by a button at the bottom of the plunger controlled by the operator's thumb. The wire is advanced by compressing the plunger on the syringe-like device.

Table 27–9. Location of 12 Occluded Vessels

Common iliac artery	2
External iliac artery	2
Superficial femoral artery	8*

*Length of occlusion 8–15 cm

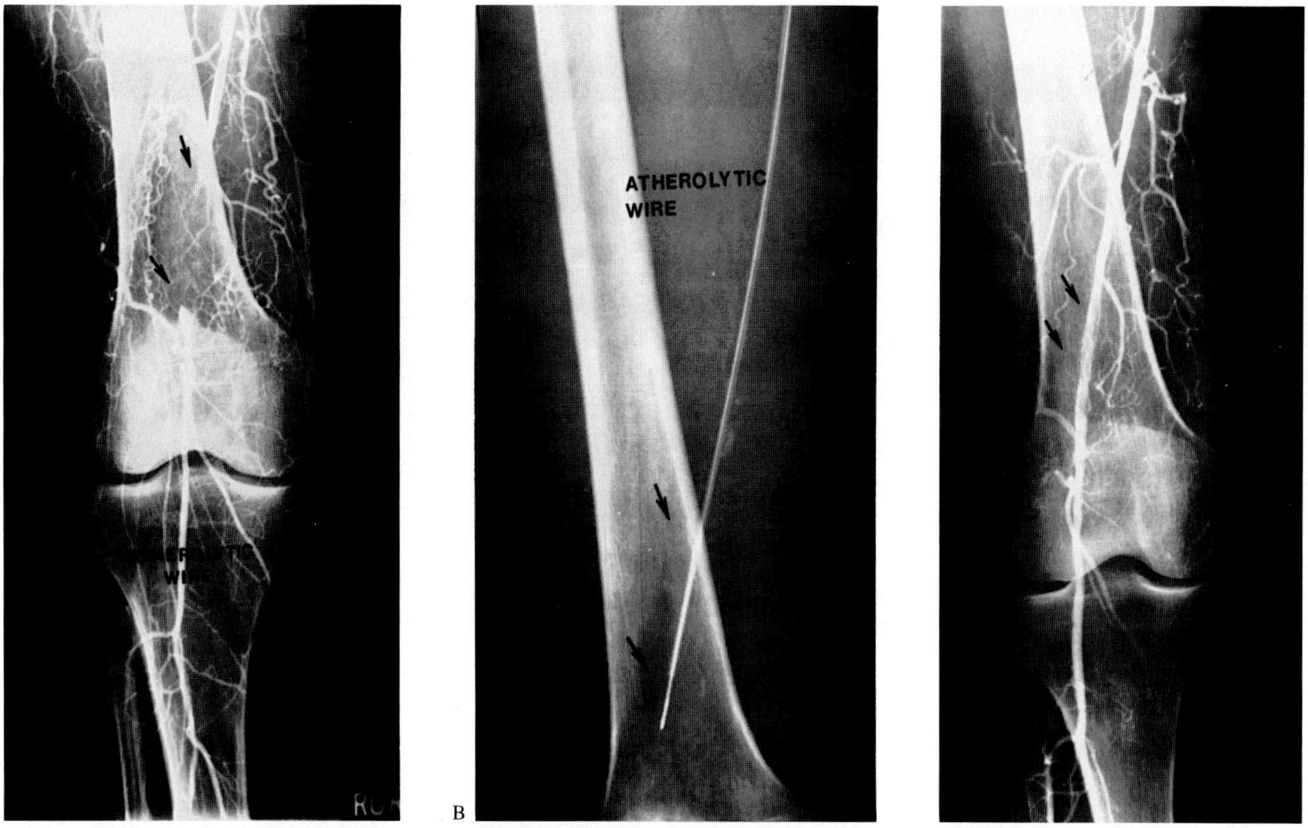

A B C

Figure 27–11. Occluded distal superficial femoral artery (SFA)/proximal popliteal artery (PA). **A:** Angiogram shows long segment occlusion of distal SFA/proximal PA (arrows) with reconstitution of distal PA by collaterals. **B:** The atherolytic wire has crossed the occluded segment. **C:** Angiogram following balloon angioplasty over atherolytic wire shows normal lumen dimension of previously occluded segment.

Table 27–10. Technical Results with Atherolytic Wire

Recanalization	8/12 (75%)
Failure to recanalize	4/12 (25%)

Table 27–11. Complications with Atherolytic Wire

Limited dissection*	3/12 (25%)
Extensive dissection*	1/12 (8%)

*all 4 patients had rigid occlusive disease which could not be recanalized

Table 27–12. 1-Year Clinical Follow-Up

Continued patency	6/8 (75%)
Reocclusion	2/8 (25%)

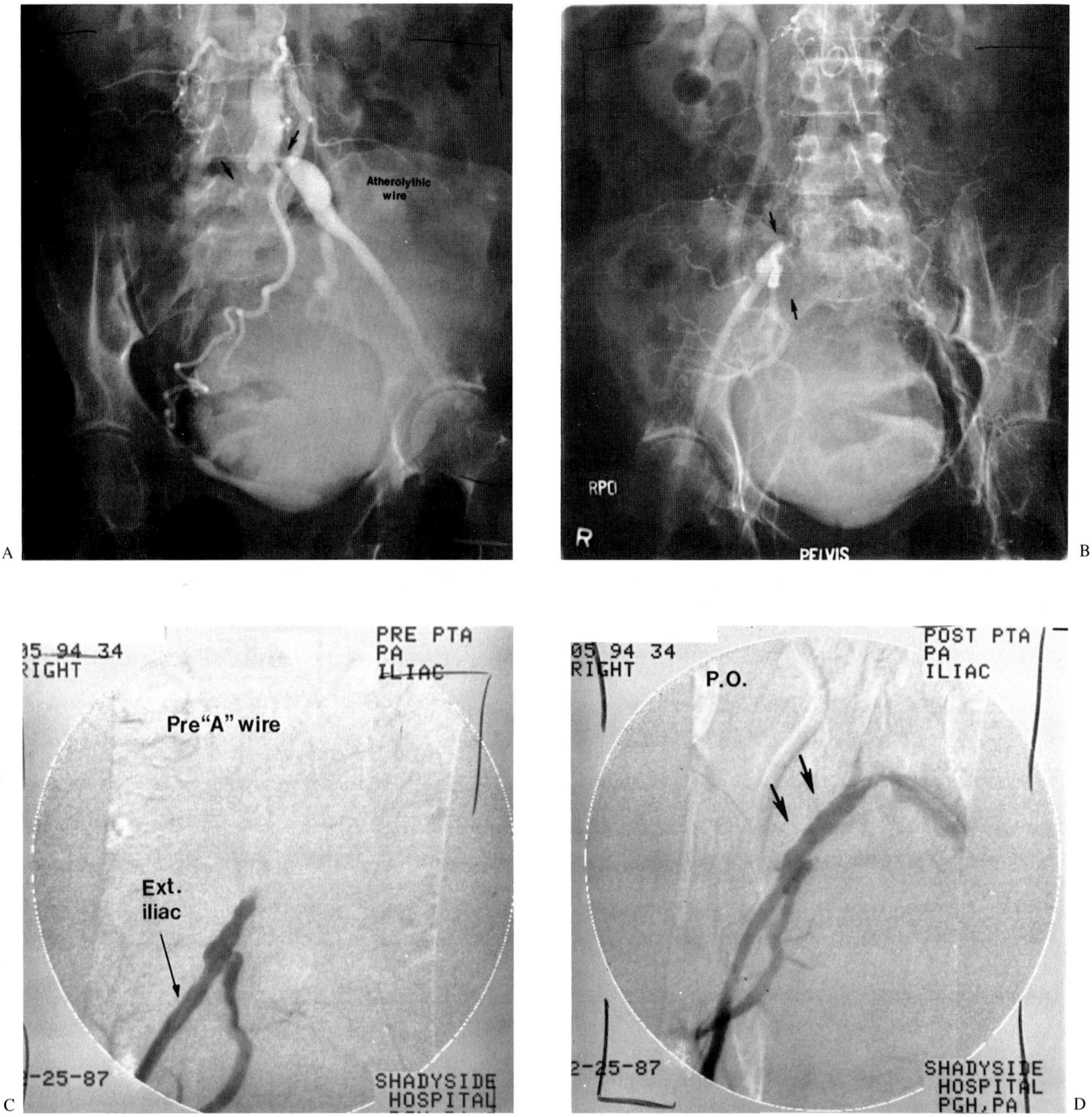

Figure 27–12. Occluded right common iliac artery (CIA). **A:** Aortogram shows occlusion of heavily calcified right CIA at its origin (arrow) and high-grade stenosis of left CIA at its origin (arrow). **B:** Later film from aortogram shows reconstitution of right CIA near its bifurcation (arrows). **C:** Digital subtraction angiogram (DSA) of reconstituted distal right CIA. An atherolytic wire was subsequently passed through the occluded right CIA segment from a retrograde left common femoral artery approach. **D:** DSA following balloon angioplasty over atherolytic wire shows normal dimension to previously occluded right CIA.

perforation, embolization of atherosclerotic material, and hematoma formation at the puncture site did not occur in our series.

Clinical Results

One year clinical follow-up was obtained in the eight patients with successfully recanalized occlusions. Doppler studies and angiography (four patients) demonstrated continued patency in six patients and reocclusion in two patients (Table 27-12).

CURRENT STATUS OF THE ATHEROLYTIC REPERFUSION WIRE DEVICE

The atherolytic wire device remains an investigational device. A modification of the wire is under development, which would allow passage of a 0.014 inch torque-controlled coronary wire through the 0.035 inch wire. This would allow more precise positioning within the lumen of an occluded vessel and reduce the incidence of vessel dissection.

REFERENCES

1. Hofling B, Backa D, Lauterjung L, et al. Percutaneous removal of atheromatous plaques in peripheral arteries. Lancet 1988;1:384–5.
2. Johnston KW, Rae M, Hogg-Johnston SA, et al. 5-year results of a prospective study of percutaneous transluminal angioplasty. Ann Surg 1987;206:403–13.
3. Hinohara T, Semon MR, Robertson GC, et al. Directional atherectomy: new approaches for treatment of obstructive coronary and peripheral vascular disease. Circulation 1990;81 (suppl III):III-79–91.
4. Bates ER, O'Neill WW, Topol EJ. Percutaneous atherectomy catheters. Cardiol Clin 1988;6:373–82.
5. Perez JA, Hinohara T, Quigley PJ, et al. In-vitro and in-vivo experimental results using a new wire concentric atherectomy device. (Abstr.) Circulation 1988;78 (Suppl II):II-21.
6. Wholey MH, Jarmolowski CR. New reperfusion devices: the Kensey catheter, the atherolytic reperfusion wire device and the transluminal extraction catheter. Radiology 1989;172:947–52.
7. Graor RA, Whitlow PL. Transluminal atherectomy for occlusive peripheral vascular disease. J Am Coll Cardiol 1990; 15:1551–8.
8. Selmon MR, Robertson GC, Simpson JB. Restenosis in peripheral transluminal atherectomy. (Abstr.) Circulation 1988;78 (Suppl II):II-269.
9. Godlewski P. Restenosis rates in peripheral TEC-alone cases: a comparative analysis of the effect of change in the cutter manufacture procedure. Interventional Technologies, October 16, 1990.
10. Wholey MH, Smith JAM. Newer atherectomy and reperfusion devices for the peripheral circulation. In Taveras JM, Ferrucci JT (eds): Radiology: Diagnosis-Imaging-Intervention. Philadelphia: JB Lippincott, 1990:1–12.
11. Wholey MH. A newly designed directionally controlled guidewire. Cathet Cardiovasc Diagn 1986;12:66–70.

28 The Auth Rotablator: Percutaneous Transluminal Rotational Ablation in Peripheral Vascular Disease

Patricia E. Thorpe, M.D., Catherine A. Kusnick, M.D., Lewis Wexler, M.D., John T. Mehigan, M.D., Robert S. Ginsberg, M.D., Noni Jenkins, R.N., Richard Baxter, M.D., Alan Wright, M.D.

An over-the-wire rotary ablation catheter designed to restore luminal patency to occluded vessels leaving a smooth, polished endoluminal surface was described by Hansen.[2–5] David Auth pioneered the Rotablator (Heart Technology) design and, with his colleagues, conducted critical studies in the laboratory.[2–11]

Data from the Stanford University clinical trials, which focused on the treatment of severe and end-stage peripheral vascular disease, are presented in this chapter along with recent data pertaining to additional peripheral trials and coronary use presented at the American Heart Association meeting in November 1990.

TECHNICAL DESCRIPTION

An elliptical abrasive burr is available in sizes from 1.5 to 4.5 mm in diameter. The front half of the brass burr is covered with more than 1000 microscopic diamond chips (Fig. 28-1). The tip is rotated between 150,000–180,000 rpm. The drive shaft is housed in a 4 F Teflon sheath and driven by an air turbine. Only the abrasive rotating burr is exposed to the vessel wall. The Rotablator's speed of rotation is controlled from the control panel. An automatic pump infuses sterile saline into the plastic sheath to cool the rotating drive shaft and burr. The burr and drive shaft track coaxially over a 0.009 inch platinum tip guide wire that helps to maintain the intraluminal position of the burr during ablation. The guide wire is fixed in a stationary position during rotation of the drive shaft by an automatically activated brake, but it can remain in position or be advanced in the artery following withdrawal of the device (Fig. 28-2).

MECHANISM OF ACTION

Ablation of the atheromatous obstruction is achieved by removing small pieces of atheromatous material by the elliptical burr spinning at 180,000 rpm, leaving a smooth lumen that at angioscopy is like a polished surface without intimal flaps[12] (Figs. 28-3, 28-4).

The length of time needed to pass the device through a lesion depends on several factors, including degree of calcification, length of the lesion, diameter of the artery, percent of stenosis, and operator experience. In our series, focal, shorter lesions in the superficial femoral artery (SFA) averaged between 3 and 5 minutes application. Longer lesions can range from 5 to 15 minutes for complete ablation.

PRINCIPLE OF DIFFERENTIAL CUTTING

The advantage of the Rotablator design is a cutting mechanism based on the principle of differential cutting (Fig. 28-5). The diamond crystals take advantage of the inelastic nature of atherosclerotic plaque.[13] A common example of differential cutting is shaving. The inelastic whisker is cut by a sharp razor blade, while the soft skin surrounding the whisker is not injured. By cutting preferentially the hard atherosclerotic material is ablated without damaging the media.[14] Therefore the design may contribute to a decreased incidence of restenosis and a lower incidence of complications than documented in follow-up percutaneous transluminal angioplasty (PTA) studies.[15–20]

As opposed to angioplasty the Rotablator does not stretch the vascular wall nor displace the plaque. It transforms the plaque into millions of tiny particles that are removed by the reticuloendothelial system. The abrasive burr creates a smooth surface channel as long as the device is advanced slowly and gently. When an adequate lumen is thus created, the barotrauma associated with balloon dilation can be avoided. The characteristics of barotrauma render balloon dilation undesirable prior to application of the rotational ablation catheter because of the increased risk of passing the guide wire out of the true lumen.

PARTICLE SIZE

The average particle size has been shown to be 2 μm; 90% of the particles produced are under 8 μm.[21] As with other rotating-ablating devices, the size of the particles is determined by the diameter, speed of advancement, and forward pressure applied to the advancing burr. The degree of fragmentation can therefore be modified by adjusting the diameter of the burr, the speed of advancement across the lesion, and the pressure at the application site.[22,23]

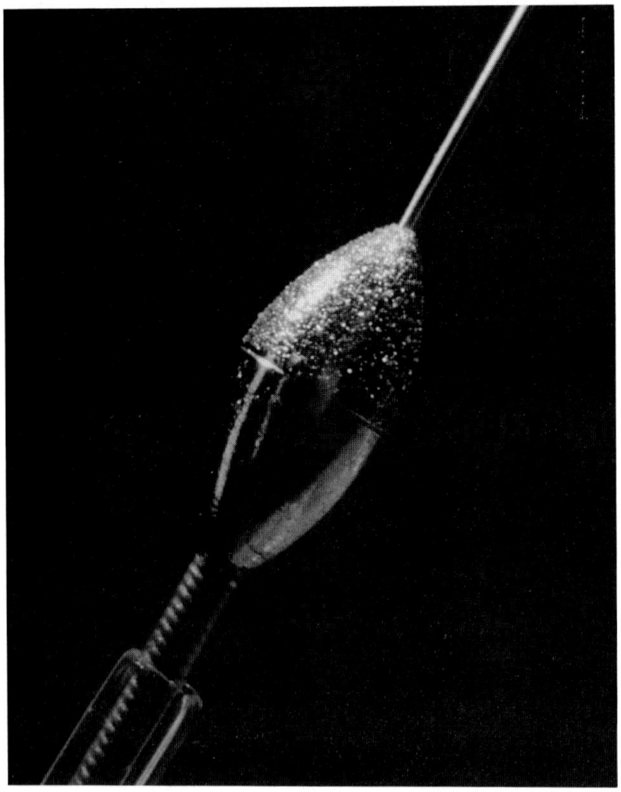

Figure 28–1. Close-up enlargement of the Rotablator burr as it tracks over its 0.009 inch guide wire. Hundreds of microscopic chips are embedded in the burr. When the burr rotates, each chip scoops out a microscopic amount of plaque.

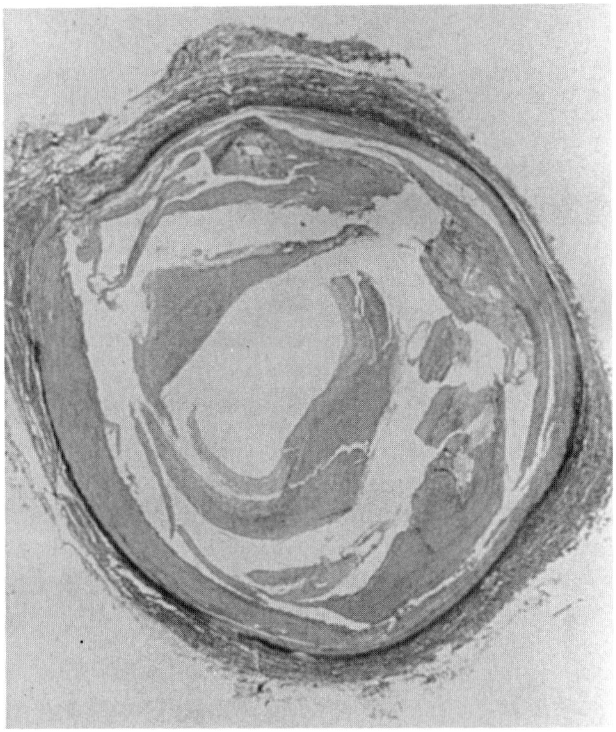

Figure 28–3. Photomicrograph of vessel cross-section following balloon angioplasty showing a rough intraluminal surface with multiple flaps. Results such as these stimulated David Auth, of the University of Washington, to develop a device that would remove the plaque without damaging the wall of the artery.

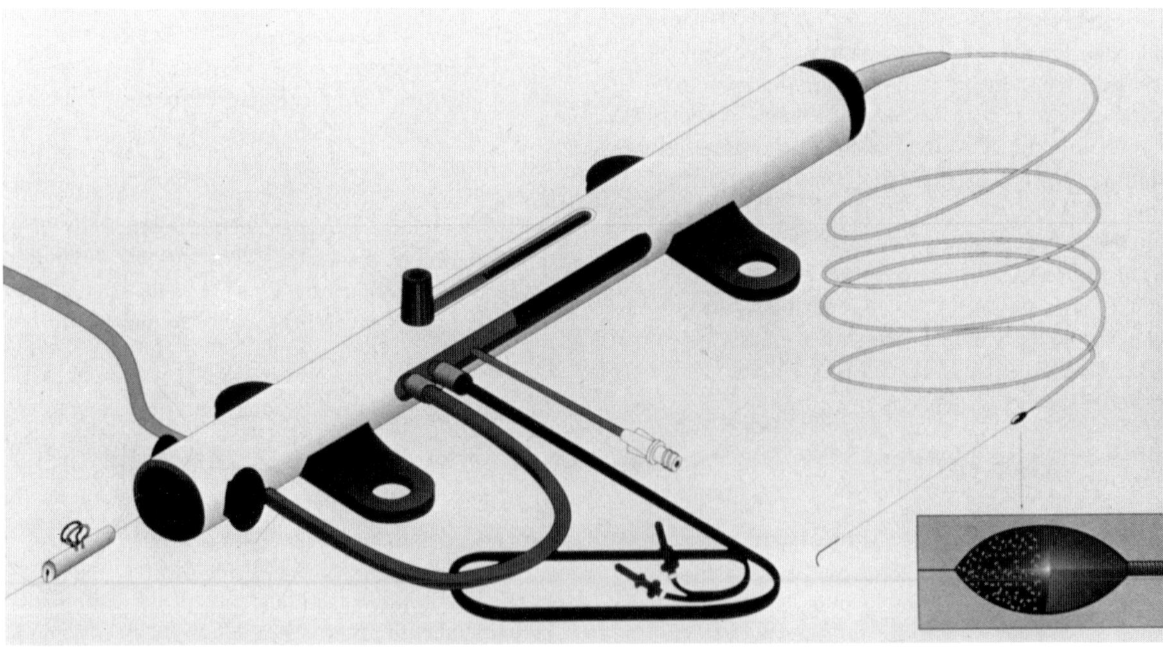

Figure 28–2. The Rotablator system showing the burr advancer unit, guide wire, sheath, and burr. Everything shown is disposable. Not shown is a small console used to control and monitor the burr revolutions and an air source.

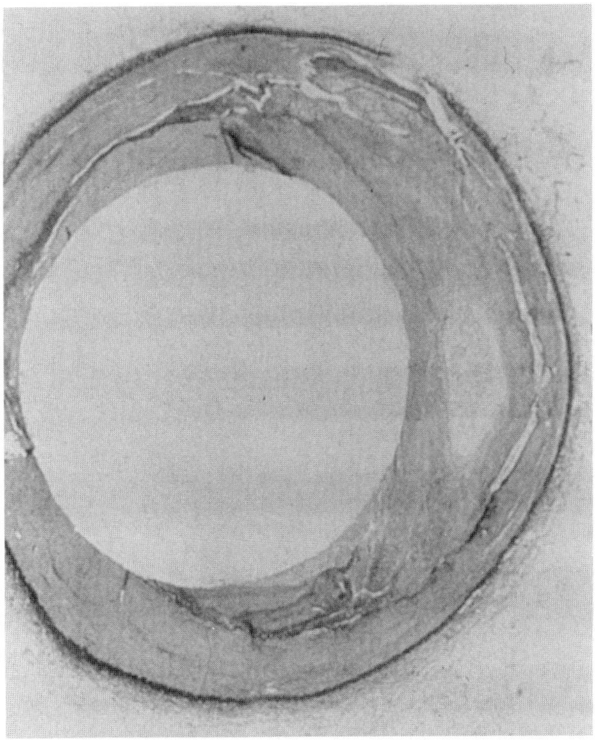

Figure 28–4. Photomicrograph of vessel cross-section following treatment with the Rotablator. Note the smooth, polished surface.

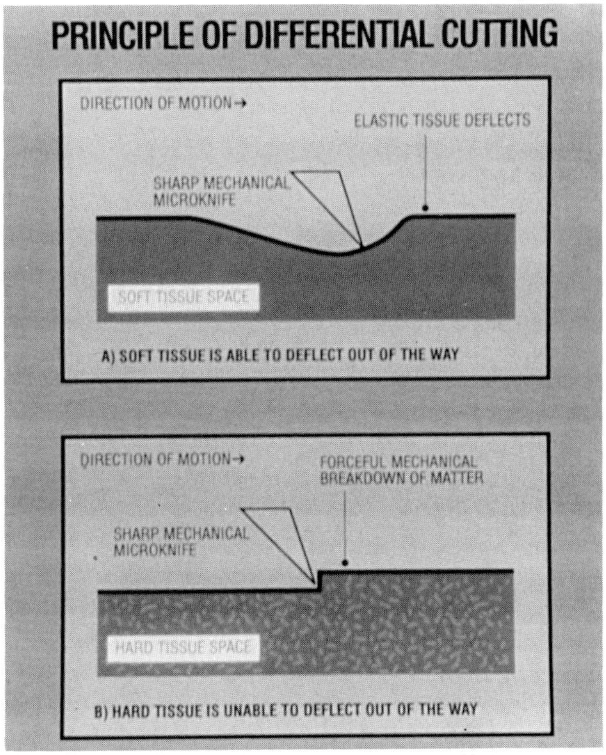

Figure 28–5. The Rotablator operates on the principle of differential cutting, like a cast saw. It rapidly removes inelastic plaque whether it is calcified, fibrous, or fatty. The normal vessel wall, being elastic, moves away from the rotating burr. This schematic shows how the Rotablator treats eccentric plaque in the bend of an artery. Animal and clinical studies have shown that the plaque is ablated to particles much smaller than a red blood cell. These pass out of the body via the reticuloendothelial system.

media and adventitia. The transition from the treated to the nontreated segments was smooth and tapered.[24] These same findings were found in in vivo studies on humans, which demonstrated removal of fibrous or calcified plaque with the ablated surface being smooth and free of thrombus. Damage to the endothelium of the adjacent normal vessel wall was shown, but no evidence of damage to the media or adventitia was present and no perforations were found. It is not advised to operate the ablation catheter at speeds below 75,000 rpm, because dehiscence of the intima and media, as well as surface irregularities, were seen with rotational speeds well below the normal operating parameters.[25]

MATERIALS AND METHODS

A total of 37 patients were included in the Stanford trials (Tables 28-1, 28-2, 28-3). The rotational ablation catheter was designated for use in patients with symptomatic stenosis or occlusions in a total of 44 procedures, including 49 infrainguinal sites and two iliac lesions. Of the initial 44 procedures, 37 were unilateral, three bilateral and four procedures were performed on patients who returned for a second atherectomy. Of these four patients, one had recurrent symptoms related to a new lesion and three had restenosis at the original atherectomy site. Indications were significant claudication in 22 (59%), severe claudication (less than 100 feet) in four (11%), and rest pain or limb threat in 11 (30%) patients. Preoperative evaluation prior to percutaneous ablation indicated that 24 (65%) patients were good candidates, and 13 (35%) poor candidates for conventional surgical bypass. Baseline evaluation should include noninvasive ultrasound studies and diagnostic angiography. After percutaneous transluminal rotational ablation (PTRA) angiography is important for recording the degree of residual stenosis. Because many people will not consent to follow-up angiography, particularly if they are clinically improved, it is necessary to obtain follow-up noninvasive duplex studies at 24 hours, 1-, 3-, 6-, and 12-month intervals during the initial postatherectomy period, to monitor the patient's recovery and diagnose new lesions or restenosis.

The most lesions treated (24 of 51, 47%) were in the distal SFA. (In two cases the device was not attempted because initial guide wire access was not possible.) The next largest group (15 of 51, 29%) were below the knee vessels. The remaining 12 lesions involved the popliteal artery in ten (20%) and one each in the profunda femoris and the iliac artery. A retrograde approach was used in ten patients; in

Table 28–1. Patient Demographics

Number of patients	37
Number of cases	44
Number of lesions	51
Males	25
Females	12
Mean age	67
Patients with at least one prior vascular procedure	21

Table 28–2. Patient Profile Successful Procedures

PATIENT NUMBER	SEX	AGE	PREVIOUS VASCULAR SX	DIABETIC	SMOKER	HPTN	REST PAIN	ULCER	GANGRENE
1	F	50	+	+	—	+	—	+	—
2	F	82	+	—	—	+	+	—	—
3*	F	80	+	—	—	+	—	+	—
5	M	71	+	—	—	+	—	—	—
6*	M	79	+	—	—	+	+	—	—
9*	F	73	—	—	+	+	—	—	—
11	M	62	—	—	—	+	—	—	—
15	F	67	—	+	—	—	+	+	—
16*	M	54	+	+	—	—	+	+	—
19	M	53	—	—	—	+	+	+	—
21	M	71	+	—	+	—	—	—	—
22	M	68	+	—	+	+	—	—	—
23	M	69	—	—	—	+	+	—	—
24	M	73	—	+	—	—	—	—	+
25	M	52	—	—	+	+	—	—	—
28	M	48	+	—	—	—	+	+	+
29	M	72	—	+	+	—	—	—	—
30	M	66	—	—	+	—	—	—	—
32	F	56	—	—	—	+	—	+	—
33	F	79	+	+	—	—	—	+	+
34	M	48	—	—	—	—	—	+	+
35	F	46	+	+	—	+	+	—	—
37	F	64	—	—	—	—	—	—	—
			11/24 (46%)	**8/24 (33%)**	**6/24 (25%)**	**14/24 (58%)**	**9/24 (37.5%)**	**9/24 (37.5%)**	**4/24 (17%)**

24 CASES/24 PATIENTS

*Repeat procedure

Mean age all patients = 67.95, M = 16, Male mean age = 67.38, F = 8, Female mean age = 69.28

Table 28–3. Patient Profile of Procedure Failures

PATIENT NUMBER	SEX	AGE	PREVIOUS VASCULAR SX	DIABETIC	SMOKER	HPTN	REST PAIN	ULCER	GANGRENE
5	M	71	+	—	—	+	—	—	—
4	M	56	+	+	+	+	—	+	—
8	F	64	—	—	—	—	—	—	—
10	F	67	+	—	—	+	—	+	—
12	M	43	—	—	+	+	—	+	—
13	M	61	—	+	+	+	—	—	+
14	M	85	+	—	—	—	+	—	—
17	M	64	+	—	—	+	—	—	—
18	F	63	+	—	+	+	—	—	—
20	M	53	+	+	+	—	—	—	—
21	M	71	+	—	+	—	—	—	—
26	M	74	—	—	—	+	+	—	—
27	F	70	—	—	—	+	—	—	—
31	M	64	+	—	—	+	—	—	—
35	M	65	+	+	—	—	+	+	—
36	M	69	—	+	—	+	—	+	+
			10/16 (63%)	**5/16 (31%)**	**6/16 (37.5%)**	**11/16 (69%)**	**3/16 (19%)**	**5/16 (31%)**	**2/16 (12.5%)**

16 CASES/16 PATIENTS

Mean age all patients = 65, M = 12, Male mean age = 64.56, F = 4, Female mean age = 66

four procedures, the Rotablator was advanced over the bifurcation for treatment of SFA or profunda femoris disease. In the remaining procedures (37 of 42, 88%) an antegrade approach from the ipsilateral superficial femoral artery was used. 26 of 51 (51%) lesions represented stenosis versus occlusion (25 of 51, 49%). Twenty-three of the 44 procedures were performed in the radiology angiography suite, and 21 procedures were completed in the operating room with surgical exposure of the SFA. The indications for this approach include patient obesity and relative requirement for anesthesia monitoring and adequate sedation. Ideally, a room that combines good radiographic equipment while maintaining a sterile environment would provide the best circumstances for performance of either a percutaneous or nonpercutaneous approach. Surgical exposure of the vessel does not significantly increase the duration of the procedure and, in certain ways, minimizes the incidence of procedural complication, particularly with obese patients. Also, a surgical approach does not compromise one's ability to anticoagulate the patient or to use direct thrombolytic therapy during the procedure.

The use of balloon angioplasty was equally divided among patients who had a good or poor clinical outcome. Adjunctive balloon dilation was performed in 21 (48%) patients. In 18 cases, balloon angioplasty followed initial atherectomy to augment the luminal diameter, and in three cases the dilation was performed before atherectomy. In these three instances, a small balloon was used with the thought of facilitating passage of the Rotablator. However, in retrospect, this is not necessary or desirable because the risk of a subsequent subintimal tract is increased. The large percentage of adjunctive PTA procedures reflects the fact that only small ablative burr sizes (1.5 mm to 3.0 mm) were available at the time of the clinical trial; they created a pilot lumen with insufficient reduction of lesion bulk to provide an adequate angiographic or hemodynamic result. Therefore, balloon dilation was necessary to augment the arterial lumen. Currently, larger burr sizes can most often preclude the necessity of adjunctive PTA. In two procedures, balloon dilation was used to optimize the result when a small subintimal flap (probably caused by guide wire manipulation) was recognized. In this respect, the "balloon rescue" was advantageous and resulted in a good clinical outcome, which might otherwise not have occurred.

TECHNIQUE

Following diagnostic angiography, the preferred approach to the lesion is selected. An antegrade puncture is favored over a retrograde contralateral approach in most atherectomy procedures. Even though the Rotablator catheter is flexible and capable of tracking over the bifurcation with relative ease, a retrograde approach is preferred for iliac lesions. The angle of the sheath placement is critical for prevention of hematoma formation or hemorrhage during the procedure. An optimal angle of placement also facilitates insertion and operation of rotational devices. Although, as mentioned before, even though the Rotablator is a flexible instrument, if the angle of entry into the vessel is too acute, it is difficult to advance the device or balloon catheters. In obese patients, an open surgical/radiology procedure is preferred. A femoral cut-down procedure can be performed in the angiography suite with local anesthesia. This portion of the procedure requires approximately 15 minutes for adequate exposure of the SFA. Surgical exposure of the vessel is also needed for the placement of the 14 F sheaths required for introduction of the 4.5 mm Rotablator burr.

When surgical exposure of the vessel is provided, placement of the sheath through the arteriotomy site is performed using the Seldinger technique followed by serial dilation of the vessel. This permits placement of the sheath without damage to the vessel wall, which can occur if the sheath is positioned without the appropriate series of steps. It is important to make the arteriotomy puncture with the Seldinger needle in the distal aspect of the surgically exposed vessel. This affords maximum working room above the sheath. If the puncture is made in the middle of the exposed vessel, it is frequently necessary to extend the surgical incision cephalad, in order to create adequate working space. Positioning the arteriotomy site in the distal aspect of the exposed vessel also decreases the angle of entry of the atherectomy catheter. This is relative in the use of rotational devices in which the entire working length of the catheter includes rotating mechanisms that are subject to damage if acute angulation occurs at any point along the shaft.

The placement of large sheaths can cause impairment of blood flow in patients in whom significant collateralization has not been developed via the profunda femoris branches. The decrease in antegrade flow through the superficial femoral artery can result in thrombosis during the atherectomy or angioplasty. This requires the physician to minimize the time of arterial occlusion.

As such, the systemic administration of 10,000 U of heparin during the procedure helps to minimize acute thrombosis. After placement of the introducer sheath, an 8 F guiding catheter is introduced over a 0.035 inch angled Terumo wire or Bentson guide wire. A Tuohy-Borst adaptor is placed on the end of the guiding catheter. This enables intermittent contrast injection for fluoroscopic visualization. A 5 F straight end-hole catheter is then advanced over the guide wire to the proximal aspect of the lesion. At this point, the tapered steerable guide wire is manipulated in order to pass through the residual lumen. Frequently, this lumen is not visible angiographically until the guide wire has passed through the lesion. The guide wire should not be forced but turned gently in multiple directions in order to seek the residual lumen. If the guide wire cannot cross the lesion, a 50,000 IU bolus of urokinase can be administered into the proximal aspect of the lesion. The bolus of urokinase can be repeated several times, if necessary, to remove or soften the chronic thrombus. Again, the guide wire should not be forced, because this increases the risk of subintimal tracking. On occasions, a short infusion of urokinase (250,000 IU in 50 cc of D5W) might be necessary.

Once the lesion is crossed, the 5 F end-hole catheter is advanced distally. The position of the distal tip of the guide wire should be 5 to 10 cm below the distal end of the lesion. With the 8 F guiding catheter positioned proximal to the occlusion site and the 5 F catheter across the lesion, the access guide wire is exchanged for the 0.009 inch exchange length PTRA guide wire which accompanies the Rotablator device. This guide wire is positioned across the lesion and the 5 F catheter is removed. The Rotablator device is front loaded onto the guide wire and advanced to a position distal to the lesion. With the larger burr sizes, a guiding catheter is not used. An optional and preferred method is direct placement of the 0.009 inch guide wire through the lesion via the proximally positioned 5 F end-hole catheter. Primary access with the 0.009 inch wire is desirable because this eliminates an exchange step and permits direct use of the ablation catheter.

Operation of the rotational ablation catheter is initiated with the foot pedal and controlled with the console. Continuous saline irrigation is mandatory during operation. Visual guidance is seen with fluoroscopy. The audio feedback from the device passing through the lesion is an excellent indication of the progress made by the burr during the ablation process. Calcified lesions result in a different tone than organized thrombus. The change in pitch is due to forward progress and "loading" of the burr. The burr is loaded in forward motion and unloaded as one backs off in a pulsed fashion. This is particularly effective when advancing through calcified material. The device is moved slowly but evenly throughout uncalcified plaque and thrombus. Heavily calcified lesions require longer periods for successful ablation. As opposed to other artherectomy devices, the motor drive in the ablation catheter is continuously "on" during ablation.

Selection of burr sizes needed is similar to the selection of balloon size for angioplasty, although one does not oversize the burr for the artery. The diameter of the vessel is measured proximal and distal to the lesion location. Following the initial successful passage of the first burr, a second larger abrasive tip can be used until the lesion is reduced to less than 30% residual narrowing. During exchanges of Rotablator burrs, the guide wire remains in place. Following lesion ablation, the device is removed, leaving the guide wire in position. Through the guiding catheter or sheath, contrast can be injected to evaluate the results of the ablation with digital imaging.

If necessary, balloon angioplasty should be performed at this time. When an optimal burr size has been used, and the residual luminal narrowing is less than 20 to 25%, additional balloon dilation is not indicated.

If distal spasm occurs, due to manipulation of the guide wire or rotational ablation, intra-arterial nitroglycerin or papaverine may be administered to reverse the spasm. Acute thrombus at the atherectomy site is managed by the direct infusion of 50,000 to 250,000 IU of urokinase. This is usually adequate to restore blood flow, and/or to totally lyse the thrombus. A digital angiographic study is performed to exclude the presence of intimal flaps or subintimal dissection that could cause acute reocclusion if not treated. Intimal flap can be removed with the Simpson atherectomy device or remodeled by balloon dilation. Because of the principle of differential cutting, the rotational ablation catheter is less able to remove subintimal flaps because they are generally elastic in nature. The creation of subintimal flaps with preablation balloon angioplasty should be avoided.

Heparinization should be maintained with partial thromboplastin time between 50 and 90 seconds. Continuous postprocedure heparinization is recommended following the ablation of small (less than 3 mm) vessels. Before and after the procedure, the patient is given one coated aspirin per day; other antiplatelet medications are not routinely used. If hemoglobinuria occurs, aggressive hydration and lasix administration are recommended. It almost always resolves within 24–36 hours without sequelae.

RESULTS

Evaluation of a new device needs to include assessment of device performance as well as overall procedure. We decided to analyze the results in four categories (Table 28-4):

1. Procedure success and device success
2. Procedure success, but device failure
3. Procedure failure, but device success
4. Procedure failure and device failure

The definition for procedure success requires immediate angiographic and hemodynamic success as indicated by a greater than 0.15 unit increase in ankle-brachial index (ABI) or newly palpable foot pulses as well as angiographic images demonstrating less than 20% residual stenosis. The hemodynamic success must persist for greater than 24 hours for a procedure to be classified as a success. Loss of distal pulses,

Table 28–4. Immediate Device Success

PATIENT NUMBER	SITE	LENGTH	% STENOSIS	PRE ABI	POST ABI	0–12 MONTHS FU ABI	1 YR. PATENCY CLINICAL STATUS
1	R SFA	3 cm	100%	—	.73	.73	Improved/Deceased
2	R SFA	3 cm	100%	.47	.75	.83	Improved/Mild Claudication
3	L Pop	3 cm	100%	.37	.86	.50	Restenosis/Redo
5	L Pop/PT	5 cm	100%	.65	.86	—	Improved/Deceased
6	R SFA	2 cm	95%	.56	.72	.42	Restenosis/Redo/Deceased
	R SFA	4 cm	100%	.41	—	.32	
7	L Pop	3 cm	95%	.56	—	—	Worse/Deceased (PF Disease)
8	L Tib/Per	3 cm	99%	—	—	—	Improved/Deceased
9	L SFA	30 cm	99%	.34	.41	.24	Restenosis/Redo
11	L SFA	30 cm	100%	.53	—	1.0	Improved
15	L SFA	15 cm	100%	.38	.55	.39	Improved/Mild Claudication
16	R PF	2 cm	90%	.31	.90	.58	Worse/New Lesion/PF OK
19	R SFA	20 cm	70%	—	—	—	Improved
21	R SFA	7 cm	100%	.71	.71	.96	Improved/No Claudication
22	R SFA	20 cm	90%	.37	.68	.55	Improved/No Claudication
23	R SFA	10 cm	100%	—	.91	.96	Improved
24	L Pop	2 cm	95%	.45	.65	—	Improved Initially/BKA 6 mo
25	R Pop	4 cm	100%	.65	—	.56	Improved
28	R SFA	13 cm	100%	.56	.72	.36	Restenosis
29	L Pop/AT	10 cm	100%	.45	.65	—	Improved
30	R Pop	4 cm	100%	.26	.39	.25	Stable
32	R SFA	5 cm	100%	—	.52	.71	Improved
33	L AT	2 cm	100%	—	—	—	Improved Initially/BKA 6 mo
34	L SFA	1 cm	99%	—	.83	.96	Improved
37	L SFA	5 cm	100%	—	—	—	Improved/No Claudication
3* RS+	L Pop	5 cm	100%	—	—	—	Improved
6* RS+	R Per	2 cm	100%	.42	.60	—	Improved
9* RS+	L SFA	20 cm	99%	—	—	—	Improved
16* NEW	R Pop	2 cm	95%	.58	.70	.75	Improved

* = Redo, + = Restenosis

24 PATIENTS, 30 SITES, 28 PROCEDURES

indicating thrombosis, occurring within 24 hours was deemed a procedure failure even if the exact cause of failure was not determined. Diagnostic angiography at the time of failure was not always obtained because of the decline in clinical status. Device success is defined as the ability to pass the ablation burr through the stenosis or occlusion without resulting in perforation, irreversible spasm, or immediate thrombosis resulting in compromise of the clinical outcome. Device failure is defined as inability to pass the Rotablator through the lesion or the occurrence of perforation, irreversible spasm, or immediate thrombosis at the atherectomy site. Subintimal dissection resulting from misplacement of the guide wire is not considered a device failure.

As noted in Table 28-5, procedure failure was recorded in all cases in which clinical decline occurred during the procedure or within 24 hours following ablational atherectomy. In the majority of these cases, the clinical decline was related to technical events unrelated to performance of the device. Sheath flaps, intimal dissections, and thrombosis (perhaps due to an appreciated subintimal dissection with guide wire) comprise the majority of clinical failures. Although characterized by loss of distal pulses and ensuing ischemic changes, most of these patients underwent successful application of the device and the decline of their vascular status can be attributed to the severity of the disease or technical problems not related to actual device application.

In the Stanford clinical trials, there were two cases of initial failure of the guide wire to cross the lesion. Therefore, an 83.3% technical success was achieved in terms of the device performance (Table 28-6, 28-7). The Rotablator traversed the stenosis or occlusion without complication and achieved the goal of desired clinical and angiographic results. However, in seven of these procedures, although rotational ablation was initially successful, the procedure failed due to technical complications unrelated to device performance (Table 28-8). In the procedures where the device failed to cross the lesion, a subintimal position of the guide wire was responsible for the inability to perform the atherectomy successfully. In two procedures, the device incompletely traversed the lesion, but balloon angioplasty was performed and a good clinical outcome was achieved.

The majority of the cases in which device success was achieved were SFA lesions. The relative rate of success decreased significantly with lesions involving trifurcation results (Table 28-9). Of the patients in whom the initial guide wire passage failed, in 75% the lesions were below the knee and 31% had tandem lesions (Fig. 28-6). In the group of procedure failures, 19% of the lesions were greater than 7 cm and 81% of these lesions were less than 7 cm in length. Therefore length, per se, does not appear to correlate with predictable outcome (Fig. 28-7A–B). Location, as will be discussed, is a more critical factor. As with balloon angioplasty, lesions below the knee represent a high-risk group for revascularization and successful outcome. If one asks if initial technical success depends on stenosis versus occlusion, analysis shows that there is no relative advantage in

Table 28–5. Procedure Failure

PATIENT NUMBER	SITE	LENGTH	% STENOSIS	PRE ABI	POST ABI	FU ABI	OUTCOME
5	R PT	3 cm	99%	.57	—	—	Subintimal Balloon Rescue
4*	R AT	2 cm	100%	.56	.81	—	Below Knee Amputation
8**	R SFA	3 cm	100%	—	—	—	No Change
10*	R Per	3 cm	90%	.65	.89	—	Sheath Flap
	R SFA	10 cm	90%	—	—	—	
12*	R SFA	4 cm	100%	.81	.49	—	Graft
13	L Per/AT	4 cm	100%	—	—	—	Graft
	L Per	2 cm	100%	—	.48	—	
14	L Per	1 cm	90%	.43	—	—	Below Knee Amputation
17	R Iliac	10 cm	100%	—	—	—	Aorto-Femoral Graft
18*	R SFA	30 cm	90%	—	—	—	Sheath Flap
20	R Pop/R Tib	3 cm	100%	.21	.58	.93	Subintimal Balloon Rescue
21**	L SFA	15 cm	100%	—	—	—	Graft
26*	L SFA	8 cm	100%	.48	.48	—	Thrombosis <7d, clinically no change
27*	L SFA	2 cm	100%	.62	—	—	Sheath Flap
31*	R SFA	20 cm	90%	—	—	—	Graft
35	R Per	2 cm	90%	—	—	—	Graft
36	R AT	20 cm	90%	—	—	—	Graft

*7 Rotablator successful but procedure failure

**2 Guidewire not successful

19 Sites, 16 Patients, 16 Procedures, 3 Multiple lesions, 6 Rotablator not successful 2° subintimal guidewire

Table 28–6. Early Trial Results/Stanford 1987–1989*

	DEVICE SUCCESS	DEVICE FAILURE	
Procedure Success	28/42 (67%)	2/42 (5%)	30/42 (72%)
Procedure Failure	7/42 (16%)	5/42 (12%)	12/42 (28%)
	35/42 (83%)	7/42 (17%)	TOTALS

*Note that the % success is slightly lower when using total procedures, not sites, as the denominator.

Table 28–7. Device Success: Distribution per Atherectomy Site

	VESSEL				
DEVICE	*SFA**	*POP***	*Tibial*	*PF/Iliac°*	TOTAL
Success	22	9	5	1	37/51 (73%)
Failure	2	1	10	1	14/51 (27%)

*Superficial Femoral Artery; **Popliteal; °Profunda Femoris
+ Initial guidewire access not successful

Table 28–8. Rotablator Successful but Procedure Failed

PATIENT NUMBER	VESSEL	LENGTH	% STENOSIS	PROBLEM	OUTCOME	COMMENTS
4	R AT	20 cm	100%	Thrombosis <7d	Vein graft-BKA	Poor Runoff/No Coumadin
10	R Tib Per	3 cm	90%	Sheath flap	Venous Patch	Technical Problem
	R SFA	10 cm	90%			
12	L SFA	4 cm	100%	Thrombosis	Graft	Residual Stenosis > 20%
18	R SFA	30 cm	90%	Sheath flap	Endarterectomy	Technical Problem
26	L SFA	8 cm	100%	Thrombosis <7d	Clinically No Change	Refused New Procedure
27	L SFA	2 cm	100%	Sheath flap	Graft	Technical Problem
31	R SFA	20 cm	90%	Thrombosis	Graft	Residual Stenosis 40% Distal Emboli ?

Table 28–9. Distribution of Technical Percutaneous Transluminal Rotational Ablation Success**

VESSEL	OCCLUSION	STENOSIS	TOTAL
SFA	11*/12	11/12	22/24 (92%)
POP	6/7	3/3	9/10 (90%)
TRI	1/5	4/10	5/15 (33%)
PF	0/0	1/1	1/1 (100%)
ILIAC	0/1	0/0	0/1 (0%)
TOTAL	**18/25 (72%)**	**19/26 (73%)**	**37/51 (73%)**

*Failure of initial guidewire access

**Defined as passage of device across occlusion or stenosis

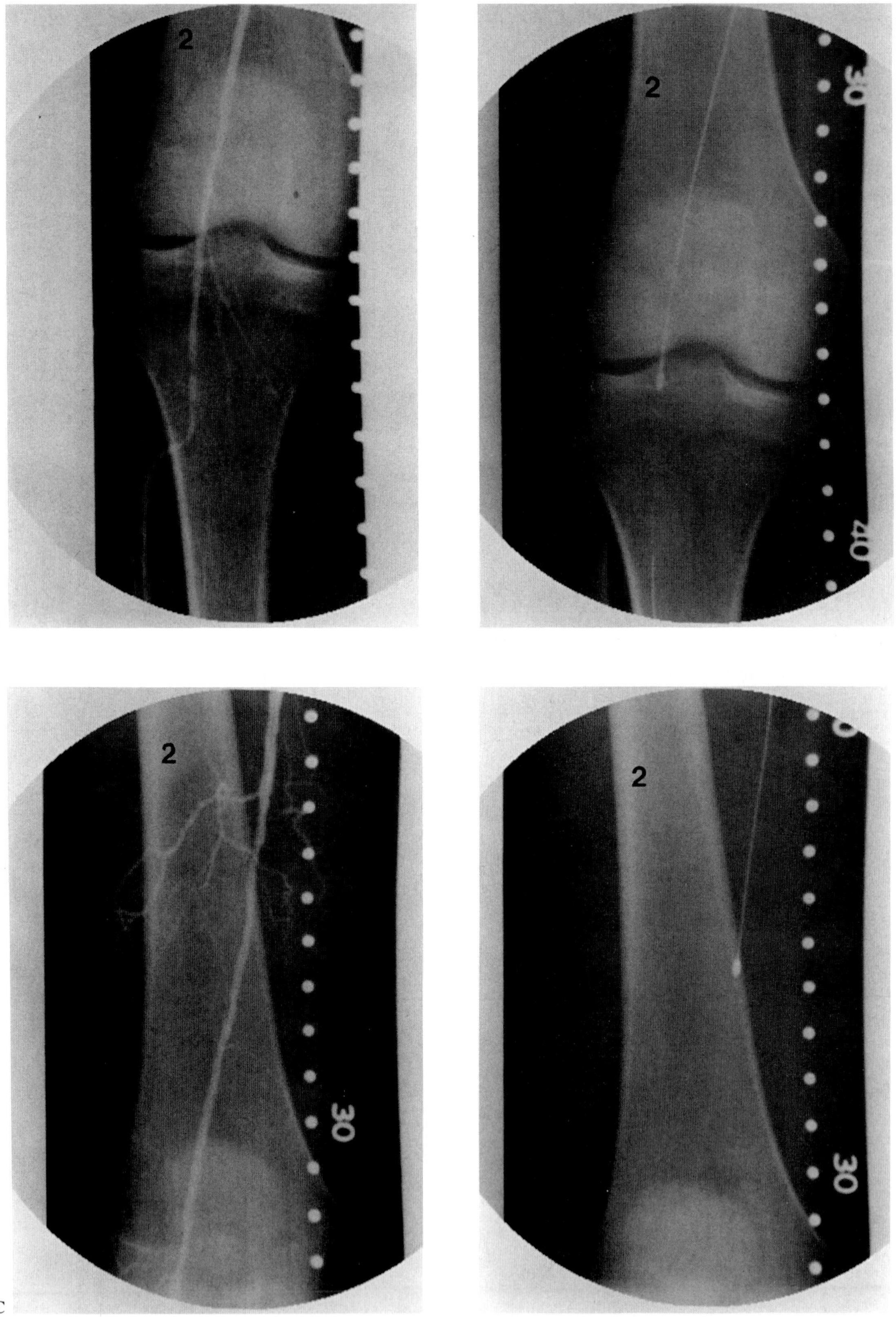

Figure 28–6. An 82-year-old woman with rest pain. **A:** High-grade stenosis of distal popliteal artery. **B:** Spot film during the Rotablator advancement. **C:** A 60 to 70% stenosis in the distal superficial femoral artery. **D:** Spot film of Rotablator.

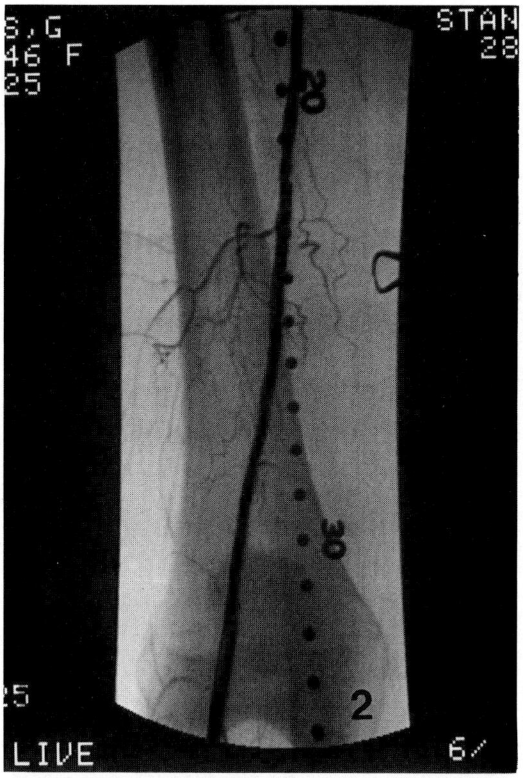

E

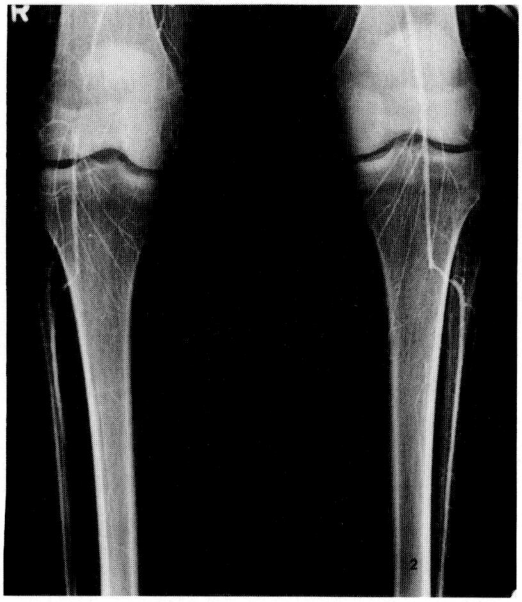

F

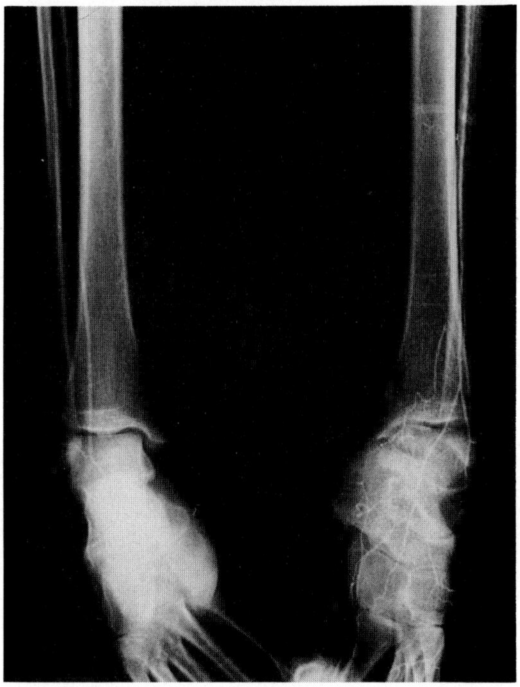

G

Figure 28–6. (*Continued*) **E:** Follow-up femoral arteriogram: widely patent lumen at site of ablation. **F:** Site of ablation on distal right popliteal artery is widely patent. **G:** One vessel runoff in the calf is patent.

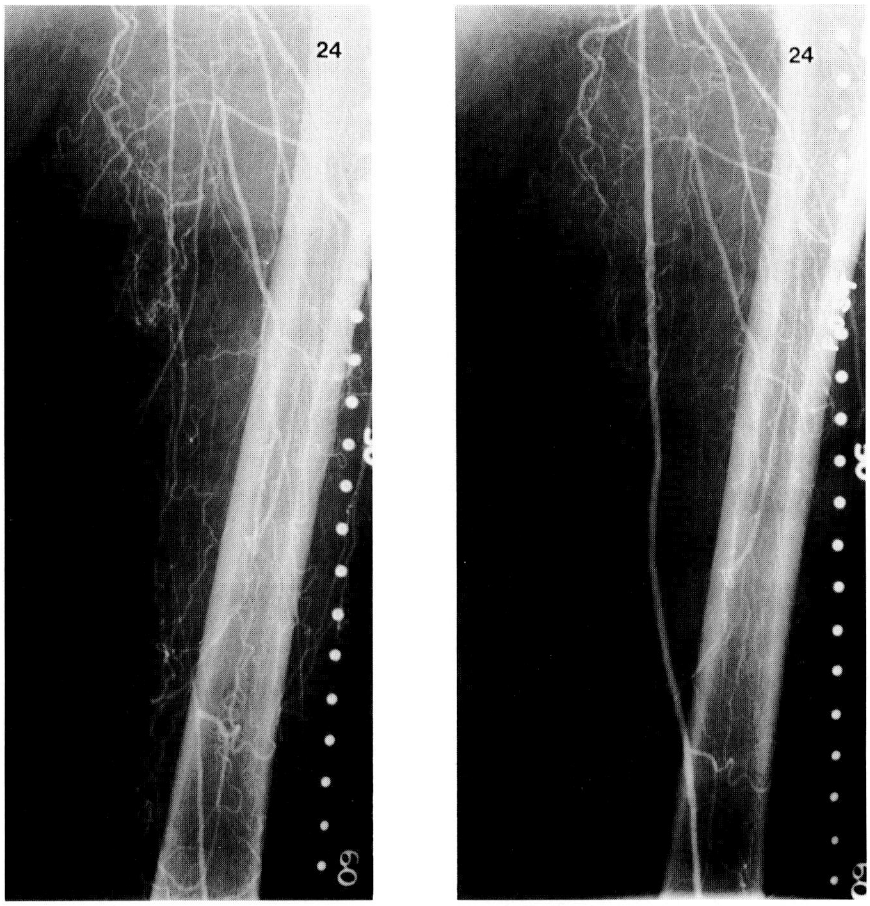

A B

Figure 28–7. A 73-year-old man, with diabetes and a heavy smoker. **A:** Diffuse disease of the entire superficial femoral artery. **B:** After passage of the Rotablator. Note the clean, smooth lumen.

subocclusive disease. Seventy-two percent of occlusions and 73% of stenoses were successfully traversed by the Rotablator. The site of the lesion and the presence or absence of tandem disease, as well as the quality of runoff below the knee are important factors in determining success of atherectomy or angioplasty. In the Stanford series, 24 (50%) of all lesions were in the superficial femoral artery. In the group of immediate technical failures, including procedural complications as well as device failure, 10 of 17 (59%) of the lesions were located below the knee. However, in the initial success group only 4 of 24 (17%) of the lesions involved tibial and peroneal vessels, whereas 80% of the lesions were in the superficial femoral and popliteal arteries. If one eliminates the procedures in which technical difficulties caused procedure failure, and only considers the instances in which the Rotablator was unsuccessful or resulted in immediate clinical failure, five of seven (71%) of these lesions were below the knee. The other two lesions in this category included one popliteal and one iliac lesion.

Evaluation of cases in which the Rotablator failed to traverse the lesion shows that subintimal position of the guide wire, as mentioned before, was the primary reason for failure (Table 28-10). The incidence of subintimal dissection can be reduced by adjunctive thrombolytic therapy to transform occlusions to high-grade stenosis and the use of steerable platinum-tipped guide wires. Technical complications resulting in procedure failure are decreased by experience.

Of those patients who underwent a below-knee amputation, within 12 months of PTRA, the disease pattern varied

Table 28–10. Technical Complications

Distal emboli	1
Known subintimal dissection++	4
Sheath related flaps*	3
Perforation	1
Hematoma*	2
Thrombosis	4
Spasm	1
Pseudoaneurysm*	1
TOTAL	**17**

*Not directly related to device.

++Subintimal guidewire

from short focal occlusion to long occlusions or diffuse disease. In addition, 4 of 5 (80%) of these patients were diabetic or had single vessel runoff. The profunda femoris artery was patent in each patient and collateral arteries were developed despite the presence of small vessel disease related to diabetes. Of note, the ablation site was a tibial or peroneal vessel in four of six lesions (67%) and the SFA and popliteal were each involved in a single instance. Two of the patients had previously undergone contralateral below-knee amputation, and four of the patients presented with nonhealing ulcers, indicative of severe ischemia. Among the group, three patients required amputation immediately after the failed rotational ablation procedure, because of acute thrombosis. Each of these patients had extremely advanced and complex disease. Therefore the Rotablator, per se, cannot be solely implicated in the decline in clinical status. Compromised flow, due to severe disease, contributed to thrombosis subsequent to vascular intervention. Only two of these patients experienced a successful procedure and were able to have an interval of clinical improvement before progressive disease resulted in clinical deterioration and ultimate amputation. In Figure 28-8, a successful ablation of a focal popliteal stenosis shows re-narrowing at 6 months. This is consistent with intimal hyperplasia and indicates the importance of close follow-up in patients who can benefit from a second procedure to treat the restenosis. Whether or not restenosis occurs at the site or overall progression of distal disease causes further clinical decline cannot be distinguished without follow-up diagnostic angiography or duplex evaluation.

Objective follow-up data such as angiography are difficult to obtain in patients who have clinical improvement following a procedure. Geographic disbursement of the Stanford patients also made acquisition of follow-up Doppler studies difficult. However, clinical follow-up by telephone conversation with the patient, their family, or their physician was obtained in all patients who have continued to exhibit improved clinical status since ablational atherectomy. The summary follow-up data are shown in Table 28-11. At 6 months, 75% of the 24 patients who underwent successful ablational atherectomy showed clinical improvement. During the first 6 months, four patients were noted to have recurrent symptoms. In three patients, repeat angiography demonstrated restenosis (2) and thrombosis (1). These patients underwent repeat procedures with favorable clinical outcome. When evaluated at 12 months following ablational atherectomy, 15 patients (63%) still showed improved or stable clinical status. During this period, two patients who showed initial improvement, subsequently experienced clinical decline and underwent below-knee amputations. One patient returned with recurrent symptoms and was found to have a new lesion that was treated with the Rotablator. An

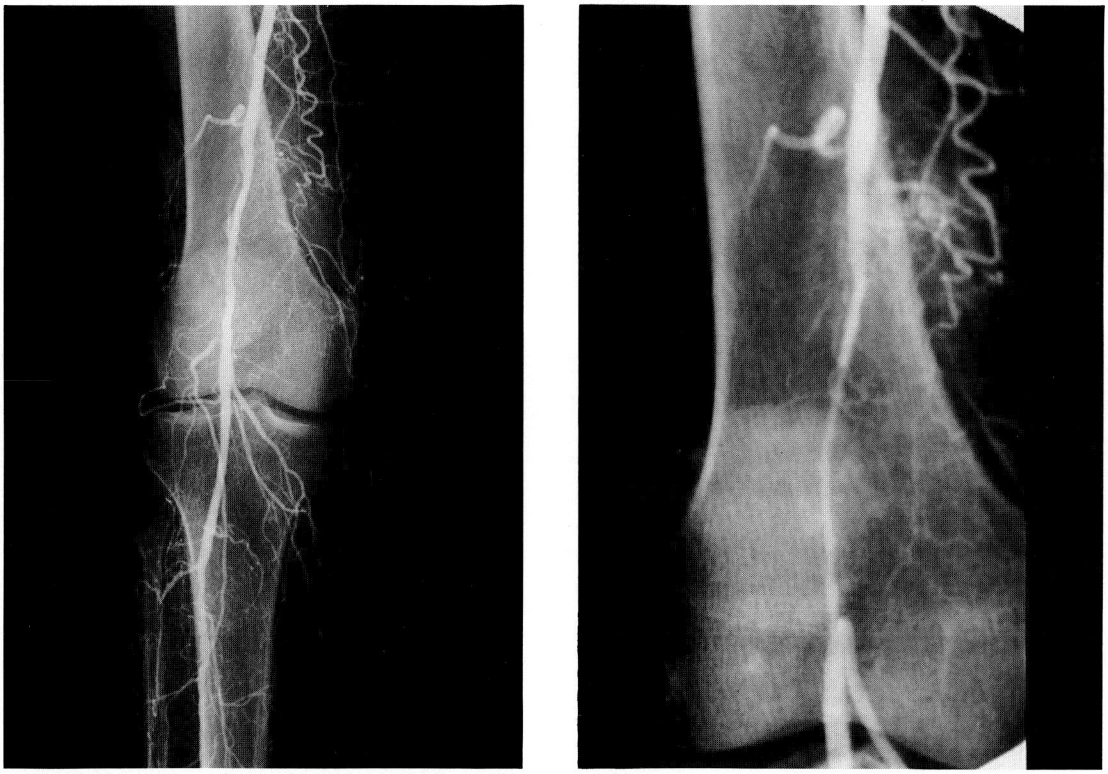

A B

Figure 28–8. A 73-year-old man with a history of hypertension and smoking. **A:** Follow-up angiogram after ablation of high-grade stenosis of the mid popliteal artery. Residual 30% stenosis. **B:** Six-month follow-up shows recurrence of disease at site of ablation and a long segment of narrowing distally.

Table 28–11. Stanford Data: 0–24 Months Clinical Follow-up Successful Percutaneous Transluminal Rotational Ablation

CLINICAL STATUS	0–6 MONTHS	6–12 MONTHS	12–24 MONTHS
Improved	18 (75%)	15 (62%)	9 (37%)
Worse			
No Angiogram	1	0	0
Angiogram			
Restenosis	2*	1	0
New Lesion	0	1*	0
Thrombosis	1*	0	0
BKA	0	2	0
Deceased**	2 (8%)	2 (8%)	5 (21%)
LTFU++	0	1	3

*Repeat procedure

**9/24 (37%) Deceased at 2 years

++4/24 (17%) Lost to follow-up at 2 years

additional case of documented restenosis was treated with a bypass procedure. At the end of 2 years, a total of nine patients (38%) still showed improved clinical status in the extremity treated with the Rotablator. However, within the second 12-month follow-up period, five patients died of causes unrelated to vascular disease. A total of nine patients (38%) of the 24 patients in whom a successful procedure had been performed were deceased within 24 months. An additional four patients (17%) were lost to follow-up during the initial 2-year follow-up. Our data indicate that restenosis is most likely to occur within the first 12 months following ablational atherectomy. However, longer follow-up with a greater number of patients is needed to confirm this impression. Without documenting patency or restenosis by angiography, one can only hope to infer that continued clinical stability indicates patency at the site of atherectomy. However, we know that restenosis can occur in association with collateral recruitment and therefore clinical stability can be maintained despite decreased patency at the site of previous angioplasty or atherectomy.

Evaluation of the patient profile reveals an even distribution of female to male representation among patients grouped according to procedure success or failure. A slightly higher number of patients in the failure group had a history of multiple vascular procedures prior to attempted rotational ablation. This indicates the severity of the disease encountered in the Stanford trials. The presenting signs and symptoms of vascular insufficiency are also similar among the two groups; the incidence of diabetes (approximately 33%) parallels patient data noted in other series of peripheral vascular therapy. Of note is the relatively low percentage of patients currently smoking. In truth, almost invariably, all patients with the degree of vascular disease we noted have smoked at one time. The patient profile reflects those currently smoking at the time of interview. In evaluating patients for hypertension, it is important to note whether or not the hypertension has been long-standing, and whether or not it is well controlled with medication. The incidence of associated renal vascular disease was not recorded.

PERIPHERAL VASCULAR LITERATURE REVIEW

Ahn et al[24] reported results in 68 cadaver arteries with atheromatous lesions involving the superficial femoral, popliteal, and tibial arteries. Obstructive lesions were removed in 36 of 37 stenotic lesions (97%) and 18 of 31 complete occlusions (58%) for an overall efficacy of 79%.[24] The reasons for failure are not discussed, however, but our experience suggests that failure is most commonly related to inability to pass the guide wire in the true lumen. Zacca et al[23] reported success on all six patients attempted, with a residual stenosis of less than 30% of the normal lumen and 100% patency at 3.5 months mean follow-up was found by Doppler and clinical evaluation in five patients with eight atherectomized lesions. Ahn and colleagues[25] have also reported on their intraoperative experience with the Rotablator. They had arteriographic success in 92% of cases. Early thrombosis caused failure in 5 cases reinforcing the need to combine thrombolytics and heparin with atherectomy. Their low two year patency, 12%, is multifunctional and includes treatment of long segmental lesions in tibial vessels. Intimal hyperplasia is not precluded and appears to be a factor with all similar interventions.

Dorros et al[26] recorded success on 85 of 96 (89%) lesions, 69 of 77 stenoses and 16 of 19 occlusions. The arterial obstruction was significantly reduced in stenoses from 85 to 0% and in occlusions from 100 to 15%. Complications included gross hemoglobinuria in 40 patients (65%), groin hematoma in ten (16%), arterial spasm in 12 (20%), arterial perforation in five (8%), and subsequent arterial bypass in two patients (3%) (unpublished data).[26] These data do not exclusively represent peripheral vascular cases. Furthermore, the incidence of complication in early trials, as at Stanford, reflects a learning curve as well as patient selection.

Fourrier et al[27] reported results in 53 long superficial femoral artery lesions treated with a Rotablator. Of these, 38 were 5 to 10 cm in length, 11 were 10 to 20 cm, and four were longer than 20 cm. Overall success was 90.6% (48 of 53). Adjunctive angioplasty was required in 17 of 53 (32%). The average initial percent stenosis of 91% was reduced to 33.8% with the Rotablator alone. After adjunctive balloon angioplasty, a residual stenosis averaged 16.8%. There was only one complication requiring intervention (1.9%); a severe spasm was resolved with balloon dilation. In short, at follow-up of 2 to 5 months, 75% were clinically improved.[27]

CORONARY LITERATURE REVIEW

In the Buchbinder et al[28] series, 118 consecutive coronary patients with 140 lesions were treated: 58% eccentric lesions,

34% tortuous vessels, 29% calcified, and 25% at bifurcation points. Acute success defined as less than 50% residual stenosis was achieved in 95%. The mean stenosis was reduced from 86.5 to 40.4% post-treatment. Adjunctive angioplasty was performed in 41% of patients, reducing the stenosis to 22.6%.[27] Cheirif et al[29] studied the effects of particles liberated during rotational atherectomy in the coronary arteries in comparison to the ischemic changes induced by coronary angioplasty and found that rotational atherectomy is as effective as coronary angioplasty (PTCA) and is associated with less evidence of ischemia than PTCA. Rodriguez et al[30] reported on the use of larger burr sizes (2.25 or 2.50 mm) in 27 patients without adjunctive balloon angioplasty and described a substantial decrease in the percent of residual stenosis to values around 34.2 ± 11.0%. Transient spasm was common and one patient had an intimal dissection.[30]

COMPLICATIONS

Complications can be divided into technical complications related to the procedure and those directly related to the manipulation and operation of the device. Since the Rotablator is an over the wire system, once the guide wire successfully crosses the lesion, the incidence of device-related complications during atherectomy is very small. In the Stanford series, one instance of distal embolization was recorded and in the collective experience from the multicenter trials, distal embolization has been recorded in two cases. In our one case, two mottled toes were noted 24 hours after an ablation procedure in a long segmental SFA occlusion. The most frequent complication related to Rotablator atherectomy in the combined national series has been distal spasm. This has occurred in five cases in which papaverine was able to reverse the symptoms in two cases and in three patients, balloon angioplasty was required. In the Stanford series, irreversible spasm in the anterior tibial artery in one patient resulted in thrombosis. Subintimal tracts associated with use of the device is invariably subsequent to initial malposition of the guide wire. It is important to note that successful ablation is dependent on intraluminal guide wire placement. As such, procedure failure due to subintimal tracking is not exactly a device failure; the Rotablator performs well when the guide wire is properly positioned. In no instances did the Rotablator fail to cross a lesion when the guide wire was in the true lumen.

In the Stanford clinical trials, technical complications contributed to procedure failure in seven cases (Tables 28-8, 28-12). Sheath-related flaps accounted for three failures; such complications can be avoided by using a percutaneous technique when placing a sheath under direct visualization into a surgically exposed vessel. In two of these cases, the ablation site was unaffected. In one case the patient proceeded to have a femoral popliteal graft. In two percutaneous procedures, large hematomas occurred at the groin; one of these required transfusion and extended hospital stay. Thrombosis occurred in five patients within 24 hours after an apparently successful angiographic and hemodynamic result at the time of atherectomy. Thrombogenicity related to atherectomy as well as the possibility of a subintimal dissection cannot be excluded in these cases. One pseudoaneurysm resulted in a patient who underwent atherectomy via a percutaneous approach. Therefore technical complications were recorded in 17 (40%) of the procedures, although in six instances, the complication was not device related. In addition, hemoglobinuria was recorded in five cases. Although not noted in early applications, hemoglobinuria was most often noted in cases requiring longer time for atherectomy, even though the available burr size ranged from 1.75 to 4.0 mm. Occurrence may be related to degree of back-flow from distal collaterals, thus exposing blood to the trauma of high-speed rotation. The hemoglobinuria generally clears spontaneously and is, in itself, not clinically significant. In one case however, the related decrease in hematocrit required transfusion. In the five patients in whom hemoglobinuria was seen, the average duration of rotational ablation was greater than 10 minutes. However, some patients with long sessions did not have hemoglobinuria, whereas one focal lesion requiring only 3 minutes, 17 seconds rotational ablation did result in mild hemoglobinuria.

Table 28–12. Rotablator Unsuccessful

PATIENT NUMBER	VESSEL	LENGTH	% STENOSIS	PROBLEM	RESULT	OUTCOME
5	R Per	5 cm	95%	Could not advance	Balloon	Improved
20	R Pop	10 cm	100%	Subintimal*	Balloon	Improved
13	L AT	4 cm	100%	Perforation	Thrombosis	Graft
14	L Per	6 cm	90%	Subintimal*	Thrombosis	BKA
17	R Iliac	10 cm	100%	Subintimal*	Thrombosis	AFB
35	R Per	2 cm	90%	Subintimal*	Thrombosis	Graft
36	R AT	20 cm	90%	Spasm	Thrombosis	Graft

*Guidewire position

IMPRESSION

Analysis of the complications and modifications of the procedure have resulted in fewer difficulties in later clinical applications. Review of our experience has yielded at least three lessons, which will be listed.

Rotational ablation can be safely performed on all lesions that can be traversed with a guide wire. This includes eccentric, calcified, ostial, diffuse, tortuous, small caliber, bifurcation, or abductor lesions. The one prerequisite for successful use of the Rotablator is access across the lesion with a guide wire. The use of thrombolysis and new guide wires have improved the success of crossing vascular occlusions; the Rotablator can therefore be used in the treatment of the majority of peripheral lesions. The coaxial design and other features of the device contribute to a predictable atherectomy result and fewer complications. Long-term results regarding restenosis rate associated with rotational ablations are forthcoming. Because many patients underwent adjunctive PTA, to augment the lumen, the disadvantages of barotrauma were not completely eliminated from early studies (Table 28-13). Whether or not adjunctive balloon angioplasty will contribute to long-term patency or diminish long-term favorable outcome is a question that still has not been answered. Specifically, the incidence of restenosis associated with atherectomy, with or without balloon assistance, is a complex issue to be resolved. Additional randomized clinical trials involving patients with comparable disease are necessary to establish an answer to this question.

In summary, results suggest that length of the lesion is not a factor in determining success or failure of Rotablator ablation (Tables 28-14, 28-15, 28-16). Since many high-grade focal stenoses have superimposed thrombus, which can propagate through the entire extent of the superficial femoral artery, the length of occlusion, per se, does not accurately allow one to predict outcome. Patient selection is, however, very important. A greater number of technical and clinical failures are encountered when treating below-knee lesions. As might be expected, the pattern of the disease is pertinent as well; diffuse disease yields poorer long-term results with atherectomy as well as with endarterectomy and angioplasty. In addition, the presence of tandem disease negatively affects long-term results, as similarly documented in follow-up studies of PTA and bypass procedures. Early results reflect the fact that initial clinical trials were performed on patients with very severe disease. Many of these patients had previous vascular procedures and failed surgery as well as balloon angioplasty prior to attempted rotational ablation.

Table 28–13. Balloon Assistance

VESSEL*	OCCLUSION	STENOSIS
SFA	8/12 (67%)	3/12 (25%)
POP	5/7 (71%)	2/3 (67%)
TRI	2/5 (40%)	2/10 (20%)
PRO	0/0	1/1
ILIAC	0/1	0/0
TOTAL	**15/25 (60%)**	**8/26 (31%)**

*Superficial Femoral Artery, Popliteal, Tibial Peroneal Arteries, Profunda Femoris

Table 28–14. Stenosis: Length of Lesion

VESSEL*	<7.5 cm	7.5–15 cm	>15 cm
SFA	6	1	5
POP	0	0	3
TIB	2	0	8
PRO	1	0	0
TOTAL	**9/26 (34%)**	**1/26 (4%)**	**16/26 (62%)**

*Superficial Femoral Artery, Popliteal, Tibial Peroneal Arteries, Profunda Femoris

Table 28–15. Occlusion: Length of Lesion

VESSEL*	<7.5 cm	7.5–15 cm	>15 cm
SFA	3	4	5
POP	5	2	0
TIB	4	0	1
ILIAC	0	1	0
TOTAL	**12/25 (48%)**	**7/25 (28%)**	**6/25 (24%)**

*Superficial Femoral Artery, Popliteal, Tibial Peroneal Arteries

Table 28–16. Length of Lesion

	<7.5 cm	7.5–15 cm	>15 cm
Stenosis	9/26	1/26	16/26
Occlusion	13/25	7/25	5/25
TOTAL	**22/51 (43%)**	**8/51 (16%)**	**21/51 (41%)**

Acknowledgments. To Denise Baccus, Barbara Behring, and Dawn Schmidt for assistance in preparing the manuscript and to David Stiehr for thoughtful and astute editorial contributions.

REFERENCES

1. Hansen DD, Auth DC, Vracko R, Ritchie JL. Rotational atherectomy in atherosclerotic rabbit iliac arteries. Prog Cardiol 1987;115 (Pt 1):160–5.

2. Lai P, O'Neill WW, Auth D, et al. Non-surgical human coronary endarterectomy: use of a mechanical rotary catheter. Circulation 1985;72 (part II):II-371.
3. Hansen DD, Auth D, Vracko R, Ritchie JL. Rotating mechanical angioplasty in atherosclerotic iliac arteries in rabbits. J Am Coll Cardiol 1986;7:213A.
4. Ritchie JL, Hansen DD, Vracko R, Auth D. Mechanical thrombolysis: a new rotational catheter approach for acute thrombi. Circulation 1986;73:1006–12.
5. Hansen DD, Auth D, Vracko R, Ritchie JL. Rotating mechanical angioplasty in atherosclerotic iliac (sic) vessels in rabbits. X World Congress of Cardiology, Abstract Book 1:280, #1599, September 1986.
6. Hansen DD, Hall M, Intlekofer MJ, et al. In-vivo rotational angioplasty in atherosclerotic rabbits: comparison of angioscopy and angiography. International Symposium Interventional Cardiology, Abstract Book 1:58, September 1986.
7. Hansen DD, Vracko R, Auth D, et al. In-vivo rotational angioplasty in canine coronary arteries. International Symposium Interventional Cardiology, Abstract Book 1:106, 1986.
8. Blankenship J, Thomas W, Abrams G, et al. Non-surgical percutaneous endarterectomy using a mechanical rotational catheter in normal canine coronary arteries in vivo. J Am Coll Cardiol 1987;9:188A.
9. Culverwell M. Blades and reamers move into balloon angioplasty turf. Cardiology April 1987;74:22–25.
10. Hansen DD, Intlekofer MJ, Hall M, Ritchie JL. In-vivo rotational endarterectomy in canine coronary arteries. Lasers Surg Med 1987;7:82.
11. Hansen DD, Auth DC, Hall M, Ritchie JL. Rotational endarterectomy in normal canine coronary arteries: Preliminary report. J Am Coll Cardiol 1988;11:1073–7.
12. Hansen DD, Hall M, Intlekofer MJ, et al. In vivo rotational angioplasty in atherosclerotic rabbits: comparison of angioscopy and angiography. (Abstr 1443.) Circulation 1986;78(II).
13. Ritchie JL, Hansen DD, Intlekofer MJ, et al. Rotational approaches to atherectomy and thrombectomy. Z Kardiol 1987;76(6):59–65.
14. Fourrier JL, Stankowiak C, Lablanche JM, et al. Histopathology after rotational angioplasty of peripheral arteries in human beings. J Am Coll Cardiol 1988;11:109A.
15. Hall M, Hansen D, Intlekofer M, Auth D, Ritchie J. PTCA vs rotational atherectomy (PTRA) in rabbit atherosclerosis: early and late effects. J Am Coll Cardiol 1988;11:173A.
16. Weibull H, Bergqvist D, Jonsson K, et al. Complications after percutaneous transluminal angioplasty in the iliac, femoral, and popliteal arteries. J Vasc Surg 1987;5:681–6.
17. Hewes RC, White RI Jr, Murray RR, et al. Long-term results of superficial femoral artery angioplasty. AJR 1986;146: 1025–9.
18. Gardiner GA, et al. Complications of transluminal angioplasty. Radiology 1986;59:201–8.
19. Johnston WK, et al. 5 year results of a prospective study of percutaneous transluminal angioplasty. Ann Surg 1987; 206:903–13.
20. Rooke TW, et al. Percutaneous transluminal angioplasty in the lower extremities: A 5 year experience. Mayo Clin Proc 1987;62:85–91.
21. Zacca NM, Short HD III, Edwards T, et al. In-vitro assessment of particles generated by rotational atherectomy of human atheroma. Texas Heart Institute Cardiology & Cardiovascular Surgery: Interventions, 1987 Annual Symposium, Abstract Book, 158, October 1987.
22. Zacca N, Raizner A, Short D, et al. First in-vivo human experience with a recently developed rotational atherectomy device. Circulation 1987;76:IV-46.
23. Zacca NM, Raizner AE, Noon GP, et al. Short term follow-up of patients treated with a recently developed rotational atherectomy device and in-vivo assessment of the particles generated. J Am Coll Cardiol 1988;11:109A.
24. Ahn SS, Auth D, Marcus DR, Moore WS. Removal of focal atheromatous lesions by angioscopically guided high-speed rotary atherectomy preliminary experimental observations. J Vasc Surg 1988;7:292–300.
25. Ahn SS, Darwin E, et al. Intraoperative peripheral rotary atherectomy: Early and late clinical results. Ann of Vasc Surg Vol. 6, No. 3, 1992, pp 272–280.
26. Dorros G, Iyer SS, Zaitoun R, et al. Acute angiographic and clinical outcome of high speed percutaneous rotational atherectomy (Rotablator). 63rd Scientific Sessions Abstract Form, Dallas, Texas, November 1990.
27. Fourrier JL, Dorros G, Ginsburg R, et al. Percutaneous peripheral rotational ablation in long lesions: multi-center experience. 63rd Scientific Sessions Abstract Form, Dallas, Texas, November 1990.
28. Buchbinder M, O'Neill W, Warth D, et al. Percutaneous coronary rotational ablation using the Rotablator: Results of a multi-center study. 63rd Scientific Sessions Abstract Form, Dallas, Texas, November 1990:III-493.
29. Cheirif BJ, Heibig J, Harris S, et al. Rotational ablation is associated with less myocardial ischemia than PTCA. 63rd Scientific Sessions Abstract Form, Dallas, Texas, November 1990:III-493.
30. Rodriguez AR, Zacca N, Heibig J, et al. Coronary rotary ablation using single large burr and without balloon assistance. Circulation 82 (Suppl III):III-310.

29 An Overview of Laser Angioplasty

Andrew H. Cragg, M.D., Tony P. Smith, M.D., Flavio Castañeda, M.D.

Since the first working laser was constructed in 1960,[1] lasers have been applied to numerous disease states and their value has been well demonstrated. The use of lasers in the treatment of vascular disease, however, is a relatively recent phenomenon.

Over the past several years, there has been tremendous interest in development of new technology to treat atherosclerotic vascular disease. The impetus for this has arisen from several factors, including: (1) demonstration of the long-term efficacy of balloon angioplasty as an alternative to surgery, (2) rapid proliferation and application of angioplasty procedures to the treatment of coronary artery disease, and (3) recognition by scientists and industry that a large market existed for new technology that would improve on the results of balloon angioplasty.

With the refinement of existing catheter technology, it occurred to numerous investigators that remote delivery of laser energy via catheter-based quartz fibers could potentially allow percutaneous obliteration of atherosclerotic plaque, thereby achieving vessel recanalization without surgery or balloon angioplasty. The major potential advantage to this type of approach was that by removing plaque from the blood vessel, rather than redistributing it, as occurs with angioplasty, one would achieve a better long-term result.

During the early 1980s, a number of investigators began developing delivery systems for various laser sources in order to accomplish percutaneous laser angioplasty.[2–9] Some of this work has matured into clinical studies and Food and Drug Administration approval of laser devices. Difficulty, however, in harnessing laser energy for angioplasty has slowed development of the technique. In addition, major questions remain about the efficacy of any laser angioplasty system given the high cost and mixed results that have been obtained to date. To illustrate the present state of development of laser angioplasty, it may be useful to review briefly what is currently known about laser sources, catheter delivery systems, and experimental and clinical results.

LASER SOURCES

Argon

Argon gas is the active medium for this type of laser, which produces coherent, monochromatic light in the visible range of the spectrum, particularly 488 and 514 nm. Advantages of argon lasers as a source for laser angioplasty include the ability to lase in a blood field, the ability to easily transmit argon light down an optical fiber, and the fact that argon lasers are readily available and economical to operate. Disadvantages that have been demonstrated in experimental and clinical work to date include relatively low peak energy of the argon beam that results in thermal tissue destruction and charring at the lasing site,[10] continuous wave output that adds to the thermal effect of the laser source, and difficulty in controlling the depth of ablation, which has required shielding or capping of the argon laser output to prevent vessel perforation.

Neodymium-yttrium Aluminum Garnet

Neodymium-yttrium aluminum garnet (Nd-YAG) lasers emit light in the visible range of the spectrum (700 to 1000 nm). There is broad experience with Nd-YAG lasers in other areas of medicine, such as ophthalmology. Therefore, because of their availability, they have been fairly extensively investigated as sources for laser angioplasty. Nd-YAG lasers may be operated in both continuous and pulsed modes. Pulsed radiation seems to be preferable for atheroma ablation because thermal effects on the irradiated vessel are reduced when compared with continuous wave radiation.[11,12] This is likely due to a combination of shorter wavelength (higher energy) pulses and the fact that interpulse time allows for more efficient cooling than can occur with continuous radiation. In practice, most Nd-YAG laser angioplasty systems operate in the continuous mode. Although a higher power output is achieved than with the argon source, there is considerable thermal damage that again limits the usefulness of Nd-YAG as a free beam source.

Advantages of Nd-YAG lasers therefore include ready availability, higher power output than other sources, and relatively easy transmission down optical fibers.

Disadvantages include deep, relatively nonspecific tissue penetration and thermal effects related to continuous wave delivery.

Excimer

Excimer lasers have sparked considerable interest as a laser angioplasty source since they appear to obviate many of the disadvantages that have plagued more conventional laser sources such as argon and Nd-YAG. Common medical excimer lasers use as active media various halide-based gases, such as XeCl or XeF. The output from these media is in the ultraviolet range (200 to 400 nm) and in the pulsed mode.

With respect to direct irradiation of atherosclerotic plaque, excimer lasers appear to possess several advantages over argon and Nd-YAG laser sources. First, excimer light has a short wavelength (200 to 400 nm) and the pulsed radiation is of short duration (10 to 250 ns). These factors result in the advantageous combination high peak energy and relatively nonthermal tissue ablation. The high peak energy allows one to obliterate calcified plaque, which is generally not possible with argon and Nd-YAG sources, and the combination of high energy, pulsed radiation produces clean tissue ablation without significant thermal effects[13,14] (Fig. 29-1). In addition, excimer light appears to have a very short zone of ablation, which means that the device can be operated as a free beam laser with a lower risk of laser-induced vessel perforation than with argon or Nd-YAG sources.[15]

There are disadvantages to the excimer laser, however, which have hampered its introduction into the laser angioplasty field. The lasers are large and relatively cumbersome to operate. The high peak power can make transmission down optical fibers difficult.[16] Excimer light does not transmit well through blood, which requires a blood-free lasing field. Finally, excimer lasers are expensive, which adds to the cost of the revascularization procedure itself.

New Laser Sources

Newer laser sources such as the tunable dye or solid-state Alexandrite lasers hold promise as relatively powerful, compact systems that can be operated in the pulsed mode. If laser delivery systems are refined to the point of efficacy, these types of sources may allow laser angioplasty to be simple and inexpensive enough to achieve clinical utility.

LASER DELIVERY SYSTEMS

Early laser angioplasty systems consisted of an argon or Nd-YAG source coupled to a bare quartz silica fiber. The fiber was directed to the lasing site by passing it through the lumen of a conventional angiographic catheter. As the results of research were compiled, it became apparent that there were two major limitations of the technique.

First, the perforation rate using a bare fiber was unacceptably high and, second, the amount of plaque ablated was insufficient to use the technique as sole therapy.[17,18] As such, most research into development of laser delivery systems over the past several years has focused on solution of these two problems, particularly the problem of vessel perforation. A brief review of the results of several different laser delivery systems follows (Fig. 29-2).

Bare Fibers

Quartz silica fibers, which form the basis of all laser angioplasty systems, are quite efficient at delivering laser energy from the source to the target. Given a 20 to 30% power loss at the distal tip of the fiber, it is still possible to generate high fluences at the target site or plaque. Because the cone angle or degree of beam divergence at the fiber tip is quite small, however, laser light delivered in this fashion is very concentrated, which means that a relatively small hole is created in the target tissue by the incident beam. In addition, since the power of the beam is concentrated in a small area, the depth of penetration tends to be difficult to control. These difficulties have been demonstrated in experimental studies that have generally shown an inability to remove completely an atherosclerotic stenosis without an unacceptably high perforation rate.[19,20] These findings were confirmed in preliminary clinical trials with a bare fiber delivery system that demonstrated a 50% recanalization rate and an 18% perforation rate.[21] These initial poor results prompted most investigators, in collaboration with industry, to pursue fiber

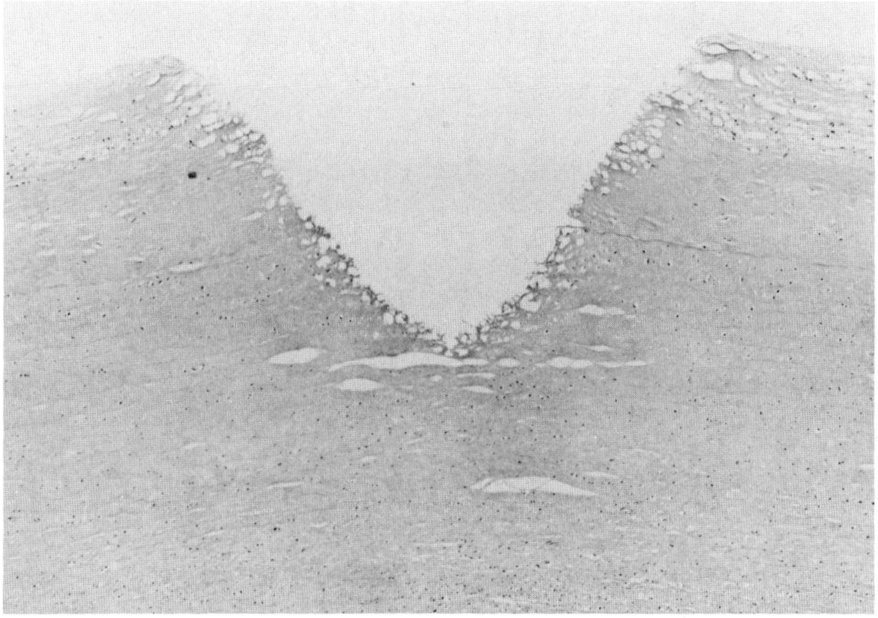

Figure 29–1. Photomicrograph of atherosclerotic plaque after irradiation by excimer laser demonstrates relatively athermal ablation with precise crater formation and lack of tissue vacuolization.

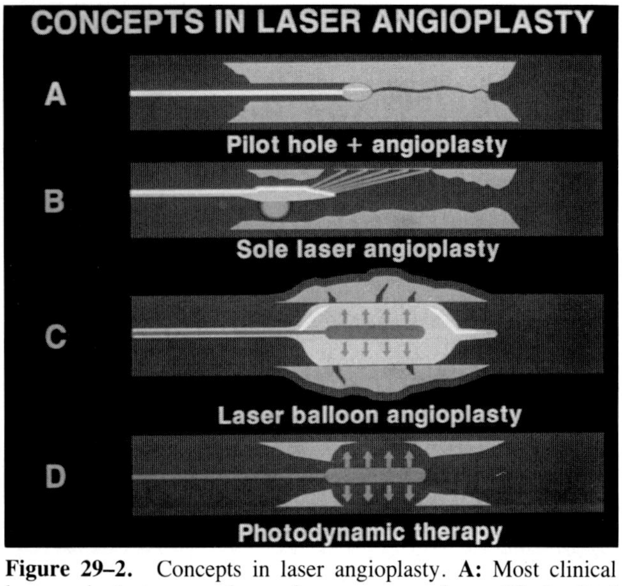

Figure 29–2. Concepts in laser angioplasty. **A:** Most clinical laser angioplasty research now focuses on use of a modified optical fiber to create a small pilot hole in an obstructed vessel prior to balloon angioplasty. The efficacy of this concept is unproved. **B:** More favorable laser sources, such as excimer or tunable dye, may allow plaque ablation without the need for modification of the fiber tip or subsequent balloon angioplasty. **C:** Laser irradiation through an inflated balloon causes "welding" of fractured plaques and decreased elastic recoil. Potential, but unproved, advantages include decreased abrupt closure and lower restenosis rates compared with conventional balloon angioplasty. **D:** Chemical modification of plaque may allow more rapid and selective laser angioplasty. This technique could theoretically produce plaque regression in diffusely diseased vessels. (Reprinted with permission from Radiology 1989;172:925–35.)

tip modification as the means of improving the safety and efficacy of laser angioplasty.

Recently, however, several vendors have instituted clinical trials with only slightly modified bare fiber delivery systems. These systems use excimer and tunable dye sources, which investigators hope will prove to be safer and more efficacious than previously used argon and Nd-YAG sources (Fig. 29-3). At the time of this writing, no detailed report of the clinical results of these systems was available.

Fiber Tip Modification

To reduce the risk of vessel perforation, which occurred frequently with bare fibers, numerous modifications of the distal fiber tip have been proposed. The best known of these is the "hot tip" device in which a metal cap is crimped on the end of a fiber.[22] The laser light then is absorbed by the metal cap, which causes rapid heating of the cap. In air, the cap can reach 300° to 500°C; however, tissue temperatures are generally between 100° and 200°C.[23] When contact is made with noncalcified plaque, the probe is capable of thermally ablating tissue within a narrow zone of the tissue probe interface.

The purpose of this device is to recanalize occluded peripheral blood vessels that cannot be traversed with conventional guide wire and catheter techniques. As such, the device represents an adjunct to conventional balloon angioplasty.

Sanborn et al[24] have reported good clinical results with this device. Primary angiographic and clinical success was achieved in 21 of 22 stenoses (95%) and 78 of 107 occlusions (73%). Others, however, have reported less favorable results. Perler et al[25] reported a 15-month patency of 7% in 47 laser-treated femoropopliteal occlusions. Matsumoto et al[26] recently reported their results using an argon or YAG hot tip laser to treat 148 lesions in 137 patients. They reported an overall immediate success rate of only 53%. Their success rate in treating stenoses and segmental occlusions was 61%. Their perforation rate was 6% and amputation rate, 10%. These results are inferior to conventional guide wire and balloon angioplasty. Interestingly, Morgenstern et al[27] have recently reported a 91% technical success rate for treatment of femoropopliteal occlusions with guide wire and balloon therapy, which is as good or better than results reported with laser-assisted balloon angioplasty. This seems to confirm the anecdotal experience of most experienced angiographers, that most occluded peripheral vessels can be recanalized successfully with a catheter and guide wire alone. As such, the value of laser recanalization in this setting is dubious.

Other investigators have studied the effect of sapphire contact probes. Recanalization of occluded femoropopliteal segments has been reported in 74 to 88% of cases[28] without a clear difference between the metal and sapphire tips.[29] Still other tip modifications such as quartz optical assemblies to increase beam divergence have been successfully used to recanalize occluded vessel segments in association with conventional balloon angioplasty.[30]

Plaque Modification

The concept of modifying the spectral properties of atherosclerotic plaque to allow selective ablation by laser light is an intriguing one that has been investigated by several groups. Murphy-Chutorian et al[31] showed that physiologic levels of tetracycline would be preferentially taken up in plaque. Since tetracycline selectively absorbs light in the red range (peak, 355 nm), a laser that operates at or near this wavelength will be more strongly absorbed by tetracycline-treated plaque. This finding has been confirmed by our group using an excimer laser operating at 351 nm.[32] Other plaque modifiers such as hematoporphyrin derivative (HPD) and exogenous carotenoids have shown promise for selective plaque destruction; however, clinical application of these drugs has not been successful.[33,34]

Laser Balloon

The application of laser energy to the blood vessel wall in a radial fashion through an inflated angioplasty balloon has been postulated to have several important, potentially beneficial effects.[35,36] Thermal "welding" of the dehisced plaque elements could reduce the incidence of acute closure after

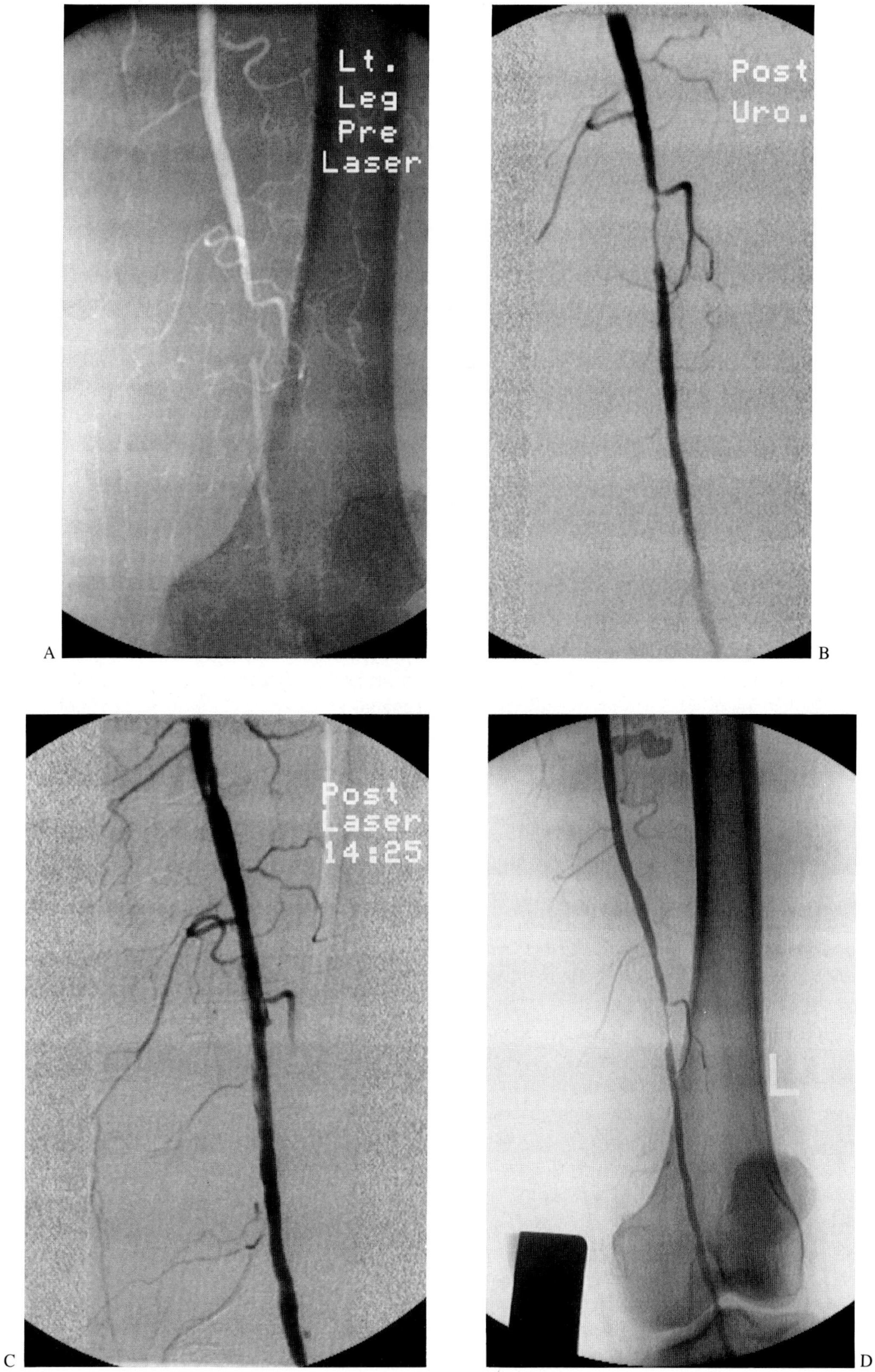

Figure 29–3. A 55-year-old diabetic woman with a nonhealing left foot ulcer. **A:** Note 3 cm occlusion of distal superficial femoral artery. Patient had runoff via a widely patent anterior tibial artery. **B:** After recanalization with a guide wire and infusion of 250,000 U urokinase, a small channel has been opened. **C:** After 14 minutes 25 seconds of lasing with an excimer laser (351 nm, 20 mJ/pulse, 100 Hz), the artery is widely patent, although somewhat irregular. The patient's ulcer healed and she remained asymptomatic 6 months after the procedure; however, a follow-up angiogram revealed restenosis at the laser site **(D).**

conventional balloon angioplasty, elastic recoil of the dilated vessel may be reduced due to medial coagulation, and atherogenesis may be reduced by thermal destruction of smooth muscle cells. These concepts have been tested experimentally with favorable results[37] and they are now being investigated in clinical trials. We have investigated the same principle using hot water in the angioplasty balloon with similar results.[38]

SUMMARY AND FUTURE DIRECTIONS

A discussion of the state-of-the-art of laser angioplasty in 1990 would not be complete without reference to the technical limitations of present laser systems and the political ramifications of laser angioplasty.

During the past 10 years or so, there have been great changes in the American medical system which have altered the way that physicians treat patients with vascular disease. For most physicians and administrators, medicine is now a market-driven, competitive industry that responds quickly to the demands of the consumer (the patient). The cardiovascular market is one of the most profitable and competitive markets in medicine today. The boom in cardiovascular intervention really began when cardiologists began performing coronary angioplasty. The explosive growth of this technique spurred the development of numerous industries to support this procedure.

As with any competitive and lucrative market, new technology formed the cornerstone of any company that wished to enter the market or stay competitive. Patients have benefited from this competition by innovation and refinement of vascular technology. Because of media attention, it is often the patients themselves who demand new, sometimes unproven, technology in their treatment.

As the American medical system becomes more competitive, physicians now find themselves in direct competition with their colleagues for patients. This competition, which is, in part, driven by a surplus of physicians and changes in reimbursement patterns, has become fierce among cardiovascular specialists and has resulted in "foraging" of one specialty into the domain of another in order to garner new patients.

Unfortunately, the laser angioplasty industry has developed in this atmosphere and has to a large extent come to embody the negative aspects of this competitive environment. This has occurred for several reasons.

First, the technologic potential of medical lasers is indisputable. This fact has been quite effectively communicated to the public and there now exists an "aura" about lasers that patients find irresistible. This fact, in combination with the demand for technical innovation in the cardiovascular market, has created a powerful incentive for development of laser angioplasty.

Second, early development of laser angioplasty systems did not meet expectations of the investigators who developed them. The hope that laser light could "clean out" a blood vessel quickly and efficiently has not been realized. This has created a great deal of skepticism on the part of many individuals in the cardiovascular field.

Third, early laser devices, which received FDA approval based on demonstration of safety, have demonstrated little efficacy in the hands of most practitioners. Despite this, however, the devices have found their niche as a marketing tool to garner patients. This has created tremendous cynicism about lasers and, in concert with the general climate of competition in the cardiovascular field, it has fueled the estrangement of the previously collegial specialties of cardiology, interventional radiology, and vascular surgery.

Despite the problems that exist between cardiovascular specialists today, it seems clear that the role of interventional vascular therapy will continue to expand. Cardiovascular laser therapy is in its infancy and it is not yet clear what role it will play. Ethical investigation of the merits of any new technology should continue to be the gold standard by which we practice.

REFERENCES

1. Maiman TH. Stimulated optical radiation in ruby. Nature 1960;187:493–4.
2. Abela GS. Laser recanalization: a basic and clinical perspective. Thorac Cardiovasc Surg 1988;36:137–41.
3. Choy DSJ. History and state-of-the-art of lasers in cardiovascular disease. Laser Med Surg News Adv 1988;June:34–38.
4. Grundfest WS, Litvack F, Hickey A, et al. The current status of angioscopy and laser angioplasty. J Vasc Surg 1987;5:667–72.
5. Isner JM, Clarke RH. Laser angioplasty: unraveling the Gordian knot. J Am Coll Cardiol 1986;7:705–8.
6. Lee G, Chan MC, Reis RL, et al. Potential applications of lasers in the management of cardiovascular diseases. J Intervent Cardiol 1988;1:59–74.
7. Litvack F, Grundfest WS, Papaioannou T, et al. Role of laser and thermal ablation devices in the treatment of vascular diseases. Am J Cardiol 1988;61:81G–6G.
8. Sanborn T. Laser angioplasty: what has been learned from experimental studies and clinical trials? Circulation 1988;78:769–74.
9. Spears JR. Percutaneous laser treatment of atherosclerosis: an overview of emerging techniques. Cardiovasc Intervent Radiol 1986;9:303–12.
10. Grundfest WS, Litvack IF, Goldenberg T, et al. Pulsed ultraviolet lasers and the potential for safe laser angioplasty. Am J Surg 1985;150:220–6.
11. Deckelbaum LI, Isner JM, Donaldson RF, et al. Reduction of laser-induced pathologic tissue injury using pulsed energy delivery. Am J Cardiol 1985;56:662–7.
12. Gibson PH, Holten D, Smith SC, et al. Absence of thermal tissue injury using a pulsed mode Nd-YAG laser. (Abstr.) Circulation 1985;72(suppl 3):1605.
13. Grundfest WS, Litvack F, Forrester JS, et al. Laser ablation of human atherosclerotic plaque without adjacent tissue injury. J Am Coll Cardiol 1985;5:929–33.
14. Grundfest WS, Litvack F, Doyle L, et al. Comparison of in vitro and in vivo thermal effects of argon and excimer lasers for laser angioplasty. (Abstr.) Circulation 1987;74(suppl 2):813.

15. Cross FW, Bowker TJ. The physical properties of tissue ablation with excimer lasers. Med Instrum 1987;21:226–30.
16. Forrester JS, Litvack F, Grundfest W, et al. The excimer laser: current knowledge and future prospects. J Intervent Cardiol 1988;1:75–80.
17. Anderson HV, Zaatari GS, Roubin GS, et al. Steerable fiberoptic catheter delivery of laser energy in atherosclerotic rabbits. Am Heart J 1986;111:1065–72.
18. Anderson HV, Zaatari GS, Roubin GS, et al. Coaxial laser energy delivery using a steerable catheter in canine coronary arteries. Am Heart J 1987;113:37–47.
19. Crea F, Abela GS, Fenech A, et al. Transluminal laser irradiation of coronary arteries in live dogs: an angiographic and morphologic study of acute effects. Am J Cardiol 1986;57:171–4.
20. Isner JM, Donaldson RF, Funai JT, et al. Factors contributing to perforations resulting from laser coronary angioplasty: observations in an intact human postmortem preparation of intraoperative laser coronary angioplasty. Circulation 1985; 72(suppl 2):191–9.
21. Ginsburg R, Wexler L, Mitchell RS, Profitt D. Percutaneous transluminal laser angioplasty for treatment of peripheral vascular disease: clinical experience with 16 patients. Radiology 1985;156:619–24.
22. Lee G, Ikeda RM, Chan MC, et al. Dissolution of human atherosclerotic disease by fiberoptic laser-heated metal cautery cap. Am Heart J 1984;107:777–8.
23. Welch AJ, Bradley AB, Torres JH, et al. Laser probe ablation of normal and atherosclerotic human aorta in vitro: a first thermographic and histologic analysis. Circulation 1987; 76:1353–63.
24. Sanborn TA, Cumberland DC, Greenfield AJ, et al. Percutaneous laser thermal angioplasty: initial results and 1-year follow-up in 129 femoropopliteal lesions. Radiology 1988;168:121–5.
25. Perler BA, Osterman FA, White RI Jr, Williams GM. Percutaneous laser probe femoropopliteal angioplasty: A preliminary experience. J Vasc Surg 1989;10:351–7.
26. Matsumoto T, Okamura T, Rajyaguru V. Laser arterial disobstructive procedures in 148 lower extremities. J Vasc Surg 1989;10:169–77.
27. Morgenstern BR, Getrajdman GI, Laffey KJ, et al. Total occlusions of the femoropopliteal artery: high technical success rate of conventional balloon angioplasty. Radiology 1989; 172:937–40.
28. Lammer J, Pilger E, Karnel F, et al. Austrian multicenter trial for laser angioplasty: 2-year results. (Abstr.) Radiology 1988;169(P):139.
29. Lammer J, Karnel F. Percutaneous transluminal laser angioplasty with contract probes. Radiology 1988;168:733–7.
30. Nordstrom LA, Castañeda-Zúñiga WR, Young EG, Von Seggern KB. Direct argon laser exposure for recanalization of peripheral arteries: early results. Radiology 1988;168:359–64.
31. Murphy-Chutorian DM, Kosek J, Mok W, et al. Selective absorption of ultraviolet laser energy by human atherosclerotic plaque treated with tetracycline. Am J Cardiol 1985; 55:1293–7.
32. Smith TP, Cragg AH, Landas SK. Plaque modification with tetracycline: enhanced tissue ablation during excimer lasing. (Abstr.) 75th Scientific Assembly and Annual Meeting of the Radiological Society of North America, November 1989.
33. Spears JR, Serur J, Shropshire D, Paulin S. Fluorescence of experimental atheromatous plaques with hematoporphyrin derivative. J Clin Invest 1983;71:395–9.
34. Prince MR, Deutsch TF, Shapiro AH, et al. Selective ablation of atheromas using a flashlamp-excited dye laser at 465 nm. Proc Natl Acad Sci USA 1986;83:7064–8.
35. Ward H. Laser recanalization of atheromatous vessels using fiber optics. Lasers Surg Med 1984;4:353–63.
36. Spears JR. Percutaneous transluminal coronary angioplasty restenosis: potential prevention with laser balloon angioplasty. Am J Cardiol 1987;60:61B–4B.
37. Jenkins RD, Sinclair N, Anand R, et al. Laser balloon angioplasty: effect of tissue temperature on weld strength of human postmortem intima-media separations. Lasers Surg Med 1988;8:30–9.
38. Gleason T, Cragg AH, DeJong SC, Smith TP. Results of thermal balloon angioplasty in a canine model. (Abstr.) 75th Scientific Assembly and Annual Meeting of the Radiological Society of North America, November 1989.

30 Laser Physics and Spectrum of Available Lasers and Laser Safety

Edward J. Grogan, C.C.E.

In 1960, Theodore H. Maiman and associates at Hughes Aircraft Company in Culver City, California, developed the first laser device utilizing ruby crystals as their lasing medium.[1] Since that date, lasers have been developed for numerous applications. This chapter seeks to present a basic understanding of laser physics as well as some insight into the functional design of current laser systems utilized for angioplasty. In addition, I shall discuss general guidelines to ensure safe application of this new technology in the patient care environment.

LASER PHYSICS

Atomic Theory

The structure of an atom is such that at any given time the atom exists in an energy state dependent on the number of orbiting electrons and their distance from the nucleus of the atom. As the distance between nucleus and orbiting electron increases, so does the atom's defined energy state. The lowest energy level is defined as the resting or ground state of the atom. It is in this state that the radius of electron orbit is at its minimum.

Electrons orbiting about the nucleus of an atom may change energy levels by atomic absorption or emission of energy. If an orbiting electron absorbs energy, $\Delta E_{0 \rightarrow 1}$, in the form of heat, light, or an electric field, a transition will occur so that it will make a "quantum leap" into a more distant orbit. The atom, once in its resting energy state, E_0, will assume an excited state with an increased energy level, $E_1 = E_0 + \Delta E_{0 \rightarrow 1}$ (Fig. 30-1). Within a short period of time (on the order of 10^{-8} second), however, the electron will spontaneously drop to a lower level; the atom no longer remains in its excited state with energy, E_1, but seeks to return to its ground state, E_0. The atom emits, in the form of a photon, a bundle of energy, $\Delta E_{1 \rightarrow 0}$, equal in magnitude to the absorbed energy (Fig. 30-1). This is known as spontaneous emission of radiation by an atom and was hypothesized by Bohr in the 19th century.

Spontaneous emission may also occur between two excited levels so that a bundle of energy, $\Delta E_{2 \rightarrow 1}$, is emitted (Fig. 30-2).

In the early 1900s, Albert Einstein hypothesized that if atoms in their excited states ($E_1 = E_0 + \Delta E_{0 \rightarrow 1}$) prior to spontaneous decay were bombarded by photons of precisely the same energy, $\Delta E_i = \Delta E_{0 \rightarrow 1}$, as was initially absorbed to achieve excitation, that excited electrons would move to a lower state and emit a photon of energy $\Delta E_{1 \rightarrow 0}$, equal in magnitude to ΔE_i. The stimulating photon, rather than being absorbed, would instead also be propagated to produce a net result of two photons of equal energy traveling in the same spatial and temporal phase (Fig. 30-3). This is known as stimulated emission of radiation and is the principle on which the laser (or light amplification by stimulated emission of radiation) is based.[1–3]

Laser Beam Production

For a sustained stimulated emission to occur, and thus a sustained production of laser light to be produced, a "population inversion" must be achieved so that a majority of atoms exist in their excited state. This condition is produced by "pumping" energy into a laser medium so as to produce spontaneous emissions of photons that then collide with other atoms in their excited state, stimulating them to emit an additional photon. These photons then collide with other transitional atoms and a chain reaction of stimulated emission occurs. To maintain this state, energy must be continually supplied to the laser media being excited. Gas lasing mediums use electric power (direct current or radiofrequency electric fields), whereas liquid or solid lasing mediums

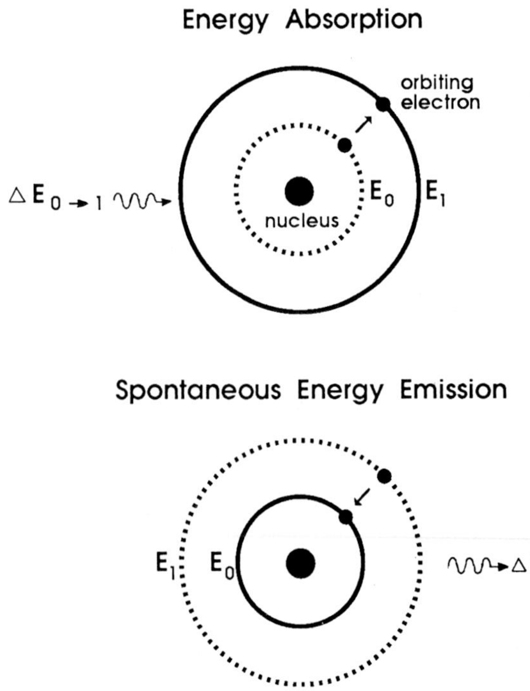

Figure 30–1. Spontaneous emission of radiation.

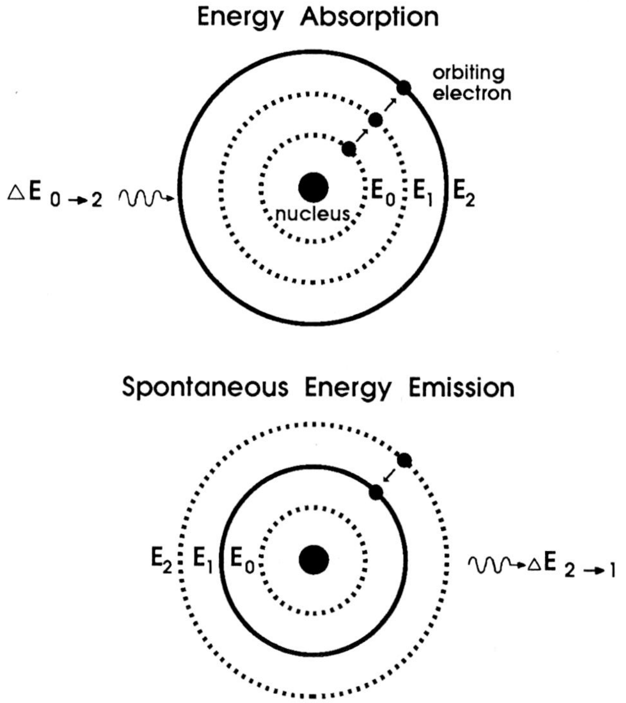

Figure 30–2. Spontaneous emission of radiation.

require optical power produced by a xenon flash lamp or other lasers.

Since a fine beam of laser light is desired, the random directional movement of spontaneous and stimulated emissions must be changed to a uniform direction. This requires an amplification scheme (Fig. 30-4) incorporating a laser tube (optical or resonant cavity) designed so that photon

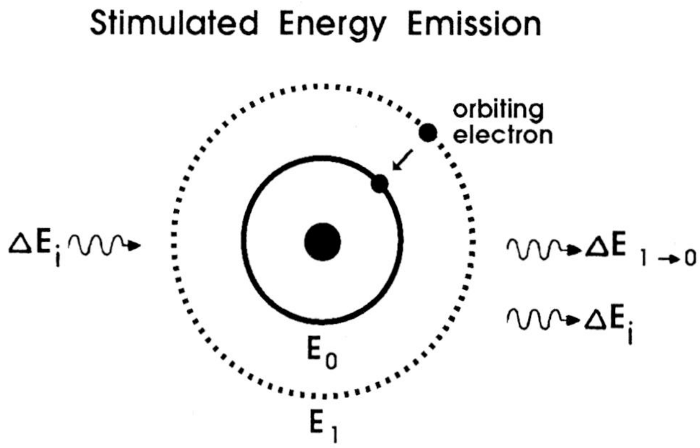

Figure 30–3. Stimulated emission of radiation.

propagation parallel to the axis of the tube is reflected back through the axis of the medium causing more atoms in their excited state to emit photons. Carefully aligned mirrors are placed at both ends of the laser tube. The lasing effect is amplified with photons resonating back and forth along the axis of the optical cavity. One of the mirrors is designed to be 100% reflective and the other is designed to partially transmit the laser beam out of the resonant tube. The energy from spontaneous photon emissions nonparallel to the axis of the tube is lost in the form of heat. Air or water cooling systems will often be incorporated into the design of the laser system to dissipate this lost energy and to prevent laser tube damage.

Optical delivery systems that are used to transmit laser energy from the output of the laser tube to the point of application are currently of two primary designs: flexible delivery systems utilizing a focusing lens and fiberoptic bundles, and rigid delivery systems utilizing a hollow

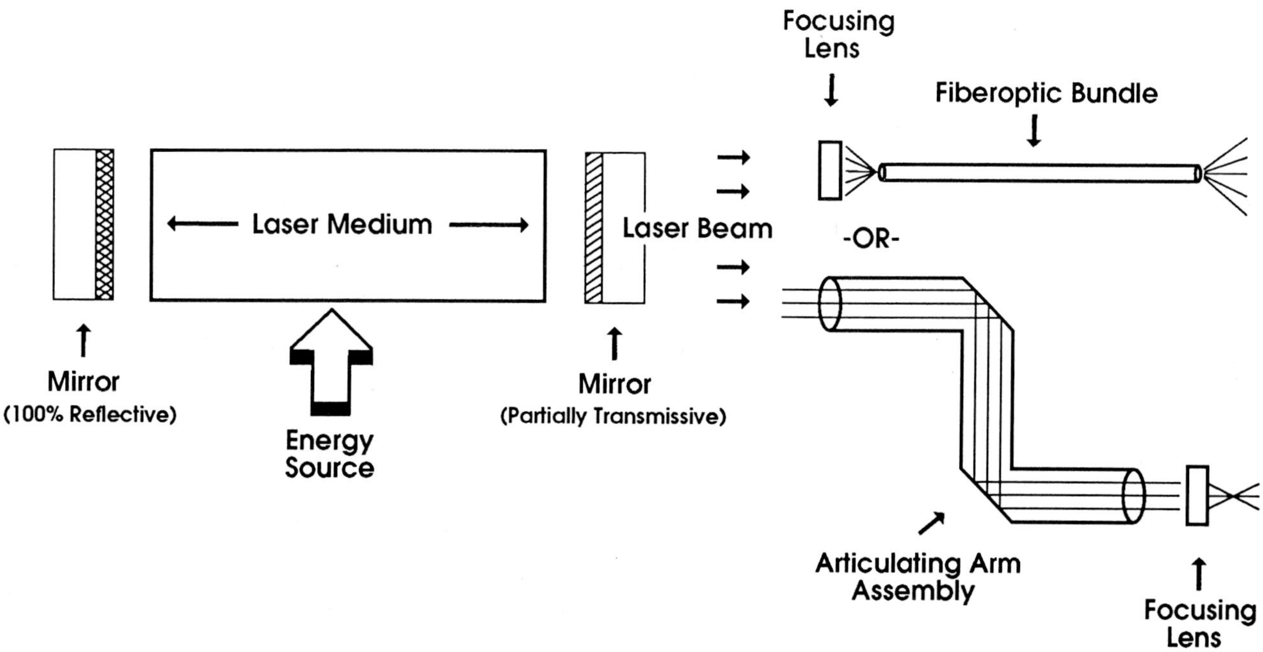

Figure 30–4. Basic laser system design.

waveguide or an articulating arm assembly consisting of a series of mirrors, hollow tubes, and elbow joints.[1–3]

Properties and Characteristics of Laser Energy

Laser radiation possesses three unique characteristics: coherence, collimation, and monochromaticity.

Coherence refers to the phenomenon that all electromagnetic radiation in the form of photons emitted from the laser tube are in phase with each other both in time and in space. Thus, the effect on the amplitude of the waves is additive, and superimposing individual photons provides for maximum power yield.[4,5]

Collimation refers to the fact that photons exiting the laser cavity do not appreciably diverge from one another as they travel outward. The path of the laser beam is such that all photons travel parallel to one another at the output of the laser tube. This accounts for the remarkable directionality of laser light. For example, the National Aeronautics and Space Administration has fired a high power neodymium (Nd):glass laser from the earth to the moon, producing a spot size about ½ mile in diameter. This divergence is small in comparison to the approximate 240,000 mile distance between the earth and moon.[4]

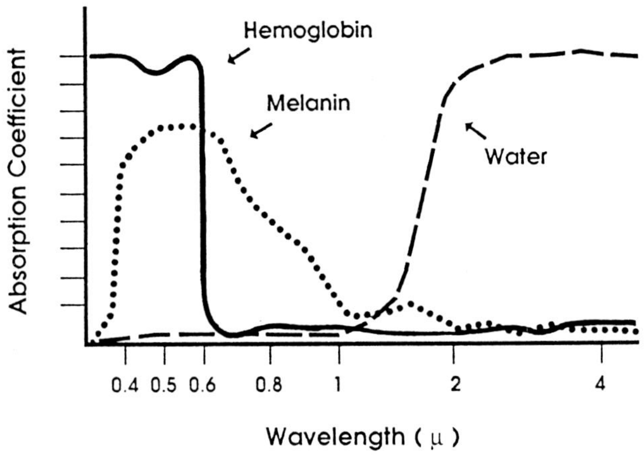

Figure 30–5. Absorption characteristics versus wavelength. (Courtesy of Sharplan Lasers, Inc., Allendale, NJ.)

Table 30–1. The Electromagnetic Spectrum*

RADIATION	WAVELENGTH
Cosmic	10^{-8} μm
X-ray	10^{-4} μm
Ultraviolet	10^{-2} to 0.4 μm
HeCd	0.325 μm
Excimer	
XeCl	0.308 μm
XeF	0.351 μm
Optical	0.4 to 0.7 μm
Argon	0.488 μm (blue)
	0.514 μm (green)
532 YAG	0.532 μm (green)
Krypton	0.531 μm (green)
	0.568 μm (yellow)
Tunable dye (optical spectrum)	0.4 μm to 0.7 μm
Coumarin	0.480 μm (blue)
Helium neon	0.630 μm (red)
Gold vapor	0.630 μm (red)
Krypton	0.647 μm (red)
Ruby	0.694 μm (red)
Infrared	1.0 to 10^2 μm
Nd:YAG	1.064 μm
Ho:YLF	2.06 μm
Er:YAG	2.94 μm
CO_2	10.6 μm
Microwave	10^4 μm
TV, FM radio	10^6 μm
Shortwave radio	10^7 μm
AM radio	10^9 μm

HeCd: helium cadmium; XeCl: xenon-chloride; XeF: xenon fluoride; YAG: yttrium aluminum garnet; Nd: neodymium; Ho: holmium; Er: erbium; CO_2: carbon dioxide; TV: television; FM: frequency modulation; AM: amplitude modulation.

Monochromaticity signifies that all emitted laser photons are of discrete wavelengths because all photons originate from discrete energy level transitions.[5] Whereas white light from a regular light bulb emits photons of numerous wavelengths, the unique characteristic of monochromaticity provides that a laser can be selected for a discrete wavelength to have a designated tissue effect during a medical procedure. Current medical lasers presently operate in the ultraviolet to infrared portion of the electromagnetic spectrum[3,6] (Table 30-1).

Laser Energy Interaction with Tissue

Electromagnetic radiation interacts with objects in primarily one of four manners: transmission, reflection, scattering, or absorption. It is important to note that for laser energy to exert any effect on tissue, the energy must be absorbed. Reflection or transmission, although important in various applications, will not render any significant effect on incident tissue. Scattering will result in absorption over a larger area so that its effect is more diffuse than direct absorption.[4]

The way in which tissue absorbs laser energy, and thus the net effect of interaction, is determined by the characteristics of the laser beam (wavelength, energy density, fluence) as well as the characteristics of the incident tissue. Let us look at these considerations in detail.

Wavelength

Absorption characteristics vary with wavelength for different tissues. An analysis of absorption versus wavelength for water, hemoglobin, and melanin (substances most abundant in various tissues) is illustrated in Figure 30-5. Generally, the greater the degree of absorption, the greater the tissue effect. Likewise, the degree of "scattering" is also wavelength dependent.

Energy Density

Energy density is a most important factor in determining tissue effect of incident laser energy. Generally speaking, the greater the energy density of the laser beam, the greater the tissue effect.[5] The energy density of the laser beam is determined by two factors, exposure time and power density, and is determined as follows:

$$\text{Energy density} = \text{exposure time} \times \text{power density}$$

As we see, tissue effect may be increased by increasing the exposure duration or by increasing the power density. Power density, termed irradiance, refers to the amount of power per unit surface area directed toward tissue during a single pulse. Power density is calculated as follows:

$$\text{Power density} = \text{power/cross-sectional area}$$

Greater tissue effect may be obtained by either increasing the power setting on the laser or by decreasing the cross-sectional area of the incident beam.

In those angioplasty applications in which laser energy is incident on tissue, it is important to understand this concept of power density and its effect on tissue. Optical delivery systems most common to laser angioplasty applications require delivery of laser energy via fiberoptics incorporated into the design of flexible catheters. Laser energy propagates through the fiberoptic bundle from the output of the laser tube via a series of numerous reflections off the sides of the fiberoptic strand and eventually exits the catheter at some point with its output beam not in collimated form, but in a divergent manner (Fig. 30-6). It is important to note that for a given power setting on the laser, tissue effect will decrease as the distance from catheter to tissue to be lased increases, since the cross-sectional area of the laser beam necessarily increases (and thus the power density decreases) due to the divergent nature of the laser beam output.[7]

Fluence

The term "fluence" refers to the rate in which laser energy is delivered to tissue, and it also has great bearing on tissue effect. In general, the higher the fluence, the more precise tissue effects will be realized. For example, since energy density equals power density multiplied by exposure time, 100 J of energy per cm^2 delivered at different rates could yield different tissue effects, as illustrated in Figure 30-7.

We see that increased peak power (fluence) results in decreased effect on underlying tissue and increased effect on incident tissue.

Laser energy may be delivered to tissue not only in a continuous mode of operation, but it may also be delivered in a pulsed mode (Fig. 30-8).

Let us define several concepts associated with pulsed laser energy:

- Activation time (t) = duration of pulse
- Cycle time (T) = interval between onset of consecutive pulses
- Frequency (f) = number of pulses per second = 1/T
- Duty cycle (%) = percent "on" time of laser = (t/T) × 100%
- Peak power (P_{pk}) = maximum power during energy application
- Average power (P_{av}) = P_{pk} × duty cycle

$$\text{Average power} = \text{peak power} \times \text{pulse width} \times \text{pulse frequency}$$

Just as with single pulse delivery, maximum precision may be realized in pulsed mode (with a given average power available) by maximizing the fluence via selection of output with highest peak power at the shortest pulse width.

To summarize, in order to determine tissue effect resultant from incident laser energy, we need to know not only the tissue type to be lased, but also the following characteristics of the laser energy to be applied:

1. Wavelength, to determine tissue absorption
2. Energy density, determined by exposure time, peak power, and cross-sectional area of the incident laser beam
3. Fluence, determined by peak power density, pulse width, and pulse rate

Modes of Absorption

Three basic mechanisms of absorption of laser energy have been observed: photothermal, photoplasma, and photochemical.

The photothermal mechanism is the most commonly observed for continuous wave and low peak power pulsed lasers in the optical and infrared spectrum. In this mechanism, absorbed photons are converted to heat and the temperature of the tissue rises to 60°C, whereby protein denaturization and cell necrosis occurs. As laser energy continues to be applied, temperature rises until it exceeds 100°C, where vaporization begins to occur and tissue is ablated. The photothermal mechanism presents perhaps the least precise mode of absorption in that thermal conduction may result in damage to surrounding tissue.

The photoplasma mechanism is observed, resultant from the use of very high peak-power pulsed lasers such that a dielectric breakdown of material occurs producing a local plasma and resultant shock-wave effect resulting in precise tissue ablation.

The photochemical mechanism is observed from the use of high peak-power short pulse ultraviolet wavelengths such

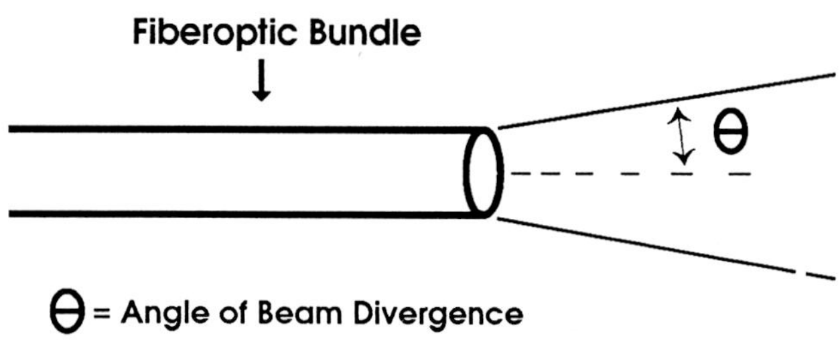

Figure 30–6. Beam divergence from a fiberoptic bundle.

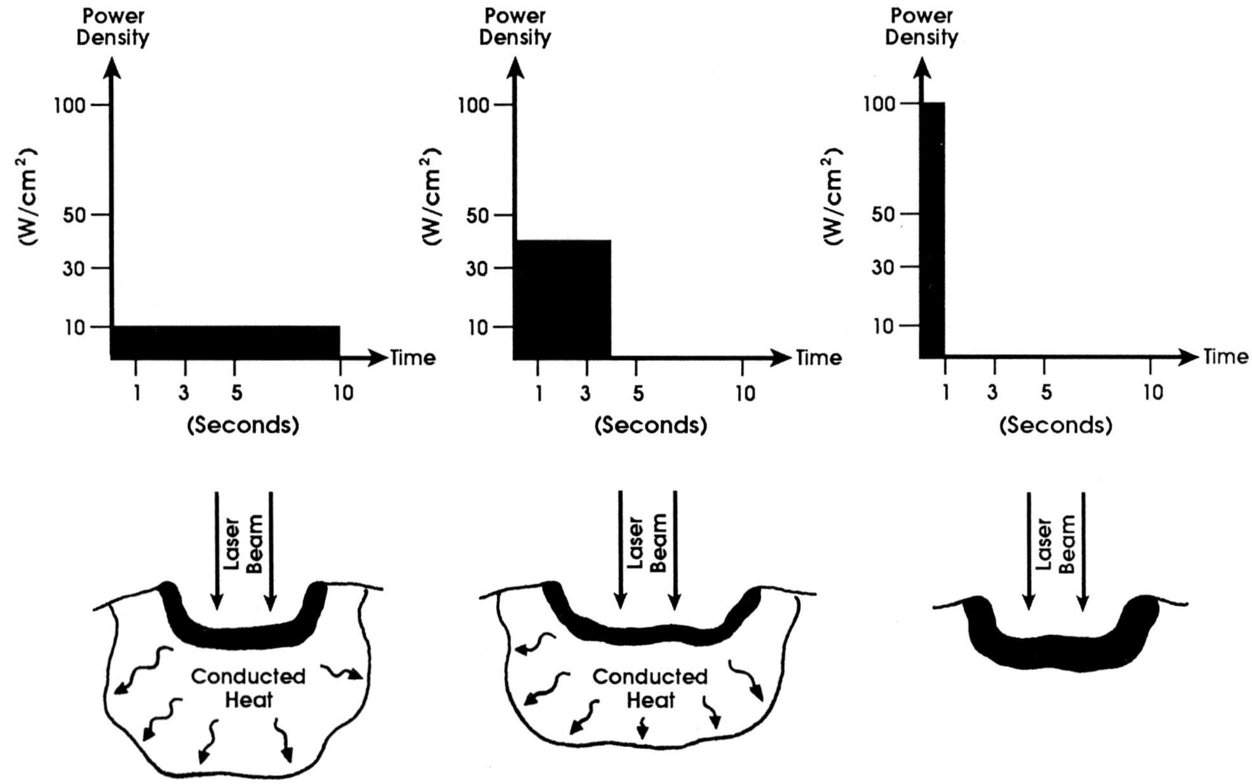

Figure 30–7. Effects of fluence. (Courtesy of Sharplan Lasers, Inc., Allendale, NJ.)

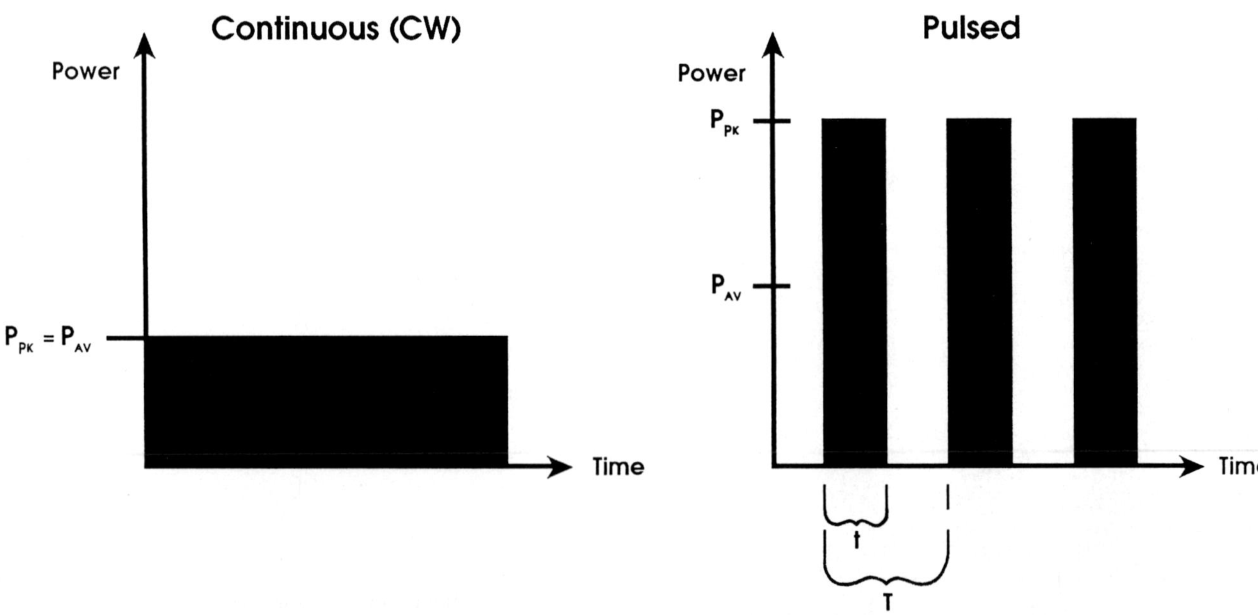

Figure 30–8. Continuous versus pulsed mode of energy delivery.

that molecular bonds are directly broken, resulting in precise tissue ablation.[6]

SPECTRUM OF AVAILABLE LASERS

Although the Food and Drug Administration (FDA) has approved the use of a limited number of laser systems for angioplasty applications at the time of this writing, the vast majority remain investigational. It is important to keep in mind that what is written today about the spectrum of available lasers may become outdated within a short period of time as technology evolves rapidly in an effort to develop a useful tool for the percutaneous treatment of vascular disease.

Argon Laser Systems

A very high electrical current is passed through the argon gas lasing medium to produce excited argon ions and stimulated emission of photons with wavelengths in the blue-green portion of the optical spectrum. Specifically, argon lasers are designed to produce primarily two discrete wavelengths of 0.488 and 0.514 μm. These discrete wavelengths are highly absorbed by hemoglobin and melanin, and exhibit an intermediate scattering effect. Argon systems are currently designed to deliver laser power up to 20 W continuous wave (CW) in continuous or pulsed fashions via fiberoptics. Generally, because the argon laser is highly inefficient in production of optical energy, special electrical hookups are required for operation. In addition, elaborate water-cooling systems are often required to prevent excessive heat build-up (and consequent damage) to the laser tube.[2,3]

At present, two argon laser systems have been approved by the FDA for general use in the peripheral vasculature (still investigational in coronary vessels). One system (Trimedyne Optilase 900) incorporates use of a 12 W argon laser source and utilization of two types of delivery systems. The Laserprobe and LaserCath (Fig. 30-9) catheters incorporate an optical fiber coupled to a metallic cap in which laser energy (4 to 12 W) is applied to heat the metal cap in order to ablate tissue thermally.[8,9] The Spectraprobe catheter (investigational) combines thermal and optical delivery by incorporating an optical fiber coupled to a metallic cap with a recessed sapphire crystal that enables 18% of the total energy to be emitted through a small window at the distal end of the catheter.

The other approved argon laser system (GV Medical Lastac System II) incorporates use of a 20 W argon laser source coupled to a control monitor and an optical fiber control handle. The delivery system (Fig. 30-10) incorporates an optical quartz fiber, a balloon, an irrigating lumen, and an optical assembly at the distal tip which diverges the delivered laser energy (multiple 10 W exposures for 2 to 10 seconds) to a 40° cone angle (in a clear fluid medium). Whereas a bare fiber might diverge the beam 5° (to produce a 10° cone angle) in a clear fluid medium, the increased divergence of the Lastac system more quickly increases the diameter of area of ablation and dissipates the intensity of the beam as distance from catheter tip increases so that beyond 3 mm from the fiber tip, power density falls below the threshold for tissue ablation. The centering, dilating balloon coaxially aligns the fiber tip within the arterial lumen and the delivery of a heparinized saline irrigating solution clears blood and contrast media from the fiber tip.[10]

One other argon laser system is currently undergoing investigation. This system provides for thermal angioplasty in a temperature-controlled manner, utilizing a 16 W argon laser source (HGM 20-S) and a delivery system (HGM PLAC) incorporating an optical fiber coupled to a metallic tip (a platinum/iridium sphere) with a thermocouple junction to allow continuous monitoring and adjustment of tip temperature (typically set from 300° to 400°C).

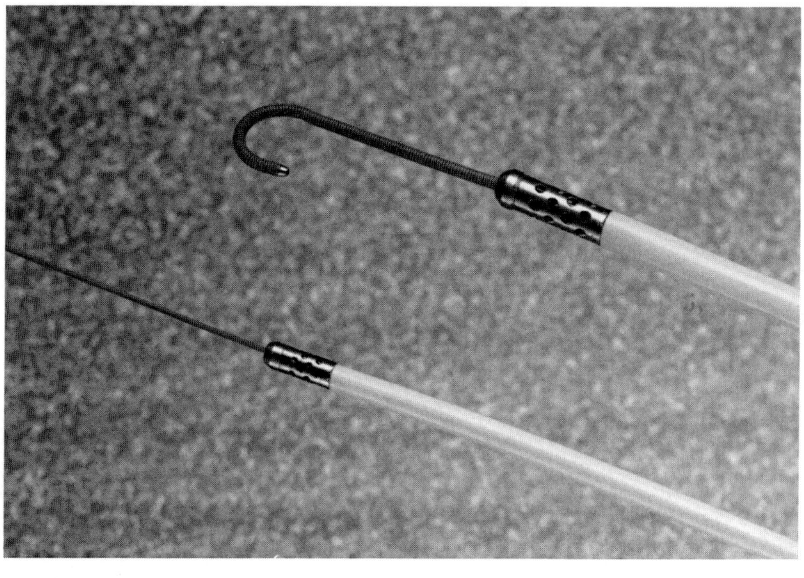

Figure 30–9. Trimedyne 1.7 and 2.5 mm "LaserCath-PLR" Catheters. (Courtesy of Trimedyne.)

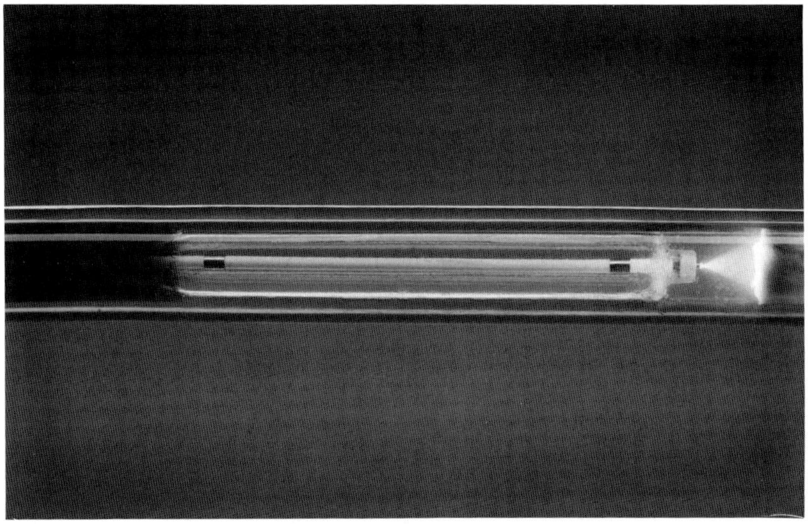

Figure 30–10. GV Medical "LASTAC" delivery system. (Courtesy of GV Medical, Inc., Minneapolis, MN.)

Excimer Laser Systems

The excimer laser, or rare gas halide laser, operates in the ultraviolet region of the electromagnetic spectrum. The high-power pulsed output is achieved via a high-voltage, pulsed electric discharge through a gas mixture containing one inert gas (helium, neon, or argon), another inert rare gas (xenon or krypton), and a halogen compound (hydrogen chloride or fluorine). The term "excimer" is derived from "excited dimer" and refers to an ionic bond that is created by the halogen ion and the inert rare gas ion in their excited states. The wavelengths produced by the various excimer lasers include 0.193 μm (ArF), 0.222 μm (KrCl), 0.308 μm (XeCl), and 0.351 μm (XeF). Peak powers of up to several hundred kilowatts per pulse are delivered in pulse durations ranging from 10 to 250 nsec. These high bursts of energy account for the photochemical molecular dissociation mechanism observed in tissue interaction, as use of the excimer laser allows for precise ablation of incident tissue without thermal conduction to surrounding tissue.[6] Figure 30-11 illustrates the precise effect of an ArF excimer laser on a strand of human hair.

At present, only the "long-pulse" XeCl excimer laser produces laser energy of sufficient magnitude to ablate tissue efficiently, and which also may be transmitted through high-purity silica-based flexible fiberoptics and, thus, is the only excimer laser currently undergoing investigation. This "long-pulse" XeCl excimer laser system (AIS Dymer 200+) provides direct irradiation with laser energy of high fluence (peak power to hundreds of kilowatts, pulse width of 200 nsec) and energy density of 35 to 60 mJ/mm^2/pulse, at a repetition rate of 20 to 30 Hz. For total occlusions, a delivery system is available in which an external balloon is utilized to center the fiber within the vessel. Contact ablation within the blood field prevents the propagation of laser light from the region of the fiber end, thereby preventing laser ablation of any part of the vessel not in direct contact with the fiber tip.[11]

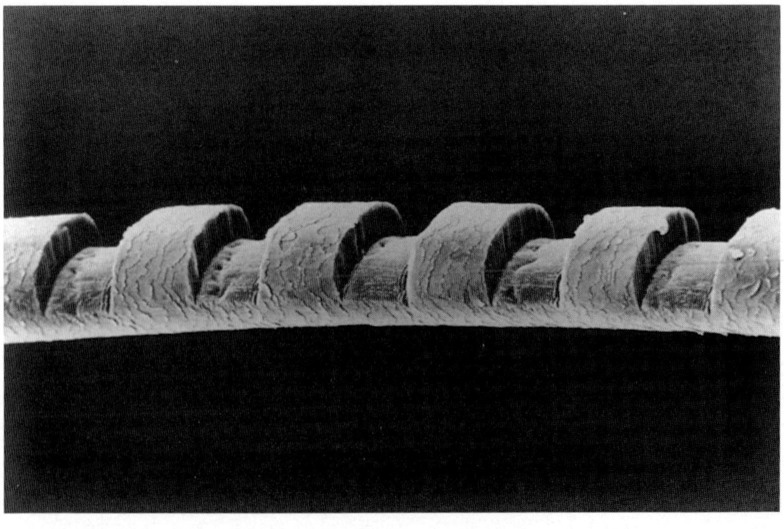

Figure 30–11. Human hair cut with an ArF excimer laser. (R. Srinivasan, IBM Research.)

Pulsed Dye Laser Systems

A pulsed dye laser system utilizes a liquid lasing medium in which optical energy (via the use of a flash lamp or another laser) excites the liquid dye medium, adjusted to produce a specific wavelength in the optical spectral region.[1]

One such laser (Medilase System 4000) currently undergoing investigation utilizes flash lamp excitation of a coumarin dye solution to produce high-power (150 kW), short-duration (1 μsec) pulses (energy of 150 mJ/pulse) with a wavelength of 480 nm in order to remove plaque via a combination of both photothermal and photoacoustic effect. This pulsed dye laser is guided by an integrated angioscope and aimable laser fiber system. A low-power helium-neon laser is used as an aiming beam, and a motorized catheter positioner is controlled by the system's computer to aim the laser precisely toward the obstruction as directed by the physician.[12]

Neodymium:Yttrium Aluminum Garnet Laser Systems

The solid lasing medium for the Nd:yttrium aluminum garnet (YAG) laser consists of a yttrium aluminum garnet crystal doped with 1 to 3% Nd ions. The active medium (Nd) is excited with a xenon flashlamp to provide laser energy in the near infrared spectrum (wavelength, 1.06 μm). This wavelength is highly absorbed by tissue protein and exhibits a relatively high scattering effect when delivered in CW or low peak power pulsed modes of operation. Nd:YAG "solid-state" CW lasers are currently designed to deliver, via fiberoptics, laser power up to 140 W in continuous mode or pulsed fashion. Like the argon laser, the CW Nd:YAG laser is very inefficient in its production of laser energy, and oftentimes requires a specialized electrical hook-up as well as an elaborate water-cooling system for its laser tube. A low-power (2 to 5 mW) helium-neon gas laser with output wavelength in the visible spectrum (0.63 μm) is typically aligned with the Nd:YAG laser at its output to serve as an aiming beam.[2]

At present, CW Nd:YAG lasers are utilized in varying investigational angioplasty techniques. One system (Trimedyne Cardiolase 4000 or Optilase 1000), approved by the FDA for general use in the peripheral vasculature (still investigational in coronary vessels), utilizes an Nd:YAG laser source (40 W for Cardiolase 4000; 60 W for Optilase 1000) together with the Laserprobe and LaserCath delivery systems (the Spectraprobe delivery system is still investigational) in much the same manner as with Trimedyne's Optilase 900 argon laser system, as previously discussed.

Two Nd:YAG laser systems are currently investigational. One system utilizes a 60 W Nd:YAG laser source (SLT CL-60) together with a delivery system incorporating an optical fiber coupled to a focusing sapphire tip (Surgical Laser Technologies). This focusing tip protects the laser fiber from charring, as frequently occurs during laser emissions in blood, and provides for precise tissue ablation.[13,14]

A second investigational application involves the use of a CW Nd:YAG laser (Quantronix System 1500) with a delivery system (USCI/Bard Spears Laser Balloon) in which laser energy is transmitted radially through a balloon transparent to the laser's wavelength (Fig. 30-12). Laser energy is applied during final balloon inflation of an otherwise conventional balloon angioplasty procedure to coagulate tissues thermally within the artery wall in order to achieve two primary tissue effects: to fuse disrupted tissue elements such as plaque-arterial wall separations and to reduce elastic recoil.[15]

"Smart Laser" System

One major concern in utilizing laser technology in the coronary vessels is the risk of vessel perforation. One firm (MCM Laboratories) is addressing this concern via development of a "Smart Laser" System (Fig. 30-13) consisting of a treatment laser used in conjunction with a diagnostic laser, optical delivery and feedback system, and computer to provide for safe application of laser energy in order to avoid damage to the vessel wall. The diagnostic laser (a helium cadmium gas laser with ultraviolet wavelength of 325 nm, and low power of 2 mW) is pulsed through a fiberoptic channel, causing target tissue to fluoresce. The evoked fluorescence is transmitted back through the same fiber, where a beam splitter directs it to an optical analyzer, enabling determination of tissue type. The treatment laser (currently investigating the use of various high fluence, pulsed solid state lasers in the near infrared spectrum) is then enabled if the optical analyzer determines incident tissue does not represent normal vessel wall. Both the diagnostic and treatment lasers are pulsed in alternate fashion to assure safe delivery of laser energy.[16]

Future Developments

Two presently available laser systems—the carbon dioxide (CO_2) and the super-pulsed Nd:YAG—might find application in angioplasty applications in future years given advancements in fiberoptic technology development.

CO_2 gas lasers are currently designed to deliver laser power to 100 W in CW mode at a wavelength of 10.6 μm in the infrared region of the electromagnetic spectrum. A low-powered helium neon gas laser is aligned to the output of the CO_2 laser to serve as an aiming beam. Although CO_2 lasers are currently used in other medical specialties for precise tissue ablation (the 10.6 μm wavelength is highly absorbed by water and exhibits a relatively low scattering effect), the CO_2 laser's wavelength cannot be efficiently transmitted through presently available flexible fiberoptics.[1]

Nd:YAG lasers have also been designed to produce "super pulses" of laser energy via "Q-switching." These systems generally incorporate an intracavity fast shutter between the lasing medium and one of the mirrors. With the shutter closed, the energy contained in the lasing medium will be pumped to a level far above the lasing threshold with the

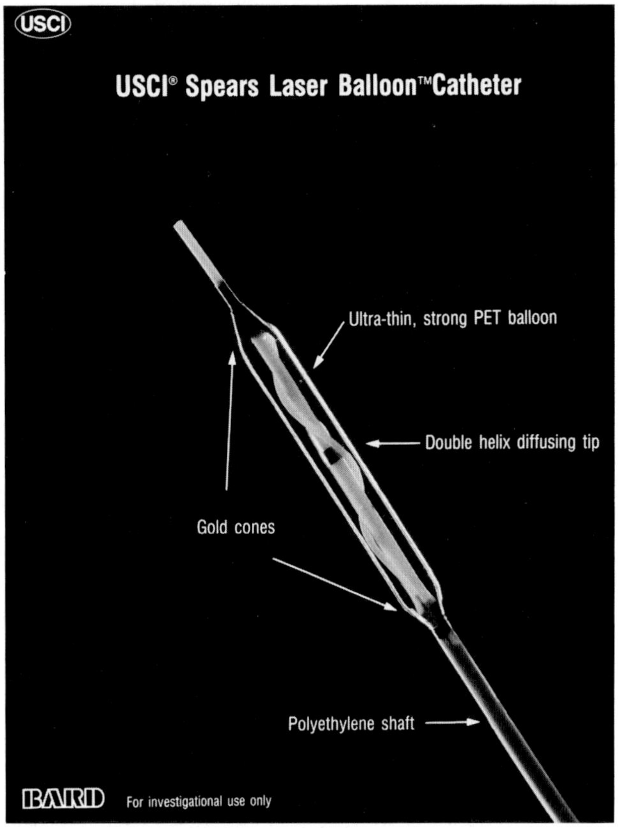

Figure 30–12. Spears "Laser Balloon" delivery system. (© 1990, USCI Division of C.R. Bard, Inc.)

shutter open, and the population inversion can be made much larger than before. The result, on releasing the shutter, is a single, short (10 to 20 nsec duration) high-power pulse on the order of up to 1 MW of power. This high-power pulse produces a photoplasma effect when incident on tissue and results in high precision tissue ablation. Unfortunately, the same dielectric effect that precisely ablates tissue also damages fiberoptics, and so the laser energy cannot presently be delivered to tissue via flexible catheters.[1,17,18]

Laser systems undergoing current development (in addition to those already mentioned) include the holmium-yttrium lithium fluoride (Ho:YLF), the erbium-YAG (Er:YAG), and other solid-state lasers. The Ho:YLF laser produces a wavelength of laser energy in the near infrared spectrum at 2.06 μm, which can be transmitted through currently available silica-based fibers. Energy is emitted as high-power pulses with pulse durations of approximately 100 μsec. Efficiency of plaque ablation is superior to current argon and CW Nd:YAG lasers because the absorption coefficient for plaque at this wavelength is greater and increased fluence leads to improved precision. The Er:YAG laser produces energy with a wavelength also in the near infrared spectrum at 2.9 μm, with high-power pulses delivered in 100 μsec bursts. The wavelength produced provides excellent ablation efficiency, but cannot be efficiently transmitted via flexible silica fibers.[19]

A relatively new breakthrough in quantum physics research has led to the development of a prototype "free electron" laser that could potentially be tuned to a broad

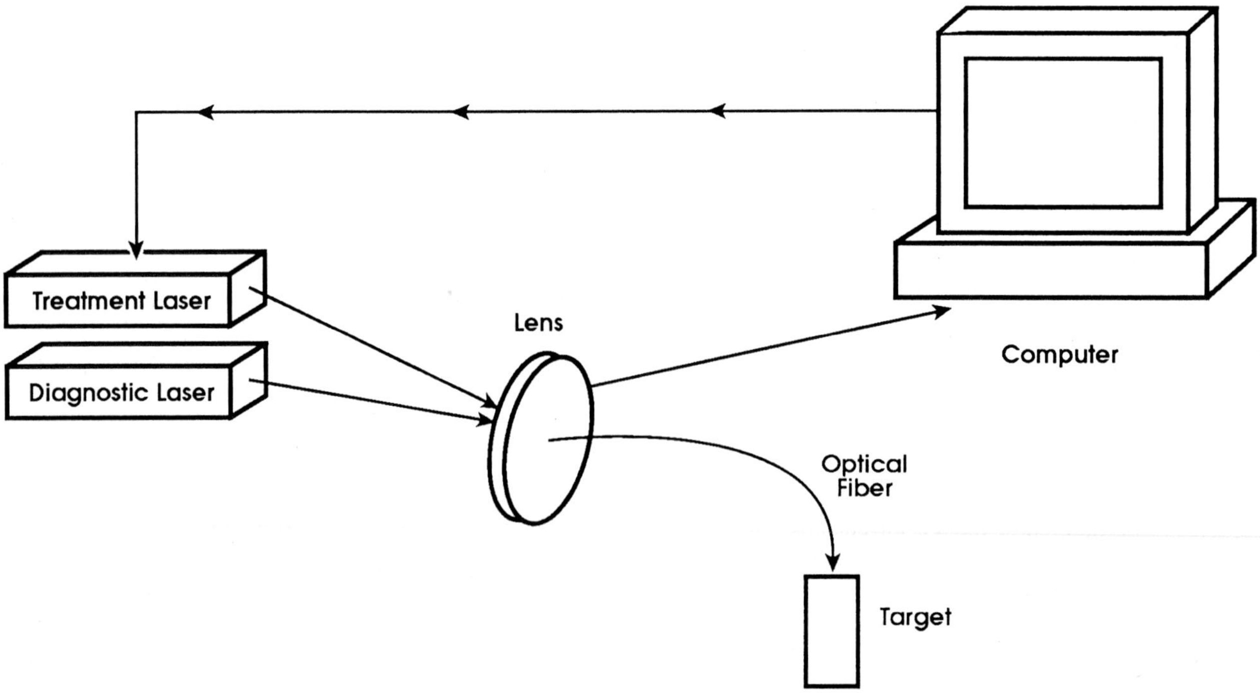

Figure 30–13. MCM Laboratories "Smart Laser" System Design. (Courtesy of MCM Laboratories.)

range of discrete wavelengths enabling use of one device for ablation, welding, coagulation, etc., of numerous tissue types. Development of this versatile product into a useful clinical tool is projected into the 21st century.[20]

Research and development efforts in the near future will focus primarily on delivery systems that will enable safe and effective utilization of medical lasers for angioplasty applications. Research will continue in the development of fibers that will more efficiently transmit laser energy in the ultraviolet and infrared spectrums to enable investigation of the use of the ArF, KrCl, and XeF excimers, CO_2, and Er:YAG lasers. Development of specialized optical lens tips will provide for the ability to focus or defocus the laser energy at the output of the catheter. Modifications to catheter design will enable better placement of the catheter tip within the vessel.

Research will also focus on improvements to the "smart laser" design concept. Multifiber catheters could be designed in which individual fibers are responsible for fluorescence plaque identification and subsequent laser ablation for a given tissue zone, providing for selective topographic vaporization of sclerotic plaque.[19] Incorporation of ultrasound technology into "smart laser" catheter tip design may provide for increased safety, because information would be provided not only about the surface of incident tissue but also about tissue depth. Such information may prove valuable when the laser beam is removing tissue close to the vessel wall and would enable production of three-dimensional images of the artery during the angioplasty procedure.[19]

LASER SAFETY

The American National Standards Institute (ANSI) has developed guidelines for the safe design and use of medical laser systems.[21,22] This section will briefly summarize these guidelines as they apply to the angioplasty suite.

Hazard Classification

The Radiation Control for Health and Safety Act (RCHSA) and the Federal Laser Product Performance Standard established a classification scheme (Table 30-2) for lasers in which the laser's class determines the kind of controls, performance features, and labeling requirements. The manufacturer is responsible for properly classifying their products.

Table 30–2. Hazard Classification

CLASS	CONTROL MEASURES	MEDICAL SURVEILLANCE
1	Not Applicable	Not Applicable
2a	Applicable	Not Applicable
3a	Applicable	Not Applicable
3b	Applicable	Applicable
4	Applicable	Applicable

Administrative Controls

Institutional administrative controls are required to assure safe implementation. These include the designation of a laser safety officer (LSO) responsible for the establishment and surveillance of appropriate laser safety control measures and the formation of a Laser Use Committee to govern laser activity and establish use criteria. Committee membership would consist of a physician representative from each specialty utilizing laser technology, the designated LSO, and other support personnel. The committee typically approves all facility users after receipt of a formal protocol and standard operating procedures.

Equipment Controls

Manufacturers are required to incorporate equipment controls in the design of their class 3 and class 4 laser systems. These include incorporation of a protective housing for the laser tube to limit laser radiation exposure, interlocks on equipment covers to guard against electrical and optical hazards, a keyswitch master interlock, a guarded footswitch, and application of warning labels. Beam delivery disconnect features are required so that disconnection of a delivery system (i.e., optical fibers) from a laser source shall not permit excess laser radiation to exit directly from the laser system. A beam stop attenuator is required to prevent output emission when the laser system is on standby. (Note: It is important to disable output emission by turning off the footswitch enable control or by closing the mechanical safety shutter during interims when laser energy is not required for treatment.) An audible or visual warning associated with delayed emission of laser radiation is also required.

Laser Treatment Controlled Area

A laser treatment controlled area is to be defined in which certain safety measures are to be implemented. This typically would include the procedure suite and possibly any remote viewing areas. The controlled area is defined by the limits of the nominal hazard zone (NHZ) as determined by the LSO. The NHZ describes the area within which the level of direct, reflected, or scattered radiation, during normal operation, exceeds the maximum permissible exposure limit, and may be determined by information supplied by the manufacturer, by measurement, or by using the NHZ equations referenced in the ANSI standard.

Laser treatment controlled areas for class 3b and class 4 laser systems require the following:

1. Posted with appropriate warning signs.
2. Supervised and only occupied by authorized personnel.
3. Under the direct supervision of an individual knowledgeable in laser safety.
4. Located so that access to the area by spectators is limited and requires approval.

5. Have any potentially hazardous beam terminated by a beam stop of an appropriate material.
6. Have only diffusely reflective materials in or near the beam path, where feasible.
7. Have personnel who regularly require entry adequately trained, provided with appropriate protective equipment, and required to follow all applicable administrative and procedural controls.
8. Have all windows, doorways, etc., either covered or restricted in such a manner as to reduce the transmitted laser radiation to levels at or below the appropriate ocular maximum permissible exposure (MPE) limit.
9. Require storage or disabling (removal of the key) of the laser system when not in use to prevent unauthorized use.
10. Assure that the shutter mechanism is closed during stand-by periods.
11. Provide an emergency shutoff switch to enable rapid shutdown of the laser system.

Personal Protective Equipment

Eye protection must be worn by all persons within the NHZ (including the patient) to prevent possible exposure to hazardous laser radiation. Corneal or retinal burns, depending on wavelength, are possible from acute exposure; and corneal or lenticular opacities, or retinal injury may be possible from chronic exposure to excessive levels.[23]

Per the standard, the optical density (OD) of lens filters must meet or exceed that specified by the laser manufacturer for all applicable wavelengths of emitted laser energy. In addition, all laser protective eyewear should be clearly labeled with the optical density and wavelength for which protection is afforded, should be comfortable, and should prevent exposure to hazardous peripheral radiation. Periodic inspection should be made of protective eyewear to ensure satisfactory condition, including inspection of attenuation material for pitting, crazing, cracking, or discoloration, inspection of frame for mechanical integrity, and inspection for light leaks that could permit hazardous intrabeam viewing. An appropriate protocol would be to require that applicable eyewear be worn anytime the mechanical beam stop is in its open position to enable laser energy output.

Where personnel may be exposed to levels of radiation that clearly exceed the maximum permissible exposure for skin, consideration should be given to the use of protective clothing. Where personnel may be subject to chronic skin exposure from scattered ultraviolet radiation, skin protection should be provided even at levels below the MPE for skin.

Warning Signs

Warning signs are placed at all entrances to the laser treatment area. The design of the sign should be in accordance with Figure 30-14.[22] Position 1 should indicate precautionary instructions, such as "Laser in Use—Eye Protection Required," and in addition, the following: "Laser Radiation—Avoid Direct Eye Exposure" (class 3a laser systems); "Laser Radiation—Avoid Direct Exposure to Beam" (class 3b laser systems); "Laser Radiation—Avoid Eye or Skin Exposure to Direct or Scattered Radiation" (class 4 laser systems). Position 2 should indicate type of laser or emitted wavelength, pulse duration if appropriate, and maximum output. Position 3 should indicate the class of the laser system.

Laser Safety and Training Programs

All laser support personnel (technicians, nurses, service personnel) shall receive adequate training appropriate to their

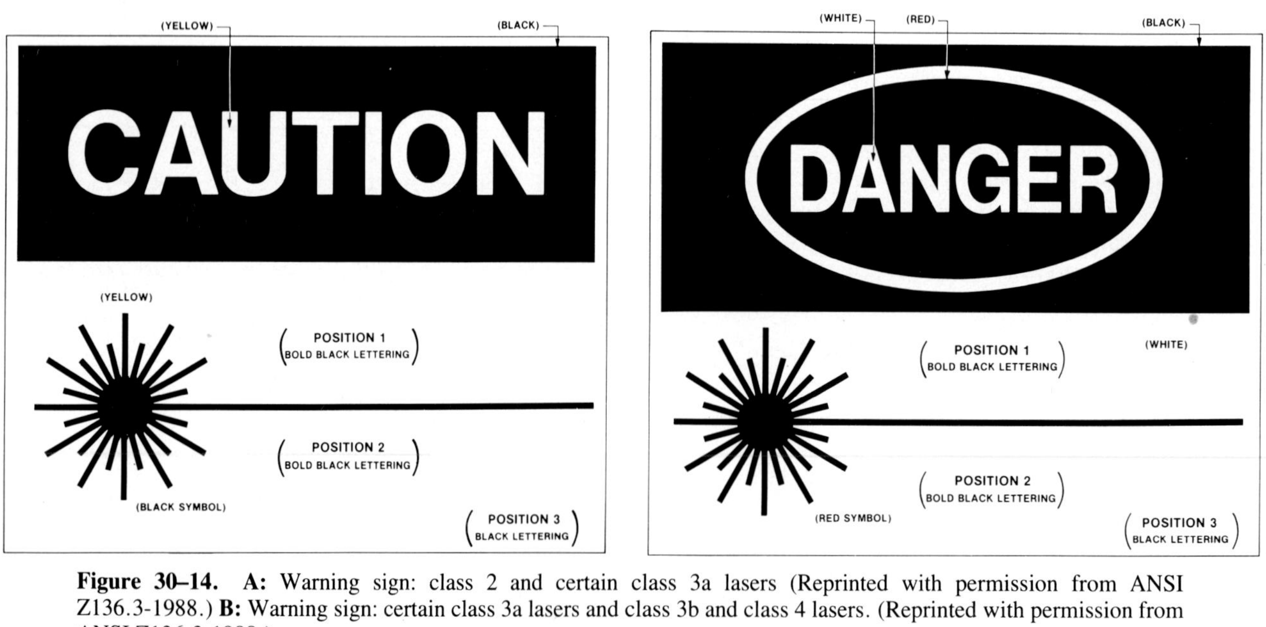

A B

Figure 30–14. **A:** Warning sign: class 2 and certain class 3a lasers (Reprinted with permission from ANSI Z136.3-1988.) **B:** Warning sign: certain class 3a lasers and class 3b and class 4 lasers. (Reprinted with permission from ANSI Z136.3-1988.)

role to include basic laser physics, laser safety considerations, and operation of the applicable laser systems.

Physician credentialling requires attendance at a laser principles and safety course to include basic laser physics, laser tissue interaction, discussions of the clinical specialty field, and hands-on experience with lasers. In addition, preceptorship training is required in which the physician observes and assists an experienced operator in the specialty area involved.

Medical Surveillance

Health care personnel who work routinely in a laser system environment should have a baseline eye examination prior to working in the laser environment, to include an ocular history and inspection of visual acuity, macular function, and contrast sensitivity. Should ocular function in any of the tests prove abnormal, then a funduscopic examination would be required. Incidental health care personnel whose work makes it possible (but unlikely) that they will be exposed to laser energy should have a baseline eye examination to include an ocular history and inspection of visual acuity. Eye examinations should be performed prior to working with lasers, immediately after a suspected abnormal exposure of the eye, for specific eye complaints possibly related to laser energy exposure on an individual basis, and at the termination of work in the laser environment. The results of all eye examinations should be discussed with the employee, and complete eye examination records should be retained for a minimum of 30 years.

Electrical Safety

It is recommended that the laser system be accepted, certified, listed, labeled, or otherwise determined safe by a qualified testing laboratory, such as, but not limited to, Underwriters Laboratories or Factory Mutual Corporation.

Fire Safety

The laser shall not be used in the presence of flammable or combustible chemicals such as anesthetics, preparation solutions, drying agents, ointments, methylmethacrylate, or other plastic resins. Only nonflammable, flame-resistant surgical drapes should be used.

Toxic Gases

The majority of medical lasers in use today that utilize gas lasing mediums require gas sources that do not pose a hazard to operating personnel in terms of toxicity. (As with most pressurized gas cylinders, there always exists the hazard of displacement of room air in a nonventilated room.) Excimer lasers, however, do require a toxic gas source. The "long-pulse" XeCl excimer laser requires use of hydrogen chloride (HCl), an extremely corrosive gas with strong fumes. Inhalation of HCl can cause pulmonary edema and skin contact causes severe tissue irritation. The established Occupational Safety and Health Administration threshold limit value for exposure is 5 ppm.

Control measures include, but are not limited to, meticulous handling (the most important), the use of a specialized gas cabinet enclosure for storage and gas delivery, the installation of exhaust fume hoods with direct venting to outside the facility located directly above the storage of HCl, points of HCl gas hookup to the laser, or locations where the HCl cylinders are changed, storage of HCl gas mixtures in a dedicated room with direct ventilation to the outside, and separate from the storage of gases that are flammable or oxidizing agents (fire code), and the use of a gas mask (with a halogen filter) and gloves when changing HCl cylinders.[24]

Acknowledgment. The author would like to thank Ric Colegrove, a graphic artist from Tampa, Florida, for contributing this chapter's technical illustrations.

REFERENCES

1. Vassiliadis A. Lasers and Tissue Effects. Colorado Springs: Xanar, 1982:4–22.
2. Fuller TA: The physics of surgical lasers. Lasers Surg Med 1980;1:6–10.
3. Huether SE: How lasers work. AORN J 1983;38:207–13.
4. Absten GT. Fundamentals of Laser Surgery. Paul Rogers Company, 1983:7–9.
5. Janssen WD: Fundamentals of Laser Surgery, Grant Hospital Laser Center, p 7, 11–12.
6. Laudenslager JB. Laser fundamentals. In White RA, Grundfest WS (eds): Lasers in Cardiovascular Disease. Chicago, Year Book Medical Publishers, 1987:7–29.
7. Ready JF. Laser technology: the new energy source. Lastext 1988;1(2):6.
8. Sanborn TA, Haudenschild CC, Garber GR, et al. Angiographic and histologic consequences of laser thermal angioplasty: comparison with balloon angioplasty. Circulation 1987;75:1281–6.
9. Sanborn TA, Greenfield AJ, Guben JK, et al. Human percutaneous and intraoperative laser thermal angioplasty: initial clinical results as an adjunct to balloon angioplasty. J Vasc Surg 1987;5,1:83–90.
10. Nordstrom LA, Castañeda-Zúñiga WR, Young EG, et al. Direct argon laser exposure for recanalization of peripheral arteries: early results. Radiology 1988;168:359–64.
11. Laudenslager JB. Excimer lasers adapt to angioplasty. Laser Focus/Electro-Optics, May 1988.
12. Company Profile: Medilase, Inc., Angioplasty Technology Update Newsletter, 1990;1(1):3–4.
13. Geschwind HJ, Blair JD, Mongkolsmai D, et al. Development and experimental application of contact probe catheter for laser angioplasty. J Am Coll Cardiol 1987;9:101–7.
14. Fourrier JL, Brunetaud JM, Prat A, et al. Percutaneous laser angioplasty with sapphire tip. Lancet 1987;1:105.
15. Spears JR: Percutaneous transluminal coronary angioplasty restenosis: potential prevention with laser balloon angioplasty. Am J Cardiol 1987;60:61B–4B.
16. Miller DL. Fluorescence-guided laser angioplasty: the probe and treat laser system. Vascular Interventional Laser: Physics, Safety, and Clinical Applications Course, SCVIR Annual Meeting, 1989.
17. Wyard SJ. Solid State Biophysics, New York, McGraw-Hill, 1969:377–84.

18. Young M. Optics and Lasers: An Engineering Physics Approach. New York: Springer-Verlag, 1977:151–66.
19. Leon MB, Smith PD, Bonner RF. Laser angioplasty delivery systems. In White RA, Grundfest WS (eds): Lasers in Cardiovascular Disease. Chicago: Year Book Medical Publishers, 1987:51–60.
20. Gallivan M. "Star wars" laser may alter the future of surgery. Hospitals 1986;60(18):90.
21. *American National Standard for the Safe Use of Lasers*. ANSI Z136.1-1986. Toledo: The Laser Institute of America, 1986.
22. *American National Standard for the Safe Use of Lasers in Health Care Facilities,* ANSI Z136.3-1988, Toledo: The Laser Institute of America, 1988.
23. Smith JF (ed): Laser Safety Guide. Toledo: The Laser Institute of America, 1988:1.
24. Lorenz AK. Gas handling safety for laser makers and users. Lasers Appl March 1987.

31 Laser-Tissue Interaction

A.J. Welch, Ph.D., Martin J.C. van Gemert

The response of tissue to laser irradiation is highly dependent on the characteristics of the laser source. Therefore in this chapter we will describe various laser parameters and their influence on the tissue response. Certainly, basic parameters for establishing dosimetry requirements for any laser procedure are power and time of irradiation for continuous wave (CW) lasers or energy per pulse and number of pulses for pulse lasers. Yet the wavelength and spot size of the laser beam are just as important.

The spectrum of commercially available lasers for medical applications stretches from 193 nm to 10.6 μm. Both CW and pulse lasers are available in ultraviolet (UV), visible, and infrared (IR). The penetration of laser light in tissue is highly wavelength dependent, as shown in Figure 31-1. As the collimated beam passes through the tissue, it is attenuated by absorption and scattering. If scattering dominates absorption, the scattered light forms a diffuse fluence around the exponentially decreasing collimated beam. Heat is generated wherever collimated or diffuse light is absorbed. Details of the optical and thermal responses are described in the following paragraphs. We examine many of the events that are involved in the response of tissue to laser irradiation. Particular emphasis is placed on events that provide some insight into the thermal response during treatment procedures.

The events depicted in Figure 31-2 comprise a coupled optical, thermal, and damage model for laser-tissue interaction. Optical and thermal parameters are not constants, but depend on the condition of the tissue, which is a function of temperature, hydration, and thermal damage. The distribution of light (fluence rate, watts per square meter) within laser-irradiated tissue is a function of: (1) the laser beam power, wavelength, and spatial irradiance profile; (2) the local optical properties (absorption, scattering, and phase function) of the tissue that are wavelength dependent; and (3) the index of refraction of the media (i.e., air, quartz fiber, etc.) delivering the laser beam and indices of refraction of the tissue. Generally, an approximation of the transport equation is used to estimate the fluence rate within tissue.[1] The rate of heat generation at a particular location is governed by absorption of photons by local chromophores and is numerically represented as the product of the fluence rate and the tissue absorption coefficient at that location.[2] The rate of heat transfer is dependent on thermal conductivity, thermal diffusivity, and heat transfer coefficients. Tissue temperature is determined by the rate of heat generation and rate of heat transfer to cooler regions by conduction and convection. Sufficient temperature increases cause coagulation or ablation. An analytical description of the optical-thermal response of tissue to laser irradiation requires a reasonable geometric representation of the tissue that may require multiple layers and a realistic distribution of absorbing elements representing tissue chromophores.

The interaction of laser light with tissue is highly dependent on the method for delivery of the light energy to a selected target. For example, if the laser beam is delivered through air to tissue, as depicted in Figure 31-3, a portion of the beam is reflected at the surface due to the difference in the index of refraction n_1 of the air and the index of refraction n_2 of the tissue. The fraction of light that is directly reflected from the surface depends on the angle of incidence of the laser beam. Even when the laser beam is perpendicular to the tissue, a small fraction is reflected. The angular dependence of specular reflection at an air-tissue interface is shown in Figure 31-4 for n(air) = 1.0 and n(tissue) equal to either 1.33 or 1.5. These curves are calculated using the Fresnel relationship for specular reflection R_s:

$$R_S = \frac{1}{2}\left[\frac{\tan^2(\theta_1 - \theta_2)}{\tan^2(\theta_1 + \theta_2)} + \frac{\sin^2(\theta_1 - \theta_2)}{\sin^2(\theta_1 + \theta_2)}\right] \quad (1a)$$

For a unit irradiance, the light transmitted into the tissue is:

$$T = 1 - R_s \quad (1b)$$

For a smooth flat surface, the reflected beam has the same angle as the incident beam. The angle of the transmitted beam is given by Snell's law as

$$n_1 \sin\theta_1 = n_2 \sin\theta_2 \quad (2)$$

In addition to describing reflection and transmission of a laser beam at the surface of tissue, equations 1 and 2 govern the behavior of internal reflections of light in tissue. If light within the tissue strikes the surface with an angle greater than θ_{2c}, the light is internally reflected. The critical angle θ_{2c} is given by:

$$\sin\theta_{2c} = \frac{n_1}{n_2} \sin 90° \text{ for } n_1 < n_2 \quad (3)$$

Also, these equations govern the path of light transmitted via delivery tips and shields. For example, consider light delivered to tissue via a fiberoptic with a quartz or sapphire tip. The index of refraction of quartz is 1.4 and the index of refraction of sapphire is 1.76. The direction of light that is transmitted to the air from the tip is given by equation 2. However, if the angle of incidence is greater than the critical angle θ_{2c}, then the light is totally internally reflected. Thus, the surfaces of tips can be designed to either concentrate or scatter laser light. Consider the quartz-pointed tip probe illustrated in Figure 31-5A. The mismatched index of refraction between the quartz and air concentrates the laser light at

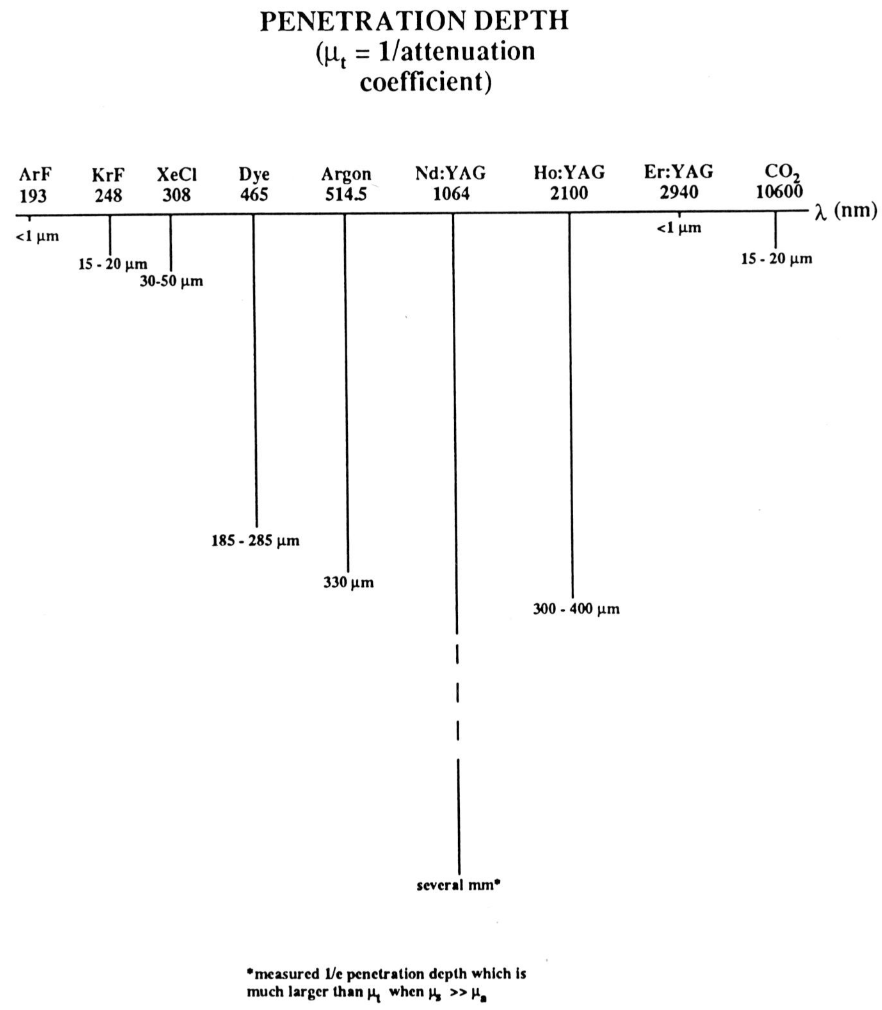

Figure 31–1. Penetration depth of laser light in soft noncolored tissue as a function of wavelength. Penetration depth is defined as $1/\mu_{tr}$, where μ_{tr} is the reduced attenuation coefficient (m^{-1}) $\mu'_t = \mu_a + (1 - g)\mu_s$.

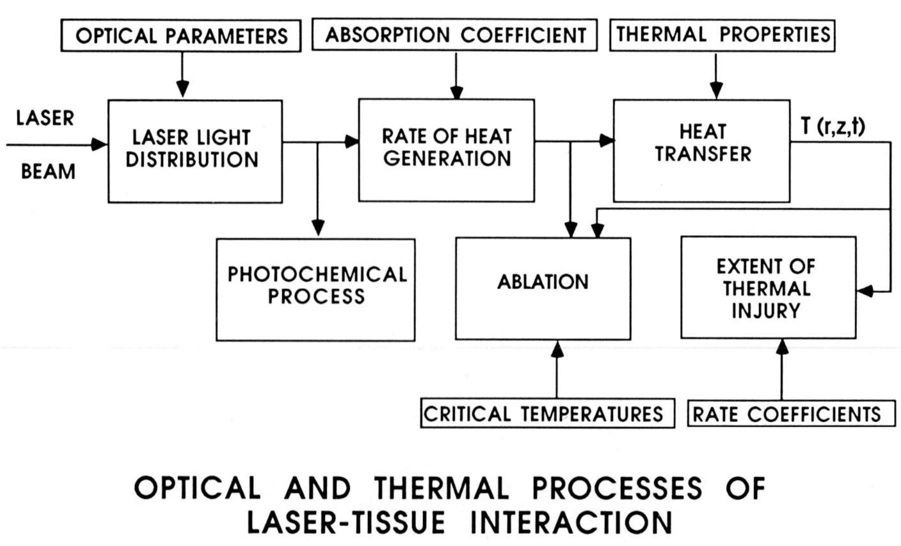

Figure 31–2. Diagram of optical-thermal interaction.

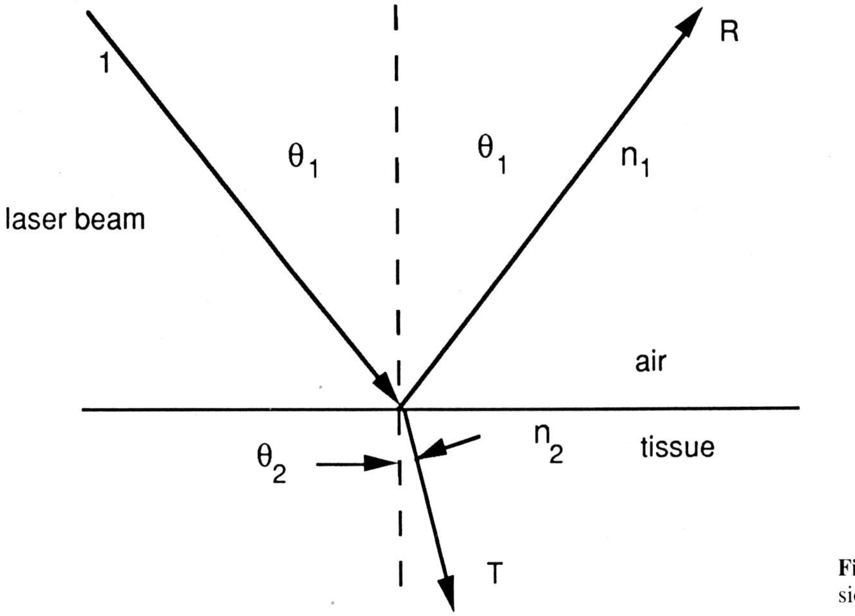

Figure 31–3. Reflection and transmission at interface where there is a mismatch in the index of refraction.

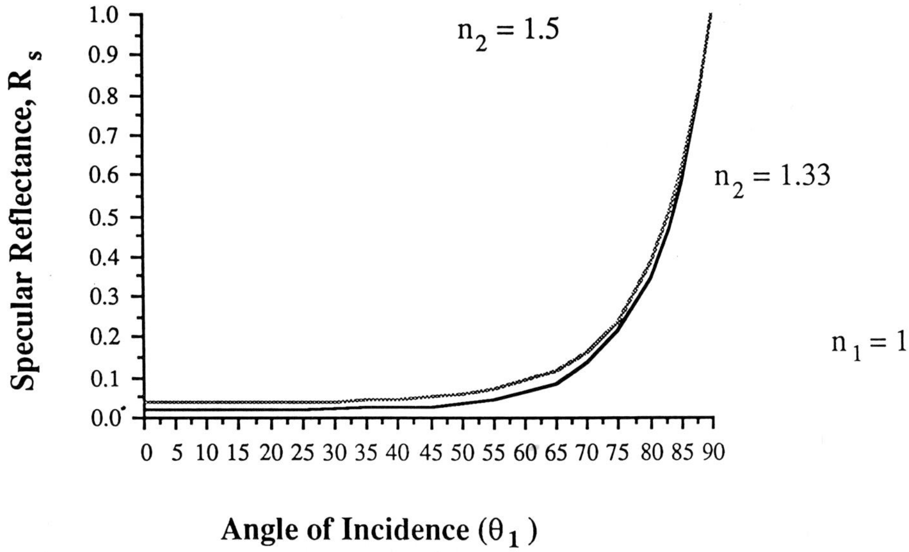

Figure 31–4. Angular dependence of specular (Fresnel) reflection for $n_1 = 1$ and $n_2 = 1.33$ and 1.5.

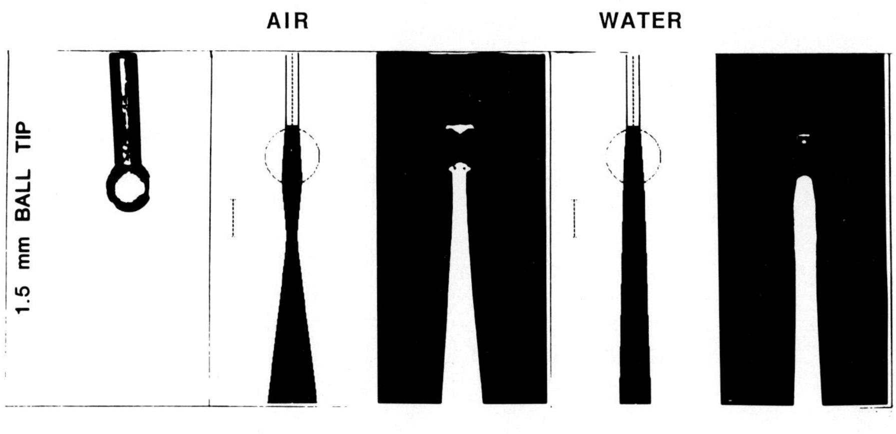

Figure 31–5. Light distribution for quartz tip probe in air and in water. (Reprinted with permission from Verdaasdonk.[14])

the tip of the probe, which produces a tip configuration that is excellent for cutting tissue. However, if the tip is placed in water (or into tissue), the mismatch of index of refraction is greatly reduced and now light passes through the side of the tip as shown in Figure 31-5B. The radiation pattern of the delivered beam is similar to the pattern produced by a standard fiberoptic probe. Tips constructed from a high index of refraction material such as sapphire will still alter the path of the light at their surfaces when they are inserted in water or against tissue.

Light entering tissue is subject to scattering and absorption. The collimated laser beam is attenuated by absorption and scattering according to Beers' law:

$$\phi_c(z) = \phi_o e^{-(\mu_a+\mu_s)z} \quad (4)$$

where $\phi_c(z)$ is the collimated fluence rate in the tissue (W/m^2), ϕ_o is the collimated irradiance transmitted to the tissue (W/m^2), μ_a is the absorption coefficient (m^{-1}), and μ_s is the scattering coefficient (m^{-1}).

The sum of μ_a and μ_s is designated as the attenuation coefficient, μ_t. The penetration depth δ of the collimated beam is defined as the depth that $\phi_c(\delta) = \phi_o e^{-1}$, that is, 0.37 ϕ_o. Thus, penetration depth is equal to the reciprocal of the attenuation coefficient:

$$\delta = \frac{1}{\mu_t} \quad (5)$$

where $\mu_t = \mu_a + \mu_s$.

DOMINANT ABSORPTION

Typically, absorption dominates scattering in cardiovascular tissue for wavelengths either below 300 nm or above 1.5 μm and the magnitude of light scattered is small with respect to the fluence rate of the collimated beam. As a result, equation 4 is a reasonable estimate of the total amount of light distributed in the tissue. For many wavelengths of interest for angioplasty, such as excimer at 248 nm, holmium:yttrium aluminum garnet (Ho:YAG) at 2.1 μm and erbium (Er):YAG at 2.94 μm, scattering can be neglected.

DOMINANT SCATTERING

The spectrum between 600 nm and 1.2 μm is often referred to as a "window" for light penetration in tissue. Within this window the absorption associated with tissue chromophores is low relative to the scattering properties in the tissue. The attenuation of the laser beam is still governed by equation 4, but the exponential decrease is primarily due to scattering, not absorption. Multiple scattering of the light prior to absorption or transmittance from the tissue produces a diffuse light that propagates beyond the decaying beam of collimated light. Multiple scattering produces the unexpected phenomenon of a larger fluence rate (W/m^2) within the tissue than the irradiance at the surface of the tissue.[1]

The magnitude of the diffuse light can be estimated by solving equations based on the transport equation for light propagation in a turbid medium.[1] Essentially, the equation states that the gradient in light radiance ($W/m^2/sr$) at position **r** travelling in direction **s** is:

gradient in radiance (r, s) = losses due to absorption and scattering plus gain of light scattered from all other directions into the s direction

The fluence rate (W/m^2) at the position **r** is found by integrating the radiance at **r** over all solid angles.

Solutions for light propagation based on the diffusion approximation or Monte Carlo simulations can provide estimates of the fluence rate (W/m^2) of the diffuse light in tissue.[2] By combining the diffuse and collimated light, the distribution of the laser light in tissue can be approximated. As the scattering coefficient increases, the penetration of the collimated light is decreased (see equation 4) and the magnitude of the diffuse light is increased. The fluence rate as a function of depth in the tissue is strongly influenced by the spot size of the laser beam. If the diameter of the laser beam is large with respect to the depth of penetration of the diffuse light, then scattering is effectively in the axial direction except at the edges of the beam. Thus, over most of the beam, a one-dimensional solution can be used to calculate the distribution of the diffuse light. For example, at 476 nm the absorption coefficient μ_a, scattering coefficient μ_s, and anisotropy factor g for human aorta are 6 cm^{-1}, 414 cm^{-1}, and 0.91, respectively. The anisotropy factor is the average cosine of the scattering angle. A value of g = 1.0 represents complete forward scattering and a value of g = 0 represents isotropic scattering. The solution for a large beam diameter irradiance of 1 W/cm^2 at 476 nm is shown in Figure 31-6A. Notice that except at the edges the solution does not vary in the radial direction. As the beam diameter is decreased, radial scattering affects the entire distribution (Fig. 31-6B, C). The fluence rate as a function of depth for beam diameters of 0.2, 1.0, and 4.0 mm was determined by Monte Carlo simulations.[2] For the large spot, the fluence rate at the center just below the surface is 2.4 times the surface irradiance. However, when the beam diameter is reduced to 0.2 mm, this center fluence rate below the surface is reduced to 1.2 W/cm^2 for a surface irradiance of 1.0 W/cm^2.

For a uniform irradiance, the decrease in fluence rate with depth in the diffusion region (greater than 5 optical depths below the surface) is exponential. That is, it has the form:

$$\phi(z) = A_1 e^{-\mu_{eff} z} \quad (6)$$

where A_1 is a constant and μ_{eff} is the effective scattering coefficient. Wherever the diffusion approximation is a reasonable estimate of the fluence rate of the diffuse light:

$$\mu_{eff}^2 = 3\mu_s [\mu_a + (1 - g)\mu_s] \quad (7)$$

Typically, optical properties change during laser irradiation. Both dehydration and carbonization can produce changes. The most dramatic is the local increase in μ_a at locations of carbonization. The effective penetration depth for neody-

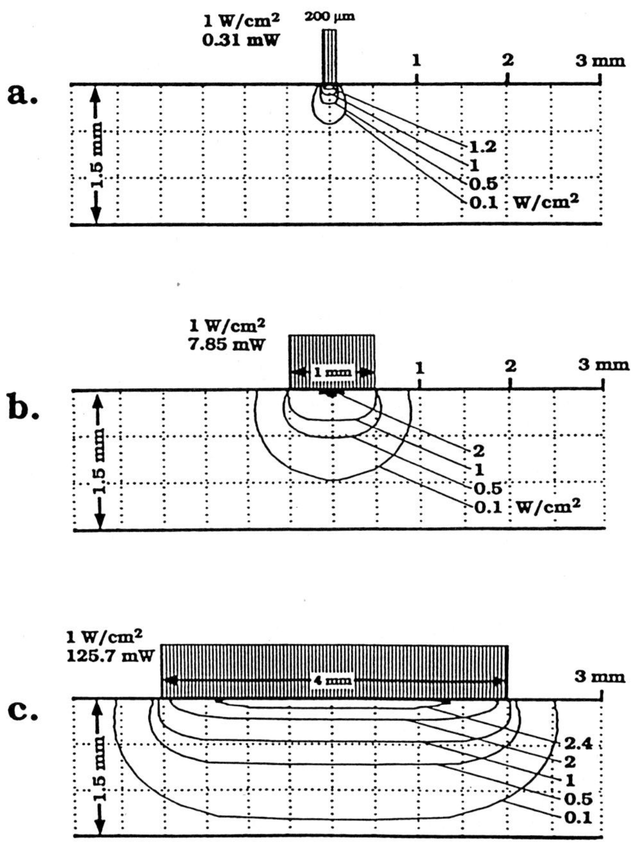

Figure 31–6. Monte Carlo simulation of light distribution in tissue for a uniform collimated beam with diameters of 0.2 mm **(A)**, 1.0 mm **(B)**, and 4.0 mm **(C)**. The optical properties of the tissue are $\mu_a = 6.0\ \text{cm}^{-1}$, $\mu_s = 414\ \text{cm}^{-1}$, and g = 0.91. (Reprinted with permission from Keijzer et al.[2])

mium (Nd):YAG at 1.06 µm radiation can change from a few millimeters to a few micrometers once a local region carbonizes.

RATE OF HEAT GENERATION

The absorption of laser light by tissue produces heat. The magnitude of the local rate of heat production **S(r)** (W/m^3) is the product of the absorption coefficient and the fluence rate, that is:

$$S(\mathbf{r}) = \mu_a(\mathbf{r})\phi(\mathbf{r}) \tag{8}$$

For a gaussian beam and dominant absorption, the rate of heat production in cylindrical coordinates (r,z) for uniform tissue with an absorption coefficient μ_a is:

$$S(r,z) = \mu_a\phi_0 e^{-(\mu_a + \mu_s)z}\, e^{\frac{-2r^2}{w_0^2}} \tag{9}$$

where w_0 is the $1/e^2$ radius of the gaussian beam.

For dominant scattering, most of the heat production is from the absorption of the diffuse light, not the collimated beams. The rate of heat production in a uniform tissue with absorption coefficient μ_a is:

$$S(r,z) = \mu_a[\phi_d(r,z) + \phi_c(r,z)] \tag{10}$$

where ϕ_d is the diffuse fluence rate and ϕ_c is the collimated fluence rate. Note that for the aorta tissue irradiated at 476 nm, the rate of heat generation is obtained by multiplying the curves of Figure 31-6 by μ_a.

THERMAL RESPONSE OF TISSUE TO LASER PULSES

The absorption of laser light by tissue generates heat at the absorption sites and increases the local temperature. Heat is conducted to cooler regions, creating a temperature field that is a function of time and space. The rate of temperature change $\frac{\delta T}{\delta t}$ at a position **r** indicates changes in the local storage of heat and is influenced by heat conduction and the local rate of heat generation **S(r)**. Solutions of the conduction of heat in laser-irradiated tissue are described in Birngruber,[3] Carslaw and Jaeger,[4] and Welch.[5] During the early moments of laser irradiation prior to heat conduction, temperature increases are proportional to the local rate of heat production and the time of irradiation. Pulse durations less than 1.0 msec are typically much shorter than the thermal relaxation time of the volume of tissue that is heated.[6] When this condition is met, the local temperature rise reaches a maximum value at the end of a laser pulse that can be approximated by:

$$\Delta T(\mathbf{r}) = \frac{\phi(\mathbf{r})\mu_a(\mathbf{r})t_0}{\rho c} \tag{11}$$

where ΔT is the temperature rise [°C], **r** is the position vector (x,y,z) [m], ϕ is the fluence rate at **r** (W/m^2), μ_a is the absorption coefficient at r (1/m), t_0 is the pulse duration [s], and ρc is the volumetric heat capacity ($J/m^3 \cdot °C$).

The product $\phi(\mathbf{r})t_0$ is the fluence (J/m^2) of the laser light at position **r**. The laser pulse appears to be an impulse to the tissue when irradiation time is shorter than the thermal relaxation time. After the optical energy is converted to internal thermal energy, peak temperatures decrease as heat is conducted to cooler regions. The decrease in temperature field for $t > t_0$ is called the impulse response. The time course of the temperature relaxation is governed by the heat conduction equation. Two important parameters in the thermal relaxation response are the volume of tissue that is heated and the thermal diffusivity $\gamma = k/\rho c[m^2/s]$.

The diffusion time of heat in laser-irradiated tissue is a function of the beam diameter (w_0), penetration depth (δ), and diffusivity (γ). The diffusion time is defined as:

$$\tau_d = \frac{\ell^2}{4\gamma} \tag{12}$$

where ℓ^2 is a characteristic length. van Gemert and Welch[7] have shown that a similar term called the thermal time constant τ can be defined as:

$$\frac{1}{\tau} = \frac{1}{\tau_r} + \frac{1}{\tau_z} \tag{13}$$

where:

$$\tau_r \sim w_0^2 \qquad (14)$$

if w_0 is in millimeters and τ_z in seconds and:

$$\tau_z \sim \left(\frac{3}{\mu_{tr}}\right)^2 \qquad (15)$$

if μ_{tr} is mm^{-1} and τ_z is seconds. The attenuation coefficient μ_{tr} is:

$$\mu_{tr} = \mu_a + (1 - g)\,\mu_s \qquad (16)$$

and $1/\mu_{tr}$ provides a measure of penetration depth in the presence of forward scattering.

For penetration depths much less than the spot radius, as pictured in Figure 31-7, heat conduction is in the direction of the laser beam. The transient time is governed by τ_z. When the penetration depth is much larger than the spot radius, heat conduction is perpendicular to the direction of the bar. In this case, the transient is governed by τ_r.

If the laser pulses come close together in comparison with the thermal relaxation period and individual pulses do not ablate tissue, then individual temperature responses are superimposed and the resulting thermal behavior for a long sequence of pulses approximates that of tissue subjected to CW irradiation at the same wavelength and average power.[8]

Many of the denaturation processes can be modeled by Arrhenius rate reactions,[5,9,10] and the rate of denaturation is approximated by:

$$\frac{d\Omega}{dt}(\mathbf{r},t) = Ae^{-\frac{E}{RT}} \qquad (17)$$

where $\Omega(\mathbf{r},t)$ is an empirically defined accumulated damage constant. The physical significance of Ω is that it is the log of the ratio of the initial concentration of undamaged tissue, C(0), to the remaining undamaged tissue C(t):

$$\Omega = \ln\left[\frac{C(0)}{C(t)}\right] \qquad (18)$$

We specify that $\Omega > 1.0$ represents irreversible damage. A and E are, respectively, the experimentally determined integration constant [1/sec] and activation energy (J/M), and R is the universal gas constant (J/M · K). For most laser-induced thermal reactions in tissue, the degree and extent of damage is a nonlinear function of both temperature and time. Values for A and E for aorta have been determined by Agah[11] by applying constant temperatures to tissue samples for fixed periods of time and determining the temperature-time pairs associated with threshold damage and Ω set equal to 1.0. Note that in equation 15 damage is linearly related to time at an elevated constant temperature but exponentially related to a varying temperature. For transient temperature responses, damage at position **r** is associated with the maximum temperature at position **r** and the time within 1 or 2 degrees of this temperature.

ABLATION

Since tissue is 75 to 80% water, it is tempting to describe ablation in terms of the vaporization of water. If water is at some temperature T_i, vaporization requires heating the water to a critical temperature T_c (usually 100°C for water) and then additional heating for vaporization. That is, the threshold radiant energy density W_{th} is:

$$W_{th} = \rho c(T_c - T_i) + \rho H\left[\frac{J}{cm^3}\right] \qquad (19)$$

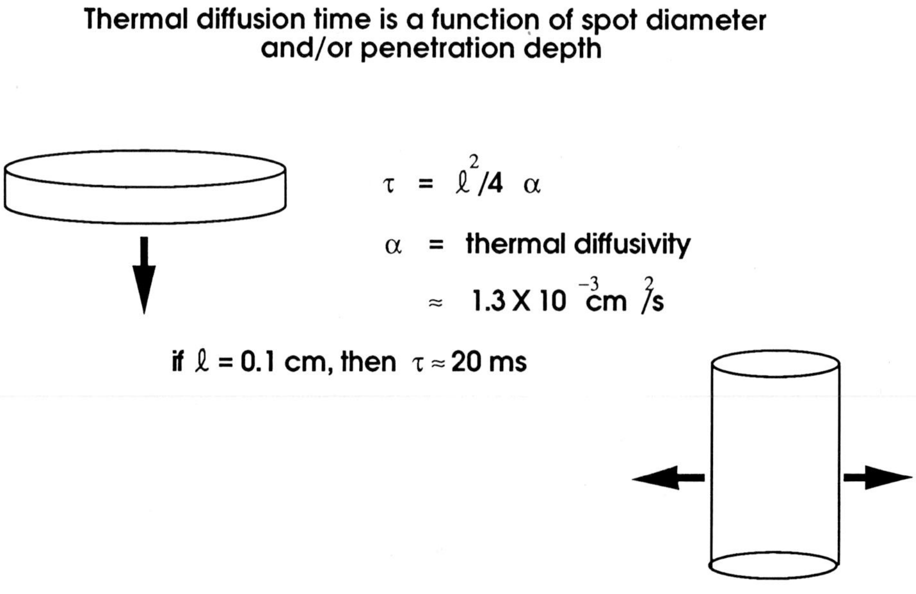

Figure 31–7. Dependency of diffusion time (time constant) on penetration depth and radius of laser beam. ℓ is termed the characteristic length. The value of ℓ is the smaller of the penetration depth or the beam radius. If penetration depth is much less than beam radius, then heat conduction is first in the axial direction. If beam radius is much less than penetration depth, then conduction is initially in the radial direction.

where ρ: density (g/cm^3), c: heat capacity (J/gm − °C), T: temperature (°C), H: heat of vaporization (J/gm).

For water at 37°C, and vaporization at 100°C, $\rho c(\Delta T) \approx 0.25\ kJ/cm^3$ and $\rho H \approx 2.25\ kJ/cm^3$. So approximately 2.5 kJ/cm^3 are required to vaporize water. A generalization of the fluence required to vaporize water can be formulated by assuming that the laser beam has a uniform irradiance profile, ϕ_0 and pulse duration t_0 with area A, and the laser energy is uniformly distributed to an optical penetration depth δ, which is also assumed to be the ablation depth. With these assumptions, the threshold fluence ψ_{th} (J/cm^2) for vaporization:

$$\psi_{th} = W_{th}\delta = 2500\delta = \phi_0 t_0 \tag{20}$$

and the energy delivery requirements are:

$$Q_{Laser}\ [J] = \psi_{th}A \tag{21}$$

A crude estimate of the irradiance or fluence requirements for vaporization of tissue as a function of pulse duration can be obtained from equation 20. Although tissue is not water, the 2.5 kJ/cm^3 is a reasonable benchmark. Also, optical penetration depth and ablation depth for a single pulse is a generalization for which there are many counter-examples.

One counter-example is tissue ablation with a CW laser. Typically, a large portion of the heat generated by the laser light is conducted axially and radially into the tissue. The radial component produces an increase in temperature that is beyond the radius of the ablation crater. Although ablation with pulsed lasers is growing in prominence, the events associated with CW ablation provide clues for understanding the mechanisms of pulse ablation. By using a moderate irradiance from an argon laser and measuring surface temperature with a thermal camera, it is possible to document the initial surface heating and explosive ejection of tissue (popcorn effect). This process is illustrated in Figure 31-8 for argon laser irradiation of aorta. The rather low irradiance used in this experiment permits a clear visualization of these thermal events. The onset of ablation occurs above 100°C, and as heated tissue is removed, a cooler layer is exposed to the laser irradiation. The temperature remains at approximately 100°C as the laser irradiation dehydrates the tissue. The removal of water decreases the local thermal conductivity, reducing heat conduction to the surrounding area. Continued radiation rapidly increases the tissue temperature until it reaches about 300°C.

The thermal response is further complicated by changes in the optical and thermal properties of tissue as a function of dehydration and thermal damage, as described in Figure 31-9. Irradiation that produces temperatures at or above 100°C causes rapid drying of the tissue, which decreases the density and thermal conductivity.[4] Significant reductions in thermal conductivity will retard heat flow to cooler regions; consequently, peak temperatures will increase, and at approximately 285° to 350°C, nucleation sites carbonize and burn.

The ablation process is strongly influenced by the wavelength-dependent penetration depth of the laser beam and its fluence. The penetration depth at any wavelength is governed by the chromophores that absorb the laser light. In the UV region, the important absorbers are proteins and amino acids, whereas water is the dominant chromophore for IR wavelengths above 1.3 μm. In between, the color of tissue and blood governs the absorption process. Typical penetration depths for several of the lasers considered for angioplasty are presented in Figure 31-1. It is important to realize that for every penetration depth associated with a UV wavelength, there is at least one IR wavelength that will give exactly the same penetration depth.

Let us examine the ablation process of the Er:YAG laser that has a macropulse of approximately 200 μsec. For example, consider the response of tissue such as aorta to Er:YAG irradiation at 2.94 nm. Each macropulse from the laser contains approximately 10 micropulses of approxi-

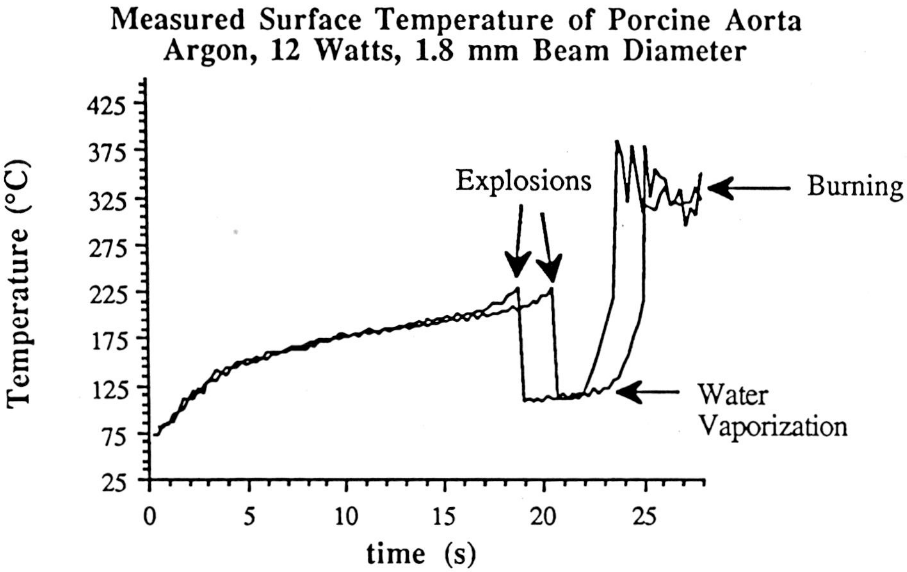

Figure 31–8. Surface temperature measurement during argon laser ablation of aorta. Laser power was 8.0 W and the spot size was 2.0 mm.

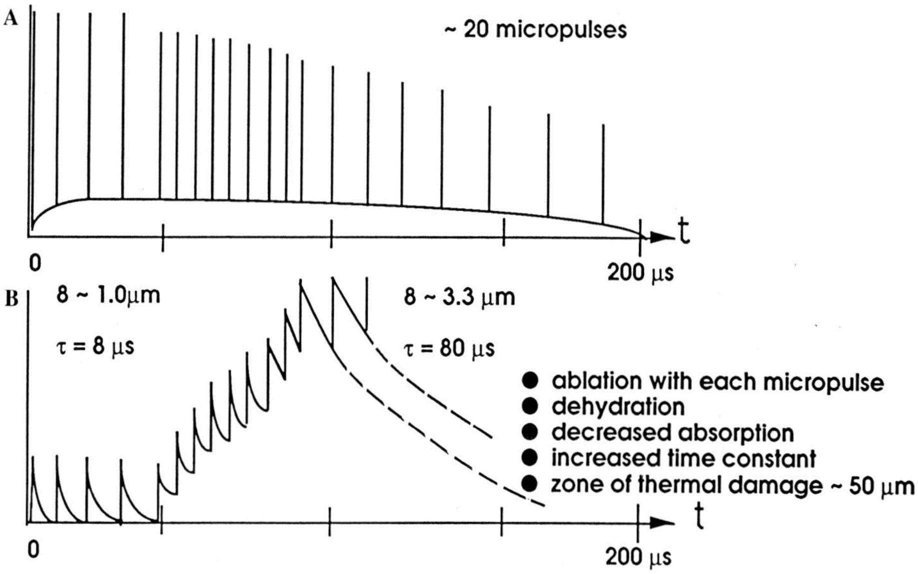

Figure 31–9. **A:** Cartoon of the structure of an Er:YAG (2.94 nm) macropulse. **B:** Cartoon of the temperature response of the tissue due to each micropulse. The temperature time constant of normal tissue for a short (1 μsec or less) pulse is approximately 8 μsec. As the tissue dehydrates, the penetration depth increases and the time constant may increase to 1.0 msec.

mately 1.0 μsec duration[12] and typically there are at least 100 msec between macropulses. The micropulses are not uniformly spaced but cluster together near the beginning of the pulse, as illustrated by the measurements of Joseph Walsh,[12] which are shown in Figure 31-9. Er:YAG irradiation is absorbed within 1 μm in tissue because of the high absorption of water at 2.94 nm. The thermal relaxation time associated with this penetration depth is about 9 μsec.[7] On the average, there should be sufficient time separation of the micropulses that the response of each pulse is almost independent of the previous micropulse and any residual thermal damage should be on the order of a few micrometers. Yet, Walsh has noted a depth of thermal damage on the order of 50 μm, which is much deeper than would be expected for the 1 μm penetration depth of this wavelength. This depth of damage would be associated with penetration depth of 20 to 30 μm and diffusion times on the order of 1.0 msec.

Whenever a micropulse causes some dehydration, the penetration depth of the next micropulse is increased and the diffusion time is increased by the square of the new penetration depth. Furthermore, if some of the micropulses are bunched together, as suggested in Figure 31-10A, then the increased time constant (diffusion time) may lead to superposition of individual temperature responses, as illustrated in the graph of Figure 31-9. If dehydration from micropulses or macropulses increases the penetration depth to 20.0 μm, the thermal response would be similar to that of a pulsed carbon dioxide laser at 10.6 μm.

When the laser light penetrates more than a few micrometers into the tissue, the ablation process is more of a subsurface explosive event than a surface phenomenon. The tissue is superheated and then ablated; the resulting crater formation ejects fragments of tissue and may lift portions of the torn rim above the normal surface level. Far more tissue

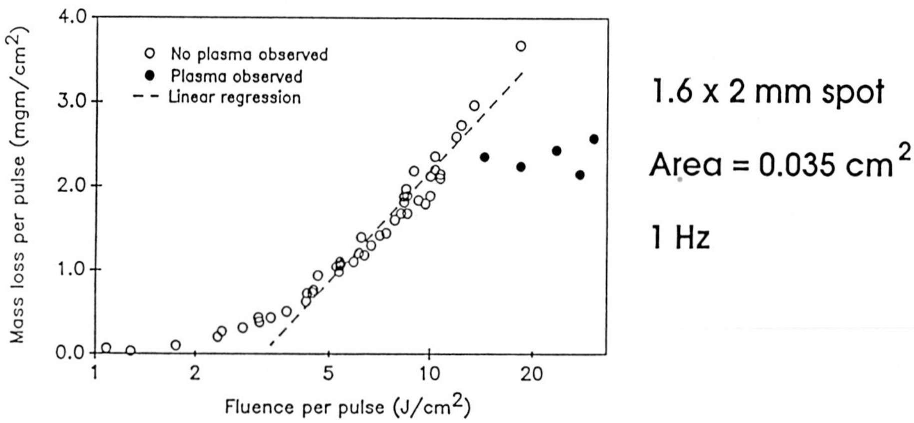

$$M = \frac{\rho A}{\mu_a} \ln (F_0 / F_{th})$$

Figure 31–10. Pulsed carbon dioxide laser ablation depth in pig skin as a function of fluence. The spot area was 0.32 cm^2 and the pulse rate was 1 Hz. (Reprinted with permission from Walsh and Deutsch.[13])

may be removed in this process than suggested by predictions based on the vaporization of water. When the penetration depth is reduced to 1 μm or less, very smooth ablations can be achieved, as is evident from craters formed by the argon fluorine excimer laser at 193 nm.

Further increases in pulse energy beyond the ablation threshold may lead to plasma formation at a focal point or at an absorption site. The resulting superficial plasma layer traps the laser radiation and reduces or stops heat generation inside the tissue. The efficiency and rate of ablation of soft tissue is adversely affected by plasma formation, yet the associated shock waves may be advantageous for fragmentation of kidney and gallstones and calcified plaque. The influence of plasma formation on ablation depth is illustrated in Figure 31-10. The slope of mass loss per pulse versus fluence per pulse is almost zero once a plasma is formed.[13]

CONCLUSIONS

The response of tissue to laser irradiation is highly dependent on irradiation time, irradiance (W/m^2) or fluence (J/m^2) for CW or pulsed irradiation, respectively, and the wavelength-dependent optical properties of tissue. For wavelengths between 600 nm and 1.2 μm, the laser beam is highly scattered and significant heat may be generated beyond the collimated laser beam. These are rather poor wavelengths for ablation. Efficient, rapid ablation is associated with wavelengths where absorption dominates scattering. Noteworthy are the excimer UV wavelengths at 248 and 308 nm and IR wavelengths in the region of the water absorption peaks at 1.9 and 2.9 μm. Short (less than 1.0 msec), high fluence pulses for ablation produce less thermal damage than CW irradiation. However, if the pulse irradiance is too high (larger than 10^8 W/cm^2), a plasma is formed and shock waves are produced. Although these acoustic waves may dislodge and crack calcified plaque, they may also damage normal tissue at some distance from the site of irradiation.

No single wavelength, pulse duration, or fluence produces optimum ablation results. There appear to be advantages and disadvantages to all of the wavelengths being considered for angioplasty.

REFERENCES

1. Ishimaru A. Wave Propagation and Scattering in Random Media, vol. 1. New York: Academic Press, 1978.
2. Keijzer M, Jacques SL, Prahl SA, Welch AJ. Light distributions in artery tissue: Monte Carlo simulations for finite-diameter laser beams. Lasers Surg Med 1989;9:148–54.
3. Birngruber R. The thermal modeling of biological tissue. In Lasers in Biology and Medicine. New York: Plenum Publishing Corp., 1980:77–97.
4. Carslaw HS, Jaeger JC. Conduction of Heat in Solids, 2nd ed. Oxford: Oxford University Press, 1959.
5. Welch AJ. Laser irradiation of tissue. In Shitzer A, Eberhart RC (eds): Heat Transfer in Medicine and Biology, vol. 12. New York: Plenum Press, 1985:135–84.
6. Furzikov NP. Different lasers for angioplasty: thermo-optical comparison. IEEE J Quant Elect 1987;QE-23:1751–5.
7. van Gemert MJC, Welch AJ. Time constants in thermal laser medicine. Lasers Surg Med 1989;9:405–21.
8. Deckelbaum LI, Isner JM, Donaldson RF, et al. Reduction of laser-induced pathologic tissue injury using pulsed energy delivery. Am J Cardiol 1985;56:662–7.
9. Henriques FC. Studies of thermal injury: V. The predictability and the significance of thermally induced rate processes leading to irreversible thermal injury. Arch Pathol 1947;43:489–502.
10. Cheong WF, Welch AJ. A model for optical and thermal analysis of laser balloon angioplasty. IEEE Trans Biomed Elect 1989;BME-36:1233–43.
11. Agah R. Quantitative characterization of arterial tissue thermal damage. Masters Thesis, University of Texas, Austin, 1988.
12. Walsh JT, Flotte TJ, Deutsch TF. Er:YAG laser ablation of tissue: effect of pulse duration and tissue type on thermal damage. Lasers Surg Med 1989;9:314–26.
13. Walsh JT, Deutsch TF. Pulsed CO_2 laser tissue ablation: measurement of the ablation rate. Lasers Surg Med 1988;8:264–75.
14. Verdaasdonk RM. Laser angioplasty with modified fiber tips. Ph.D. dissertation, University of Utrecht, The Netherlands, 1990.

32 Mechanisms of Laser Recanalization

Cres P. Miranda, M.D., Masahito Moriuchi, M.D., Michael McRae, M.D., Larry-Stuart Deutsch, M.D., Michael Berns, Ph.D., Walter Henry, M.D., Jonathan M. Tobis, M.D.

Although laser angioplasty has tremendous potential in expanding the ability to treat obstructive atherosclerotic disease, serious complications such as vasospasm,[1–3] thrombogenicity,[4] and vessel perforation[5–8] have diminished the initial enthusiasm. A better understanding of the biologic tissue response to laser and thermal energy will help minimize these complications and act as a guide of this novel form of energy. This chapter will review the effects of various methods of laser angioplasty on vascular tissue. In addition, we will discuss the predominant mechanism of recanalization of atherosclerotic obstructions, which is relevant to all the methods of laser ablation.

BASIC MECHANISMS

The interaction between vascular tissue and laser energy depends on a multitude of factors:

1. Laser wavelength
2. Optical properties of the tissue
3. Fluid medium through which the laser must traverse to the tissue
4. Delivered power and energy of the laser
5. Area of the tissue irradiated
6. Laser pulse duration

The delivery of laser energy to the irradiated tissue is described by the following terms. Fluence is the energy per pulse divided by the area irradiated (joules/mm^2). Fluence rate is the power (W) divided by the irradiated area (W/mm^2). Pulse power is obtained by dividing the pulse energy by the pulse duration (J/sec).

The interaction between laser energy and tissue is similar to any electromagnetic wavefront coming in contact with a different medium, which produces reflection, scattering, and absorption.[9] Once the photons are absorbed, the tissue responds in one of four different ways. A familiar pattern is that the absorbed energy can again be released as light, or fluorescence, of a longer wavelength from the tissue, since there is some loss of energy in the interaction. Another way the laser energy can be absorbed in the tissue is with the production of an intense electrical field creating a liquid plasma with resultant tissue destruction; this is called a photoplasma.[10] In addition, the laser can be absorbed with an increase in movement and collisions of atoms resulting in heat production, or photothermal energy. In this localized area of heating, protein denaturation and tissue coagulation occurs above 60°C, water vaporization occurs above 100°C, and carbonization occurs later.[11] This is the major mechanism of tissue destruction by continuous wave lasers. Lastly, the absorbed photoenergy can be of such magnitude that it actually cleaves and dissociates molecular bonds, breaking large molecules into smaller ones, a photochemical process.[12] This is the major mechanism proposed for the excimer laser.

A model developed by Garrison and Srinivasan[13] of the ablation of polymethyl methacrylate by ultraviolet radiation lends support to this theory of photochemical disruption. The photon energy of an excimer laser at 193 nm is 6.4 eV, whereas a peptide bond energy is 3 eV;[12] thus, this laser has enough energy to disrupt chemical bonds. The resulting photodecomposition products occupy a larger volume than the original polymer.[13] These photoproducts remove some of the thermal energy from the target site as they are released.[11] In contrast, higher wavelength photons in the visible and infrared regions do not have enough energy to break molecular bonds, but instead cause vibratory movements of the atoms, producing heat and subsequent thermal injury. Grundfest and associates[14] compared the thermal effects of an argon laser (wavelength 418 or 514 nm) with a pulse duration of 10 msec to a 308 nm excimer laser with a pulse duration of 85 nsec. They recorded the surface temperature of the irradiated site, cadaver atherosclerotic aorta, with an AGA 782 thermographic camera. The temperature at point of impact for the argon laser was 160°C and only 63.5°C for the pulsed excimer laser.[14]

Further studies have shown that it may not only be the wavelength of the laser that is most important in initiating tissue destruction with a minimum of thermal injury, but also the frequency with which it is delivered.[15,16] Murphy-Chutorian and colleagues[15] varied xenon fluoride (XeFl) excimer laser pulse energy (wavelength, 351 nm) and frequency on isolated normal and atherosclerotic aorta. They found that precise tissue ablation occurred at low frequencies, but as the pulse repetition rate was increased from 10 to 75 Hz, the pulse interval consequently decreased proportionately, and histologic features of vacuolization consistent with thermal injury occurred. Localized heat is dissipated by tissue conductivity and the thermal sink of the surrounding fluid. This localized cooling requires a finite period of time to occur. It is estimated that a minimum of 50 to 100 msec was required for adequate cooling.[15] If the time between pulse intervals is shortened, there will be an accumulation of heat and thermal injury will occur. This thermal phenomenon has been observed regardless of wavelength, as demonstrated by thermal measurements with the excimer laser exposing cornea tissue at 193 nm.[17]

HISTOLOGIC ANALYSIS

Argon, neodymium:yttrium aluminum garnet (Nd:YAG) and carbon dioxide (CO_2) continuous wave lasers all produce severe thermal vascular injury.[18] The targeted tissue is melted and destroyed by photothermal energy and a residual cone-shaped crater is surrounded at its periphery with concentric zones of charred and carbonized tissue, the eosinophilic coagulum of protein denaturation and vacuolization that represents acoustic damage caused by the rapid vaporization of water (Fig. 32-1). Abela and coworkers[18] studied the effects of CO_2, Nd:YAG, and argon lasers on atherosclerotic coronary arteries obtained at necropsy and showed that crater diameter and the depth of these three surrounding zones varies with laser wavelength, pulse duration, the medium bathing the tissue (saline or blood), and predominantly with the energy delivered (power times duration of exposure). Litvack and associates[19] visually documented the photothermal ablation process with the use of high-speed film analysis (500 frames/sec) and described five distinct phases. Initially, the tissue blanches, presumably from denaturation of protein, followed by melting of the tissue, then boiling with bubbles on the molten surface, the crater then increases in size and carbonization occurs at its edges, and finally, the tissue adjacent to the crater expands.[19] Vascular aneurysm formation and complete vessel wall disruption have been documented with the use of argon bare laser fiberoptics.[6,7]

Delivery of laser energy through pulsed modes may provide the combination of microscopically precise tissue ablation with a predictable effect and minimization of thermal injury to adjacent tissue.[20,21] This mode of laser energy delivery has been shown to reduce signs of thermal injury by gross and microscopic analysis.[14,21] The histologic findings of pulsed excimer irradiated vascular tissue have shown incisions with sharp borders, no evidence of charring or carbonization, and absence of lacunae or coagulation necrosis (Fig. 32-2).[14,22] This absence of thermal injury may be conducive to healing of the vascular endothelium.[11]

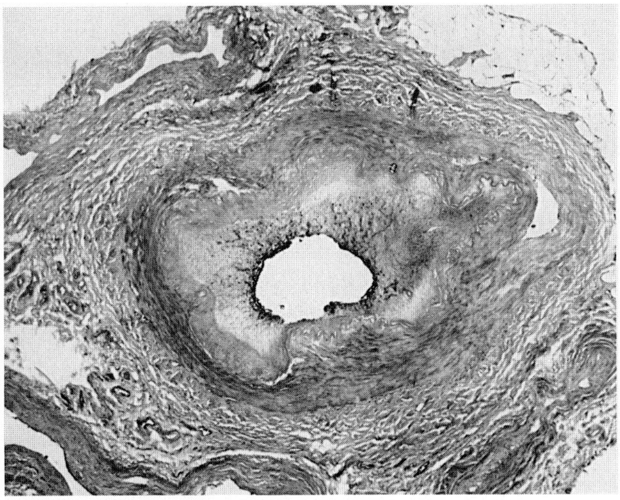

Figure 32–1. Histologic section of a human tibial artery that was completely occluded with atherosclerosis. The central lumen has been created by direct application of argon laser energy through a fiberoptic conduit. Around the perimeter of the ablated tissue is a dark band due to the charring effect of the argon laser.

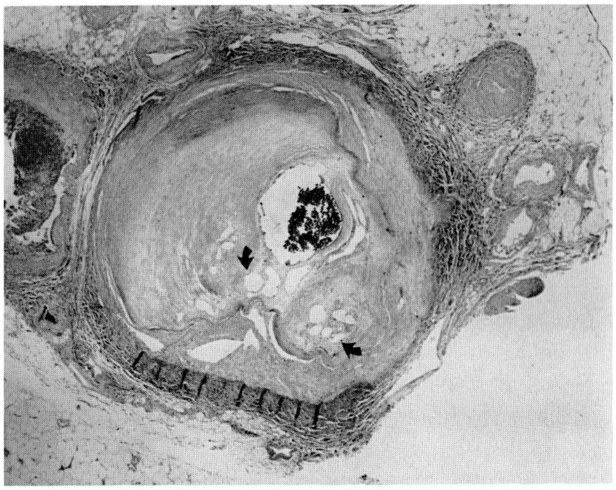

Figure 32–2. Excimer laser energy (308 nm) was applied to this occluded iliac artery using a 400 μm quartz fiber. The central lumen was created by passing the excimer laser followed by a 6 F catheter. A silk thread was then tied to the quartz fiber and drawn back through the artery section to document the channel created by the excimer laser. In addition, there are multiple smaller holes (arrows) due to excimer laser ablation as the fiber was moved back and forth in the atheroma in an attempt to increase the volume of tissue ablated.

FLUID EFFECTS ON LASERS

Before the laser energy comes in contact with the vascular wall, it must first traverse a fluid medium, saline or blood (unless it is a direct contact method). The fluid not only alters the dispersion angle and penetrating depth of the laser beam, which changes the size of the area irradiated, it also modifies the transfer of heat to the vascular tissue, diminishing thermal injury. Fenech and colleagues[23] studied the effects of saline solution and blood in vitro on the argon laser irradiation of arterial tissue. They found that blood, compared with saline, increased the divergence angle and reduced the forward projection of the laser beam, and this effect increased proportionately with increasing concentrations of blood.[23] When lasing perpendicular to the vascular tissue, through saline, the size of the crater produced was similar in size to the optical fiber. When blood was substituted, the resulting crater diameter was significantly increased at the same energy levels, and increasing distances between laser and tissue produced more injury through blood than saline. The authors theorized that since the argon ion laser wavelength was similar to the absorption spectra of hemoglobin,[24] blood was a more efficient heat conductor than saline, carrying more energy over a longer distance despite the greater beam divergence.[23] They also noted that lasing through blood created gas bubbles at the targeted site, and the generation of these bubbles may have contributed acoustic injury to the tissue, as well as increased laser energy delivery because gas is a more efficient medium for laser energy conduction than fluid.[18,24,25]

LASER-LIBERATED PHOTOPRODUCTS

In order to identify the photoproducts of laser ablation, Isner and associates[26] irradiated atherosclerotic plaque in vitro with an argon laser. The liberated photoproducts were collected and analyzed with gas chromatography, mass spectrometry, and absorbance spectroscopy. Analysis by these methods demonstrated that hydrogen, water vapor, light hydrocarbon fragmentation products of acetylene, ethylene, ethane, propylene, and butadiene, were released during laser ablation. Trace amounts of hydrogen cyanide and carbon monoxide were also demonstrated. There was no significant difference in liberated photoproducts from more extensively calcified arterial segments or experimentally induced rabbit aortic atherosclerosis with a predominance of foam cells instead of collagen.[26] This suggests that laser angioplasty, with continuous wave laser in the visible and infrared wavelengths, proceeds via an incomplete thermal combustion mechanism with liberation of small protein fragments and light hydrocarbon fragments.

RESIDUAL DEBRIS

One of the initial concerns with lysis of atherosclerosis by lasers was the production of residual debris that could embolize and compromise the arterial supply distal to the targeted lesion. Isner et al[26] collected, filtered, and x-rayed the postirradiation aqueous media and found no evidence of residual particulate matter. In vivo animal studies by Abela and colleagues[27] and studies in man by Ginsburg and associates[1] disclosed no angiographic documentation of emboli produced by laser angioplasty. Abela and coworkers[28] also performed laser recanalization on totally occluded superficial femoral arteries and found that there was minimal liberation of residual debris.

POSTLASER HEALING

Abela and colleagues[29] evaluated the immediate and short-term healing response to argon laser radiation of the aorta and iliofemoral arteries of dogs and monkeys. Vascular perforation was a common complication, but there were no aneurysms or dissections by angiography. Three hundred seventy-three arterial sites were irradiated in 12 atherosclerotic arteries of four monkeys and lasing induced thrombosis in three arteries. No thrombosis was noted in the normal canine arteries. Within 1 hour after lasing, the impact crater had a layer of coagulated elements, few adherent platelets, and cellular debris. Early healing noted at 2 to 4 days showed no polymorphonuclear leukocytes and only a minimal mononuclear phagocytic response. By 7 days, there was a low-grade cellular infiltration of smooth muscle cells and undifferentiated mesenchymal cells, probably fibroblasts. An endothelial lining was noted at days 7 to 14 with complete reendothelialization by 30 days and total healing at 60 days. Gerrity and colleagues[30] using a CO_2 laser on hypercholesterolemic swine documented a similar healing response. An interesting note is that despite continual feeding with a hypercholesterolemic diet to the monkeys, there was no reappearance of foam cells or cholesterol deposits up to 60 days after lasing.[29,30] One theory advanced for this phenomenon is that the vasa vasorum are cauterized at the lased sites and they may be a necessary component for the production of atherosclerosis.[31] It has been shown that the vasa vasorum are increased in relation to atherosclerosis, and it has been postulated that this neovascularization may be a necessary component for the formation of atheromatous plaques.[32]

Prevosti and associates[33] irradiated normal canine femoral arteries with a 308 nm excimer laser. At 10 days postirradiation, reendothelialization was well underway without evidence of thrombus. At 6 weeks, there were no aneurysms and the target craters were barely visible due to fibrointimal growth and granulation tissue.[33] Forrester and coworkers[34] compared argon with excimer irradiation of normal canine aortas. With argon lasing, they found medial necrosis at 24 to 72 hours, and medial scarring with transmural necrosis at 4 weeks. In contrast, the excimer laser showed no acute thermal injury and at 4 weeks healing was so complete as to be unrecognizable from normal tissue.[34,35] The resultant smooth intimal topography may be less thrombogenic and reduce the risk of restenosis.[11]

LASER ENERGY DELIVERY SYSTEMS

Not only are there various lasers of differing wavelengths, continuous and pulsed, but there are many ways to deliver this energy to the targeted site: bare fiberoptics;[18] metal-capped hot-tip thermal probe;[36] a combination laser-thermal "hybrid" probe in which part of the laser energy is emitted out the end of the probe as ablative light surrounded by a thermal metal cap;[37] two types of laser-balloon combinations, one in which an inflated balloon holds the laser in place coaxially for the emission of an argon laser beam,[38] and another in which the balloon itself is directly heated by Nd:YAG laser to thermally seal the dilated segment;[39] a sapphire-tip laser;[40] a circumferential array of laser fiberoptics surrounding the central guide wire lumen;[41] and a "smart" laser that utilizes the optical spectrum differences between atherosclerotic plaque and normal tissue to direct its ablative laser beam.[42] Differing mechanisms of recanalization may dictate different levels of success and complications with each system. In the final analysis, randomized clinical trials between standard interventional methods and the various laser-assisted techniques must be performed to determine the clinical utility of these laser devices.

Metal-Capped Thermal Probe

Sanborn and associates[36] placed a metal cap on the end of a 1 mm in diameter optical fiber connected to an argon laser (laser probe, Trimedyne, Santa Ana, CA) and compared it directly with the bare fiberoptic itself. They had greater success in dilating a stenosis with the laser probe and there was less perforation compared with the bare fiberoptic.[36] Histologically, the bare fiberoptic caused thermal injury as previously described,[18] extending through the intima and into the media of the artery. Histologic examination of the arteries tested with the laser probe showed an even and circumferential distribution of thermal injury around the lumen. However, removal of the laser probe disclosed atheroma adhering to the metal tip resulting in tearing and a functional endartherectomy that remained patent on follow-up angiography.[36,43]

Several clinical studies were performed with the laser-mediated thermal probe in which recanalization was attempted in complete occlusions of the superficial femoral and popliteal arteries.[44,45] If these initial results were successful, the thermal probe might be applicable in the coronary circulation to reopen occluded vessels. Early studies demonstrated satisfactory results with the success rate dependent on the length of the lesion, tortuosity of the vessel, and the presence of calcification in the atheroma (Fig. 32-3).[45] For femoropopliteal or straight iliac artery occlusions with a mean length of 6.8 cm, the angiographic success rate was 81% and decreased to 61% for lesions with a mean length of 11.7 cm.[46] These initial results were encouraging and the Food and Drug Administration (FDA) approved the clinical use of the Trimedyne Laserprobe and the Argon laser, which became the first laser device approved for treatment of atherosclerotic disease. The FDA approval implied satisfaction with the safety of the Laserprobe but did not require a controlled study to demonstrate that the Laserprobe was any better than traditional methods of recanalization, such as with guide wires and catheters. As many centers began to gain experience with the thermal probe, it became clear that there was an incidence of arterial perforation greater than that predicted by the initial clinical trials.[47]

Because of the concerns about arterial perforation during human in vivo trials, Tobis and colleagues[45] studied the mechanism of recanalization with guide wires and with the argon laser-mediated thermal probe in vitro on 25 human peripheral arterial segments obtained at necropsy or after limb amputation. Atherosclerotic human arteries were used because animal models produce fat-laden foam cell atheroma, which might respond differently than densely fibrotic and calcified arteries found in humans with peripheral vascular disease. The thermal probe was compared with purely mechanical recanalization using a 0.035 inch guide wire and a 6 F multipurpose catheter or a balloon dilation catheter, and

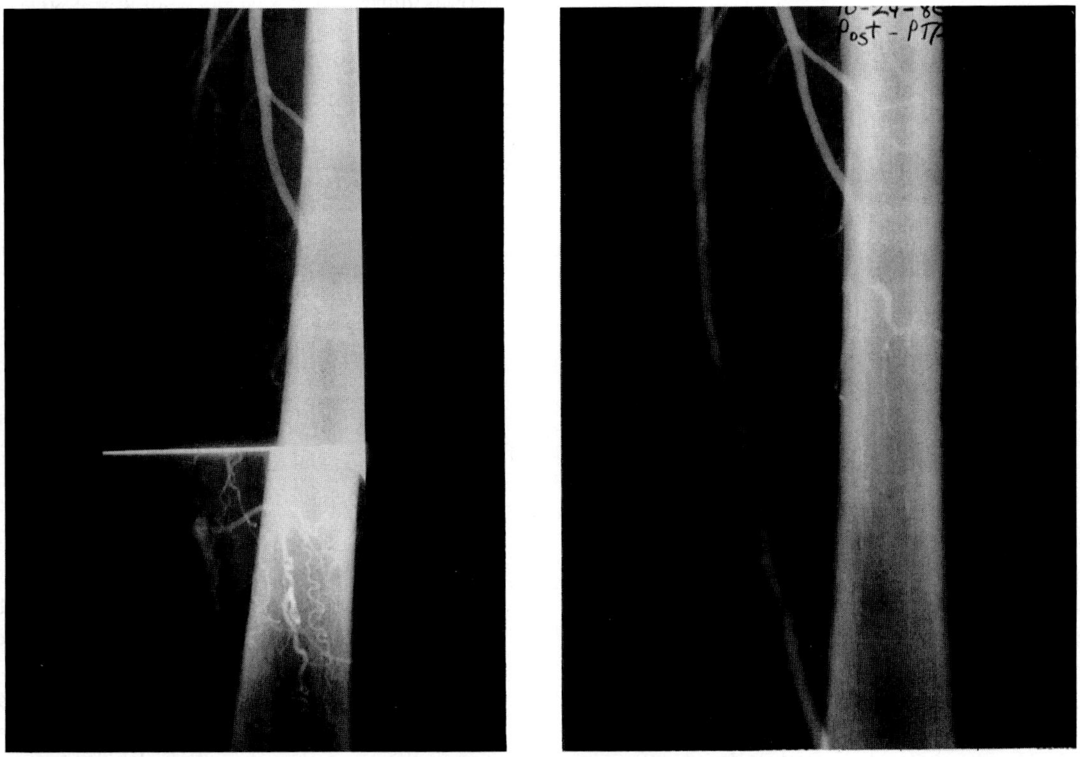

A B

Figure 32–3. Femoral angiograms. **A:** A 10 cm long occluded left superficial femoral artery with reconstitution of the distal portion from collateral vessels of the femoral profundus artery. **B:** The result after laser recanalization and balloon dilation. The proximal residual dissection was created by the balloon dilation. The Laserprobe was not used over the portion of the artery that developed the dissection.

with the nonheated Laserprobe itself. All three modes, the guide wire, the heated Laserprobe, and the nonheated Laserprobe, predominantly followed the path of least resistance and were deflected away from the hard, fibrocalcific plaque (Fig. 32-4). Instead of following the path of the true lumen, the devices advanced in the plane between the intima and the media (Fig. 32-5). This plane between the internal elastic lamina and the atheroma plaque is the same dissection plane that is created during mechanical endartherectomy to lift up and remove the plaque. In addition, two of ten arteries were perforated with the guide wire, one of four were perforated with the nonheated Laserprobe, and 10 of 11 arteries were perforated with the heated Laserprobe ($p < 0.01$). Once the device was in this dissection plane, it could take one of three pathways (Fig. 32-6). The guide wire or probe could continue within the dissection plane until the end of the artery section; it could continue within the dissection plane until the atheroma became thin again more distally, at which point the device could potentially reenter the true lumen; or it could continue laterally and perforate the arterial wall. The presence of a heated Laserprobe at 200°C within this dissection plane would explain the higher perforation rate with the heated probe than with the nonheated devices. In fact, to take advantage of this process of mechanical recanalization, Meier and colleagues[48] have developed a guide wire designed specifically for this purpose (Magnum wire, Schneider Europe). It is a 0.021 inch solid steel wire with a distal flexible spring wire and an olive-shaped ball tip of 1 mm in diameter. Using this wire in 17 patients with chronic total coronary occlusions that were refractory to conventional techniques, 8 (47%) were successfully crossed with the Magnum wire.

Moriuchi and associates[49] extended these observations by comparing the excimer laser as well to the heated Laserprobe and the mechanical guide wire. They found that the excimer laser maintained a pathway through the atheroma in only 8 of 21 arterial segments (38%), and in the other 13 it was deflected by the fibrocalcific plaque to follow a plane between the internal elastic membrane and the media. External perforation occurred in 7 of these 13 arteries (54%). In all of the perforated arteries, extensive calcification of the atheroma was noted.

The following case history demonstrates that this mechanism of mechanical recanalization indeed occurs clinically and is not isolated to peripheral artery occlusion. Figure 32-7 displays a series of coronary angiograms from a patient 3 days after a myocardial infarction with recurrent angina who had a complete occlusion of the left anterior descending artery. The occluded artery was successfully reopened with relief of the angina using a standard mechanical method with an 0.018 inch guide wire and a 3.0 mm angioplasty balloon dilation catheter. A follow-up angiogram 2 months later (Fig. 32-7C) demonstrated wide patency at the level of previous dilation with adequate flow down the distal anterior descending artery. Because of the presence of left main and triple vessel coronary artery disease, it was decided to send the patient electively for coronary bypass surgery. The patient had a perioperative inferior wall infarction and died. The histologic section of the left anterior descending artery at the level of the previous balloon angioplasty is shown in Figure 32-7D. The guide wire in this clinically successful mechanical recanalization did not push through the central portion of the atheroma to reenter the distal lumen. The histologic sections demonstrate that the mechanically recanalized lumen (which remained patent for 2 months), had been created by the guide wire and catheter after they were deflected from the resistant fibrous plaque and tracked between the media and the intima. There is disruption of the media and internal elastic membrane secondary to the balloon distention.

The results of these studies and observations suggest that the major mechanism of action of the metal-capped Laserprobe during recanalization is a mechanical process. In fact, the mechanism of successful recanalization of occluded arteries by most devices is a mechanical process of dissection between the atheroma and the internal elastic membrane. Neither the Laserprobe nor standard guide wires inherently seek the "true lumen" of a chronically occluded artery. Evidence that the pathway of recanalization is a mechanical process around the atheroma plaque and within the periintimal dissection plane has recently been provided by the new methodology of intravascular ultrasound imaging. In this technology, a 20 MHz ultrasound transducer has been miniaturized and adapted on the end of a 1.2 mm catheter with the ultrasound beam directed perpendicularly to the long axis of the catheter. Early in vitro studies demonstrated that high-quality cross-sectional arterial images could be obtained of the lumen and arterial wall (Fig. 32-8).[50]

More recent clinical studies with mechanically rotating catheters that yield real-time images at 30 frames/sec, provide exquisite in vivo images of microanatomic structures and tissue characteristics such as fibrosis and calcification. In one study during Laserprobe recanalization, the Laserprobe successfully recanalized a 20 cm long occlusion of the superficial femoral artery.[51] This was accomplished without turning the laser on, that is, the probe was used as a nonheated mechanical device (Fig. 32-9A, B). The ultrasound imaging catheter was placed in the track created by the Laserprobe and the cross-sectional images revealed that the probe started within the true lumen of the vessel (Fig. 32-9C) but was quickly deflected after 3 cm of penetrating the occlusion and entered the dissection plane between the internal elastic membrane and the atheroma (Fig. 32-9D, 9E). The probe continued in this plane in a retrograde fashion from the adductor canal to the bifurcation of the superficial femoral artery with the common femoral artery. At the point where the atheroma thinned out, the Laserprobe penetrated the residual atheroma and reentered the true lumen of the common femoral artery. Balloon dilation extended the dissection plane and reestablished flow between the common femoral and popliteal arteries (Fig. 32-9F). Representative intravascular ultrasound images following balloon dilation

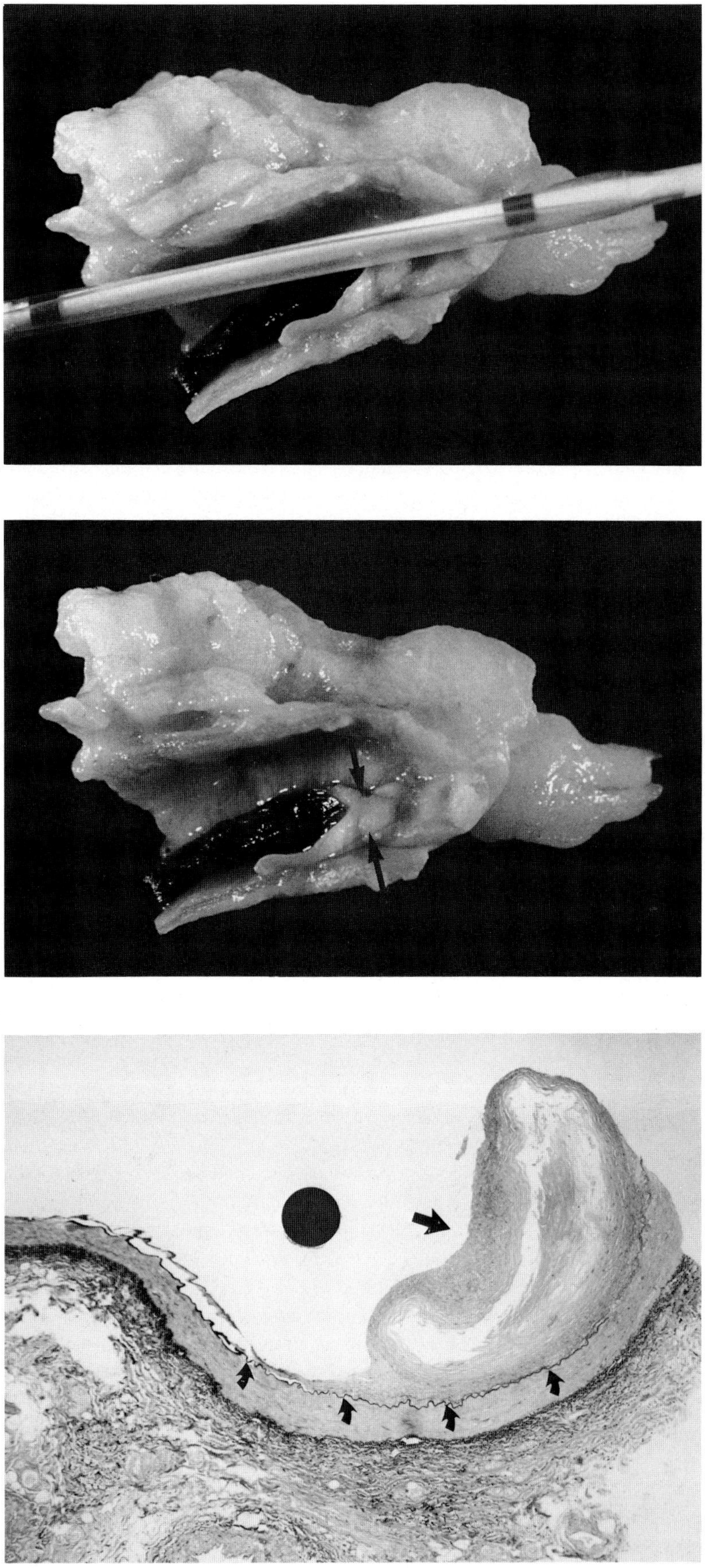

A

B

C

Figure 32–4. This completely occluded arterial segment was recanalized with an 0.018 inch guide wire and a 3.0 mm diameter angioplasty balloon. The artery was opened longitudinally prior to histologic section. **A:** The path of the balloon is demonstrated. **B:** With the balloon removed, the obstruction was noted to consist of a preexistent thrombus that funneled into a fibrous plaque and occluded the artery. The guide wire did not pass through the clot or the central atheroma but was observed at the periphery of the plaque. **C:** This histologic cross-section was taken at the level of the arrow in **B.** The guide wire and balloon were deflected from the central atheroma and advanced along a plane (represented by the circle) that was just central to the internal elastic membrane (small arrows) but was still within the intima. The inflation of the balloon indented the atheroma laterally from its side (thick arrow) and stretched the external arterial circumference.

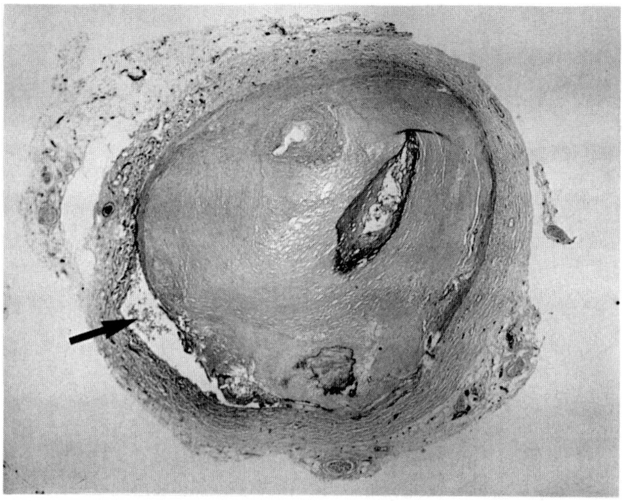

Figure 32–5. The path of the Laserprobe is demonstrated in this histologic section of a completely occluded human right coronary artery. The Laserprobe has created a new lumen in a peripheral portion of the artery, as documented by the residual suture material (thick arrow). The channel created by the Laserprobe lies outside of the fibrotic native lumen. The silk thread fibers are adjacent to the internal elastic membrane in a plane between the plaque and the media.

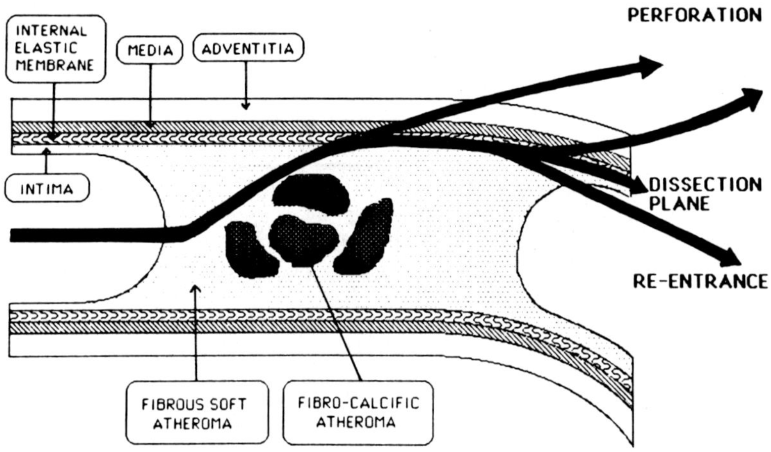

Figure 32–6. Schematic diagram of the laser fiber and catheter pathways. When there is a densely calcified or fibrotic atheroma, the laser catheters are deflected around the atheroma and advanced into a less resistant dissection plane between the internal elastic membrane and the atheroma plaque. Eventually, these devices may reenter the native lumen when the atheroma becomes thinner; they may remain within the dissection plane, or they may perforate externally. (Reprinted with permission.)

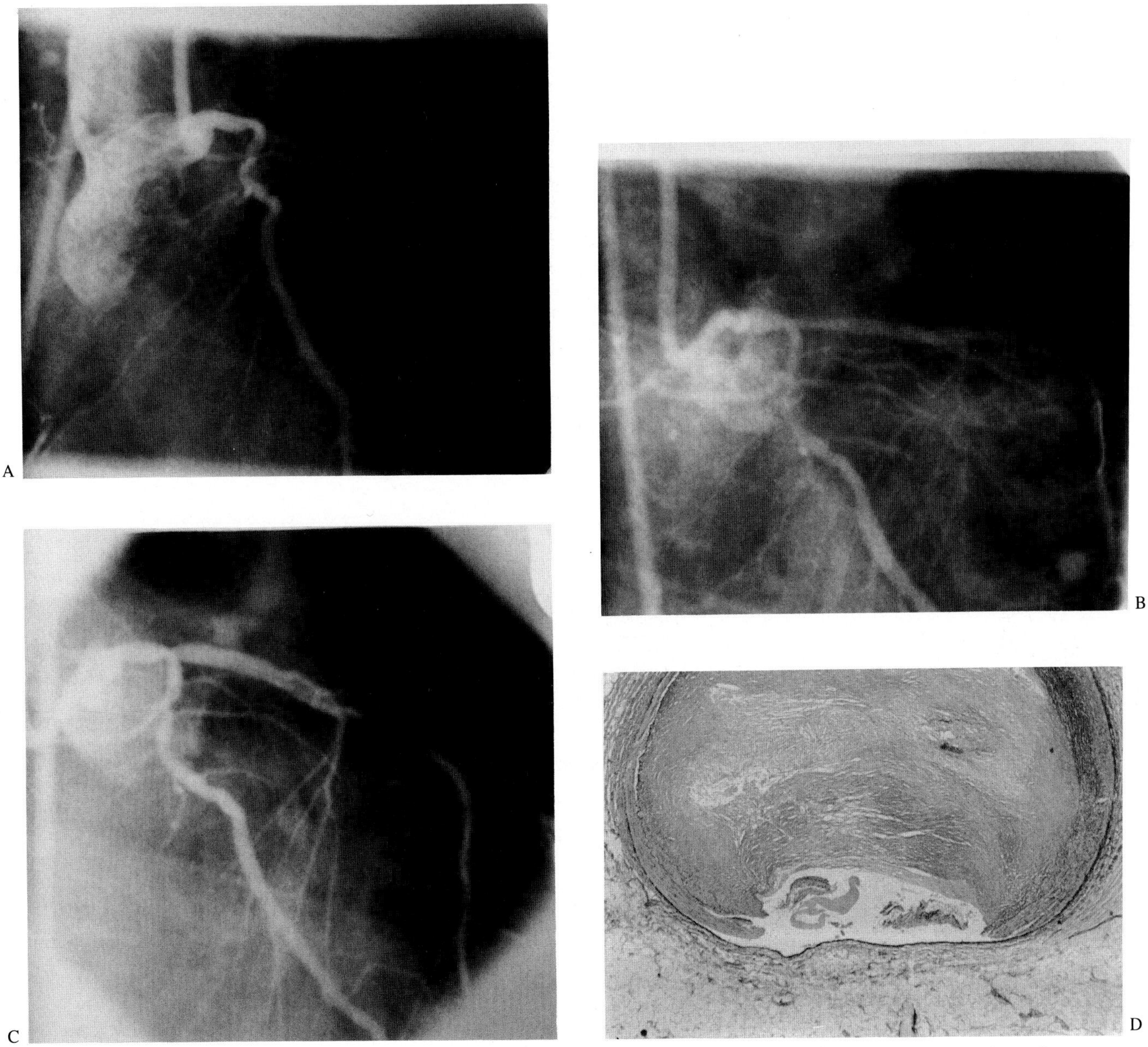

Figure 32–7. **A:** A coronary angiogram in the right anterior oblique projection from a patient with a recent anterior wall myocardial infarction demonstrates complete occlusion of the left anterior descending artery. **B:** The artery was mechanically probed with an 0.018 inch guide wire and the proximal portion of the artery was dilated with a 3.0 mm angioplasty balloon. This injection performed over the guide wire (visible in the distal segment) demonstrates patency of the distal lumen following successful recanalization. **C:** An angiogram obtained 2 months later revealed continued patency and adequate antegrade flow in the anterior descending artery. There is moderate residual disease in the left main and proximal circumflex. **D:** Histologic sections were taken every 5 mm throughout the length of the coronary arteries. This section was taken from the segment of the left anterior descending artery that had been mechanically recanalized and dilated. There is disruption of the media and internal elastic membrane with the recreated lumen constituted in the plane between the adventitia and the atheromatous plaque. There is minimal compression of the plaque.

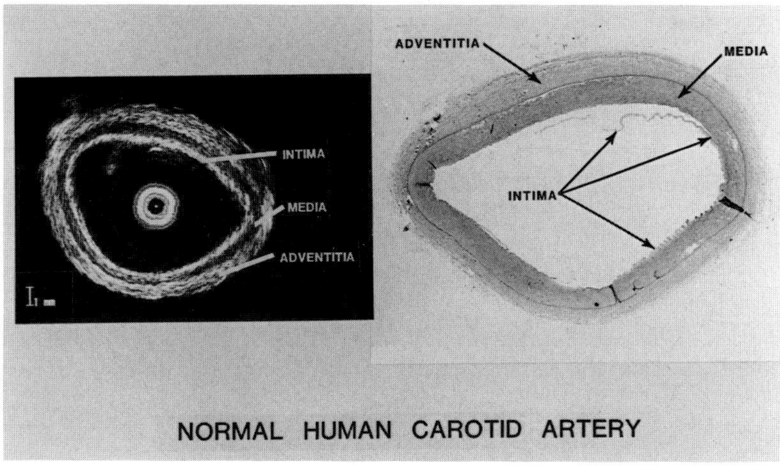

Figure 32–8. In this intravascular ultrasound image of a normal human carotid artery, a characteristic three-layer appearance is seen. The muscular medial layer of the artery is relatively echolucent and provides a reference point in the arterial cross-section separating intima from adventitia. The intima is seen extending from the lumen-tissue interface to the echolucent media. The adventitia consists of all echoes originating peripherally to the media. The corresponding histologic section demonstrates a thin intima that is in part artificially separated from the media. The dense echoes on the ultrasound image overestimate the intimal thickness. The media appears thicker on the histologic section than on the ultrasound image. The images are not at the same scale. (Reprinted with permission.)

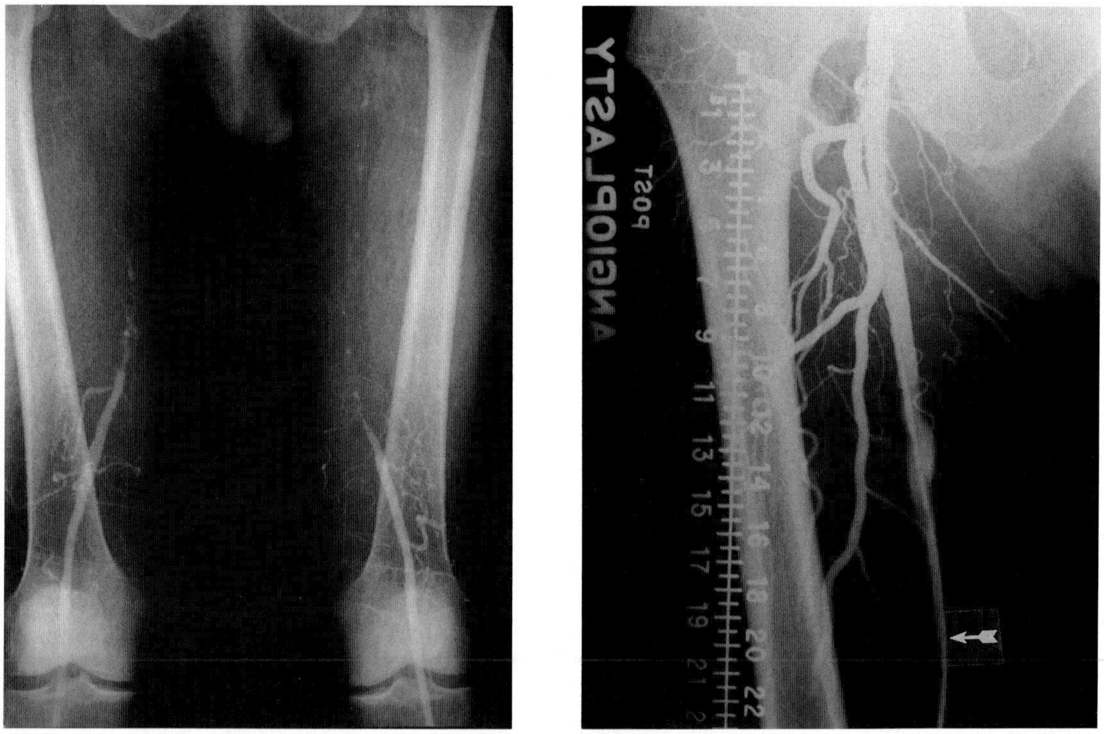

A B

Figure 32–9. A: Baseline angiogram of lower extremities showing complete bilateral occlusion of the superficial femoral artery with reconstitution at the adductor canal. **B:** Angiogram following mechanical recanalization with the nonheated Laserprobe. From a retrograde approach, continuity was established between the popliteal and common femoral artery. The catheter pathway can be seen at the arrow.

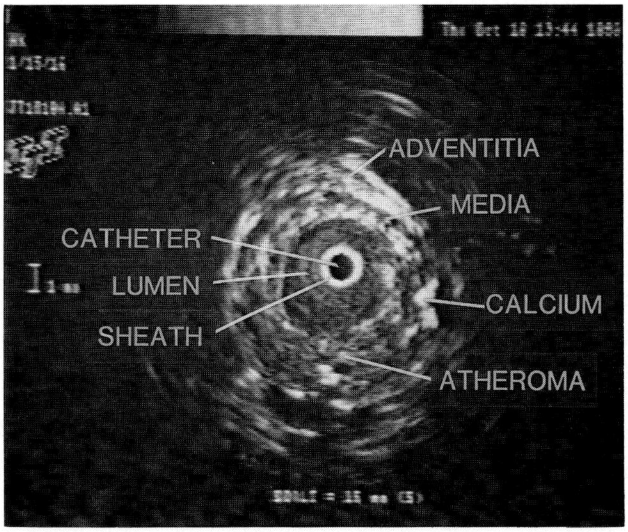

C

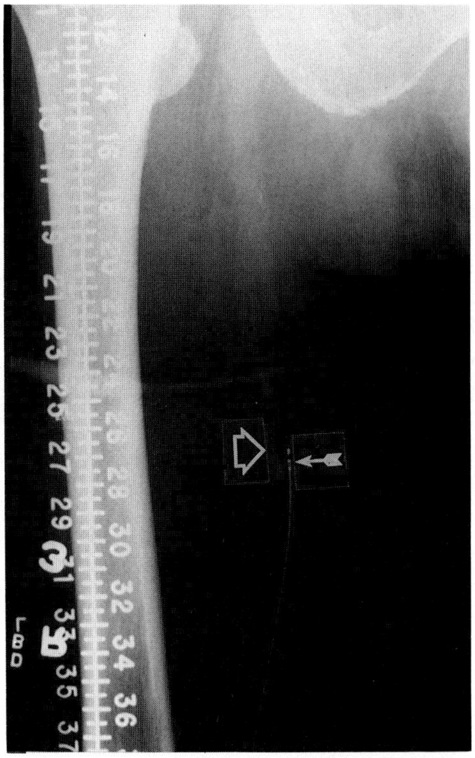

D

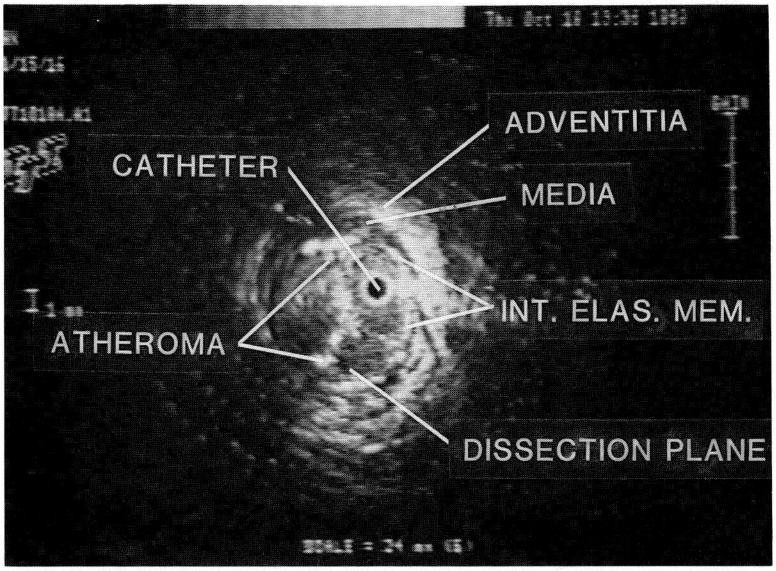

E

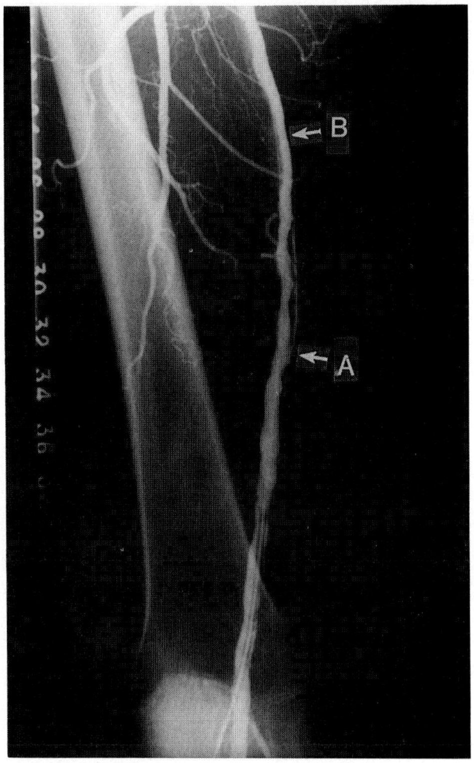

F

Figure 32–9 *(continued)*. **C:** Intravascular ultrasound image in the distal superficial femoral artery (SFA) prior to entering the area of recanalization. The central black area is due to the catheter itself; around this is the white echoreflection from the plastic sheath. In a radial distribution is the echolucent lumen, then a thick atheroma with variable echoreflections, depending on the amount of collagen within the plaque or the presence of calcium. **D:** Radiograph showing position of the ultrasound catheter parallel to a slightly radiopaque area of residual contrast and atheroma. **E:** The path of the Laserprobe is documented in this ultrasound image, in which the ultrasound catheter was passed over a guide wire along the same pathway. Instead of recanalizing the artery through the central atheroma, the catheter is in a dissection plane between the atheroma and the internal elastic membrane. **F:** Angiogram of SFA after balloon angioplasty shows a patent vessel with areas of dissection. The ultrasound images obtained at levels A and B are demonstrated in Figures 32-10 and 32-11, respectively.

are demonstrated in Figures 32-10 and 32-11. The ankle to arm index increased from 0.6 to 1.0 following the recanalization procedure.

These studies suggest that the laser-heated thermal probe acts predominantly as a mechanical guide wire, and it may be effective in that capacity even as a nonheated probe to recanalize occluded arteries. The only randomized controlled study to test this hypothesis was recently published.[52] Forty patients with an occlusion of the superficial femoral artery (mean length 16 ± 10 cm) were randomly treated by standard guide wire and catheter mechanical recanalization (20 pts), or by the laser probe (20 pts). The laser probe was used initially as a mechanical, nonthermal device and was successful in 13 of 15 patients (87%) *without* turning on the laser. In the 5 patients where the cold laser probe did not reopen the artery, the laser was then activated. This resulted in a successful result in an additional 2 patients, but also induced an arterial perforation in the other 3 patients. The overall success rate for the laser probe was 15 of 20 (75%). This was not significantly different from the success rate with the standard mechanical technique (19 of 20 pts, 95%).

The results of this randomized trial do not support the hypotheses behind the use of the thermal laser probe. Contrary to the assumption that the application of laser and thermal energy is necessary, this study demonstrates that the laser probe functions primarily as a mechanical device. The thermal activation does not significantly improve the success rate without increasing the risk of perforation. This small additional benefit does not justify the large cost of current thermal laser devices. This controlled study also demonstrates a higher success rate in long occlusions than in previous reports of mechanical balloon recanalization. This is due to a combination approach of retrograde and anterograde probing of the occluded segment.

This study underscores the necessity of performing randomized, controlled studies to test the claims of laser enthusiasts in the treatment of atherosclerosis. The use of historical controls to compare current techniques is not appropriate. These lessons have yet to be appreciated in the current claims of excimer laser energy for the treatment of coronary artery stenosis.

CONCLUSION

Knowledge gained up to this time has contributed greatly to our understanding of the responses of biologic tissue to laser angioplasty and has pointed us in the right direction to overcome the complications associated with laser photoablation of atherosclerosis. The studies cited in this chapter indicate that a guidance system that can consistently maintain coaxial alignment of the laser delivery catheter must be devised to seek the true lumen. All guidance systems must take into account the significant contribution of the mechanical force behind any laser catheter device. This mechanical force can be effective in helping to reopen occlusions; however, the user must understand the high likelihood that any device is likely to seek the path of least resistance and enter the dissection plane adjacent to the atheroma. Until better guidance systems are developed, the application of laser energy in atherosclerosis will be to enlarge stenotic lumen with coaxial fiberoptics that pass over a central guide wire. The intravascular ultrasound imaging device may provide the type of guidance that is necessary to exert control over the ablative power of laser energy. However, attempts at recanalization of complete occlusions with presently configured laser devices result in an unacceptable incidence of arterial perforation.

Acknowledgment. This study was supported in part by National Institutes of Health (NIH) grant PR01192, NIH HL31318, and SD1084-88-C-0025.

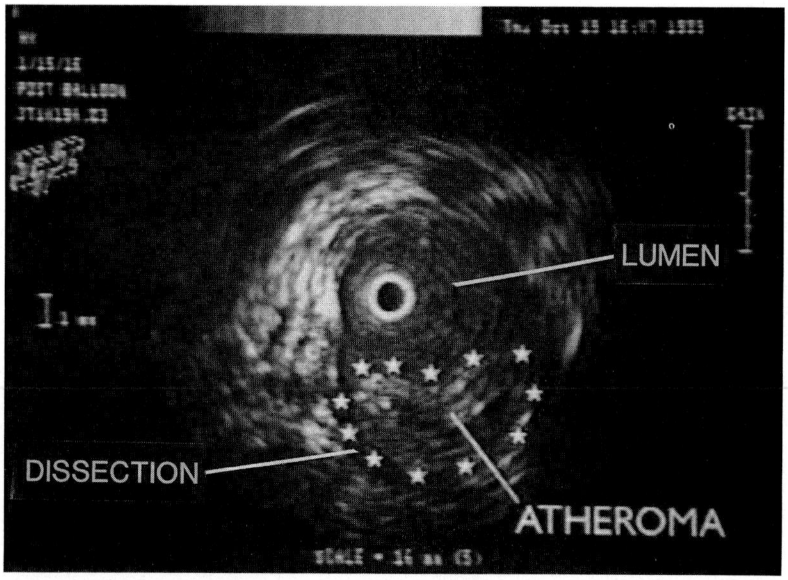

Figure 32–10. Ultrasound image at level A in Figure 32-9F following balloon angioplasty shows an eccentric atheroma that has been deformed by the balloon. In addition, there is a dissection around the capsule of the atheroma that separates the atheroma from the media.

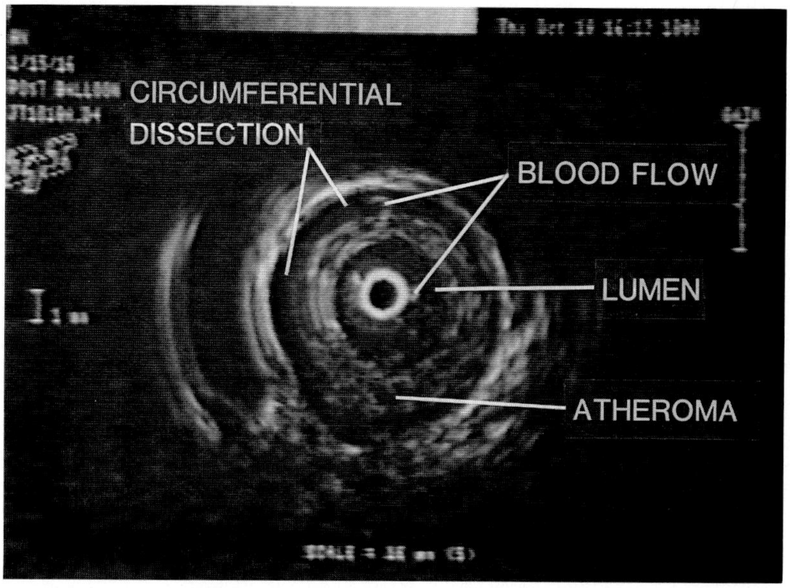

Figure 32–11. Ultrasound image at level B of Figure 32-9F shows concentric atheroma that has not been torn at this level but has been separated from the media almost circumferentially. In real-time, the ultrasound images demonstrated blood pulsating in the dissection plane as well as in the lumen.

REFERENCES

1. Ginsburg R, Wexler L, Mitchell RS, Profitt D. Percutaneous transluminal laser angioplasty for treatment of peripheral vascular disease: clinical experience with 16 patients. Radiology 1985;156:619–24.
2. Isner JM: Spasm. In Isner JM, Clarke R (eds): Cardiovascular Laser Therapy. New York: Raven Press, 1989:121.
3. Cumberland DC, Starkey IR, Oakley GDG, et al. Percutaneous laser-assisted coronary angioplasty. (Letter.) Lancet 1986;2:214.
4. Ragimov SE, Belyaev AA, Vertepa IA, et al. Comparison of different lasers in terms of thrombogenicity of the laser-treated vascular wall. Lasers Surg Med 1988;8:77–82.
5. Lee G, Ikeda RM, Chan MC, et al. Limitation, risks, and complications of laser angioplasty: a cautious approach warranted. Am J Cardiol 1985;56:181–5.
6. Lee G, Ikeda RM, Theis JM, et al. Acute and chronic complications of laser angioplasty: vascular wall damage and formation of aneurysms in the atherosclerotic rabbit. Am J Cardiol 1984;53:290–3.
7. Crea F, Abela GS, Fenech A, et al. Transluminal laser irradiation of coronary arteries in live dogs: an angiographic and morphologic study of acute effects. Am J Cardiol 1986;57:171–4.
8. Grundfest WS, et al. The current status of angioscopy and laser angioplasty. J Vasc Surg 1987;5:667.
9. Welch AJ. The thermal response of laser irradiated tissue. IEEE J Quantum Electronics 1984;QE-20:1471–81.
10. Alexopoulos D, Sanborn TA. The biological response to laser angioplasty. Cardio 1989;6:95–7.
11. Wollenek G, Laufer G. Laser angioplasty in the treatment of peripheral vascular disease. State of the art 1988. Herz 1989;14:29–38.
12. Cross F, Bowker T, Langley A, et al. Evidence for non-thermal ablation from emission spectroscopy of photoproducts. (Abstr.) Circulation 1986;74(suppl II):II-361.
13. Garrison BJ, Srinivasan R. Microscopic model for the ablative decomposition of polymers by far-ultraviolet radiation (193 nm). Appl Phys Lett 1984;44:849–51.
14. Grundfest WS, Litvack F, Doyle L, et al. Comparison of in vitro and in vivo thermal effects of argon and excimer lasers for laser angioplasty. (Abstr.) Circulation 1986;74(suppl II):II-204.
15. Murphy-Chutorian D, Selzer PM, Kosek J, et al. The interaction between excimer laser energy and vascular tissue. Am Heart J 1986;112:739–45.
16. Grundfest RS, Litvack IF, Goldenberg T, et al. Pulsed ultraviolet lasers and the potential for safe laser angioplasty. Am J Surg 1985;150:220–6.
17. Berns MW, Liaw LH, Allison O, et al. An acute light and electron microscopic study of ultraviolet 193nm excimer laser corneal incisions. Ophthalmology 1988;95:1422–33.
18. Abela GS, Norman S, Cohen D, et al. Effects of carbon dioxide, Nd:YAG, and argon laser radiation on coronary atheromatous plaques. Am J Cardiol 1982;50:1199–1205.
19. Litvack F, Grundfest W, Fishbein M, et al. A standardized method for study of laser tissue interaction (Abstr.) Circulation 1984;70:II-35.
20. Steg PG, Astier R, Meyer G, et al. In vitro pulsed laser angioplasty of human atheromatous coronary arteries. Laser 1986;2:156.
21. Abela GS: Laser recanalization: a basic and clinical perspective. Thorac Cardiovasc Surg 1988;36:137–141.
22. Isner JM, Donaldson RF, Deckelbaum LI, et al. The excimer laser: gross, light microscopic, and ultrastructural analysis of potential advantages for use in laser therapy of cardiovascular disease. J Am Coll Cardiol 1985;6:1102–1109.
23. Fenech A, Abela GS, Crea F, et al. A comparative study of laser beam characteristics in blood and saline media. Am J Cardiol 1985;55:1389–92.
24. Apfelberg DB, Maser MR, Lash H, Rivers J. The argon laser for cutaneous lesions. JAMA 1981;245:2073–5.
25. Gessman L, Reno C, Maranho V. Transcatheter dissolution of human atherosclerotic plaques: a model for testing catheters and techniques. Cathet Cardiovasc Diagn 1984;10:47–54.
26. Isner JM, Clarke RH, Donaldson RF, Aharon A. Identification of photoproducts liberated by in vitro argon laser irradiation of atherosclerotic plaque, calcified cardiac valves and myocardium. Am J Cardiol 1985;55:1192–6.

27. Abela GS, Norman SJ, Cohen DM, et al. Laser recanalization of occluded atherosclerotic arteries in vivo and in vitro. Circulation 1985;71:403–11.
28. Abela GS, Seeger JM, Barbier D, et al. Laser angioplasty with angioscopic guidance in man. J Am Coll Cardiol 1986;8:184–92.
29. Abela GS, Crea F, Seeger JM, et al. The healing process in normal canine arteries and in atherosclerotic monkey arteries after transluminal laser irradiation. Am J Cardiol 1985; 56:983–8.
30. Gerrity RG, Loop FD, Golding LAR, et al. Arterial response to laser operation for removal of atherosclerotic plaques. J Thorac Cardiovasc Surg 1983;85:409–21.
31. Abela GS, Barbieri E, Conti CR. Laser therapy in cardiovascular disease. Prog Cardiol 1987;15:155–68.
32. Barger AC, Beeuwkes R, Lainey LL, Silverman KJ. Hypothesis: vasa vasorum and neovascularization of human coronary arteries. A possible role in the pathophysiology of atherosclerosis. N Engl J Med 1983;310:175–7.
33. Prevosti LG, Leon MB, Dodd JT, et al. Early and late healing responses of canine arterial wall to excimer laser irradiation (Abstr.) J Am Coll Cardiol 1987;9:85A.
34. Forrester JS, Litvack F, Grundfest W. Vaporization of atheroma in man: the role of lasers in the era of balloon angioplasty. Int J Cardiol 1988;20:1–7.
35. Litvack F, Doyle L, Grundfest W, et al. In vivo excimer laser ablation: acute and chronic effects on canine aorta. (Abstr.) Circulation 1986;74(suppl II):II-360.
36. Sanborn TA, Faxon DP, Haudenschild CC, Ryan TJ. Experimental angioplasty: circumferential distribution of laser thermal energy with a laserprobe. J Am Coll Cardiol 1985; 5:934–8.
37. Abela GS, Seeger JM, Barbier E, et al. Laser angioplasty with angioscopic guidance in humans. J Am Coll Cardiol 1986; 8:184–92.
38. Spears JR. Percutaneous transluminal coronary angioplasty: potential prevention with laser balloon angioplasty. Am J Cardiol 1987;60:61B–4B.
39. Nordstrom LA, Castañeda-Zuñiga WR, Young EG, Von Seggern KB. Direct argon laser exposure for recanalization of peripheral arteries: early results. Radiology 1988;168:359–64.
40. Geschwind HJ, Kern MJ, Vandormael MG, et al. Efficiency and safety of optically modified fiber tips for laser angioplasty. J Am Coll Cardiol 1987;10:655–61.
41. Litvack F, Grundfest WS, Goldenberg T, et al. Percutaneous excimer laser angioplasty of aortocoronary saphenous vein grafts. J Am Coll Cardiol 1989;14:803–8.
42. Leon MB, Lu DY, Prevosti LG, et al. Human arterial surface fluorescence: atherosclerotic plaque identification and effects of laser atheroma ablation. J Am Coll Cardiol 1988;12:94–102.
43. Lee G, Ikeda RM, Chan MC, et al. Dissolution of human atherosclerotic disease by fiberoptic laser-heated metal cautery cap. Am Heart J 1984;107:777–8.
44. Cumberland DC, Sanborn TA, Tayler DI, et al. Percutaneous laser thermal angioplasty: initial clinical results with a laserprobe in total peripheral artery occlusions. Lancet 1986; 1:1457–9.
45. Tobis J, Smolin M, Mallery J, et al. Laser-assisted thermal angioplasty in human peripheral artery occlusions: mechanisms of recanalization. J Am Coll Cardiol 1989;13:1547–54.
46. Sanborn TA, Cumberland DC, Greenfield AJ, et al. Peripheral laser-assisted balloon angioplasty. Arch Surg 1989;124:1099–103.
47. van Breda A. Laser Angioplasty. Radiologic Clinics of North America 1989;6:1217–22.
48. Meier B, Carlier M, Finci L, et al. Magnum wire for balloon recanalization of chronic total coronary occlusions. Am J Cardiol 1989;64:148–54.
49. Moriuchi M, Tobis JM, McRae M, et al. A comparison of excimer laser, thermal probe, and mechanical devices for recanalizing occluded human arteries. Japanese Circulation Journal 1991;55(6):591–600.
50. Tobis JM, Mallery JA, Gessert J, et al. Intravascular ultrasound cross-sectional arterial imaging before and after angioplasty in vitro. Circulation 1989;80:873–82.
51. Tobis JM, Miranda CP, Deutsch L, et al. The mechanism of peripheral recanalization by laser-assisted thermal angioplasty. Confirmation by intravascular ultrasound. AJR 1990;155: 1100–2.
52. Tobis JM, Conroy R, Deutsch LS, et al. Laser-assisted versus mechanical recanalization of femoral arterial occlusions. Am J Cardiol 1991;68:1079–86.

33 Thermo-Optical Laser Recanalization of Totally Occluded Peripheral Arteries

Gérald R. Barbeau, M.D., Phillippe P. Giacomino, M.D., James S. Seeger, M.D., George S. Abela, M.D.

EXPERIMENTAL BACKGROUND

Preliminary experimental work done in our and other laboratories has shown that atherosclerotic plaque can be vaporized effectively with argon and neodymium:yttrium aluminum garnet (Nd:YAG) continuous wave lasers transmitted by silica optical fibers.[1–5]

Various fiber-catheter devices were first used to test the feasibility of laser ablation and evaluate the acute and chronic effects on healing in normal and atherosclerotic animals[6–10] (Fig. 33-1). These studies revealed that plaque vaporization could be accomplished within blood-filled vessels, without acute occlusion by flaps or thrombosis.[7,8] Also, there was no acceleration of the atherosclerotic process when laser irradiation was performed in the peripheral arteries of atherosclerotic animals.[11–13] However, irradiation through optical fibers with bare-ended tips was associated with a small channel size and a high rate of arterial perforation.[14] The high arterial perforation rate was mainly due to stiffness and sharpness of the bare silica fiber, as well as scattering of the laser beam. Another major limitation associated with the bare silica fiber was that the radiolucent fiber could not be visualized by fluoroscopy.

In order to prevent arterial perforation, an attempt was made to improve visualization of the probe tip by the incorporation of a radiopaque metal sleeve that was crimped at the distal end of the fiber.[8] Although the direction of the fiber tip could be observed under fluoroscopy, the perforation rate did not improve due to lack of direction control and persistent beam scattering. The addition of the metal sleeve, however, served to protect the fiber tip against destruction by the reflected laser beam, thus maintaining the optical integrity of the device.

Further device modification consisted of complete encapsulation of the fiber tip using a metallic cap.[14–16] This resulted in a less traumatic probe tip when compared with the bare-ended tip and also reduced the arterial perforation rate.[14,17] Also, the availability of different probe sizes (1 to 2.5 mm) made possible the creation of channel larger than the fiber body. This device, however, became a thermal probe that could only vaporize plaque by direct tissue contact. Because the metal cap stiffened the fiber tip, this system was limited in negotiating plaque at arterial bends. Thus, the finer control of the photoablative process by the laser beam was lost.[18]

UNIVERSITY OF FLORIDA EXPERIENCE

Clinical experience at the University of Florida, College of Medicine, was initiated in 1984 with a Phase I feasibility trial, as the first Food and Drug Administration (FDA)-approved clinical trial for peripheral laser angioplasty.[19] This trial was primarily designed to evaluate the immediate effects of laser recanalization.

In a second phase, laser was used as sole therapy to recanalize peripheral occluded arteries. However, if unable to achieve a sufficient channel with less than 50% residual luminal stenosis, the artery was bypassed during the same procedure. In both Phases I and II, all procedures were performed via femoral cut-down in the operating room.

In a third phase, begun in 1986, cases were attempted percutaneously with, if necessary, balloon angioplasty as adjunctive therapy. This also included some procedures that were performed intraoperatively in patients with access problems or who required additional surgical procedures for inflow disease. Only totally occluded vessels were attempted, after standard balloon angioplasty recanalization techniques had not been successful.

A "hybrid" probe was used in all three phases of this clinical trial. This device is composed of a steel jacket at the tip of a 300 μm core silica fiber. Unlike the hot-tip probe, 20% of the input laser beam exits from the tip through a circular window incorporated at the fiber tip, and the remaining energy serves to heat the metal cap. A microlens was placed in front of the fiber to focus the laser beam[20] (Fig. 33-2). This combination provides an optically made crater and a thermally made crater (Fig. 33-3). This dual effect makes the vaporization with the hybrid probe more efficient than a pure thermal device.[18]

Phase I

During phase I, laser recanalization was performed in 11 patients with totally occluded superficial femoral arteries prior to bypass procedures. The hybrid probe was tested in two different sizes: a 1 mm steel cap composed of an open-ended ring or a 2 mm elliptical tip with a 250 μm window at the tip that allowed exit of 20% of the input laser beam.[19]

In this trial, 10 to 15 cm of the common and superficial femoral arteries were exposed before probe insertion into the

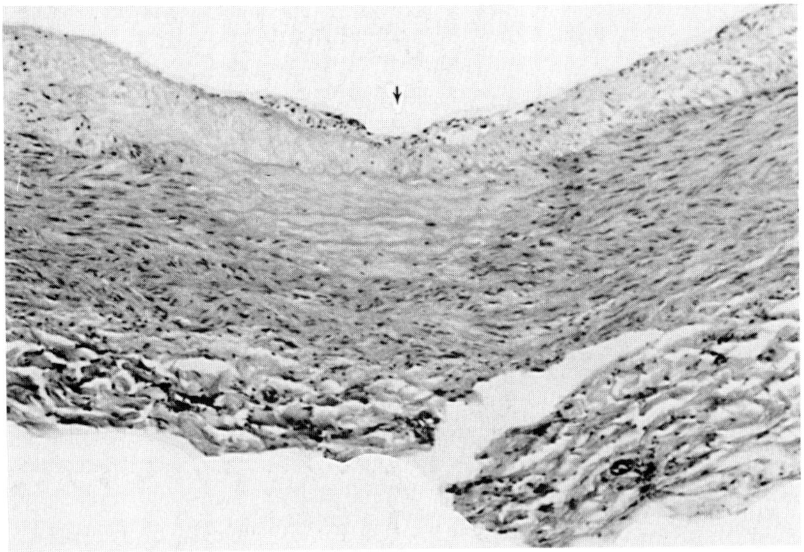

Figure 33–1. Laser crater in an atherosclerotic monkey sacrificed at 30 days following lasing (2.5 W for 1 sec). A central zone shows the area of previous lasing, which represents a crater filled with loose cellular elements with a reendothelialized surface (arrow). The reformed arterial intima at the crater site is thinner than at the adjacent unlased area of plaque. (Reprinted with permission from Abela et al.[12])

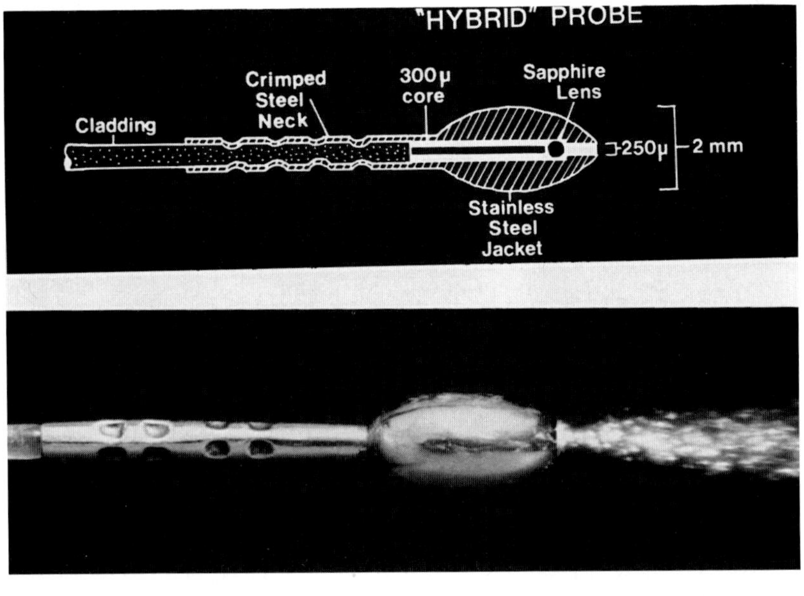

Figure 33–2. Hybrid probe (Spectraprobe PLR). **Top panel:** Schematic of a "hybrid" probe is illustrated. A metal cap 2 mm in diameter is crimped on a 300 µm core fiber. A 250 µm window allows 20% of the laser beam to exit. Behind the window a sapphire lens is used to focus the beam as it exits. **Bottom panel:** Probe with exiting argon laser beam. The beam has a waist at 1 mm from the probe tip and is defocused into a diffuse light. (Reprinted with permission from Abela GS et al.[19])

arteriotomy. Laser recanalization was attempted only in the occluded segment of the artery, using angioscopic and fluoroscopic guidance. The recanalized portion of the artery was excised and the segment perfused with saline solution at a mean pressure of 80 mmHg to measure flow rate and to collect debris generated during laser recanalization. Segments were perfusion-fixed and mounted for histology. The bypass procedure was then completed in the usual fashion.

Overall, 11 of 13 totally occluded arteries were recanalized. Perforation occurred in all of the four arteries recanalized with the 1 mm probe although only two of the nine vessels treated with the 2 mm probe were perforated. Lumen diameter of the newly created channel using the 2 mm probe was larger than the probe size (3.0 ± 0.3 mm) with a flow of 157 ± 102 ml/mm (range, 60 to 360) (Fig. 33-4). The average amount of debris collected per artery weighed less than 1 mg (Fig. 33-5).

By histologic analysis, plaque composition of recanalized segments consisted of atherosclerotic plaque, which often had calcific deposits and fresh thrombus. Although thrombus was easily transversed with the probe, a patent lumen could not be established (Fig. 33-6). Transmission electron microscopy suggested that the internal elastic lamina of the laser recanalized artery may be selectively spared from thermal damage due to transparency to argon wavelength.

Phases II and III

In phases II and III, patients with ischemic symptoms were initially screened by a nurse coordinator. During the clinic

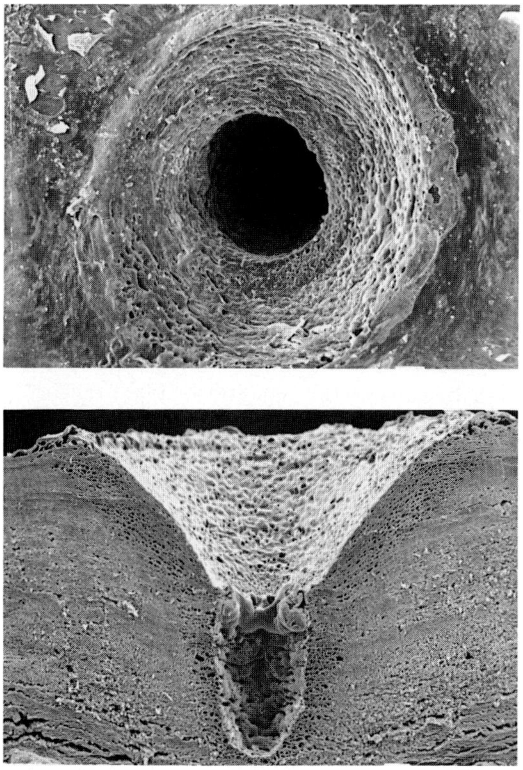

Figure 33–3. **Top panel:** Scanning electron microscope (SEM) (aerial view) of the intimal arterial surface showing the double-crater effect made by the thermal-optical, "hybrid" probe. Wrinkles on the surface correspond to the vacules seen at the tissue edges (see below). Laser power is 9 W, exposure time is 7 sec; Bar = 100 μm. **Bottom panel:** SEM (cross-section view) shows the double crater-crater effect. The deeper crater is made by the laser beam and it precedes the larger crater made by the metal probe. Bar = 100 μm. (Reprinted with permission from Hoffman et al.[18])

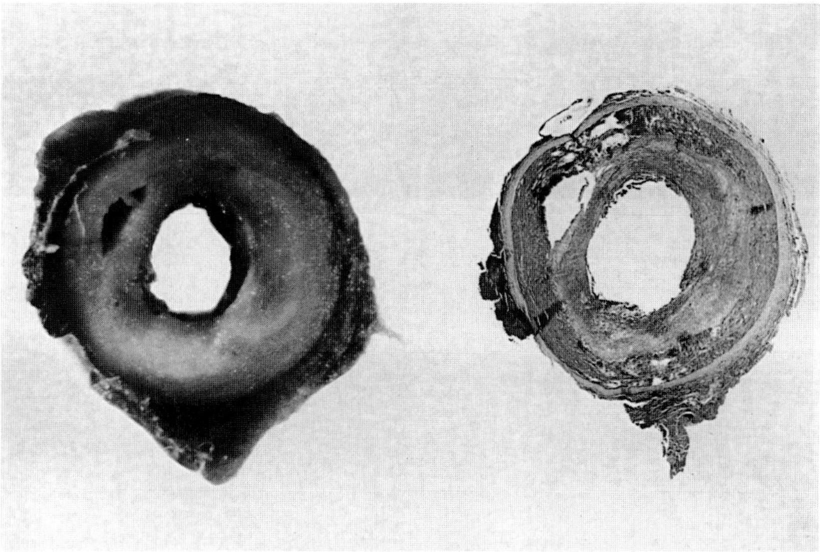

Figure 33–4. Recanalized artery. **Left,** fresh segment of superficial femoral artery after laser recanalization. The central channel was made using a 2 mm "hybrid" probe. The original lumen appears at the 11 o'clock position. **Right,** histologic cross-section of the recanalized artery illustrating a relatively smooth-walled central lumen with minimal charring and thermal injury made with the argon laser. The left upper quadrant shows the original vascular lumen. This is an example from a Phase I intraoperative recanalization procedure evaluating feasibility in humans (hematoxylin-eosin stain). (Reprinted with permission from Abela et al.[19])

visit, a complete physical examination was done and explanation of the procedure was conducted by a physician of the laser program. Clinical investigation included Doppler measurement of systolic segmental pressure at rest and following exercise. In patients considered potential candidates for laser angioplasty, an abdominal aortography with runoff arteriography was performed, unless a recent (less than 6 months) good quality angiogram was available. Only patients with totally occluded common iliac artery, superficial femoral artery, popliteal artery, or common peroneal artery were offered laser therapy.[21,22] Patients with significant stenotic lesions were referred for balloon angioplasty.

Of more than 350 patients screened, 71 patients fulfilled the inclusion criteria for laser recanalization and signed an informed consent. Patients received enteric-coated aspirin daily (325 to 650 mg) until the day of the procedure.

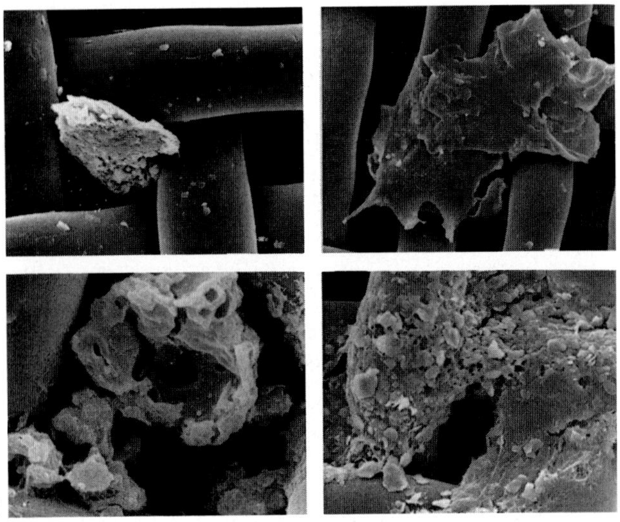

Figure 33–5. Scanning electron micrographs of debris products from patients following recanalization of the superficial femoral artery. Recanalization was done using a hybrid probe and the filtering mesh was 40 μm. Bar, 20 μm. **A:** Particulate debris of plaque is shown entrapped in the mesh. **B:** Denatured cells, possibly endothelial cells, are also shown on the mesh. **C:** Small cellular debris with remote resemblance to fused red blood cells are seen going through the mesh. **D:** Network of fused cellular fragments in smaller debris are shown adhering to mesh. (Reprinted with permission from Abela GS.[27])

Laser Procedure

Percutaneous procedures were performed in the radiology suite under local anesthesia[21] (2% lidocaine). A 7 to 9 F introducer sheath was placed in the ipsilateral common femoral artery using the Seldinger technique. Baseline angiography was obtained and served as guidance throughout the procedure. For all lesions, recanalization was first attempted by a radiologist using guide wire and balloon angioplasty techniques. A bolus of 5000 U of heparin and 200 μg of nitroglycerin were given intra-arterially prior to the introduction of the probe.

A 2 or 2.5 mm sterile disposable hybrid probe (Spectraprobe-PRL, Trimedyne, Santa Ana, CA) and a 0.016 inch guide wire were backloaded into a 7 F thin-walled catheter (Cook, Bloomington, IN), with a hemostasis valve at the hub allowing saline and contrast injections. The proximal end of the probe was attached to an argon ion laser source (HGM, Salt Lake City, UT; or Laser Ionics, Orlando, FL) and tested in saline for 3 sec irradiation at 1 W to ensure laser-fiber coupling.

After testing, probes were inserted in the introducer sheaths and advanced under fluoroscopy to the level of the obstruction. Gentle attempts were made to penetrate the obstruction mechanically with the probe. If unsuccessful, the laser was activated initially at 5 W with 1 sec exposures and 0.2 sec exposure intervals. After laser irradiation of 2 to 3 sec, probes were advanced at a rate of 2 cm/sec. Once the blockage was penetrated, laser power was held constant unless further resistance was encountered. If the probe could not be advanced, laser power was increased by 1 W increments up to 12 W. After the lesion was crossed, the guide wire was left in place and the probe was pulled back, while activated at slightly higher powers, up to a maximum of 14 W. Repeat angiogram was made to assess the result. If channel diameter appeared less than 50% of the arterial lumen above and below the obstructed segment, balloon angioplasty was performed using standard techniques (Meditech balloon, 4 to 7 mm × 5 cm).

After the procedure, hemostasis was achieved by manual compression. Heparin bolus (5000 U, intravenously) was given, followed by heparin infusion (800 to 1000 U/hr for 12 to 18 hours). Patients were kept under close monitoring for a 24-hour period. Patients were discharged the following day with enteric-coated aspirin (325 to 650 mg/day). Clinical follow-up was scheduled at 4, 12, and 24 weeks and yearly thereafter.

Intraoperative procedures were performed in the vascular operating room under regional anesthesia. Common femoral artery was exposed and clamped before the introduction of the probe through an arteriotomy. Laser recanalization was attempted under fluoroscopic guidance, using a portable fluoroscopic unit. The laser procedure was similar to the percutaneous procedure. The patient was kept for several days (mean of 4) following the procedure. Anticoagulation with heparin was used for 24 to 48 hours.

Angioscopy Procedure

In this series, angioscopy was performed at various stages of the arterial intervention.[23] Several angioscopes with an outer

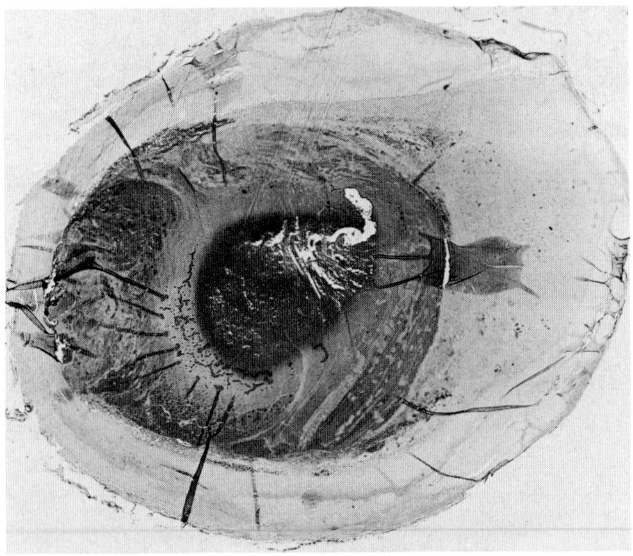

Figure 33–6. Cross-section of superficial femoral artery totally occluded by fresh thrombus after attempted laser recanalization. The central portion of the thrombus is liquified without the creation of a well-defined vascular lumen. This was obtained from a patient study in Phase I feasibility trials. (Reprinted with permission from Abela et al.[19])

diameter ranging from 0.85 to 3.2 mm were used. Illumination was provided by a xenon cold lamp (Karlstorz 487, Culver City CA, or Trimedyne model 3L9). Images were relayed to a low light sensitive RGB camera (Pulnix TMC-54) and viewed on-line using a high-resolution color monitor (Sony DVM-1910).

In intraoperative procedures, antegrade blood flow was interrupted by clamping of the artery above the arteriotomy. In percutaneous procedures, the angioscope was loaded into a guiding catheter and inserted into the introducer sheath. In order to obtain a clear field of view, one or more of the following techniques was used: pressurized flushes of saline solution or carbon dioxide gas, or balloon inflation at the catheter tip with saline injections to displace blood. The angioscope was held in a fixed position at the tip of the guiding catheter and coaxial positioning was obtained by rotation and withdraw-advance movements of the catheter.

RESULTS

In Phases II and III, 77 laser thermal-optical recanalization procedures were attempted.[24] Mean age of patients was 65 years, ranging from 38 to 81 years. Procedures were performed for ulceration of rest pain in 27 patients and for moderate-to-severe claudication in 50 patients. Occlusions were located in iliac arteries in five, in superficial femoral or popliteal arteries in 67, or below the trifurcation in five (Fig. 33-7A–D). Occlusions had a mean length of 9.4 cm, with a range of 1 to 30 cm. Intraoperative procedures were done in 25 patients and percutaneous procedures in 52.

Technical success was achieved if the obstruction could be crossed with angiographic improvement and without perforation. Technical success was obtained in 71% of the procedures, more often in lesions shorter than 15 cm. Fifteen of the 25 intraoperative procedures and 40 of the 52 percutaneous

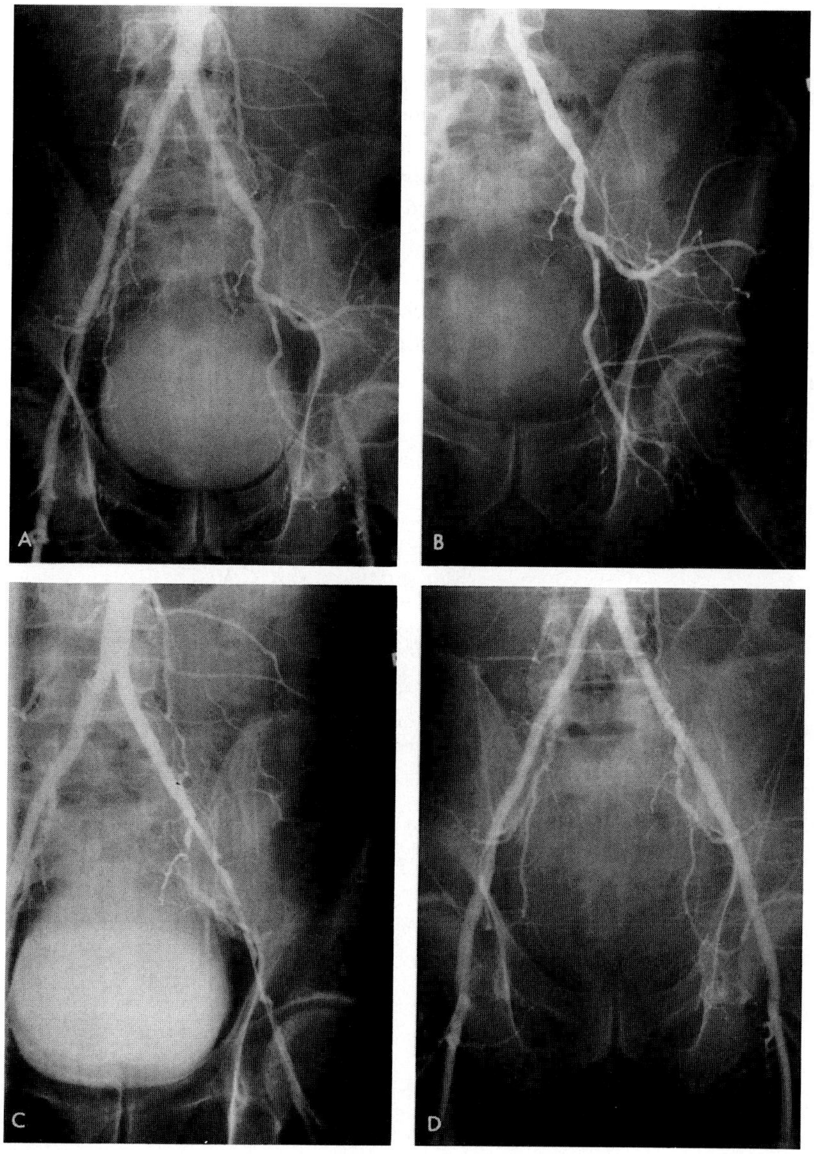

Figure 33–7. Angiogram of 65-year-old man with one block claudication of 2 years' duration. **A:** Totally occluded left iliac artery (11 cm long obstruction, white arrows). **B:** Following laser recanalization using a 2 mm Spectraprobe. Angiogram was done using a 5 F catheter across the obstruction. Contrast flow across the obstruction is not seen due to the small size of the channel and the obstruction with the catheter body. **C:** Final results showing balloon angioplasty (7 mm balloon) showing multiple sites of residual stenosis. **D:** At 6 weeks, a repeat angiogram showing further resolution of stenosis. (Reprinted with permission from Abela and Barbeau G.[28])

procedures were technically successful. Perforation or subintimal dissection occurred in 19 patients and two lesions could not be crossed. None of these perforations resulted in worsening of symptoms or blood transfusion. One additional lesion was not accessed percutaneously.

In percutaneous procedures, clinical success was defined as a residual stenosis less than 50%, increase of arm to brachial (ABI) 0.15 or more or symptom improvement and absence of complications during the hospitalization. Clinical success was obtained in 34 of the 52 percutaneous procedures (65%) using laser-assisted balloon angioplasty (30) or laser as sole therapy (4). In patients with clinical success, ABI improved from 0.54 ± 0.12 to 0.81 ± 0.14 immediately following the procedure ($p < 0.001$; two-tailed paired *t*-test).

Because of thrombosis or no improvement of their symptoms during hospitalization, six patients were considered clinical failures. In two of these patients, the artery reoccluded after lasing was used as the sole therapy. One of those patients returned to his baseline symptoms and was managed conservatively. The other patient required bypass surgery 1 week after a balloon angioplasty procedure that was complicated by dissection and acute reocclusion of a longer segment. Despite bypass, this patient eventually required partial amputation of a foot.

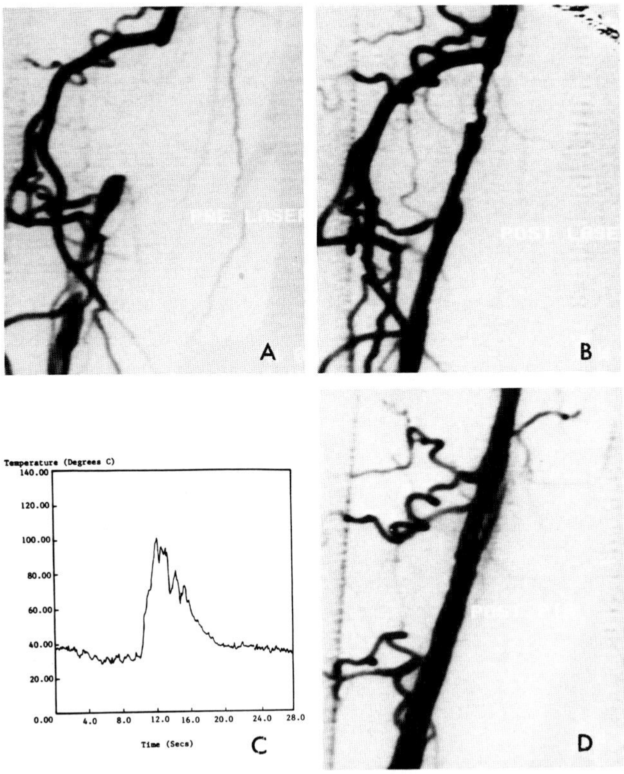

Figure 33–8. **A:** Digital angiogram of a totally occluded superficial femoral artery in a 62-year-old man. The distal portion of the artery is filled by collaterals. **B:** Irregular channel created immediately after laser recanalization with a 2 mm Spectraprobe-PLR and a K-type thermal couple at the probe tip. **C:** Recording of probe temperature during recanalization of the obstruction shown in **A.** The maximum probe temperature during recanalization was 100°C. **D:** Final result after balloon angioplasty. Arrows show a dissection plane. (Reprinted with permission from Seeger and Abela.[29])

High Risk Patients

Laser recanalization was attempted in 17 patients in whom the risk of surgical therapy was increased by severe angina (Canadian Cardiovascular Society class III and IV), infection, absent venous conduits, recent deep vein thrombosis, or complete tibial artery occlusion.[25] Recanalization was successful in nine patients and eight had relief of their symptoms. No patient with tibial artery occlusion had limb salvage. Restenosis or reocclusion developed in three patients during the first year follow-up but only one had recurrent symptoms.

Recanalization Temperature

In 21 procedures, probe temperature was monitored during recanalization.[26] A mean peak temperature of 178 ± 120°C was recorded during recanalization. Recanalization of obstruction (mean length, 5.3 ± 3.8 cm) lasted an average of 12.4 ± 14.1 seconds (Figs. 33-8, 33-9). Perforations occurred in six arteries at a peak probe temperature ranging from 73 to 502°C. Although probe temperature did not predict perforations, it suggested various mechanisms. Perforations occurred in four of six densely calcific vessels which required high probe temperature (>250°C). Probe temperature monitoring also detected probe dysfunction.

Angioscopy

Thirty-two angioscopic examinations were performed during laser recanalization, 23 in intraoperative procedures and nine in percutaneous procedures.[23] Visualization of the vascular lumen provided clear detail of the obstruction in 16 of the 23 arteries (70%) via intraoperative approach and in all nine cases via percutaneous approach.

Occluding atherosclerotic plaques were identified in 24 procedures as whitish-yellowish lesions obstructing the lumen. Fresh occlusive thrombus was visualized in six arteries and appeared as glistening red-brown, lobulated or smooth surfaces. Occasionally, older organized thrombus seemed to merge with the plaque and appeared grayish with areas of brown streaks. Angioscopy done during the arterial intervention served to place the laser probe in a coaxial position in order to avoid inadvertent irradiation of the arterial walls. However, despite the ability to visualize the relative position of the probe to the arterial wall, angioscopy did not alter the perforation rate. This was due to the inability to visualize the probe's direction once it enters the obstruction. Nevertheless, it was possible to identify bifurcations and heavily calcified plaques, which are a frequent site of perforation. Once blood flow was reestablished across the arterial obstruction, it became increasingly difficult to obtain a clear field of view.

After the laser intervention, the wall of the new channel appeared generally regular with smooth arterial lumen sur-

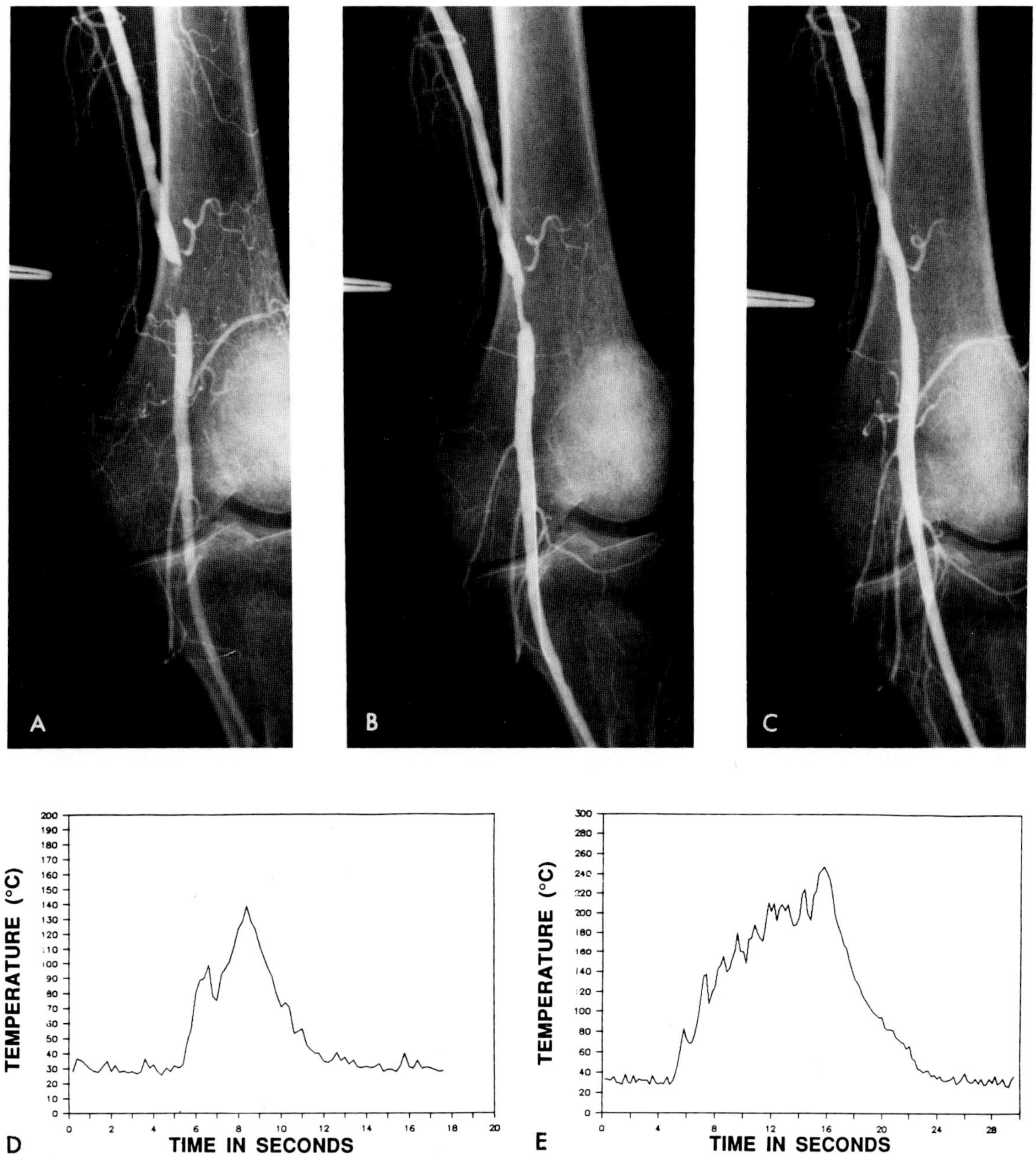

Figure 33–9. Sequential angiograms of a 73-year-old diabetic woman with a left foot ulcer. **A:** Prelaser angiogram illustrating a short segment (1.5 cm) superficial femoral artery obstruction. **B:** Following laser recanalization. A guide wire is seen across the recanalized segment. **C:** Following balloon dilation. **D:** Probe temperature peak at 138°C during recanalization. **E:** Temperature on pullback following probe crossing, attempting further lumen enlargement at a higher temperature (248°C). Of note is the sequential rise of temperature after each pulse, resulting in a saw-toothed appearance of the ascending limb of the curve.

faces. The diameter of the channel was not much wider than the diameter of the probe tip used for recanalization. Charring was present and occasionally white embedded flecks were seen, suggesting calcific deposit. Some complications of endovascular procedures could readily be assessed. In several cases, intimal flaps could clearly be identified. In two cases, large dissections were identified with the formation of a false lumen channel. In one case, a fresh occluding thrombus embedded in the arterial wall was noted.

Follow-up

An angiogram was obtained at 7 ± 4 months in 26 of the 34 clinically successful percutaneous procedures. Restenosis (more than 50% stenosis) occurred in 13 patients: nine of them were successfully treated with balloon angioplasty (6) or bypass surgery (3). The four remaining patients were treated conservatively. Clinical follow-up was obtained in the eight patients in whom angiograms were not done: five had improved or had no symptoms from the treated limb, two had claudication, and one required amputation 6 months after limb salvage by laser recanalization. Analysis of restenosis in percutaneous procedures showed that lesion length did not affect the rate of restenosis.[24]

SUMMARY

Thermo-optical laser recanalization is an effective treatment for totally occluded iliac and femoropopliteal arteries that are unmanageable by balloon angioplasty alone. Laser recanalization may provide a less invasive method for a category of patients whose only alternative to conservative therapy would have been bypass surgery, especially those who are at a higher risk for a surgical approach. Better patient selection and use of thermal systems with feedback control may contribute to achieve a high success rate and avoid some of the complications such as perforation and thrombosis.

However, because laser recanalization is nearly always completed with balloon dilation, its long-term effects may not differ greatly from those following balloon angioplasty in terms of clinical and angiographic patency.

As with any interventional techniques, laser recanalization remains very dependent on the guidance systems used. Throughout the procedure, angioscopy could provide an accurate morphopathologic analysis of the obstruction. Angioscopy allowed coaxial positioning of the probe tip in the occluded vessel and confirmed contact with the obstruction, although it did not prevent arterial perforation. Finally, the ability to visualize the complications of endovascular procedures such as intimal flaps, dissections, fresh thrombus or ulcerations confirms angioscopy as a useful adjunct to angiography for laser angioplasty.

REFERENCES

1. Lee G, Ikeda RM, Kozina J, Mason DT. Laser dissolution of coronary atherosclerotic obstruction. Am Heart J 1981;102:1074–5.
2. Abela GS, Normann S, Cohen D, Feldman RL. Effects of carbon dioxide, Nd-YAG, and argon laser radiation on coronary atheromatous plaques. Am J Cardiol 1982;50:1199–1205.
3. Choy DSJ, Stertzer SH, Rotterdam HZ, Bruno MS. Laser coronary angioplasty: experience with 9 cadaver hearts. Am J Cardiol 1982;50:1209–11.
4. Geschwind H, Boussignac G, Teisseire B, et al. Laser angioplasty: effects on coronary artery stenosis. Lancet 1983; 2:1134.
5. Abela GS, Crea F, Smith W, et al. In vitro effects of argon laser radiation on blood: quantitative and morphologic analysis. J Am Coll Cardiol 1985;5:231–7.
6. Choy DSJ, Stertzer SH. Transluminal laser catheter angioplasty. Am J Cardiol 1982;50:1206–8.
7. Abela GS, Conti CR, Normann S, et al. A new model for Investigation of Transluminal Recanalization: human atherosclerotic coronary artery xenografts. Am J Cardiol 1984; 54:200–5.
8. Abela GS, Normann SJ, Cohen DM, et al. Laser recanalization of occluded atherosclerotic arteries in vivo and in vitro. Circulation 1985;71:403–11.
9. Crea F, Fenech A, Smith W, et al. Laser recanalization of acutely thrombosed coronary arteries in live dogs: early results. J Am Coll Cardiol 1985;6:1052–6.
10. Prevosti JG, Lawrence JR, Loon MR, et al. Surface thrombogenicity after excimer laser and hot-tip thermal ablation of plaque: morphometric studies using an annular perfusion chamber. Surg Forum 1987;38:330–3.
11. Gerrity RG, Loop FD, Golding LAR, et al. Arterial response for laser operation for removal of atherosclerotic plaque. Thorac Cardiovasc Surg 1983;85:409–21.
12. Abela GS, Crea F, Seeger JM, et al. The healing process in normal canine arteries and in atherosclerotic monkey arteries after transluminal laser irradiation. Am J Cardiol 1985; 56:983–8.
13. Higginson LA, Farell EM, Walley VM, et al. Arterial response to excimer and argon laser irradiation in atherosclerotic swine. Lasers Med Sci 1989;4:85–92.
14. Sanborn TA, Faxon DP, Haudenschild CC, Ryan TJ: Experimental angioplasty: circumferential distribution of laser thermal energy with a laser probe. J Am Coll Cardiol 1985; 5:934–8.
15. Hussein H: A novel fiberoptic laser probe for treatment of occlusive vessel disease. Opti Laser Technol Med 1986; 605:59–66.
16. Abela GS, Fenech A, Crea F, Conti CR. "Hot tip": another method of laser vascular recanalization. Lasers Surg Med 1985;5:327–35.
17. Sanborn TA, Haudenschild CC, Garber GR, Ryan TJ. Angiographic and histologic consequences of laser thermal angioplasty: comparison with balloon angioplasty. Circulation 1987;75:1281–6.
18. Hoffman RG, Abela GS, Friedl SE, et al. Dosimetry of plaque ablation using thermal and thermal-optical probe systems. Proceedings of SPIE, The International Society for Optical Engineering, Optical Fibers in Medicine IV, vol. 1067:120–6, 1989.
19. Abela GS, Seeger JM, Barbieri E, et al. Laser angioplasty with angioscopic guidance in humans. J Am Coll Cardiol 1986; 8:184–92.
20. Barbieri E, Roxey T, Khoury A, Abela GS: Evaluation of optical properties and laser effects on arterial tissue using a microlens tipped optical fiber. Proceedings of SPIE, The International Society for Optical Engineering, Optical Fibers in Medicine II, vol. 713:166–169, 1986.
21. Abela GS, Seeger JM, Pry RS, et al. Percutaneous laser recanalization of totally occluded human peripheral arteries: a technical approach. Dynam Cardiovasc Imaging 1988;1:302–08.
22. Seeger JM, Abela GS, Silverman SH, Jablonski SK. Initial results of laser recanalization in lower extremity arterial reconstruction. J Vasc Surg 1989;9:10–7.
23. Giacomino PP, Abela GS, Barbeau GR, et al. Angioscopy: current techniques. Dynam Cardiovasc Imaging 1989;2:178–87.
24. Barbeau GR, Abela GS, Seeger JM, et al. Laser thermo-optical angioplasty in totally occluded peripheral arteries: immediate and intermediate results. Circulation 1989;80:II-27.
25. Seeger JM, Kaelin LD, Barbeau GR, Abela GS. Laser recanalization in high risk patients. Lasers Surg Med 1990;10:105–11.
26. Barbeau GR, Abela GS, Seeger JM, et al. Temperature monitoring during peripheral thermo-optical laser recanalization in humans. Clin Cardiol 1990;13:690–7.
27. Abela GS. Immediate and chronic effects of laser angioplasty. In Abela GS (ed): Lasers in Cardiovascular Medicine and Surgery: Fundamentals and Technique. Boston: Kluwer, 1990;113–41.
28. Abela GS, Barbeau G. Clinical experience with laser angioplasty. In Abela GS (ed): Lasers in Cardiovascular Medicine and Surgery: Fundamentals and Technique. Boston: Kluwer, 1990;257–71.
29. Seeger JM, Abela GS. Laser recanalization and treatment of peripheral atherosclerosis. In Abela GS (ed): Lasers in Cardiovascular Medicine and Surgery: Fundamentals and Technique. Boston: Kluwer, 1990;273–89.

34 Tibioperoneal and Popliteal Sole Hot Tip Laser Thermal Angioplasty

Harold A. Mitty, M.D., Timothy A. Sanborn, M.D.

Failure of femoral popliteal bypass grafts and superficial femoral artery balloon angioplasty is often related to associated compromised distal vessels. Improvement of runoff in the form of tibioperoneal and popliteal revascularization is being addressed by the interventional radiologist with small balloons and by the surgeon using distal bypass grafts. The feasibility of thermal (hot tip) laser angioplasty in these small vessels has been assessed in a clinical trial in our hospital.

The laser systems in clinical use produce a small channel so that recanalization with these devices is usually followed by conventional balloon angioplasty in larger vessels.[1–4] Thus, results obtained with laser-assisted balloon angioplasty may be difficult to interpret, since the major visible changes in the vessel lumen are due to the balloon angioplasty. The popliteal and infrapopliteal vessels are small enough so that an adequate channel could be produced with standard 1.7 to 2.5 mm thermal laser catheter probes. Since no balloon angioplasty is necessary, one then has the opportunity of evaluating the efficacy of sole laser thermal angioplasty.

PATIENTS AND METHODS

Patient Selection

Percutaneous laser thermal angioplasty without subsequent balloon angioplasty was attempted in 17 distal peripheral arterial lesions in 11 patients. In addition, one patient with diffuse disease of a small superficial femoral artery was treated by sole thermal recanalization.

In order to maximize safety, each procedure was performed over the wire. Thus, the possibility of perforation was effectively eliminated and access for balloon angioplasty was maintained should the laser probe fail to cross the stenosis or subtotal occlusion.

The average age of patients treated was 72 years. Diabetes mellitus was present in 70% of patients and 30% had a history of significant cigarette smoking. Eighty percent of patients had signs of limb ischemia in the form of rest pain, nonhealing ulcers, or gangrene. The remainder had severe claudication at less than 100 foot distances. Patient evaluation included a history and physical examination. A Doppler ankle-arm index was also obtained before the procedure. Pretreatment consisted of aspirin (325 mg once a day).

Laser Equipment

A 14 W argon laser generator (Optilase model 900; Trimedyne, Tustin, CA) was used. This was coupled to a sterile disposable laser catheter with a 2.5 mm metal cap at the distal end. One patient was treated with a laser catheter with a 1.7 mm metal cap, which became available toward the end of the study period. The central lumen of the laser catheter allowed true coaxial passage over a 0.035 or a 0.014 inch guide wire. In addition, the central lumen provides a route for injection of contrast agents or vasodilating drugs, such as nitroglycerin, should that become necessary during the procedure.

Technique

All patients had prior diagnostic arteriography so that the site of antegrade puncture of the ipsilateral common femoral artery was established. Under local anesthesia, a 5 F vessel dilator was directed into the superficial femoral artery. An initial arteriogram was performed to confirm that the extent of disease was unchanged from prior studies. At this point, an 8 F vascular sheath was inserted and its side arm constantly infused with a dilute heparin solution. Heparin, 5000 U, was then injected via the sheath so that adequate anticoagulation was produced before crossing the stenotic segments. Guide wires of 0.014 to 0.035 inch were steered across the stenotic segments. This was accomplished either by using steerable torque wires or slightly curved catheter-guide wire combinations that allowed direction change within the vessel lumen. Once a wire was across the lesion the laser catheter was advanced to the lesion. This was confirmed by injecting small amounts of contrast material through the tip of the laser catheter or by injecting a larger volume through the side arm of the vascular sheath.

Once the lesions were contacted by the tip of the laser catheter, pulses of 12 W of argon laser power were applied. This part of the procedure requires coordination between two operators. One must hold the position of the guide wire while the other applies gentle forward pressure to the laser catheter while activating the power with a foot switch. The tip of the laser catheter must be kept in motion so that cool-down can occur without the metal cap adhering to the vessel wall. This process is complete in a matter of seconds. Angiography is then performed to document the status of the vessels treated by sole thermal angioplasty. Seven of the patients in this series required laser-assisted balloon angioplasty of associated superficial femoral artery lesions.

At the completion of the procedure, all catheters and guide wires were removed and compression of the puncture site applied in the usual manner. Heparin was not continued. Patients were discharged 24 to 48 hours after the procedure with instructions to continue aspirin, 325 mg/day.

RESULTS

Results were assessed by several parameters, including angiographic success, hemodynamic success, and initial clinical success. In addition, follow-up clinical success, failures, and vessel patency were evaluated. What follows are the results of sole laser thermal popliteal and tibioperoneal angioplasty in our patients. The one patient having sole laser therapy of diffuse superficial femoral artery disease experienced reocclusion 24 hours after recanalization. In retrospect, balloon angioplasty should also have been used (Fig. 34-1).

Initial Results

Angiographic success was defined as improvement to less than 30% residual stenosis. Laser thermal angioplasty without balloon angioplasty was angiographically successful in 15 of 17 (88.2%) of infrapopliteal and below-knee popliteal vessels (Table 34-1). One failure (patient 3) was due to the fact that the 2.5 mm laser catheter would not follow the guide wire with the laser at 12 W power. This was most likely due to the relatively large diameter of the metal tip compared with the vessel diameter. The 1.7 mm laser catheters were not yet available at the time of the procedure. The second failure (patient 8) was due to a 90° angle at the origin of the anterior tibial artery. The 2.5 mm probe would not follow the 0.014 inch guide wire used to cross the lesion. As a result, balloon angioplasty was performed using a 2.75 mm balloon. The more flexible balloon catheter easily negotiated the abrupt angle of the proximal anterior tibial artery (Fig. 34-2).

Hemodynamic success was improvement of the Doppler ankle-arm index of greater than 0.15. This was the case in 8 of 11 patients (72.7%) (Fig. 34-3). The three failures were in patients in whom sole laser angioplasty was attempted just prior to expected amputation. These three patients had no distal vessels available for bypass. In one (patient 2), an anterior tibial artery was present at the ankle but there was essentially no runoff in the foot (Fig. 34-4). Amputation was required at 2 months postprocedure. The second patient (patient 5) had continued rest pain after recanalization and died of a myocardial infarction sustained during sympathectomy. The third patient remained unchanged at 4 months after the laser procedure. The overall Doppler ankle-arm ratios for the entire group of 11 patients increased from 0.43 to 0.72.

Clinical success, using Society of Vascular Surgery/International Society of Cardiovascular Surgery criteria, was initially obtained in 8 of 11 patients. In six patients with ulcers or gangrene, healing occurred and rest pain was no longer present (patients 1, 3, 4, 7, 8, and 11). Claudication was relieved in patients 6 and 9. It was not surprising that the three patients with no hemodynamic improvement due to poor distal runoff also failed to have clinical improvement.

Follow-up Results

Mean follow-up of 6 months revealed clinical improvement had been maintained in five of eight patients with initial clinical success. In patient 1 treated for rest pain, symptoms recurred 3 months after sole thermal laser angioplasty. This proved to be due to occlusion of the superficial femoral artery

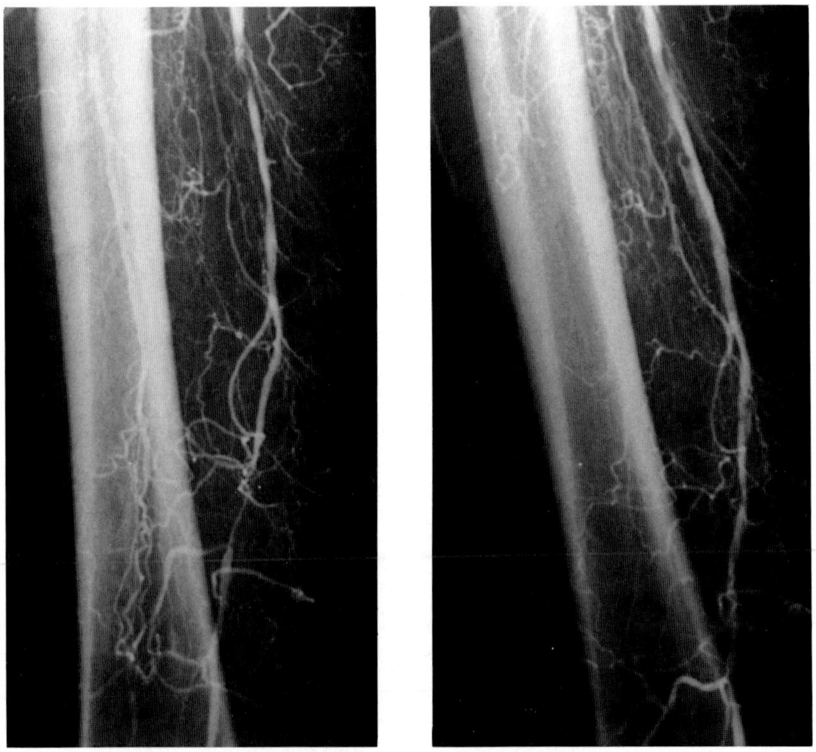

Figure 34–1. Small diameter superficial femoral artery treated by sole thermal laser angioplasty. **A:** Preangioplasty. Multiple areas of stenosis are present throughout the vessel. **B:** Following thermal laser recanalization, there is significant improvement in the angiographic appearance.

A B

Table 34–1. Sole Laser Thermal Angioplasty: Initial Angiographic and Hemodynamic Results*

PATIENT	AGE (YR)/ SEX	SVS/ISCVS CATEGORY OF ISCHEMIA	LESIONS TREATED WITH LASER ALONE	ANGIO-GRAPHIC SUCCESS	ADDITIONAL LESIONS TREATED WITH LASER AND BALLOON	DISTAL VESSEL RUNOFF (NO. VESSELS)	DOPPLER ANKLE-ARM INDEX *Before Procedure*	DOPPLER ANKLE-ARM INDEX *After Procedure*
1	60/F	4	1 cm popliteal stenosis	Yes	6 cm SFA stenosis	2	0.36	0.80
			3 cm peroneal stenosis	Yes				
2	50/F	5	1 cm anterior tibial stenosis	Yes	—	1	075†	0.83
			3 cm anterior tibial stenosis	Yes				
3	62/F	5	1 cm popliteal stenosis	Yes	—	1	—‡	0.78
			2 cm posterior tibial occlusion	No				
4	72/M	5	12 cm popliteal stenosis	Yes	6 cm SFA stenosis	1	0.56	0.81
			1 cm anterior tibial stenosis	Yes				
5	86/M	5	1 cm popliteal stenosis	Yes	—	0	0.18	0.30
6	77/M	3	1 cm anterior tibial stenosis	Yes	16 cm SFA occlusion	1	0.46	0.65
7	74/M	5	3 cm peroneal occlusion	Yes	5 cm SFA stenosis	0	0.00	0.44
8	76/F	5	12 cm popliteal stenosis	Yes	3 cm SFA occlusion	1	0.44	1.09
			2 cm anterior tibial stenosis	No§				
9	77/M	3	1 cm peroneal stenosis	Yes	12 cm SFA stenosis	1	0.64	1.00
10	81/F	5	2 cm popliteal stenosis	Yes	3 cm SFA stenosis	0	0.50	0.50
			4 cm peroneal stenosis	Yes				
11	61/F	4	3 cm anterior tibial stenosis	Yes	—	1	0.45	0.67
Mean	70.5	4.5				0.82	0.43	0.72

*SFA: superficial femoral artery; SVS/ISCVS: Society of Vascular Surgery/International Society of Cardiovascular Surgery.

†Preprocedure Doppler ankle-arm index was high due to noncompressible distal vessels.

‡Not determined due to dressing.

§Successful balloon angioplasty.

lesion that had been treated by laser-assisted balloon angioplasty. A bypass was performed, at which time patency of the popliteal and peroneal lesions treated by laser angioplasty was confirmed. Patient 6 also had a patent anterior tibial vessel demonstrated at 3 months when bypass of a reoccluded superficial femoral artery became necessary. Patient 11 had reocclusion at the angioplasty site (Fig. 34-5) 5 months after recanalization and required surgical bypass.

The three patients who never showed clinical improvement had patent sole laser thermal angioplasty sites (patients 2, 5, 10). Amputation was necessary in two due to poor runoff distal to the treated vessels. The third patient had persistent gangrene at the time of follow-up.

Complications

This small pilot series was remarkably free of complications. In particular, local vasospasm was not a problem. In no case was local intra-arterial administration of nitroglycerin necessary. No perforations, acute thrombosis, or embolizations were encountered in this group of patients. The laser catheters were prototype designs early in this study and two instances of optical fiber fracture were experienced. In each case no patient complications resulted. Change in laser catheter design has improved the device so that we have not experienced this complication in subsequent patients.

DISCUSSION

This series demonstrates the feasibility of laser thermal recanalization without balloon angioplasty in distal popliteal and infrapopliteal vessels. The one patient with diffuse superficial femoral disease who experienced early reocclusion after sole laser recanalization emphasizes that this procedure in larger vessels would require larger probes inserted at the time of surgery or some kind of expandable or directable probe inserted percutaneously.

Technical or angiographic success was obtained in 15 of 17 (88.2%) of lesions. In the case of the posterior tibial lesion that could not be crossed because the device was probably too large, clinical improvement was still obtained due to success in recanalizing an associated distal popliteal lesion. The other lesion, an anterior tibial artery stenosis, which could not be crossed by the laser catheter was successfully balloon dilated. The limitations imposed by laser catheters that were too large are being remedied in part by the newer 1.7 mm laser catheter devices (Fig. 34-5). It is of interest that the

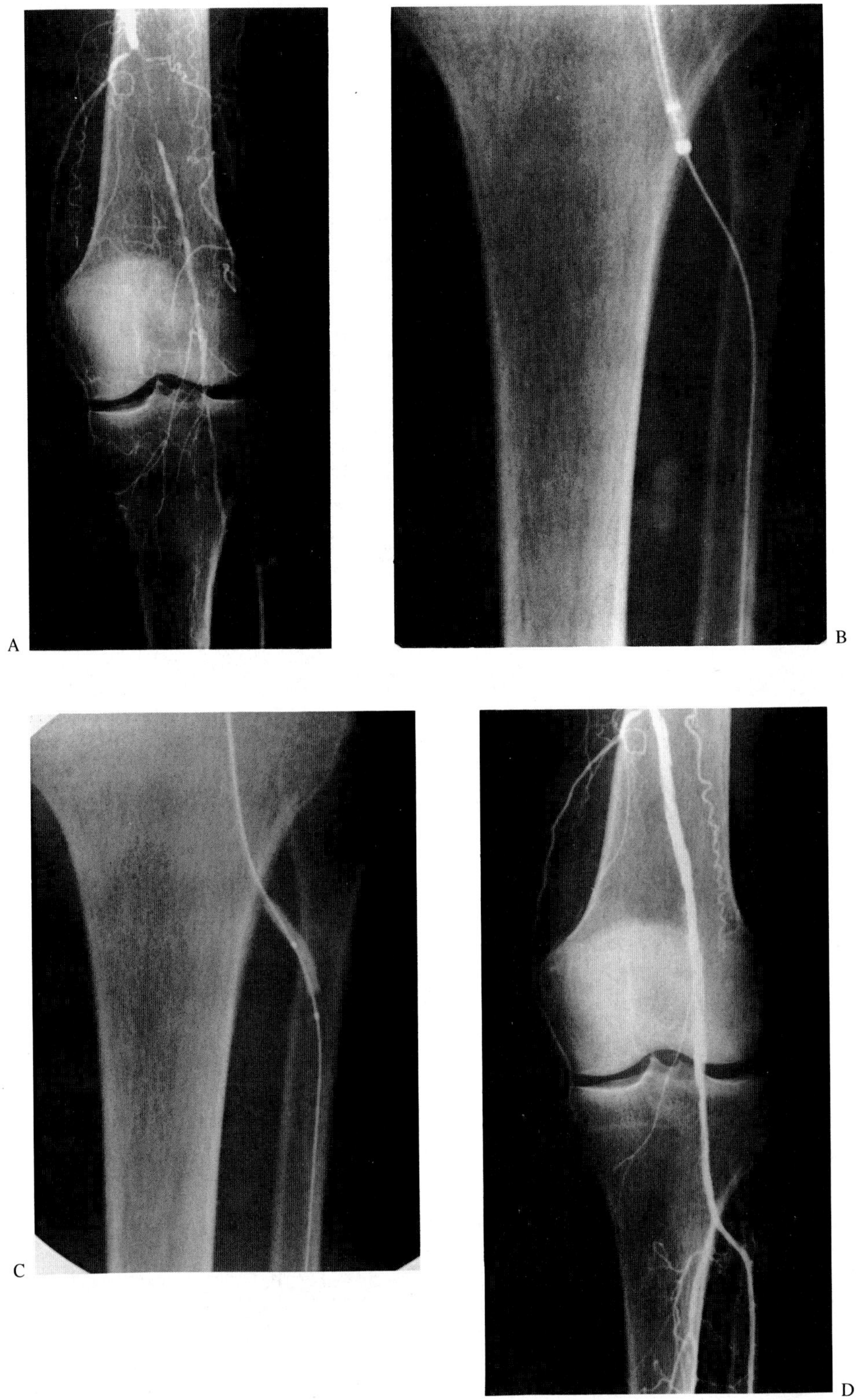

Figure 34–2. A patient with lesions of the superficial femoral, popliteal, and anterior tibial arteries treated, respectively, by laser-assisted balloon angioplasty, laser only, and balloon only. **A:** Femoral arteriogram demonstrating 4 cm distal superficial femoral occlusion and diffuse disease of the popliteal and anterior tibial arteries. **B:** Following laser-assisted balloon angioplasty of the superficial femoral artery and sole laser angioplasty of the popliteal artery, an attempt to cross the anterior tibial stenosis was made with a 5 mm laser catheter. This spot film demonstrates the point at which the laser catheter would no longer follow the 0.014 inch guide wire. **C:** Balloon angioplasty of the anterior tibial artery was performed with a 2.75 mm coronary style balloon. **D:** Final arteriogram demonstrates the patent recanalized vessels.

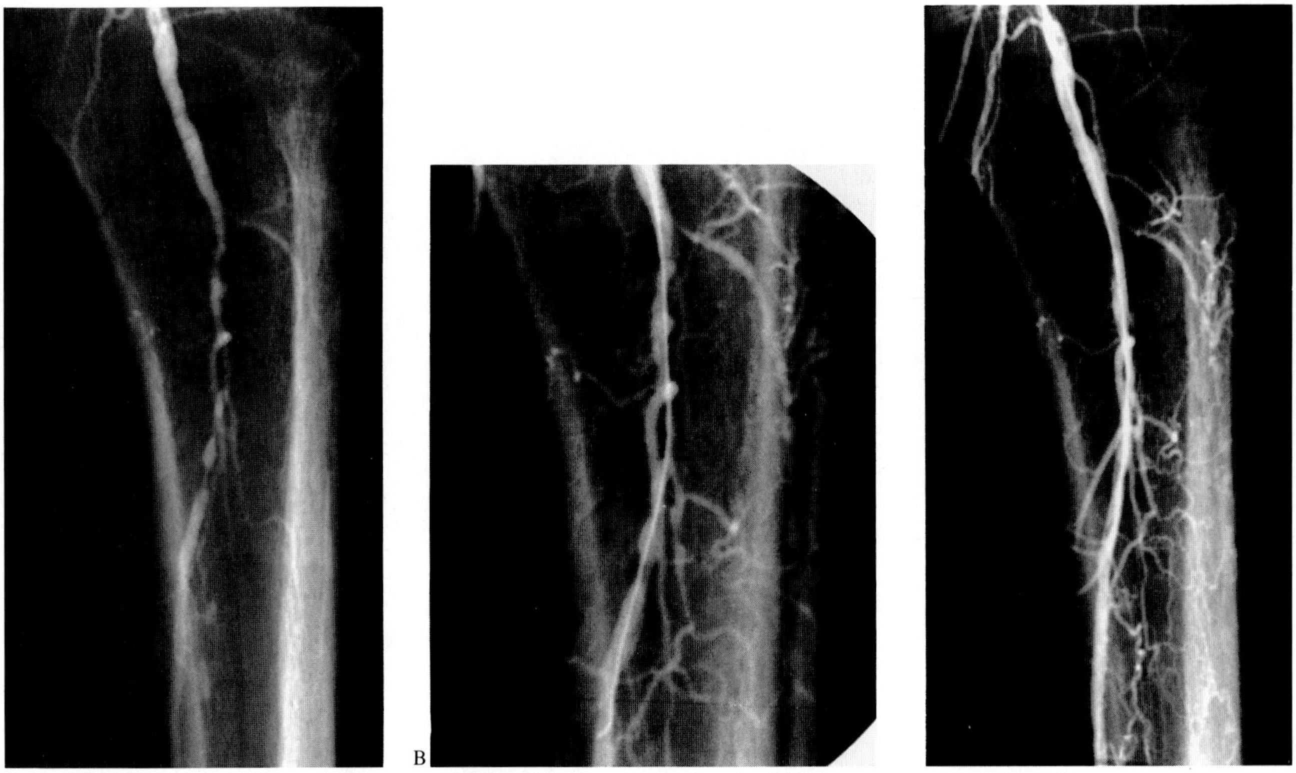

A B C

Figure 34–3. Tibioperoneal recanalization. **A:** Multiple areas of stenosis and subtotal occlusion are present. **B:** Steerable guide wire has crossed the diseased vessel. **C:** Angiogram following 2.5 mm laser catheter recanalization demonstrating a widely patent vessel. (Reprinted with permission from Sanborn et al.[7])

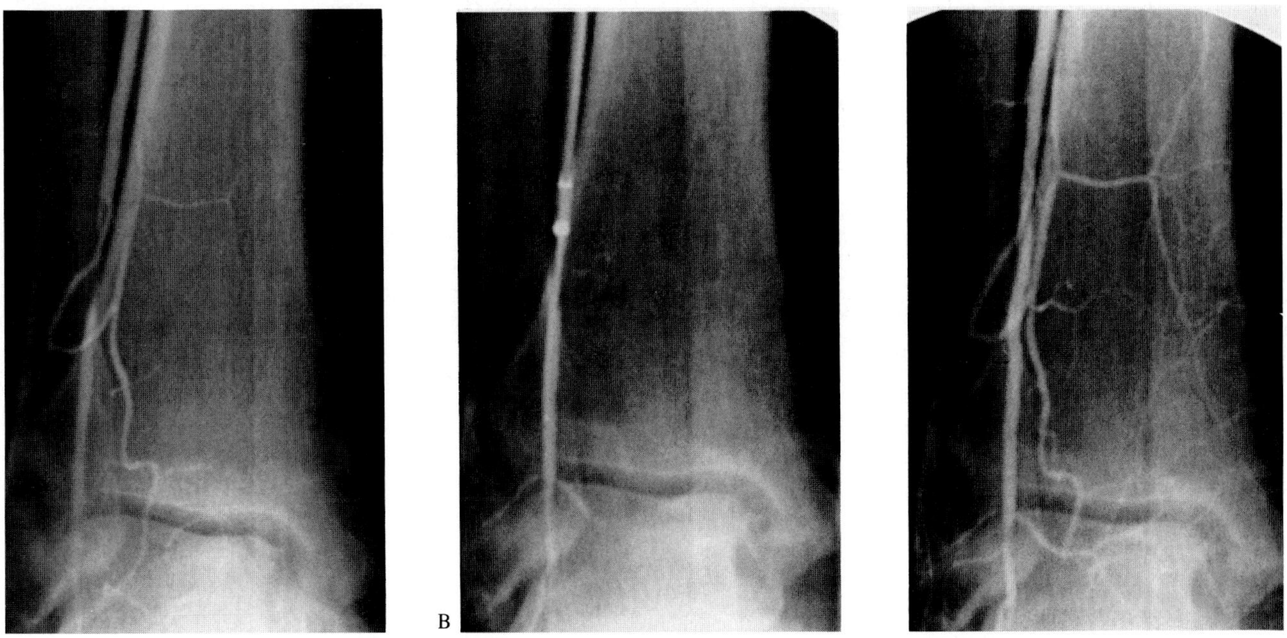

A B C

Figure 34–4. Sole laser thermal angioplasty of the distal anterior tibial artery. **A:** Angiogram reveals subtotal occlusion of the anterior tibial artery just above the ankle. **B:** Five millimeter laser catheter passing over the guide wire. **C:** Postrecanalization. The vessel is of normal caliber. (Reprinted with permission from Sanborn et al.[7])

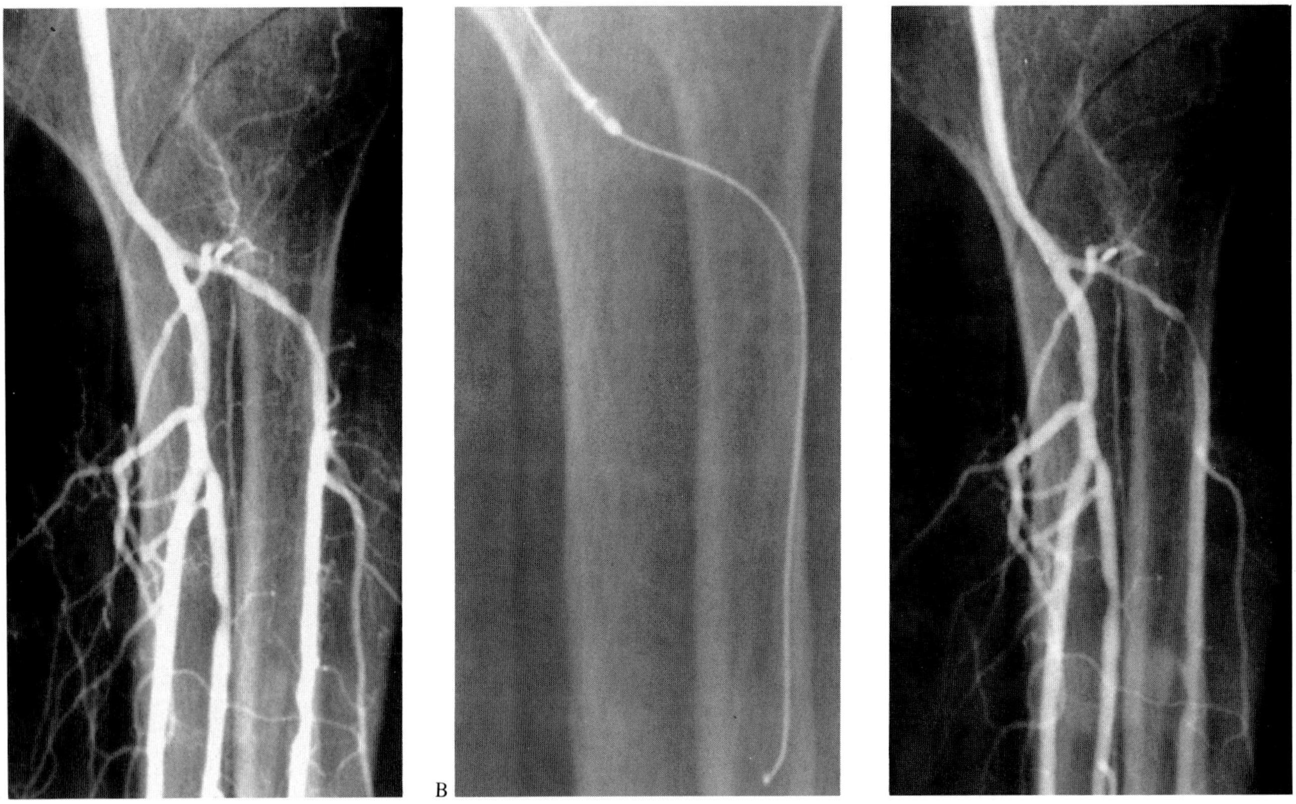

A B C

Figure 34–5. Sole laser thermal recanalization of the proximal anterior tibial artery. **A:** There is diffuse narrowing of the proximal anterior tibial artery. **B:** A 1.7 mm laser catheter is seen advancing over the wire. **C:** Postsole laser angioplasty. The stenotic segment is now of near-normal caliber. (Reprinted with permission from Mitty et al.[4])

88.2% technical or angiographic success rate that was achieved is similar to that reported for infrapopliteal balloon angioplasty. In one series[5] technical success was reported in 13 of 16 (81%) patients, and in another,[6] 141 of 145 (97%) patients.

The hemodynamic and initial clinical success experienced by 8 of 11 (72.7%) patients was gratifying. All three clinical failures were in patients not considered candidates for bypass grafts due to absence of adequate distal vessels. Patient selection and the presence of associated proximal disease all influence the eventual long-term outcome in these patients treated by sole laser thermal recanalization. In fact, balloon angioplasty of proximal lesions was required in almost 70% of this series.[7]

Comparison of sole balloon systems, other laser systems, and mechanical devices will require controlled studies. In addition, close attention to associated proximal lesions that impact on the patency of distal vessels having therapy is mandatory.

The thermal laser system, which we have employed, represents a compromise. Direct laser energy is not used and so we see the effects of indirect laser heating rather than direct photothermal or photochemical changes. Some authors have even suggested that the laser probe represents a superior shape for a "Dotterizing" device and that the same results could be expected without turning on the laser generator. This seems unlikely because we have had the experience of total resistance to passage of the probe until power is applied.

The laser catheter provides an advance in that it allows true coaxial tracking of the metal-tipped catheter over a guide wire. In addition, it represents a channel for the injection of contrast agents or spasmolytic drugs, if necessary.

Other laser systems have been in clinical evaluation. Centering balloons have been used with bare fiber argon laser systems.[2] Computer analysis of spectral characteristics of plaque versus vessel wall have also been used to determine when to activate therapeutic laser energy.[8]

We initially believed that the thermal laser procedure was valuable because it removed part of the disease and left a smoother surface that would be less apt to thrombose. There was experimental histologic and angiographic evidence to support this point of view.[9,10] More recently, attention has been turned to the excimer laser. This device appears to cause less local thrombus formation than the hot tip thermal devices. The clean interfaces between treated and untreated areas suggest that there would be less tendency to diffuse tissue injury and possibly less chance of thrombosis. A recent study at our institution on swine coronary arteries compared the effects of laser thermal angioplasty with excimer laser angioplasty.[11] Ten vessels were treated in each group using either the thermal laser or the excimer laser. Mural thrombi were seen in six of the thermal laser vessels and only one of the excimer-treated vessels. Two vessels in the thermal laser group had occlusive thrombi, whereas none of the excimer vessels occluded. Significantly, more platelet deposition was seen in the vessels treated by the thermal laser than those treated with the excimer laser. These experimental results suggest that the excimer laser may be the preferred device in small vessels. Better control is possible in newer excimer systems, which allow over-the-wire treatment. Our cardiology group has been using a xenon choride (308 mm) pulsed excimer laser generator (CVX-300, Spectranetics, Colorado Springs, CO) with a 4.5 F central lumen catheter. Thus far, this device has been used clinically as an adjunct to percutaneous transluminal coronary angioplasty or as a sole treatment modality in over 100 patients. No acute spasm, thrombosis, or perforation has been encountered. These results have been quite encouraging so that we are currently seeking permission to use this device in small vessels below the knee. This type of laser approach may replace the thermal laser probes that have been used in this group of patients.

REFERENCES

1. Sanborn TA, Cumberland DC, Greenfield AJ, et al. Percutaneous laser thermal angioplasty: initial results and 1-year follow-up in 129 femoropopliteal lesions. Radiology 1988;168:121–5.
2. Nordstrom LA, Castañeda-Zúñiga WR, Young EG, VonSeggern KB. Direct argon laser exposure for recanalization of peripheral arteries: early results. Radiology 1988;168:359–64.
3. McCowan TC, Ferris EJ, Barnes RW, Baker ML. Laser thermal angioplasty for the treatment of obstruction of the distal superficial femoral or popliteal arteries. AJR 1988;150:1169–73.
4. Mitty HA, Sanborn TA, Train JS, Dan SJ. Laser catheter thermal angioplasty: technique and early results in 34 patients. AJR 1989;153:617–21.
5. Brown KT, Schoenberg NY, Moore ED, Saddekni S. Percutaneous transluminal angioplasty of infrapopliteal vessels: preliminary results and technical considerations. Radiology 1988;169:75–8.
6. Schwarten DE, Cutcliff WB. Arterial occlusive disease below the knee: treatment with percutaneous transluminal angioplasty performed with low-profile catheters and steerable guide wires. Radiology 1988;169:71–4.
7. Sanborn TA, Mitty HA, Train JS, Dan SJ. Infrapopliteal and below-knee popliteal lesions: treatment with sole laser thermal angioplasty. Radiology 1989;172:89–93.
8. Leon MB, Lu DY, Prevosti LG, et al. Human arterial surface fluorescence: arteriosclerotic plaque identification and effects of laser atheroma ablation. J Am Coll Cardiol 1988;12:94–102.
9. Sanborn TA, Faxon DP, Haudenschild CC, Ryan TJ. Experimental angioplasty: circumferential distribution of laser thermal energy with a laser probe. J Am Coll Cardiol 1985;5:934–8.
10. Sanborn TA, Haudenschild CC, Garber GR, et al. Angiographic and histologic consequences of laser thermal angioplasty: comparison to balloon angioplasty. Circulation 1978;75:1281–6.
11. Sanborn TA, Alexopoulos D, Marmur JD, et al. Reduced coronary thrombosis with excimer vs thermal laser angioplasty. Circulation 1989;80:II-477.

35 Sapphire Probe Laser-Assisted Angioplasty

Johannes Lammer, M.D., Ernst Pilger, M.D., Günther Erich Klein, M.D.

The first experimental and clinical studies on laser angioplasty were done with continuous wave lasers and bare quartz glass fibers.[1–6] These studies demonstrated that fibrofatty arteriosclerotic plaques and thrombi can be ablated by laser energy. This led to exuberant hopes that laser recanalization might provide better initial and long-term results than conventional angioplasty. This enthusiasm was not supported by the first clinical results. Endovascular work with bare fibers produced perforation rates as high as 30%, and the channel recanalized by a 600 μm fiber was too small for antegrade flow and sometimes difficult to pass a guide wire through. Also, quartz glass fibers were easily damaged by contact with the target tissue.[3,4,6]

The development of contact probes was a major advance.[7–10] The blunt configuration of these probes reduced the perforation rate to less than 10% and the probe size created a channel 2 to 3 mm in diameter. This made laser recanalization safe and effective enough for more intensive clinical trials. Two contact probe systems were designed for laser recanalization. The metal probe or hot tip system[7,8] (Trimedyne, Santa Anna, CA) consists of a metal cautery cap clamped onto the end of a 300 μm fiber. The metal probe is heated by the laser in the center of the cautery cap. The major disadvantage of this system is that direct laser-tissue interaction does not occur, thus obviating the goal of laser treatment. The relatively slow rise and fall of the hot tip temperature caused thermal damage to surrounding tissue layers.[11]

The second contact probe system is the sapphire probe.[9] An industrial sapphire has an 80% transmittance for laser light at various visible and invisible wavelengths. Direct laser-tissue interaction increases the thermal ablation effects at the surface of the plaque.[11] This chapter presents the experimental and clinical results of laser angioplasty with sapphire contact probes since early 1986.

LASERS

Continuous wave and long pulsed lasers in the millisecond or microsecond range cause a photothermal effect due to absorption of the laser photons at the tissue surface. The quality of absorption of the surface depends on the color of the surface, the chemical composition of the tissue, and the wavelength. Carbon dioxide (CO_2) lasers are almost completely absorbed by water, making absorption at the tissue surface excellent. Unfortunately, appropriate and safe fiberoptic delivery systems for CO_2 lasers are not yet available. The absorption of argon laser light (488 nm, 514 nm), dye laser light (380 to 630 nm) and neodymium yttrium aluminum garnet (Nd:YAG) laser light (1064 nm, 1318 nm) in plaque tissue is low due to reflection and scattering at the light surface of plaque tissue. We decided to use the 1064 nm Nd:YAG laser because it is relatively inexpensive, technically mature, and can be used in other disciplines and has a low absorption in blood.

DELIVERY SYSTEM

A 2.2 mm (7 F) Teflon catheter with a central lumen for a 600 μm quartz glass fiber and flushing was used. A sapphire contact probe of 1.8, 2.2, or 3.0 mm was screwed to the tip of the fiber by a universal metal connector (Fig. 35-1). The industrial sapphire has an 80% transmittance for laser light at 1064 nm, a refraction index of 1.77, and a melting point of 2030°C. The sapphire is spherical, which focuses the laser light. The focused laser light has an increased power density in the focal area, which in turn increases the axial recanalization ability. The steep fall of the power density of the laterally scattered light minimizes the risk of thermal damage to the vessel wall.[9,11]

Experimental studies on tissue have shown that application of Nd:YAG laser light by a sapphire contact probe reduces the amount of reflected and scattered light.[9] This increases light absorption and the amount of ablated tissue while limiting the surrounding zone of thermal necrosis (Fig. 35-2). Comparisons of a bare fiber catheter, a metal probe, and a sapphire probe at equal energies revealed that the largest volume of tissue can be ablated by the sapphire probe, followed by the bare fiber and the metal probe.[11] Conversely, the metal probe caused the largest zone of surrounding thermal necrosis, followed by the bare fiber and the sapphire probe. These studies demonstrated that the sapphire probe is the most effective and safest delivery system for a long pulsed or continuous wave laser.

TECHNIQUE OF LASER-ASSISTED ANGIOPLASTY

All interventions were done percutaneously with local anesthesia. Fluoroscopy was the guidance system of choice. Angioscopy was used to confirm the result of recanalization, but did not help guide the laser catheter during the recanalization procedure. Initially, a 7 F (or 9 F) catheter introducer sheath is inserted antegradely for femoropopliteal recanalizations or retrogradely for iliac interventions. Contrast injections can be made through the side arm of the sheath during the procedure. The laser catheter is advanced up to the

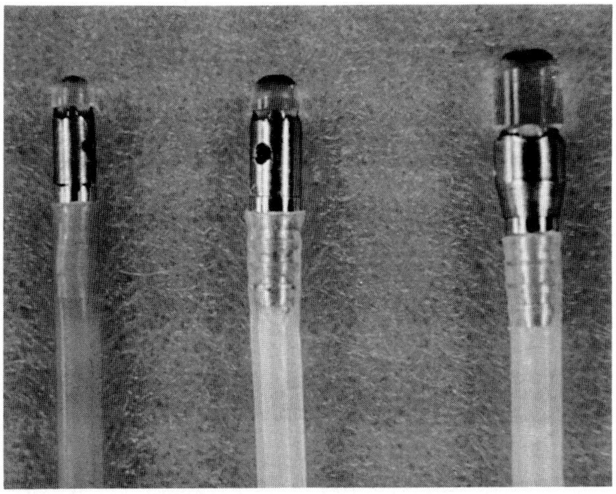

Figure 35–1. Sapphire probe laser catheters 1.8, 2.2, and 3.0 mm in diameter.

occlusion under fluoroscopic control. The laser catheter has to exert some forward pressure on the occlusion. The usual power setting is 10 W in 1-sec bursts. This short emission time was chosen to reduce heat accumulation in the arterial wall. Each burst produces an ablation of 1 mm of tissue. Mechanical recanalization has to be assumed if the laser catheter can be advanced faster. A successful recanalization opens a channel 2 to 3 mm in diameter. This channel is sufficient for antegrade flow, but still represents a hemodynamically significant stenosis for iliac or femoropopliteal arteries so that balloon dilation of the recanalized segment is indicated (Figs. 35-3, 35-4).

MANAGEMENT OF DIFFICULT SITUATIONS

If collateral arteries originate at the side of the obstruction at a flat angle, the laser probe can slide only into the collateral vessel and not into the obstructed segment. If a steerable guide wire can be manipulated into the obstructed lumen, the laser catheter can be guided over the wire (Fig. 35-5). However, if this maneuver is impossible, the procedure should be terminated before damaging the collateral artery.

Eccentric plaques tend to deflect the laser probe so that it is directed at the opposite, unaffected vessel wall. Under these circumstances, the eccentric plaque has to be ablated very slowly without too much pressure, which could deflect the probe.

Dissection into the vessel wall usually causes a burning and painful heat sensation during laser therapy. This is caused by thermal laser ablation close to the adventitial layer. Redirection of the laser catheter by a steerable guide wire or by external manual compression can help. If the laser catheter cannot be guided back into the center of the occluded artery, further attempts of laser recanalization should be discontinued (Fig. 35-6).

Perforation occurs if the warning signs such as pain and extra-axial catheter passage are ignored. It is characterized by cloudy contrast medium extravasation (Fig. 35-7). In this situation the procedure has to be stopped. Heparin anticoagulation must be reversed by protamine sulfate. Because perforations usually occur in a nonperfused segment of the artery, rapid rethrombosis will seal the leak within a few minutes.

Occlusions at the origin of the superficial femoral artery cannot be treated by an antegrade approach. In this situation a retrograde, transpopliteal approach is recommended.

INDICATIONS AND CONTRAINDICATIONS

The major *indications* for laser-assisted angioplasty are obstructions of the femoropopliteal segment, which cause limiting claudication (Fontaine stage IIb), pain at rest (Fontaine stage III), or gangrene (Fontaine stage IV). Experience with recanalization of iliac arteries is limited, but short occlusions of straight iliac arteries can be recommended for laser recanalization. Tibial vessels have been recanalized successfully, but the value of recanalization of occluded calf arteries is questionable.

There are no absolute contraindications for peripheral laser-assisted angioplasty. However, relative contraindications are acute thrombosis, which can be recanalized by intra-arterial fibrinolysis; tortuous iliac arteries, which pose a higher risk for perforation; highly calcified plaques, which cannot be ablated by low-power continuous wave lasers; obstructions longer than 15 cm; and occlusions of the popliteal artery including the trifurcation.

IMMEDIATE AND LONG-TERM RESULTS

A prospective multicenter trial was initiated in 1986 to define the clinical value of laser-assisted angioplasty with an

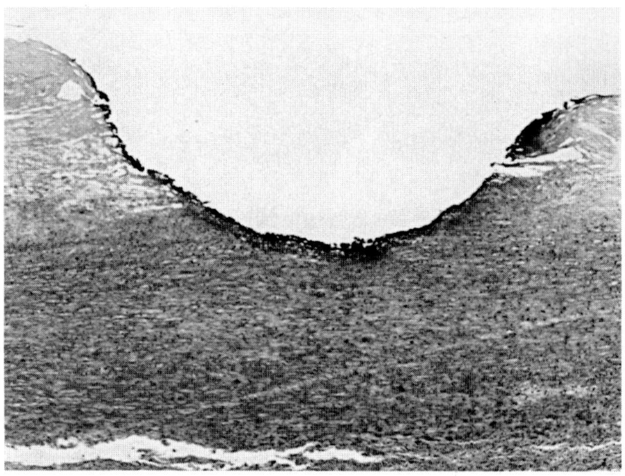

Figure 35–2. Histologic section of a laser crater caused by a sapphire probe, demonstrating the small zone of surrounding necrosis.

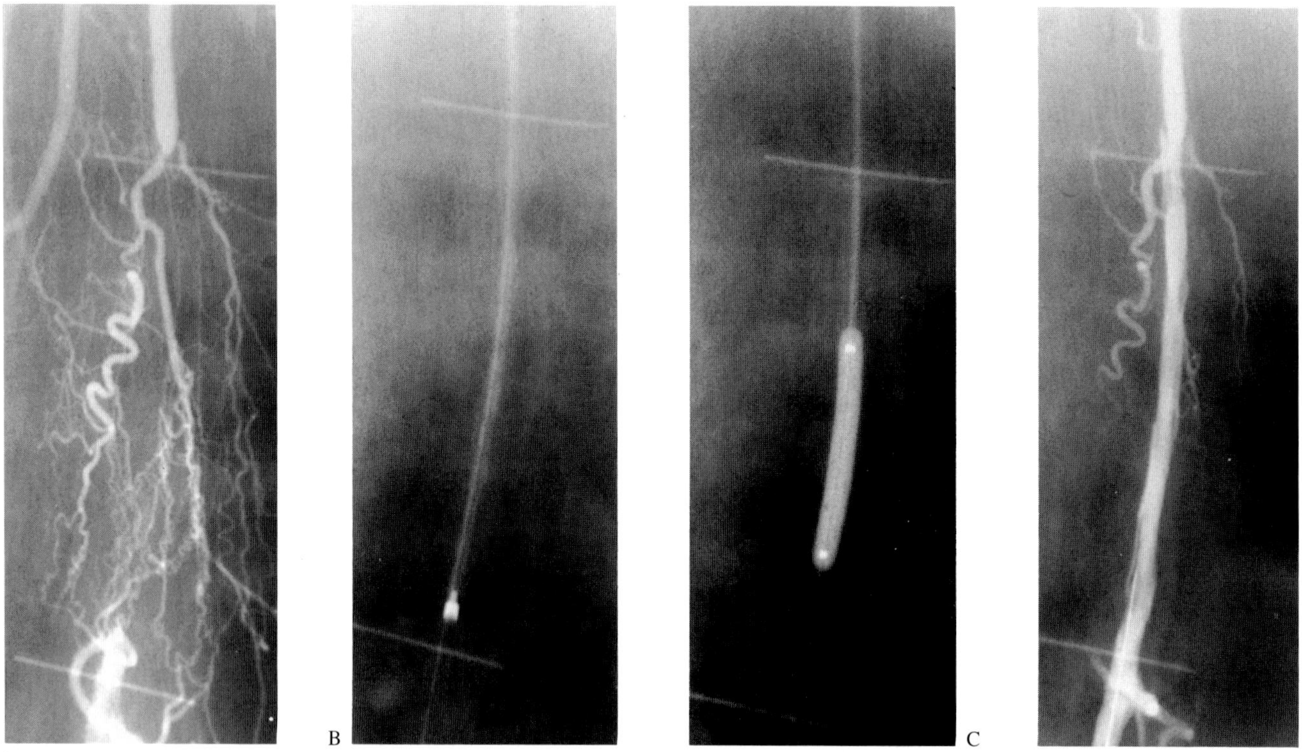

A B C D

Figure 35–3. Superficial femoral artery occlusion 9 cm in length, clinical stage IIb. **A:** Initial angiogram. **B:** Sapphire probe laser catheter during recanalization. **C:** Additional percutaneous transluminal angioplasty. **D:** Final angiogram after laser-assisted balloon angioplasty.

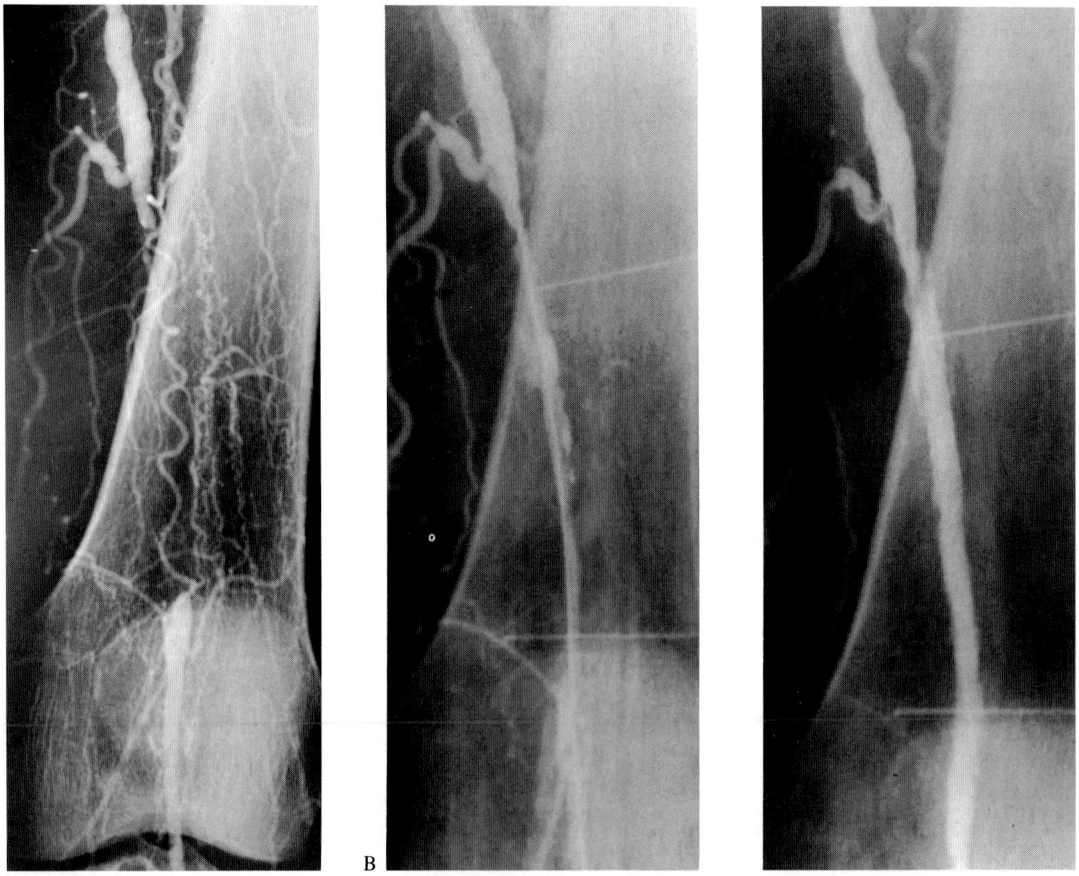

A B C

Figure 35–4. Superficial femoral artery occlusion 8 cm in length, clinical stage IIb. **A:** Initial angiogram. **B:** Channel created by 2.2 mm sapphire probe catheter. **C:** Angiogram after additional percutaneous transluminal angioplasty.

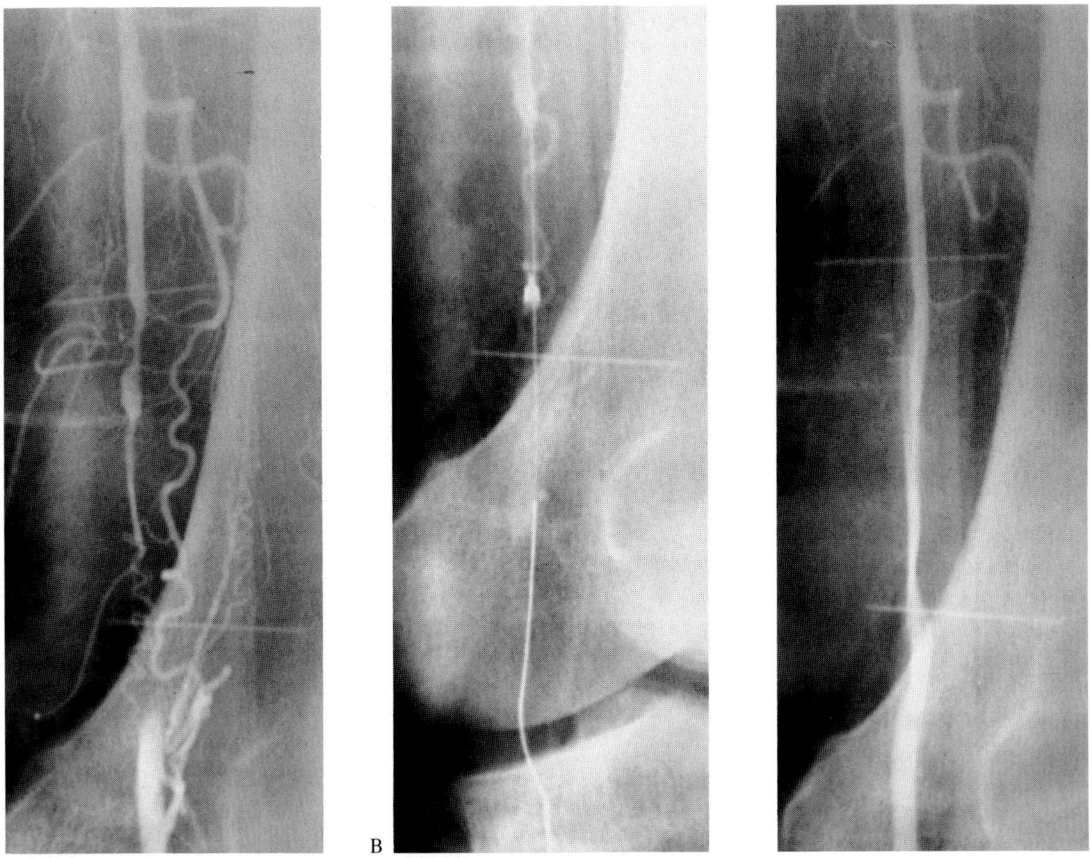

A B C

Figure 35–5. Femoropopliteal artery occlusion 7 cm in length with collateral artery originating at the occlusion site, clinical stage III. **A:** Initial angiogram. **B:** Laser catheter guided by a steerable wire to avoid damage of the collateral artery. **C:** Angiogram after laser-assisted balloon angioplasty.

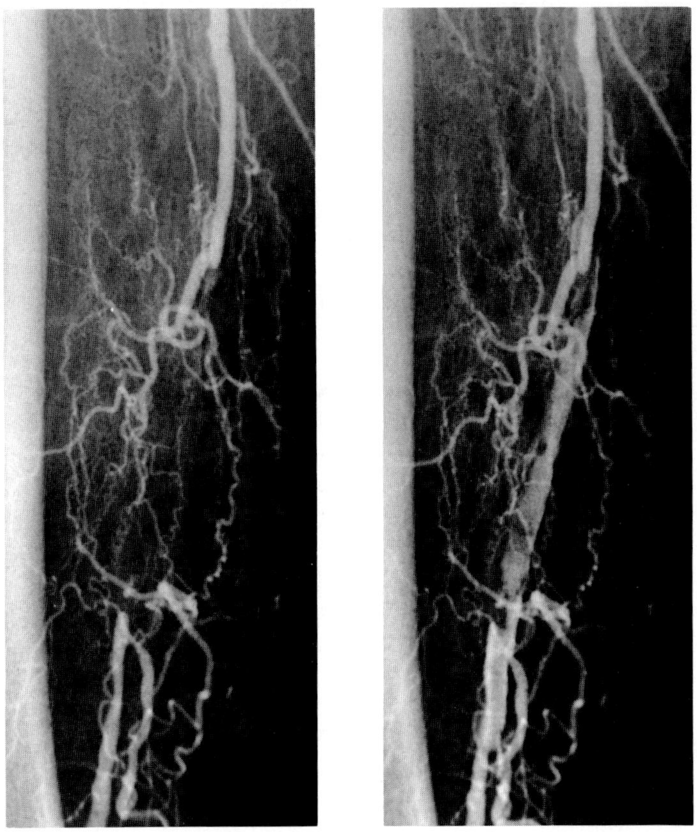

A B

Figure 35–6. Superficial femoral artery occlusion, 5 cm in length, clinical stage IIb. **A:** Initial angiogram. **B:** Dissection due to extra-axial catheter passage.

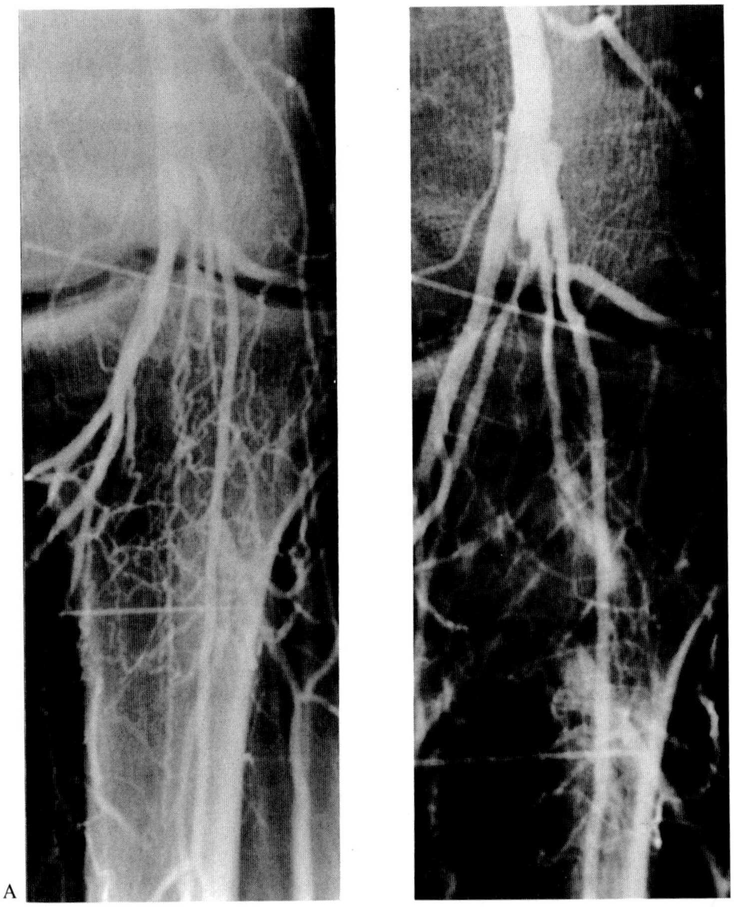

Figure 35–7. Four centimeter popliteal artery occlusion, including the trifurcation, clinical stage IV. **A:** Initial angiogram. **B:** Perforation with cloudy contrast extravasation.

Nd:YAG laser in combination with a sapphire probe catheter. The criteria for inclusion were chronic femoropopliteal artery occlusions with a length of 2 to 15 cm causing clinical stage IIb to IV disease (Fontaine). Fresh occlusions and iliac artery obstructions were excluded. A total of 338 patients were entered into this study. The mean length of the occlusions was 8.5 cm. Recanalization was successful in 288 patients (initial recanalization rate, 85%). Early rethrombosis within the first 2 weeks occurred in 10% of the patients. The long-term patency rate (life-table analysis) after 6 months, 1, 2, and 3 years, was 80%, 71%, 62%, and 57%, respectively (Fig. 35-8). The long-term patency rates were independent of the length of the occlusion and the kind of medical therapy (platelet inhibition versus anticoagulation) but significantly dependent on the outflow situation. Patients with 2 or 3 occluded calf arteries had a 3-year patency rate of only 52%, whereas patients with a normal runoff had a 3-year patency rate of 63%. About one third of the recurrent obstructions were segmental stenoses, which could be retreated easily by a second balloon dilation.

SIDE EFFECTS AND COMPLICATIONS

Perforation or dissection occurred in 9% of the patients. It was preceded by local pain in almost all cases. Peripheral emboli occurred in 3%, an arteriovenus fistula in 0.6%, a false aneurysm after previous perforation in 0.3%, and a vascular spasm in 0.6% of the patients. A serious hematoma at the inguinal puncture site was observed in 2% of the patients. The overall complication rate was 15% in 14% of the patients. Emergency surgery was required in only 5 of 338 patients (1.5%).

CONCLUSIONS

Eight years after Choy et al.'s[2] first publications about laser angioplasty, experimental series have shown that the usual human fibrofatty arteriosclerotic plaque can be ablated by low-power continuous-wave and short-pulsed lasers.[12–16] Calcified plaques are currently a serious limitation for both laser systems. Since 1985 clinical feasibility studies have shown that laser recanalization of peripheral artery obstructions with continuous wave lasers in combination with contact probes or pulsed lasers with multifiber catheters are safe procedures with clinical success rates comparable to conventional methods.[17–25] The largest prospective trial used a continuous wave Nd:YAG laser in combination with a sapphire probe catheter.[26] These results and those of other groups justify further clinical trials. These trials will have to be evaluated to see whether recanalization by laser energy

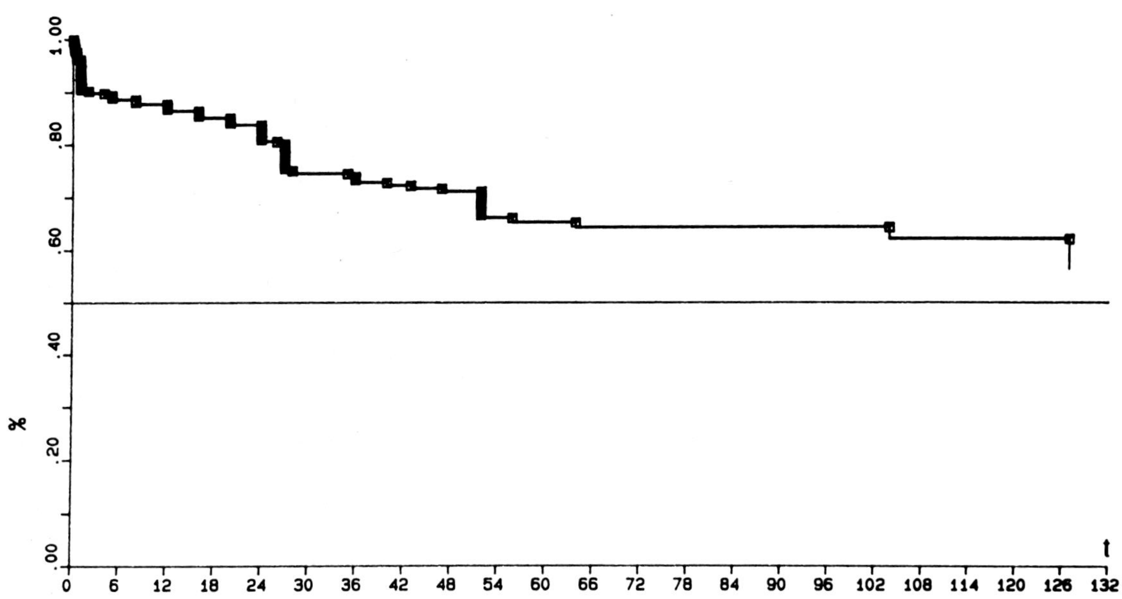

Figure 35–8. Long-term patency rate of the successfully recanalized arteries (Kaplan-Meier life-table analysis). X-axis: time in weeks; Y-axis: percentage of patent arteries.

ensures a higher recanalization and long-term patency rate than recanalization by conventional guide wire-catheter technology. The issue of whether continuous wave lasers or pulsed lasers provide better results can also be answered only by a prospective randomized trial, which is underway at the present time.[27]

REFERENCES

1. Lee G, Ikeda RM, Kozina J, Mason DT. Laser dissolution of coronary atherosclerotic obstruction. Am Heart J 1981; 102:1074–5.
2. Choy DSJ, Sterzer SH, Rotterdam HZ, et al. Transluminal laser catheter angioplasty. Am J Cardiol 1982;50:1206–8.
3. Geschwind H, Boussignac G, Teisseire B, et al. Percutaneous transluminal laser angioplasty in man. (Letter.) Lancet 1984;1:844.
4. Ginsburg R, Kim DS, Guthaner D, et al. Salvage of an ischemic limb by laser angioplasty: Description of a new technique. Clin Cardiol 1984;7:54–8.
5. Choy DSJ, Sterzer SH, Myler RK, et al. Human coronary laser recanalization. Clin Cardiol 1984;7:377–81.
6. Lammer J, Ascher PW, Choy DSJ: Transfemorale Katheter-Laser-Thrombendarterektomie (TEA) der Arteria Carotis. Dtsch Med Wochenschr 1986;111:607–10.
7. Lee G, Ikeda RM, Chan ML. Dissolution of human atherosclerotic disease by fiberoptic laser-heated metal cautery cap. Am Heart J 1984;107:777–8.
8. Sanborn TA, Haudenschild CC, Faxon DP, Ryan TJ. Experimental angioplasty: circumferential distribution of laser thermal energy with a laser probe. J Am Coll Cardiol 1985; 5:934–8.
9. Daikuzono N, Joffe SN. An artificial sapphire probe for contact photocoagulation and tissue vaporization. Med Instrum 1985;19:173–8.
10. Lammer J, Pilger E, Kleinert R, Ascher PW. Laserangioplastie peripherer arterieller Verschlüsse. Experimentelle und klinische Ergebnisse. Fortschr Roentgenstr 1987;147:1–5.
11. Lammer J, Kleinert R, Pilger E, et al. Contact probes for intravascular recanalization. Experimental evaluation. Invest Radiol 1989;24:190–5.
12. Abela GS, Normann S, Cohen D, et al. Effects of carbon dioxide, Nd:YAG, and argon laser radiation on coronary atheromatous plaques. Am J Cardiol 1982;50:1199–205.
13. Lee G, Ikeda RM, Herman I, et al. The qualitative effects of laser irradiation on human arteriosclerotic disease. Am Heart J 1983;105:885–9.
14. Lee G, Ikeda RM, Stobbe D, et al. Effects of laser irradiation on human thrombus: demonstration of a linear dissolution-dose relation between clot length and energy density. Am J Cardiol 1983;52:876–87.
15. Grundfest W, Litvak F, Forrester J. Pulsed ultraviolet lasers provide precise control of atheroma ablation. (Abstr.) Circulation 1984;70 (Suppl II):35.
16. Grundfest W, Litvak F, Forrester J. Laser injury of human atherosclerotic plaque without adjacent tissue injury. J Am Coll Cardiol 1985;5:929–33.
17. Ginsburg R, Wexler L, Mitchell RS, Profitt D. Percutaneous transluminal laser angioplasty for treatment of peripheral vascular disease. Radiology 1985;156:619–24.
18. Cumberland DC, Taylor DI, Procter AE: Use of lasers in percutaneous peripheral angioplasty. Semin Intervent Radiol 1986;3:65–8.
19. Lammer J, Pilger E, Kleinert R: Laser angioplasty by sapphire contact probe. Experimental and clinical results. J Intervent Radiol 1988;3:53–8.
20. Cumberland DC, Sanborn TA, Talyer DI, et al. Percutaneous laser thermal angioplasty: initial clinical results with a laser probe in total peripheral artery occlusions. Lancet 1986; 11457–9.
21. Sanborn TA, Greenfield AJ, Guben JK, et al. Human percutaneous and intraoperative laser thermal angioplasty: initial clinical results as an adjunct to balloon angioplasty. J Vasc Surg 1987;5:83–9.
22. Lammer J, Karnel F. Percutaneous transluminal laser angioplasty with contact probes. Radiology 1988;168:733–7.
23. Lammer J, Karnel F, Pilger E, et al. Nd-YAG Laser Angio-

plasty with Contact Probes. Pros and Cons in PTA and Auxiliary Methods. Berlin: Springer-Verlag, 1989.
24. Diethrich EB, Timbadia E, Bahadir I, et al. Argon laser-assisted peripheral angioplasty. Vasc Surg 1988;22:77–87.
25. Perler BA, Osterman FA, White RI Jr, Williams GM. Percutaneous laser probe femoropopliteal angioplasty: a preliminary experience. J Vasc Surg 1989;10:351–7.
26. Lammer J, Pilger E, Karnel F, et al. Laser angioplasty: results of a prospective, multicenter study at 3-year follow-up. Radiology 1991;178:335–7.
27. Lammer J, Pilger E, Karnel F, et al. Recanalization of arteriosclerotic occlusions with excimer laser, Nd:YAG laser, or guide wire: preliminary report of a randomized trial (WIP). Radiology 1989;173 (P):387.

36 High-Power Argon Laser Delivery in Canine Coronary Arteries

Leonard A. Nordstrom, M.D., Thomas M. Rassmussen, B.S., Diane K. Burnside, A.A.S.

Having reported our early clinical results with direct argon laser exposures for treatment of peripheral arterial obstructions,[1] we began an experimental series to investigate possible coronary applications with the same laser delivery system. Other investigators have demonstrated that 1 to 2 J of collimated, continuous wave argon laser energy are sufficient to perforate normal canine coronary arteries in vivo. However, our clinical experience in peripheral arteries suggested that higher levels of argon laser energy were necessary to ablate atherosclerotic tissue when diverged laser light was utilized.

The purpose of this study was to deliver high-power argon laser energy to normal canine coronary arteries. A second aim was to evaluate the control strategies characterizing this laser delivery system in the coronary arteries of live dogs.

Four strategies were utilized to control laser delivery: coaxial alignment, increased beam divergence, infusion of an irrigating solution during laser delivery (for this study, Ringer's solution), and surveillance of the fluorescence of a lens assembly mounted onto the optical fiber.

Laser exposures were preceded by the inflation of a multilumen balloon catheter, which contained the optical fiber within its central lumen. Inflating the balloon caused it to brace against the inner circumference of the arterial wall and axially align the optical fiber within the artery, despite systolic motion. When inflated, the balloon temporarily occluded blood flow, which would have interfered with the emitted laser beam profile,[2] from entering the lasing field. Residual blood and contrast media were then displaced by infusing lactated Ringer's solution during lasing. This infusion also convected heat from the treatment site, to limit thermal conduction to surrounding tissue.[3]

To supplement coaxial alignment, the divergence angle of the laser beam was increased by transmitting laser energy through a synthetic lens mounted at the distal tip of the optical fiber. The emitted laser beam assumed a cone profile measuring 40° in a saline medium. With a diverged laser beam, the diameter of the ablation channel was larger than otherwise possible (e.g., with a bare optical fiber transmitting collimated laser energy).[4] Increased beam divergence preserved the energy density necessary for ablation between 1 and 2 mm from the optical fiber tip; beyond this, energy density dissipated inversely by the square of increasing distance. With the focal distance of the beam foreshortened, it was possible to transmit laser energy close to the tip of the balloon catheter, rather than over a protracted distance within the artery.

As an additional strategy for controlling laser exposures, the fluorescence of the synthetic lens assembly was monitored. The wavelength of the light emitted by the lens was detectably different than the argon laser wavelengths transmitted through the lens. Lens fluorescence varied as a function of power of the incident laser beam, and the amplitude of the fluorescent signal was also inversely proportional to the operating temperature of the lens. During a laser exposure, the fluorescent light signal emitted by the lens was returned through the optical fiber to a beam splitter within the laser system. There it was filtered, amplified, and compared to known values. Whenever the fluorescence signal deviated from an assigned optimum range (±20% of a calibrated standard for normal operation of the laser), the system caused the electro-optical shutters within the laser head to close. With shutter control initiated within 500 msec and power at 10 W, this configuration yielded a 5 J laser exposure.

The optical feedback system permitted the system to recognize several potentially adverse lasing conditions as they occurred and terminate the exposure faster than would have been possible manually. Contact between the lens and tissue surfaces, or coating of the lens with blood or cellular contaminants caused the laser exposure to terminate before the selected lasing interval would have been delivered. Similarly, if the optical fiber had broken or the lens assembly detached, exposures would have terminated due to loss of the fluorescent signal.

METHODS

The study design called for performing laser exposures in coaxial alignment with the normal arterial wall, and the lasing protocol called for a maximum exposure of 10 W of power and 5 sec duration. A canine coronary model was selected for this study because of its availability; additionally, an open chest model was utilized throughout the study to allow visual confirmation of coaxial alignment. These studies were conducted from October 1986 through August 1987.

Low-power laser exposures (0.7 to 0.25 W) performed with the optical fiber coaxially aligned within the artery caused a diffused translucence along a length of the artery itself (Fig. 36-1). Conversely, an intense, focal brilliance seen through the arterial wall indicated misalignment of the laser beam (Fig. 36-2). Safety glasses providing protection from argon laser wavelengths were worn during laser exposure.

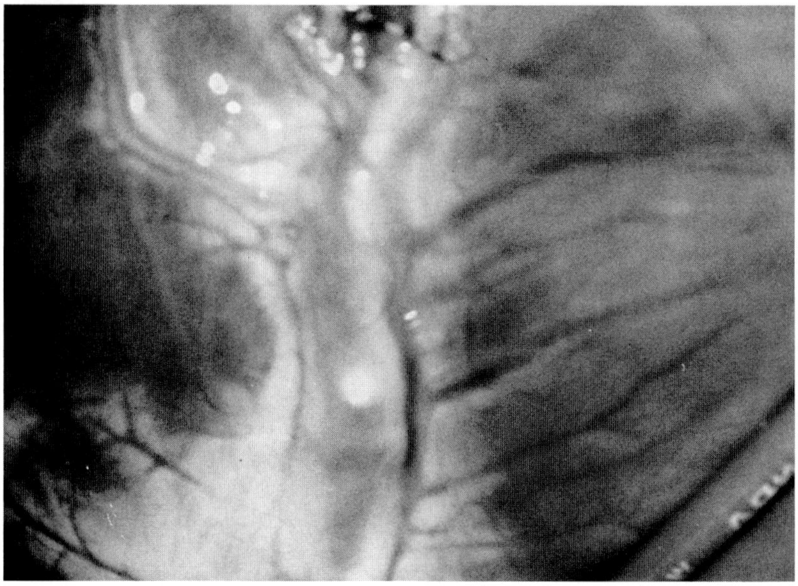

Figure 36–1. In an in vitro demonstration of transillumination, seen here in a porcine heart, a low power (0.1 to 0.25 W) exposure produced a brilliant spot on the artery wall, indicating nonaxial laser delivery. Laboratory personnel wore protective glasses sensitive to argon laser wavelengths.

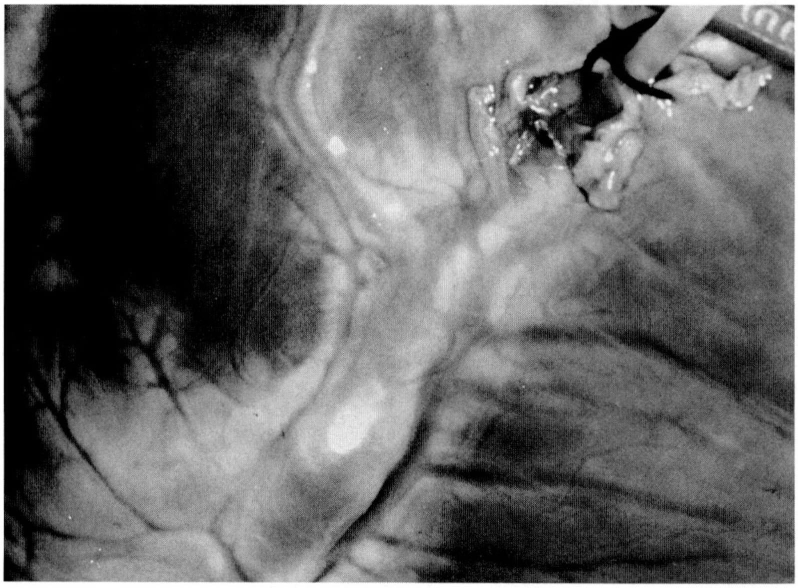

Figure 36–2. Translucence along the length of the artery confirmed coaxial alignment.

The delivery system employed in this investigation (LASTAC System, GV Medical, Inc., Plymouth, MN) applies argon laser energy directly to plaque tissue as an adjunct to angioplasty. The removal of plaque tissue is predicated on plaque tissue absorbing direct laser energy and vaporizing: the optical fiber and lens are not placed in contact with tissue while lasing.

Laser exposures were generated by an 18 W power source and were monitored continuously through a power meter integrated within the electronic circuitry of the delivery system (Fig. 36-3). A Simpson power meter and a Coherent thermal detector were used to verify the accuracy of the selected power level before and after each laser exposure.

Two balloon configurations were evaluated for this series, with both balloon designs proportionately shortened and scaled to correspond to the diameter of the coronary vasculature (Figs. 36-4, 36-5).

Treatment Protocol

Eight mongrel dogs, weighing between 27 and 40 kg each, were maintained according to National Institutes of Health animal research guidelines.[5] Dogs were anesthetized with pentobarbital (Nembutal, 25 mg/kg), and intubated. Electrocardiographic tracings were monitored throughout the procedure and arterial pressure was continuously monitored and recorded from either the left internal mammary or left carotid

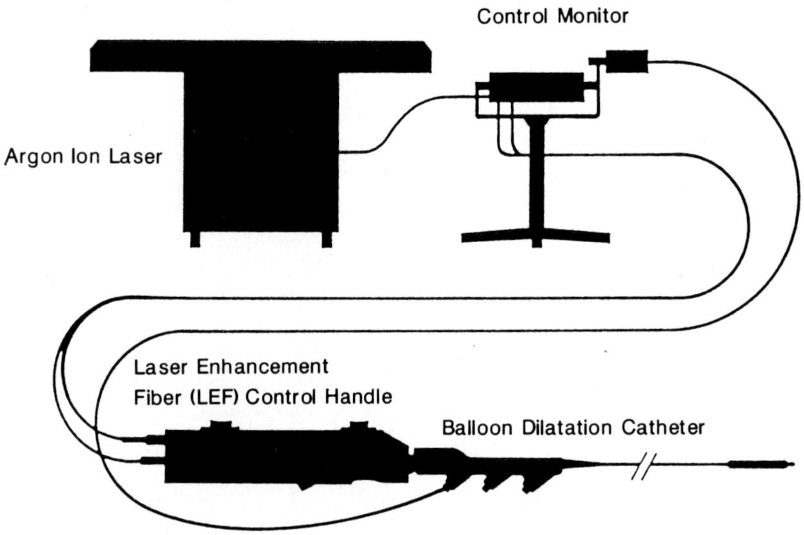

Figure 36–3. The delivery system consisted of a laser power source, a control monitor, and an integrated control handle for the optical fiber, which coupled with the balloon catheter handle. A pump infused irrigation fluid (Ringer's solution) through the multilumen balloon catheter during laser exposures.

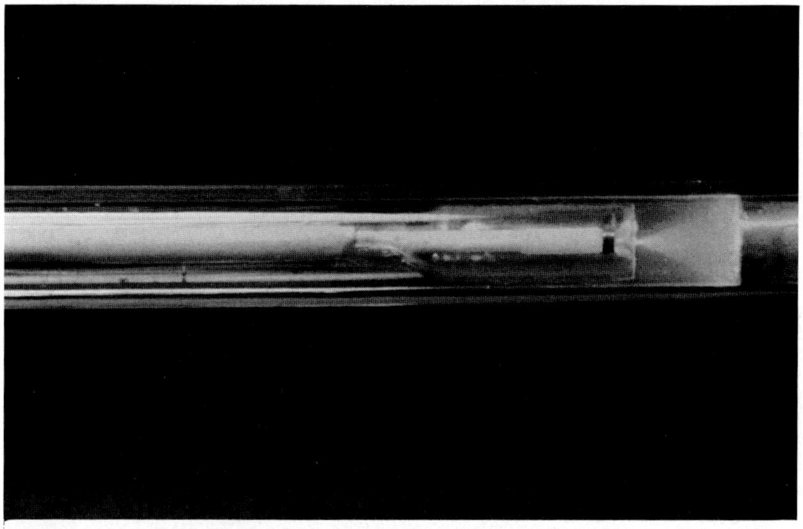

Figure 36–4. In order to occlude blood flow, coaxially align the optical fiber, and accommodate the coronary vascular bed, the balloon catheter was scaled to 1 cm × 3 mm. In this balloon design, the balloon tip was inverted with the optical fiber recessed within the cone.

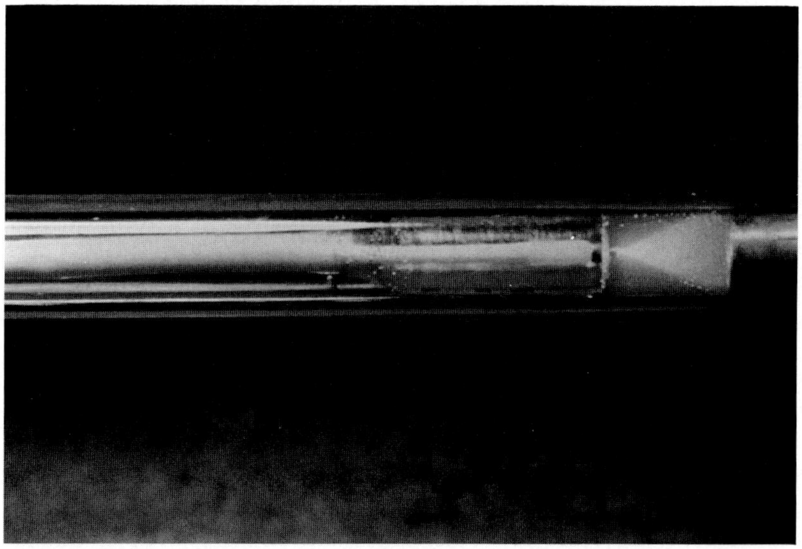

Figure 36–5. A second balloon design with a blunt tip was also investigated.

artery. A left thoracotomy was performed at the fourth intercostal space and, after careful incision of the pericardium, the heart was exposed and supported within the pericardial cradle. At this point, the right femoral artery was entered percutaneously or by surgical cut-down if necessary, and an 8.5 F introducer sheath was placed for a retrograde approach to the heart.

Prior to coronary catheterization, bretylium tosylate (Bretylol, 10 mg/kg) was diluted to a total volume of 50 ml with 9% saline solution and slowly given intravenously over 15 minutes to control arrhythmias. Heparin sodium was also administered intravenously (250 IU/kg) prior to laser treatment.

Once an 8 F coronary guiding catheter (Interventional Medical, Danvers, MA) was advanced under fluoroscopy into the left coronary ostium, either a 0.014 or 0.016 inch standard J-tipped guide wire was introduced into the left anterior descending (LAD) or left circumflex (LCx) branch of the left main coronary artery. An appropriately sized centering balloon was introduced over the guide wire until positioned within the treatment artery, whereupon the guide wire was withdrawn and exchanged for a 200 μm core quartz optical fiber with an optical assembly mounted distally. The balloon was inflated to 2 to 3 atm to occlude the artery and the optical fiber was positioned under fluoroscopy, so that the radiopaque tip of the optical fiber emerged from the balloon catheter. When properly positioned, the radiopaque tips of the balloon catheter and optical fiber formed a cruciform profile or inverted "T" configuration (Fig. 36-6).

Before laser delivery, the system synchronized an infusion of Ringer's solution through the central lumen of the balloon catheter (10 to 40 ml/min). Infusion began 5 sec before and continued for the duration of each exposure. Whenever necessary, an enhanced bolus was pumped to eliminate adherent blood or contrast media from the fiber tip. Laser exposures then commenced in distal segments of the artery, with two successive exposures attempted at each site.

Each exposure consisted of either 5 or 10 W and lasted for 0.5 to 8.5 seconds. Once treatment was completed at a given site, the optical fiber was retracted into the balloon catheter, and angiography was performed. The balloon was subsequently deflated and the catheter was withdrawn proximally, reinflated and the lasing sequence was repeated at a new site. Every effort was made to deliver at least 100 J of laser energy per site.

After laser exposures and angiography, epicardial sutures were placed just distal to the tip of the catheter to mark each lasing site for subsequent histology. Once all experimental laser treatments were completed, cine-angiography was obtained to document the integrity of the arteries treated. These films were immediately reviewed and accepted before the animal was given a drug overdose (T61: 1 ml/4.5 kg). The heart was then excised, rinsed, and fixed in formalin. Serial transverse sections 1 mm thick were taken beginning 1 cm beyond the most distal lasing site, and proceeding proximally to the coronary ostium. Sections were embedded in paraffin, sectioned serially to 4 μm and stained with hematoxylin and eosin. Examination was conducted under light microscopy, with the results fully documented in a histopathology report.

RESULTS

Sixty-eight exposures were made at 22 sites in a total of nine LAD and LCx coronary arteries; the total amount of laser energy delivered was 1550 J (Table 36-1). Eleven treatment sites sustained high-power laser exposures without thermal effects, with a mean exposure of 70 J/site (±46 J, SD). No evidence of gross or histologic perforation, charring, or related sequelae was apparent at these sites (Fig. 36-6). Nine

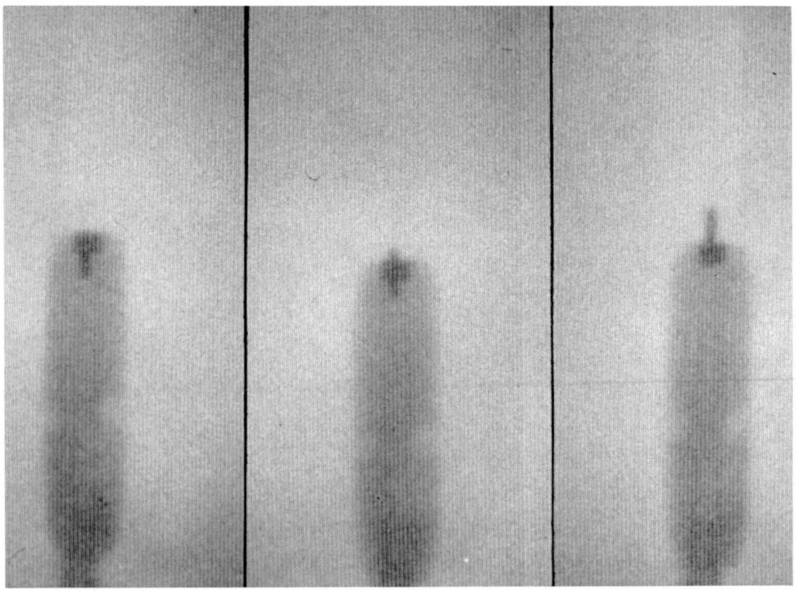

Figure 36–6. The radiopaque tip of the optical fiber is shown with fluoroscopy. The fiber is seen approaching, crossing, and extending beyond the tip of the balloon catheter, forming an "inverted T" configuration to indicate coaxial alignment.

Table 36–1. Dosimetry Summary

ARTERY	SITES (N)	EXPOSURES (N)	JOULES/SITE	JOULES/ARTERY
Left anterior descending (n = 5)				
Proximal	4	13	65 ± 50*	—
Middle	7	13	53 ± 39	—
Distal	2	10	93 ± 43	—
Summary	13	36	63 ± 45	163 ± 64
Circumflex (n = 4)				
Proximal	3	8	58 ± 33	—
Middle	4	14	74 ± 40	—
Distal	2	10	133 ± 33	—
Summary	9	32	82 ± 46	184 ± 91
All (n = 9)	22	68	70 ± 47	172 ± 78

*Standard deviation includes partial exposures terminated by the control system.

of the 11 sites sustained 10 W of laser power for up to 5 sec; the remaining two sites sustained 5 W for 2 seconds. Over the entire series, exposures averaged 89 J (±49). Partial exposures interrupted by the fluorescent feedback system were included in the total energy per site and contributed to the large standard deviation reported for the mean.

Seven perforations occurred. Two were observed directly during treatment and were also viewed on angiography as immediate extravasation of contrast dye. The first occurred in a proximal LAD segment of the LAD that had received 5 W of power for 2 sec (10 J). This laser perforation had been observed directly as a bright spot that appeared within the vessel wall. The perforation itself appeared as a charred, circular area on the arterial wall. Perivascular bleeding commenced approximately 30 seconds after the laser exposure and subsided after spontaneous formation of a periarterial hematoma. The other obvious perforation occurred at a distal segment of the LAD, on the initial laser exposure. This perforation was created by a 10 W, 5 sec exposure (50 J) and required ligation of the artery.

The remaining five perforations were not suspected clinically at the time of the lasing procedure: these microscopic perforations were only detected during histopathologic examination (Table 36-2). All perforations resulted from laser thermal injury, and each was located in the LAD, except for a single perforation in the LCx. No mechanical perforations occurred.

Histologic Findings

Mild thermal effects were evident at three sites that exhibited amorphous cellular debris, pyknotic smooth muscle cell nuclei that were associated with disruption of the internal elastic lamina, and neutrophil infiltration (Fig. 36-7). One other laser exposure penetrated halfway through the medial layer of the arterial wall (Fig. 36-8). This crater injury did not exhibit charred material on histopathologic examination, but amorphous eosinophilic material did surround the crater for approximately 0.7 mm. Thin, adherent strands of fibrinous thrombus were also present (Fig. 36-9).

Histologic features of the perforations included charring, surrounded by a vacuolized zone of tissue necrosis with amorphous material present (Fig. 36-10). Neutrophil infiltration was also observed in adjacent tissue, as was filamentous thrombi. One small clot was found adhering to an arterial segment distal to the lasing site; however, this artifact may have formed postmortem. None of these thrombi were discernible on angiography, probably due to their relatively small size, and each was tolerated by the animals until termination.

Hemodynamic Status

All animals were hypertensive prior to treatment, with normal sinus rhythm. During balloon inflations, depressed T-waves became evident in all dogs; these were resolved after release of the balloon pressure and reperfusion. All dogs remained otherwise hemodynamically stable during laser treatment.

DISCUSSION

Previous studies involving percutaneous delivery of direct laser energy to canine coronary arteries resulted in a variety of adverse sequelae, chiefly thermal perforation.[6] Among those who have prepared similar canine coronary models, Lee et al.[7] used a 400 μm bare fiber to deliver between 4 and 5.6 W for 5 to 20 seconds. Extensive vessel perforation occurred and four dogs died of complications from cardiac tamponade. Crea et al.[8] similarly reported perforations occurring with 1 W, 1 sec exposures in canine coronary arteries. Five perforations occurred in eight arteries and three dogs died from cardiac tamponade. Anderson et al.[9] coaxially aligned an optical fiber over a steerable guide wire and delivered 2 W of argon laser power for up to 40 sec before perforating. Coaxial alignment of the optical fiber did reduce the incidence of laser perforation, but one would also expect heat conduction and thermocoagulation as likely tissue effects from these low-power, long-duration exposures.

Table 36–2. Total Energy and Laser Effects Summary (Studies 1 to 7)

CORONARY ARTERY	TOTAL ENERGY (J)	EVIDENCE OF PERFORATION		THERMAL DAMAGE
		Angiographic	*Histologic*	
Left anterior descending				
Distal	135	—	−	−
	50	+	+	+
Mid	15	−	−	−
	50	−	−	+
	100	−	−	−
	10	−	−	−
	85	−	+	+
	10	−	+	+
	100	−	−	+
Proximal	10	−	+	+
	20	+	+	+
	120	−	+	+
	110	−	−	−
Left circumflex				
Distal	165	−	−	−
	100	−	−	−
Mid	25	−	−	+
	45	−	+	+
	125	−	−	−
	100	−	−	−
Proximal	20	−	−	−
	100	−	−	−
	55	−	−	+

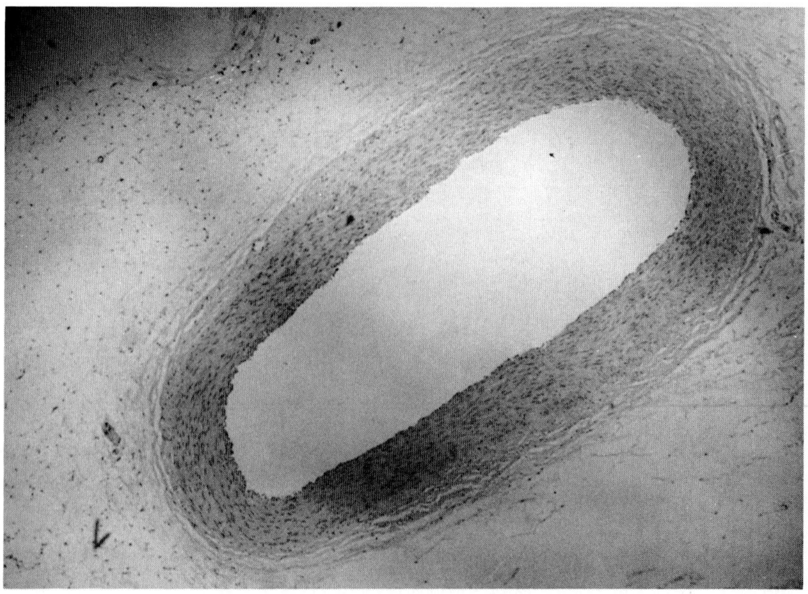

Figure 36–7. Histologic view of a mid-left anterior descending coronary artery section that received two 5 W, 5 sec exposures (50 J). No cellular shrinkage, vacuolization, or charring was evident.

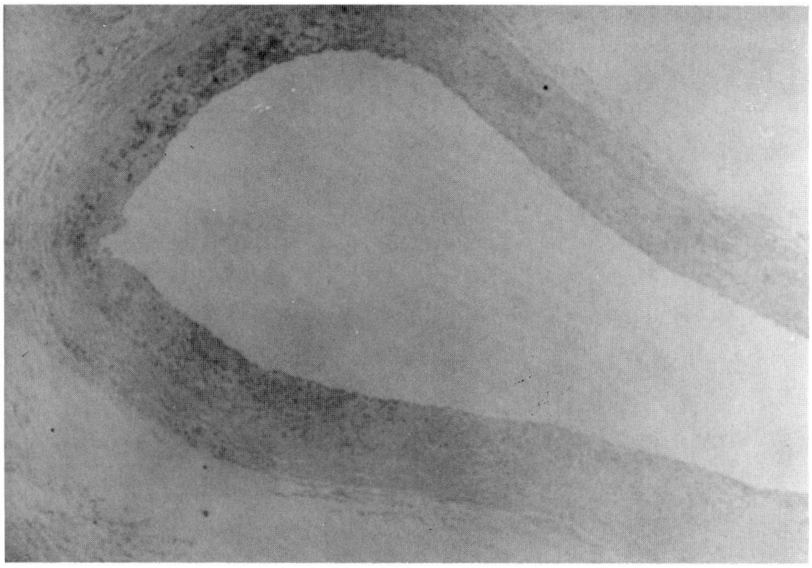

Figure 36–8. A section from a mid-left circumflex coronary artery section, which received 125 J in six exposures. Four exposures were interrupted when optical feedback became excessive; two were of 5 sec duration. Superficial epicardium contained a mild hematoma; focal thinning of the vessel with pyknotic smooth muscle cell nuclei was also evident. The luminal defect (arrow) is a sectioning artifact.

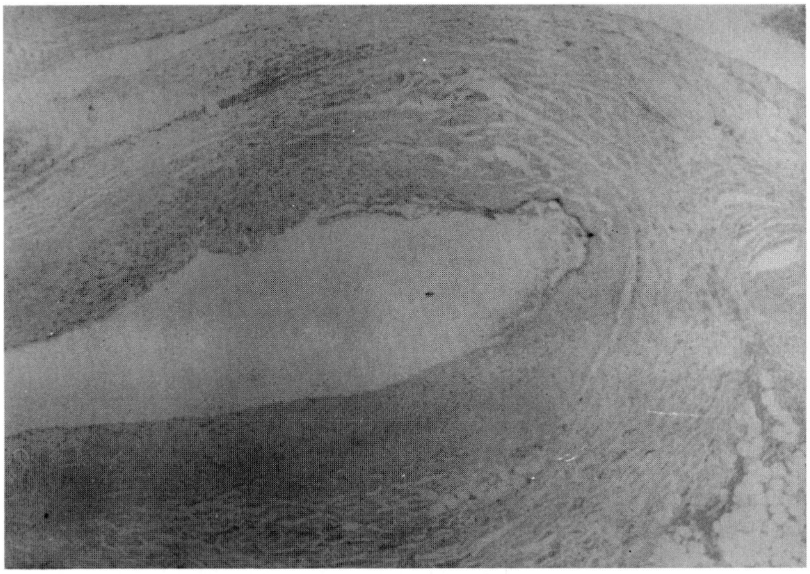

Figure 36–9. A laser injury in a mid-left circumflex coronary artery section, which received 55 J. The artery contains a focal 0.2 × 0.3 mm crater that penetrated halfway through vessel wall. Charring was absent, but amorphous eosinophilic material was present to a depth of 0.7 mm.

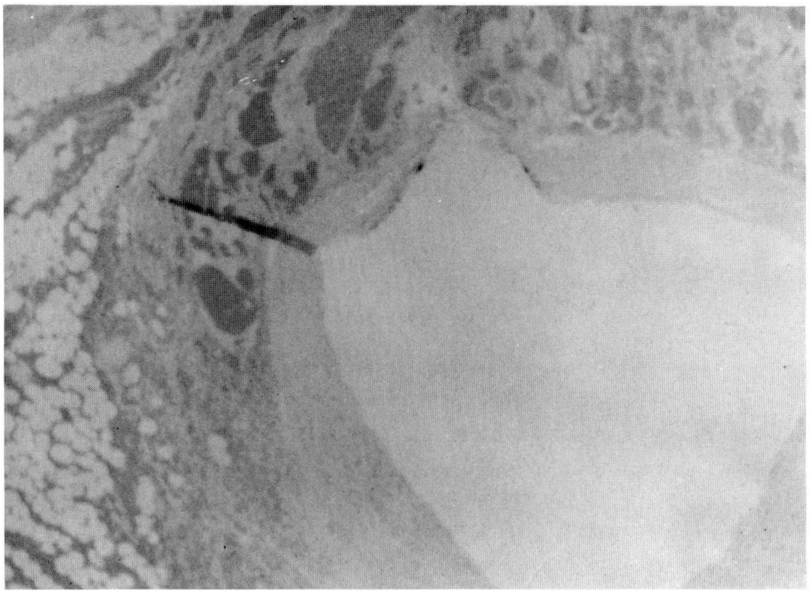

Figure 36–10. Gross perforation of a mid-left anterior descending coronary artery segment receiving 110 J. The hole is 0.4 mm at its greatest diameter; charring and vacuolization are present, as is a small epicardial hematoma.

In a study undertaken by Bowker et al.,[10] a bare optical fiber was coaxially maintained by loading it through a lumen of an inflated balloon catheter. A perforation threshold of 6 to 10 J was noted using a coaxializing balloon catheter, and 3 to 4 J without. Two perforations occurred in a total of 34 laser exposures in the 14 arteries treated. Additionally, one animal died immediately from ventricular fibrillation attributed to laser exposure.

It has been our clinical experience that little, if any, plaque would be removed by low-power argon laser energy, especially with the convective saline infusion and increased beam divergence characterizing this delivery system. In this study, the amount of power delivered was generally higher than previous investigators have delivered. An average of 70 J were delivered successfully in 11 sites, without thermal damage.

Of the seven perforations that occurred, six were located in the LAD coronary artery. Only one LCx perforation occurred in a total of 32 exposures performed at 11 sites within the four LCx arteries treated. The reasons for the predominance of perforations in the LAD coronary artery are not entirely clear, but one could speculate.

First, the LAD coronary artery of the dog tends to be smaller in diameter than the LCx. Dogs normally have a very small right coronary artery and a large circumflex, with the LAD being somewhat smaller than the latter. A smaller arterial diameter could increase the possibility of laser injury.

A second possibility would be that in dogs the middle two thirds of the circumflex coronary artery tends to be straighter than the LAD coronary artery. A relatively straight arterial segment would obviously lend itself to better coaxial placement.

As a third possibility, the fluoroscopic unit used in this study had only a fixed plane viewing capability. Thus, all judgments made in regard to proper placement of the fiber in the catheter system had to be made from fluoroscopy conducted in just one plane. The view needed to position the centering balloon properly in the LAD coronary artery proved to be a tangential (oblique) view, as opposed to perpendicular. This created the distinct possibility that the laser fiber extended too far from the tip of the balloon catheter. In an artery that was already more tortuous, the tip of the optical fiber may have come closer to the arterial wall than expected.

Two microscopic perforations were attributable to prolonged lasing intervals of 8.5 and 5 sec, respectively. With prolonged exposures at higher power levels, the thermal relaxation time in tissue is not sufficient to allow thermal energy to dissipate, thus increasing the chance of perforation. Finally, one perforation resulted after the feedback cycle interrupted two successive exposures. In this particular case, the optical fiber was either very close or in actual contact with the arterial wall during lasing; the feedback system subsequently responded properly to terminate the exposure. However, it was evident that the optical feedback cycle was too long at 500 msec. Ten W of laser power will create a 5 J exposure, which is sufficient to injure the artery.

As for the coronary balloons evaluated in this series, both had blunt, "square shoulder" profiles to aid in centering the optical fiber. In initial experiments, longer balloons that were similar to those used clinically in human peripheral arteries were found unsuitable. The canine coronary arteries either became distended along the inflated balloon profile or collapsed distally. Once the balloons were shortened, coaxial alignment could be achieved with minimal effect to the arterial wall, provided the balloon was correctly sized for the artery. By positioning and inflating the balloons before lasing, a relatively stable platform existed in situ, despite the rapid heartbeat of these dogs.

The percutaneous approach used to access treatment sites was successful in all cases. With the optical fiber and assembly sheathed within the balloon catheter, mechanical perforation did not occur. None of the dogs died or became unstable during the experimental laser treatments.

CONCLUSION

In this study, continuous wave argon laser energy (5 or 10 W) was delivered to normal canine coronary arteries, using a 200 μm optical fiber with a lens assembly to increase beam divergence, and a specially designed balloon catheter to coaxially align the optical fiber. Ringer's solution (10 to 40 ml/min) was infused during laser exposures and a shut-down mechanism terminated exposures on tissue contact. Laser exposures were attempted at 22 sites in five LAD and 4 LCx arteries; in a total of 68 exposures an average of 89 ± 49 J were delivered. Two obvious thermal perforations were detected via angiography at the time of the procedure, and an additional five microscopic perforations were subsequently revealed by histopathologic examination. One perforation required intervention (ligation); otherwise, thermal effects were either absent or mild. Eleven sites sustained no thermal damage after receiving an average exposure of 70 J (±46).

Additional recommendations from these data include limiting laser exposures to 2 sec or less and verifying coaxial placement in biplane fluoroscopic views. The 500 msec response interval for the optical feedback system was reduced after this study to 130 msec.

REFERENCES

1. Nordstrom LA, Castañeda-Zúñiga WR, Young EG, Von Seggem KB. Direct argon laser exposures for recanalization of peripheral arteries: early results. Radiology 1988;168:457–64.
2. Fenech A, Abela GS, Crea F, et al. A comparative study of laser beam characteristics in blood and saline media. Am J Cardiol 1985;55:1389–92.
3. Nordstrom LA, Castañeda-Zúñiga WR, Khoury AI. Tissue thermal profile of direct argon laser irradiation. (Abstr.) Lasers Surg Med (Suppl) 1989;1:6.
4. Nordstrom LA, Castañeda-Zúñiga WR, Lindeke CC, et al. Laser angioplasty: controlled delivery of argon laser energy. Radiology 1988;167:463–5.

5. The guide for the care and use of laboratory animals. Bethesda, MD: National Institutes of Health, publication No. 85–23, revised 1985.
6. Isner JM, Donaldson RF, Funai JT, et al. Factors contributing to perforation resulting from laser coronary angioplasty: observations an intact human post-mortem preparation of intra-operative laser coronary angioplasty. Circulation 1985;72 (suppl II):191–9.
7. Lee G, Seckinger D, Chan MC, et al. Potential complications of coronary angioplasty. Am Heart J 1984;108:1577.
8. Crea F, Abela GS, Fenech A, et al. Transluminal laser irradiation of coronary arteries in live dogs: an angiographic and morphologic study of acute effects. Am J Cardiol 1986;57:171–4.
9. Anderson HV, Zaatari GS, Roubin GS, et al. Coaxial laser energy delivery using a steerable catheter in canine coronary arteries. Am Heart J 1987:113;37–48.
10. Bowker TJ, Fox KM, Cross FW, et al. Perforation thresholds and safety factors in in vivo coronary laser angioplasty. Br Heart J 1988;59:429–37.

37 A Review of the Clinical Utility of Laser Recanalization of Peripheral Arterial Obstructions: An Analysis of Patency at 1 Year

Leonard A. Nordstrom, M.D.

Within the last few years, the intravascular delivery of laser energy has gone from basic research to clinical application. With the advent of the ruby laser 30 years ago, intravascular laser delivery was only a dream.[2] Technologic accomplishments aside, considerable discussion in the literature has more recently focused on clinical value, as interventionalists wait for laser angioplasty to develop beyond demonstrated feasibility and establish a clearer role in the treatment of atherosclerotic disease.

We believe that argon laser energy can be controlled through the use of an integrated delivery system,[3] which can be used to recanalize peripheral vascular obstructions in humans with an acceptable rate of success. Our previously reported data demonstrate that the laser procedure in peripheral arteries can be performed with a relatively low risk of perforation and distal embolization.[4]

Coronary applications, although under intense investigation by many, remain experimental. The considerable experience gained from use of lasers in the peripheral vascular bed has not necessarily translated to the coronary setting. As a consequence, it appears that the respective treatment modalities may evolve along distinctly separate paths. Coronary laser procedures are a newer entity, whereas enough time has passed to accumulate follow-up data for peripheral laser procedures. Here, evaluation of direct laser angioplasty in an extended series of peripheral procedures for a larger patient population is presented and the patency of these vessels at 1 year post-treatment is assessed.

PERIPHERAL EXPERIENCE

As of October 1989, 68 laser angioplasty procedures were performed for 63 patients at Park Nicollet Medical Center, Minneapolis, Minnesota. The diagnostic criteria that formed the basis for patient selection ranged from ischemic symptoms occurring at rest or during exercise to gangrene or nonhealing ulcers. Angiographic evidence of hemodynamically significant stenoses or occlusions was considered as a second criterion. Indications for treatment included intermittent claudication (82%), rest pain (9%), nonhealing ulcers (7%), and gangrene (2%). The mean age for these patients was 66 years, with female patients comprising 54% of the study population. Other risk factors for peripheral vascular disease included the presence of diabetes in 16% of the patients and a history of smoking in 32%. Additionally, 27% of the patients had poor distal runoff, defined as the presence of 0 or 1 patent tibial arteries.

Lesions in the iliac or femoral-popliteal arteries were included in this series. All 14 iliac arteries were totally occluded, with an average lesion length of 6.2 cm (range, 1 to 12 cm). The average length for 42 femoral-popliteal total occlusions was 9 cm (range, 1 to 37 cm). Twelve additional lesions treated in the femoral-popliteal segment were high-grade stenoses, which were selected early in the series as the procedure was evolving. In these cases, we could not traverse the lesion with the specialized centering catheter of the delivery system, even with a guide wire in place. Laser energy was therefore employed to ablate plaque, enlarge the lumen and thus facilitate eventual dilation.

All patients were evaluated angiographically pre- and post-treatment, and at follow-up if reclosure was suspected. Additionally, distal pulses and ankle-brachial indices (ABI) were evaluated and documented pre- and post-treatment, at hospital discharge, and at 1-, 2-, 6-, 12-, and 24-month follow-up examinations. The mean length of follow-up for this series was 12 months and ranged from 3 weeks to 24 months. Data were classified as follows: technical success, clinical success, and long-term patency. Technical success was determined by the angiographic appearance of recanalization, accompanied by improved distal pulses and an increase of the ABI. Clinical success was defined as patency 4 days after the treatment and was based on the alleviation of symptoms and a sustained improvement in the ABI. Long-term patency was based on the same criteria at follow-up examinations.

The delivery system used in this series was the LASTAC System (GV Medical, Minneapolis, MN), which has been previously described. To review briefly, this system transmits continuous wave argon laser energy to the vascular lesion via a 200 μm quartz optical fiber inserted into the lumen of a centering balloon dilation catheter. Ablation of plaque is accomplished without actual contact by the catheter or delivery fiber, per se. Mounted at the distal tip of the fiber is an optical assembly that diverges the light beam (Fig. 37-1). The lens tip of the optical fiber increases the divergence of the laser light and protects the optical fiber from damage.

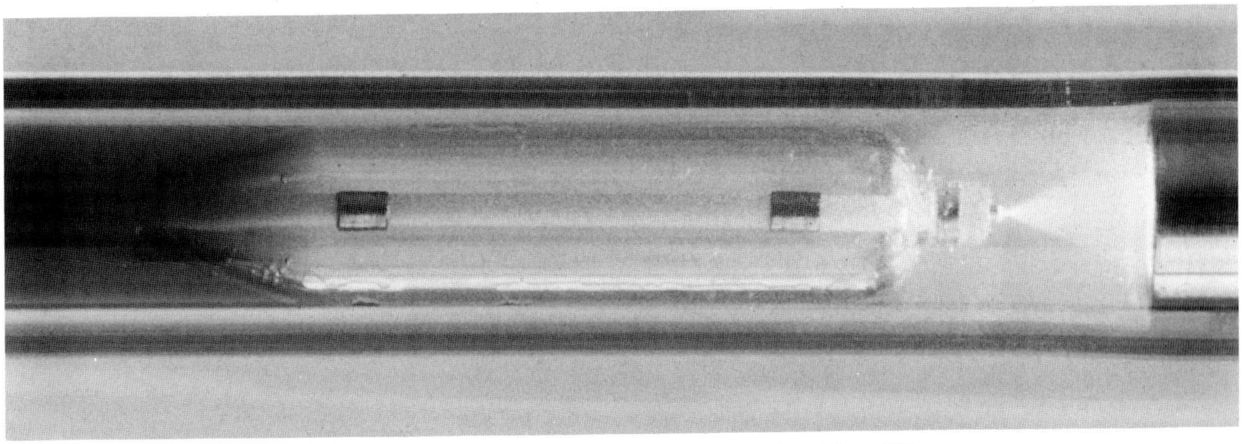

Figure 37–1. Centering balloon maintains coaxial position of fiber.

The centering balloon and optical assembly together provide the primary means of controlling beam direction. The inflated balloon aligns the fiber with the center axis of the arterial lumen, preventing a "blind" advance through the obstruction. Laser light is subsequently absorbed by plaque tissue, resulting in ablation. Because the absorption of argon laser light by plaque does not depend on actual contact with the delivery fiber, this fiber tip can be positioned 2 to 3 mm from the proximal surface of the obstruction. The optical assembly diverges the beam over this distance, increasing the diameter of the projected light spot and consequently, the area of tissue removal. With the light beam spread over a wider area, intensity is rapidly dissipated according to the inverse square law. However, the portion of the light beam in which power density (watts per square centimeter) exceeds the threshold for tissue removal remains within 3 mm of the fiber tip, where beam direction can best be controlled.[3]

Technique

All procedures were performed percutaneously, using an ipsilateral antegrade puncture to access femoral lesions and a retrograde approach for iliac. After placing an 8 F introducer sheath, 4000 to 5000 IU of intra-arterial heparin was administered, and an appropriate diameter centering balloon (3 to 4 cm long) was introduced over an 0.018 inch guide wire. Once the balloon was positioned proximal to the lesion, the optical fiber was inserted, advanced through the catheter lumen, and positioned approximately 2 mm from target tissue by visual observation. Inflating the centering balloon coaxially aligned the optical fiber and simultaneously occluded blood flow.

Laser recanalization consisted of multiple laser exposures performed at 10 W for 2 to 5 sec. Heparinized normal saline solution was infused at 10 to 30 ml/min during lasing to flush blood from the lasing field, as well as flush the fiber tip and surrounding tissue.

Tissue removal was documented by periodic contrast injections and fluoroscopy. As a channel was created through the lesion, the balloon was deflated and fiber and catheter were advanced together, with the fiber retracted within the catheter. After reinflating the balloon and repositioning the fiber, lasing was repeated until the lesion was traversed. The lesion was then segmentally dilated as the catheter was removed. In longer lesions, the centering balloon was removed altogether and a longer (10 cm) conventional balloon catheter was used to complete dilation. Conventional angioplasty was always performed after the laser procedure to increase the luminal diameter of the artery. An average of 820 J of energy were delivered per procedure.

After the treatment was completed, the sheath was removed and the heparin was either neutralized or allowed to dissipate. Post-treatment medications included aspirin and dipyridamole. Midway through the series, it was observed that patients who had either long lesions (more than 15 cm) or poor distal runoff experienced a higher rate of early reclosure postprocedure. Subsequently, patients at increased risk of early reclosure received systemic heparin for 18 to 24 hours following treatment.

Results

In this series, 59 of 68 procedures (87%) were considered technical successes. Of the 54 procedures performed in the femoral-popliteal segment, 49 were technically successful (91%). Stenoses were all successfully treated (100%). In iliac lesions, all of which were occlusions, 71% were technical successes. A summary of technical results, stratified by selected variables, is presented in Table 37-1.

Failures in the femoral-popliteal segment were attributed to the inability to ablate a sufficient amount of plaque that would have permitted the balloon catheter to advance distally. In the iliac occlusions, however, three of the four failures had actually demonstrated the angiographic appear-

Table 37–1. Lesion Characteristics and Primary Success

LESION CHARACTERISTICS			
Location	*Length (cm)*	NO.	SUCCESS (%)
Iliac occlusions	6.2*	10/14	71
Femoral-popliteal			
Occlusions	≤7	22/24	92
	>7	15/18	83
Stenoses	—	12/12	100

*Mean length.

ance of recanalization, yet when the sheath was removed, the ABI was unimproved.

Five early reclosures occurred in the entire series; the mean time to reclosure was 24 hours. Four of these reclosures occurred in the initial cohort of 36 patients.[4] In 32 subsequent procedures performed since the revised drug protocol was implemented, only one early reclosure has occurred. The clinical success rate was thus 54/68 (79%).

Complications were divided into two groups: laser-related and procedural complications of percutaneous transluminal angioplasty (PTA). Laser-related complications included two occurrences of distal embolization below the level of the knee; one was treated successfully with streptokinase and the second patient underwent several surgical procedures and, ultimately, an amputation. Three thermal perforations due to laser delivery occurred, all of which were inconsequential, clinically. Three groin hematomas that prolonged the patients' hospital stay occurred.

Compared with baseline, sustained improvement in symptoms and ABIs was observed in 39 patients at last follow-up. Fifteen arteries reclosed late, yielding a cumulative 1 year patency rate of 75%, as determined through life-table analysis. Examining long-term patency by selected variables such as lesion location and type, iliac total occlusions had a 1 year patency rate of 79%, compared with 91% for femoral-popliteal stenoses and 60% for femoral-popliteal total occlusions.

An analysis of patency, stratified by selected subgroups, is presented in Table 37-2. When all femoral-popliteal occlusions were analyzed together, patency was not affected by lesion length ($p = 0.73$), whereas the severity of disease was highly predictive of later patency ($p = 0.0003$). The patency rate for shorter lesions was, at first glance, somewhat lower than expected. The overall patency for limb salvage cases (23%) was in marked contrast to the overall patency obtained in patients treated for claudication (77%). We should, however, point out that 70% of the limb salvage cases had shorter lesions (7 cm or less), which weighted down the patency rate of shorter lesions. By controlling for the proportional difference of limb salvage cases for long and short lesions, the patency rates for the claudication group appeared more appropriate when subgrouped by lesion length. For claudicants, occlusions 7 cm or less had a 1 year patency rate of 84% and 68% for lesions longer than 7 cm.

ANALYSIS

The natural question posed by this study is whether laser-assisted balloon angioplasty offers any benefit over conventional balloon angioplasty. This question cannot be answered without examining the major limitations of balloon angioplasty itself, which are twofold. First, both the technical and clinical success of PTA are lower for total occlusions than stenoses. Second, the benefits of PTA tend to diminish predictably due to acute occlusion or later restenosis.

Compared with the results of our original series (34 patients), our technical success decreased only slightly in spite of the increased complexity of the later patients. This expanded series has produced data that differ from conventional PTA experience in several ways. In contrast to PTA of total occlusions,[5,6] our data did not show a significant difference when technical success rate was stratified according to the length of the lesions treated, which ranged up to 37 cm. One possible explanation is the design of the catheter system, which permits coaxial alignment and incremental advancement despite the varied lengths of lesions treated.[7]

In a broad context, the technical success rate for conventional PTA varies between 57[8] and 91%.[9] More specifically, our results for femoral-popliteal occlusions compare favorably with those most recently reported by Morgenstern et al,[9] and the complication rate was acceptably low. The incidence of thermal perforation, the single largest perceived risk for laser angioplasty, was actually only 4% in this series and in no case warranted emergency surgery. The incidence of distal embolization was also acceptably low (3%), and although three groin hematoma occurred that prolonged the patients' hospital stay, none required surgical intervention.

Closer comparison with historical data is fraught with many problems, such as diversity in reporting methods, patient selection, and definitions of success, to name just a few. The authors of many PTA studies have generally regarded[10] and would still maintain[11,12] that long lesions are relatively contraindicated for PTA alone. Many centers refer appropriate patients' lesions longer than 10 cm to bypass surgery, attempt thrombolysis,[13] or treat them with a combination of thrombolytic agents and PTA.[14–19]

The technical success rate for the iliac occlusions in our series was 71%. Here, comparisons with conventional PTA experience were limited because few PTA series have dealt exclusively with total obstructions in this vascular bed.[17–20]

Table 37–2. Subgroup Analysis of Patency

	PATENCY RATE AT 1 YEAR (%)			
	Claudicants	*n =*	*Limb salvage*	*n =*
All lesions (n = 35)	77	25	23	10
Occlusions				
≤7 cm	84	14	21	7
>7 cm	68	11	33	3

The reluctance to treat occluded iliac arteries as opposed to stenoses stems partially from a higher incidence of complications[19] and the relative difficulty of the procedure. Technical success rates reportedly range from 33 to 80%.

When we compared results of iliac versus femoral-popliteal arteries within our own series, the technical success rate in iliac occlusions was distinctly lower. The presence of fresh clot that failed to dilate or the "elastic recoil" phenomenon[21,22] may explain some of the technical failures in iliac occlusions. In three of the four failed cases, the lesion had been traversed using laser energy and subsequently dilated to obtain an apparent angiographic success, but despite the immediate angiographic appearance of recanalization, the ABIs remained unimproved.

Clinical success was somewhat affected by five instances of acute occlusion. In reviewing these cases two common factors were noted. The mean length of lesions treated was significantly longer: 17 versus 7.5 cm, and early reclosures tended to occur in patients with impaired runoff (one to two vessels). I believe that these factors pointed to an increased risk for acute thrombosis, so subsequently patients in those categories were treated with systemic heparin for an additional 18 to 24 hours. This change was not accompanied by an increase in complications, and in 32 subsequent procedures only one case of acute occlusion occurred. The incidence of early reclosure was thereby decreased from 11 to 3% in the expanded series ($p > 0.05$). For the entire series, the incidence of acute occlusion was 7%. That a problem with early reclosures secondary to thrombus formation was encountered is not surprising, given that angioplasty itself is known to increase the potential for thrombus formation,[23] as does impaired runoff. However, the data in this study do not answer the question of whether the laser actually intensified the thrombogenic potential.

The occurrence of such events was addressed by our definitions of success. As has been discussed previously,[24] the pathophysiologic pattern of PTA-treated arteries varies considerably over the course of time. Atheromatous plaque with or without supervening thrombus may be amenable to potential debulking by mechanical, thermal, or photoablative processes. In our series, technical success indicated the status of the artery immediately following recanalization. Once an artery is reopened, an entirely new clinical setting is faced, that of a highly thrombogenic arterial environment that may best respond to a pharmacologic approach with thrombolytic therapy.[25] One can further speculate that once a vessel is reopened with the laser, particularly in high-risk patients as described herein, it may be possible to keep it open by placing intravascular stents,[23–26] with or without subsequent thrombolytic therapy.[26–29]

Although the number of iliac procedures (10) available for follow-up analysis in this series is limited, 79% (±13) remained patent at 1 year, which compares favorably to the results obtained by Colapinto et al.[19] What Colapinto et al had observed in their series was also noted in this series: lesion length did not seem to affect long-term patency, since all four iliac lesions longer than 7 cm remained patent at 1 year. Continued patency over time would help determine the overall usefulness of the laser procedure in the iliac vascular bed.

An area of perhaps greater interest was the long-term results in the femoral-popliteal segment. The 1 year patency for femoral-popliteal occlusions was 71%. Again, the difference in patency was not statistically significant when lesion lengths were compared, but the initial review of the data pointed toward a somewhat unexpected trend: short occlusions fared slightly worse at 1 year, with a patency rate of 62%, versus 75% for lesions longer than 7 cm. Further scrutiny revealed a disproportionate number of limb salvage cases with short lesions (70%), and the poor patency (23%) experienced by these patients was fairly obvious. Although the number of limb salvage cases is small, one cannot dismiss the fact that the severity of the disease is a known predictor of poor patency[30,31] in the peripheral arteries. This assertion was supported by the patency of total occlusions treated in the claudication subgroups, which ranged from 83% for short occlusions (7 cm or less) to 86% in the long (more than 7 cm) lesions. The results within this particular subgroup compare quite favorably with the literature. Generally, patency after PTA in femoral-popliteal occlusions has been said to range from 43 to 79% at 2 years' follow-up,[32] with lower patency expected for the longer superficial femoral artery occlusions treated. Again, it is difficult to be certain whether these data represent a distinct improvement in long-term patency, given the small numbers. The results are encouraging, but ultimately need to be verified by continued long-term follow-up and duplicated in other series.

Overall, 37 of the 63 patients benefited from the procedure, with 39 of the 68 arteries patent at 1 year. Failure, whether technical, acute (prior to hospital discharge), or at a later time did not in any case jeopardize later treatment options, as others have similarly noted with conventional PTA.[33,34] Although not as durable as bypass surgery, the early results from this series suggest that laser angioplasty may at least delay the need for other therapies. The treatment does not appear to affect the underlying disease process adversely. I can say that the procedure improved symptoms for a substantial percentage of the claudicants treated.

The question of which treatment modality is appropriate for specific indications will ultimately have to be answered through controlled clinical trials. I do not take issue with the potential utility of such studies; however, a comparison of laser angioplasty with standard PTA may be premature at this time. Although laser angioplasty has made considerable strides since its inception, it still represents an immature technology. PTA in the peripheral bed has already had 15 years to develop, and there has been considerable improvement in balloon and guide wire technology that has brought balloon angioplasty to a relatively mature status. In this sense, randomized trials may succeed only in comparing an immature technology with a mature technology. I suggest that, meanwhile, the continued accumulation of long-term data and the validation of these initial results and those of others may be more realistic and pragmatic.

Acknowledgment. These results were originally presented at "MedTech '89: Advances in Interventional Cardio-Angiology" at the Second German Symposium on Laser Angioplasty, Berlin, November 4–7, 1989.

REFERENCES

1. Nordstrom LA. Direct argon laser-assisted angioplasty: one year follow-up results in peripheral arteries and initial coronary experience. Advances in Interventional Cardio-Angiology: Proceedings of the Second German Symposium on Laser Angioplasty, Berlin, November 1989.
2. McGuff PE, Bushnell D, Soroff HS, Deterling RA. Studies of the surgical applications of the laser (light amplification by stimulated emission of radiation). Surg Forum 1963;14:143–5.
3. Nordstrom LA, Castañeda-Zúñiga WR, Lindeke CC, et al. Laser angioplasty: controlled delivery of argon laser energy. Radiology 1988;167:463–465.
4. Nordstrom LA, Castañeda-Zúñiga WR, Young EG, Von Seggem KB. Direct argon laser exposure for recanalization of peripheral arteries: early results. Radiology 1988;168:359–64.
5. Henricksen LO, Jorgensen B, Holstein PE, et al. Percutaneous transluminal angioplasty of infrarenal arteries in intermittent claudication. Acta Chir Scand 1988;154:573–6.
6. Cambria RP, Faust G, Gusberg R, et al. Percutaneous angioplasty for peripheral arterial occlusive disease: correlates of clinical success. Arch Surg 1987;122:283–7.
7. Castañeda-Zúñiga WR, Nordstrom LA. Control of the optical fiber during laser-assisted percutaneous transluminal angioplasty: coaxial alignment and other critical considerations. In Zeitler E, Seyferth W, (eds): The Pros and Cons in PTA and Auxiliary Methods. Berlin: Springer-Verlag, 1989:52–9.
8. Krepel VM, van Andel GJ, van Erp WFM, Breslau PJ. Percutaneous transluminal angioplasty of the femoropopliteal artery: initial and long-term results. Radiology 1985; 156:325–8.
9. Morgenstern BR, Getrajdman GI, Laffey KJ, et al. Total occlusion of the femoropopliteal artery: high technical success rate of conventional balloon angioplasty. Radiology 1989;172:937–40.
10. Zeitler E, Richter E-I, Seyferth W. Primary results: leg arteries. In Dotter CT, Grüntzig A, Schoop W, Zeitler E (eds): Percutaneous transluminal angioplasty. Berlin: Springer-Verlag, 1983, chap. 5.
11. Deutsch LS. Techniques of percutaneous balloon angioplasty, including aortoiliac and femoropopliteal systems: indications, results, and complications. In Moore WS, Ahn SS (eds): Endovascular Surgery. Philadelphia: WB Saunders, 1989, chap. 21.
12. Schwarten DE. Aortic, iliac and peripheral artery angioplasty. In Castañeda-Zúñiga WR, Tadavarthy SM (eds): Interventional Radiology. Baltimore: Williams & Wilkins, 1988:268–97.
13. McNamara TO. Technique and results of "higher-dose" infusion. Cardiovasc Intervent Radiol 1982;S48–57.
14. Auster M, Kadir S, Mitchell SE, et al. Iliac artery occlusion: management with intrathrombus streptokinase infusion and angioplasty. Radiology 1984;153:385–8.
15. Motarjeme A. Thrombolysoangioplasty (TLA): a new approach to chronic arterial occlusions. Diagnostic angiography and interventional radiology. Proceedings of The Society of Cardiovascular & Interventional Radiology, 14th annual meeting, San Diego, 1989;155–9.
16. Motarjeme A, Keifer JW, Zuska AJ. Percutaneous transluminal angioplasty of the iliac arteries: 66 experiences. AJR 1980;135:937–44.
17. Rees CR, Palmaz JC, Garcia O, et al. Angioplasty and stenting of completely occluded iliac arteries. Radiology 1989; 172:953–9.
18. Ring EJ, Freiman DB, McLean GK, Schwartz W. Percutaneous recanalization of common iliac artery occlusions: an unacceptable complication rate? AJR 1982;139:587–9.
19. Colapinto RF, Stronell RD, Johnston WK. Transluminal angioplasty of complete iliac obstructions. AJR 1986;146:859–62.
20. Weibull H, Bergqvist D, Jonsson K, et al. Complications after percutaneous transluminal angioplasty in the iliac, femoral, and popliteal arteries. J Vasc Surg 1987;5:681–6.
21. Jenkins RD, Sinclair IN, Leonard BM, et al. Laser balloon angioplasty versus angioplasty in normal rabbit iliac arteries. Lasers Surg Med 1989;9:239–47.
22. Diethrich EB. A discussion of the applications and limitations of laser-assisted angioplasty. In Laser Applications in Cardiovascular Disease. Proceedings of The Oklahoma Heart Center and Baptist Laser Institute, October 1988.
23. Gardiner GA, Meyerovitz MF, Stokes KR, et al. Complications of transluminal angioplasty. Radiology 1986;159:201–8.
24. Sanborn TA, Nordstrom LA. Technical success, clinical success and patency in laser angioplasty. (Letter and response.) Radiology 1989;170:576–8.
25. McNamara TO. Role of thrombolysis in peripheral arterial occlusion. Am J Med 1987;83(suppl 2A):6–10.
26. Palmaz JC, Richter GM, Noeldge G, et al. Intraluminal stents in atherosclerotic iliac artery stenosis: preliminary report of a multicenter study. Radiology 1988;168:727–731.
27. Sigwart U, Puel J, Mirkovitch V, et al. Intravascular stents to prevent occlusion or restenosis after transluminal angioplasty. N Engl J Med 1987;316:701–6.
28. Günther RW, Vorwerk D, Bohndorf K, et al. Iliac and femoral artery stenoses and occlusions: treatment with intravascular stents. Radiology 1989;172:725–30.
29. Bonn J, Gardiner GA, Shapiro MJ, et al. Palmaz vascular stent: initial clinical experience. Radiology 1990;174:741–5.
30. Adar R, Critchfield GC, Eddy DM. A confidence profile analysis of the results of femoropopliteal percutaneous transluminal angioplasty in the treatment of lower-extremity ischemia. J Vasc Surg 1989;10:57–67.
31. Jorgenson B, Henriksen LO, Karle A, et al. Percutaneous transluminal angioplasty of iliac and femoral arteries in severe lower-limb ischemia. Acta Chir Scand 1988;154:647–52.
32. Becker GJ, Katzen BT, Dake MD. Noncoronary angioplasty. Radiology 1989;170:921–40.
33. Samson RH, Sprayregen S, Veith FJ, et al. Management of angioplasty complications, unsuccessful procedures and early and late failures. Ann Surg 1984;199:234–240.
34. Wilson SE, Wolf GL, Cross AP. Percutaneous transluminal angioplasty versus operation for peripheral arteriosclerosis. J Vasc Surg 1989;9:1–9.

38 Fluorescence-Guided Laser Angioplasty

Donald L. Miller, M.D.

A major problem with existing laser systems is the risk of vessel perforation during tissue ablation due to the physician's inability to determine in real-time exactly what the laser is ablating. The ideal laser system should include a sensing system capable of determining what type of tissue the laser fiber is directed at, as well as a feedback loop to keep the laser from firing when the fiber is directed at normal tissue (intima or media).

At present, three different types of sensing systems are under active development: angioscopy, intravascular ultrasound, and laser-excited fluorescence spectroscopy. Angioscopy has been used by a number of investigators but is limited to examination of the endoluminal surface of the vessel.[1–3] Intravascular ultrasound permits visualization of all layers of the vessel wall and any intramural disease.[4,5] However, at present neither of these methods permits real-time feedback between the sensing system and the mechanism controlling laser activation. Fluorescence spectroscopy is the only sensing system capable of evaluating tissue, which is actually in contact with the tip of the laser fiber, and producing data that can be used, in real-time, to control laser operation. This is the sensing system used for fluorescence-guided laser angioplasty by the Smart Laser (MCM, Mountain View, CA).

Laser-excited fluorescence spectroscopy uses a low-power ultraviolet laser to irradiate the target tissue. This causes the tissue to fluoresce, and this fluorescence is detected by the instrument. An optical multichannel analyzer is used to create a fluorescence spectrum, which displays light intensity as a function of wavelength. This spectrum can then be analyzed by computer, using algorithms that consider fluorescence intensity, spectrum peak position, and spectrum shape.[6,7] The fluorescence spectra of normal arterial wall and atheroma are sufficiently different that these tissues can be reliably differentiated with this technique, both in vitro and in vivo.[6,8–13]

COMPONENTS OF THE MCM SYSTEM

The instrument for fluorescence-guided laser angioplasty combines two lasers (a diagnostic laser and a treatment laser), an optical multichannel analyzer and a computer, in one integrated device. Both lasers fire through the same optical fiber, and both are connected to the computer.

The diagnostic laser is a low-power (2 mW), pulsed helium cadmium (HeCd) laser operating at 325 nm. Its sole purpose is to induce fluorescence in the target tissue, located at the tip of the optical fiber. This fluorescence is then conducted back along the same optical fiber, where a beam splitter directs it to the optical multichannel analyzer.

The type of laser used for tissue ablation is independent of the fluorescence guidance system. Theoretically, any pulsed laser may be used for tissue ablation. Fluorescence changes have been noted in vitro after tissue ablation with argon and excimer lasers as well as the pulsed dye laser.[6]

The treatment laser used in the MCM system is a high-power pulsed dye laser operating at 480 nm. Previous studies have shown that there is preferential ablation of pigmented atheromas (yellow atheroma, hemorrhagic atheroma) at this wavelength.[14,15] There is also preferential ablation of fibrofatty plaque and calcified plaque, compared with normal arterial wall tissue.[16] The laser uses flash-lamp excitation of a coumarin-480 dye solution. Pulses are 2 μsec in length, considerably less than the 50 μsec suggested as the maximum pulse duration for optimal selective plaque ablation.[16] Pulse energy is 35 to 50 mJ/pulse through a 200 μm optical fiber, and the pulse energy density is in the range of 1000 to 1500 mJ/mm^2/pulse. The laser produces both photothermal and photoacoustic effects. It fires through the same optical fiber as the diagnostic laser, guaranteeing that tissue characterization and ablation are performed at the same site.

Two optical delivery systems are contemplated. The first, termed a LaserWire by MCM, is a 200 μm fused silica optical fiber completely enclosed, except at the tip, within a standard type, Teflon-coated, spring coil guide wire. These optical guide wires are available in diameters from 0.018 to 0.035 inch. In use, they ablate a channel of approximately the same diameter as the guide wire, and by themselves cannot create an adequate lumen. They are intended for crossing areas of complete occlusion. The second delivery system is a catheter with a central lumen and several optical fibers arranged in a concentric circle around the central lumen. As of December 1989, this LaserCatheter is still under development and is not yet available for general use. Current plans call for a 5 F and a 7 F version. These will presumably produce channels of similar diameter to the catheter, and may be sufficient to recanalize infrapopliteal vessels without further balloon angioplasty. They may be usable by themselves for the negotiation of stenoses, but will probably require the coaxial use of a conventional guide wire or optical guide wire when used to cross occlusions.

Protective eyewear is not necessary when using either the catheter or the guide wire, since in both delivery systems the entire optical fiber, except for the tip, is enclosed within the delivery system and is completely covered and shielded. Furthermore, the treatment laser cannot be fired unless the fiber tip is in contact with atheroma or thrombus (see later) and the diagnostic laser is a very low-power instrument and is comparable in output to commercially available laser pointers.

OPERATION OF THE FLUORESCENCE-GUIDED ANGIOPLASTY SYSTEM

The MCM system permits controlled laser angioplasty, with real-time fluorescence spectroscopy and control of treatment laser operation. The system can operate in two different modes, termed "probe and display" and "probe and treat."

The probe and display mode (Fig. 38-1) is used for diagnosis and for determination of the position of the tip of the optical fiber. It does not produce tissue ablation. In this mode, only the diagnostic laser is used. It fires, and the resultant laser light travels down the optical fiber to irradiate the tissue in contact with the fiber tip. The induced fluorescence travels back up the same fiber and is directed by a beam splitter to the optical multichannel analyzer. This spectrum is displayed on a monitor screen and is also analyzed by the computer. The algorithm used with the MCM system generates a number, termed the "tissue index," which indicates tissue type: normal (intima and media), atheroma, or thrombus. The computer generates the tissue index and displays both the number and the tissue type on the monitor screen alongside the fluorescence spectrum. In clinical use, this mode of operation has been particularly helpful for both the initial evaluation of occlusions and for optical guide wire placement for ablation of these lesions.

The probe and treat mode (Fig. 38-2) produces tissue ablation. In this mode, the diagnostic laser fires first, and the entire probe and display sequence is performed. In addition, however, if the target tissue is characterized as abnormal (atheroma or thrombus) by the computer, a feedback loop then permits the computer to enable the treatment laser. If the operator has depressed a foot switch, the treatment laser will fire down the same optical fiber used for the probe and display sequence, and the target tissue will be ablated. If the computer does not characterize the target tissue as abnormal (normal or indeterminate), the treatment laser will not be enabled and will not fire even if the foot switch has been depressed.

In normal operation, the probe and display mode is used until the laser fiber is directed at abnormal tissue. The probe and treat mode is then selected, and the foot switch depressed. The diagnostic laser/computer analysis/treatment laser sequence is then carried out automatically, the entire sequence lasting 100 msec and repeated five times per second until normal tissue is reached or the foot switch is released.

Computer control over the treatment laser through a feedback loop is the basis for calling this system "smart," and is an obvious safety feature. An additional safety feature is the design of the feedback loop. Since the computer will only enable the treatment laser when a recognizable spectrum characteristic of a specific type of abnormal tissue has been identified, the risk of false-positive operation (firing of the treatment laser at normal tissue) is virtually nonexistent.

There is some risk of false-negative operation (failure of the treatment laser to fire at abnormal tissue) if the fluorescence spectrum of the target tissue is obscured by noise or is otherwise indeterminate. Theoretically, this may decrease the success rate slightly, but this is balanced by an expected decreased rate of complications. Furthermore, in over 60 patients and in over 1000 in vitro tissue specimens, the fluorescence spectroscopy system has reliably differentiated among the three basic types of tissue encountered in angioplasty: normal intima and media, thrombus and hemorrhagic atheroma, and nonhemorrhagic atheroma.[6,8,9,12,17,18]

The feedback loop is obviously effective at preventing the treatment laser from operating until the optical fiber is in contact with abnormal tissue. It is less obvious how the system keeps the laser from firing as the tip of the optical

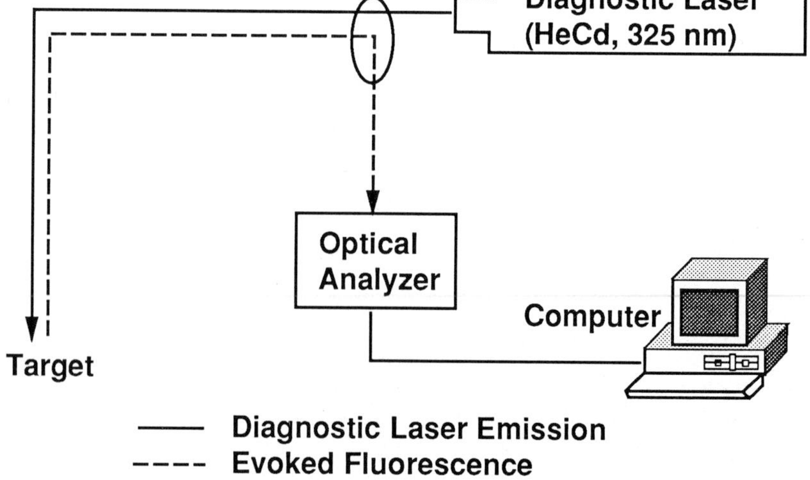

Figure 38–1. The probe and display mode of operation, used for tissue characterization, is shown diagrammatically. A low-power ultraviolet laser is used to induce fluorescence in the target tissue. The evoked fluorescence is transmitted back up the same optical fiber to an optical multichannel analyzer. A fluorescence spectrum is generated and tissue type is determined from this spectrum by a computer. The spectrum and the tissue type are displayed on a monitor screen.

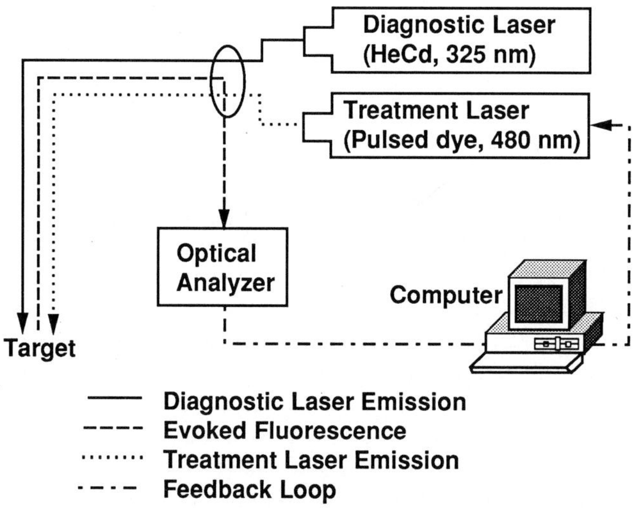

Figure 38–2. The probe and treat mode, shown diagrammatically, is used for tissue ablation. It includes a probe and display cycle. If the target tissue is classified as abnormal, the computer then enables the treatment laser, which will fire and ablate the target tissue if the operator has depressed a footswitch. This cycle may be repeated continuously as long as the operator's footswitch is depressed. The evoked fluorescence from the target tissue is monitored with each successive cycle. If the computer determines that the target tissue cannot be classified as abnormal, the treatment laser is automatically disabled. This feedback loop prevents the operator from unintentionally ablating normal tissue.

guide wire reaches the back wall of the atheroma, at the atheroma-media junction. In vitro studies in human aorta have shown that after partial ablation of an atheroma, fluorescence spectra from the shallow crater in the ablated area are unchanged from the pretreatment spectrum.[6] Fluorescence spectra recorded from deeper craters approaching the media change rapidly and become normal.[6,17,19] Histologic examination of craters of differing depths shows that fluorescence spectra begin returning to normal only when the crater base is within 100 to 200 μm of the atheroma-media junction.[6] This distance is approximately the same as the depth of ablation produced by each pulse of the treatment laser. Thus, the system prevents ablation through the back wall of an atheroma by sensing the fluorescence spectrum of the underlying normal tissue before it is actually reached by the tip of the optical guide wire.

CLINICAL EXPERIENCE

All the studies reported in this section have used the optical guide wire delivery system. The optical fiber-catheter system is still under development. Various catheter designs have been tested in vitro and in vivo, but no standard design had been adopted as of December 1989.

In the spring of 1989, MCM released figures for the first 70 clinical cases in their multicenter clinical trial. Some of these data have also been published separately.[20–23] All cases except one were performed in the femoropopliteal system (one iliac artery was also done). All procedures were performed on total occlusions, with an average length of 8.5 ± 5.6 cm (range, 1 to 27 cm). All cases involved primary recanalization of the occluded segment with the laser, followed by catheter and guide wire exchange and standard balloon angioplasty. The MCM protocol required that attempts to recanalize the occlusion with standard guide wires be made in all cases before tissue ablation with the laser was performed.

In the 70 procedures, MCM observed 57 (81%) immediate technical successes (crossing the lesion with the laser guide wire), and 53 (76%) immediate angiographic successes (residual stenosis of less than 25% after balloon angioplasty). Fifty limbs were available for follow-up at 2 months, and of these 41 (82%) were clinical successes (less symptomatic, or improved ankle-brachial indices) and 37 (74%) were combined angiographic/clinical successes. At 6 months 38 limbs were available for follow-up, and 30 (79%) were clinical successes.

National Institutes of Health (NIH) results[22] are somewhat different. The trial was conducted by Martin Leon, M.D., who has done extensive development and evaluation work on the fluorescence spectroscopy system. In all patients, a determined effort was made to negotiate femoropopliteal occlusions with standard techniques, sometimes assisted by use of the laser in the probe and display mode for guidance. Of 24 limbs initially evaluated, 9 (38%) had occlusions that were relieved without use of the treatment laser for tissue ablation. In the remaining 15 limbs, there were 3 (20%) laser failures (inability to recanalize the occlusion with the treatment laser). There were 12 (80%) technical successes (recanalization of the occluded segment with the laser guide wire), but in four of these occlusions a balloon angioplasty catheter could not be passed distal to the occlusion and thus there were only 8 (53%) angiographic/clinical successes.

In the NIH experience, the learning curve was short. Two of the three perforations created were encountered in the first three patients treated. The prototype optical guide wire was very stiff, and all of the perforations resulted from mechanical trauma to the vessel wall at a time when the optical guide wire was being advanced manually and no laser energy was being applied. None of the patients had any clinical sequelae from the perforation, probably because the optical guide wire was already several centimeters into the occluded segment at the time, and the perforations themselves were only about 0.020 inch in diameter.

All perforations occurred during attempts at recanalization of very heavily calcified vessels. Negotiation of areas of vascular calcification is a problem with this system, as with many others. Ablation of calcified lesions required substantially higher pulse energy and greater total energy per centimeter of recanalized tissue than ablation of noncalcified lesions.[21] All laser angioplasty and balloon angioplasty failures were in heavily calcified lesions.

Fluorescence spectroscopy was found to be of greatest benefit in two specific clinical situations. First, in occluded arteries where a large collateral vessel arose in close proximity to the proximal margin of the occlusion, fluorescence spectroscopy was found to be helpful for positioning the optical guide wire so that its tip was in contact with the occlusion, and not directed down the collateral channel (Fig. 38-3). Second, in the course of negotiating a long occluded segment, eccentric positioning of the optical guide wire within the occluded segment produced a change in the fluorescence pattern, indicating proximity to the media of the vessel. Early recognition of incorrect guide wire position permitted the optical guide wire to be redirected into the vessel lumen and prevented perforation of the arterial wall.

SUMMARY

The MCM Smart Laser is an innovative laser angioplasty system that combines an effective method for tissue ablation with a real-time guidance system. It is effective for recanalization of noncalcified occluded femoropopliteal arteries that cannot be negotiated with conventional (nonlaser) techniques. The probe and display mode is useful both for identifying the exact point at which an occlusion begins and for guiding both conventional and laser recanalization attempts through long occluded arterial segments. The probe and treat mode includes a feedback loop that prevents the treatment laser from ablating normal tissue. Preliminary results indicate that the guidance system functions correctly and that the system is capable of ablating abnormal tissue in vivo. A different laser system for tissue ablation may improve the success rate for ablation of calcified tissue.

As of December 1989, the largest channel this system can create unassisted is 0.035 inch (the diameter of the optical guide wire), which means that standard balloon angioplasty is required even when laser angioplasty is completely successful. Development of effective catheters incorporating optical fibers may permit unassisted laser angioplasty, but this goal has not yet been realized.

REFERENCES

1. Abela GS, Seeger GM, Barbieri E, et al. Laser angioplasty with angioscopic guidance in humans. J Am Coll Cardiol 1986;8:184–92.

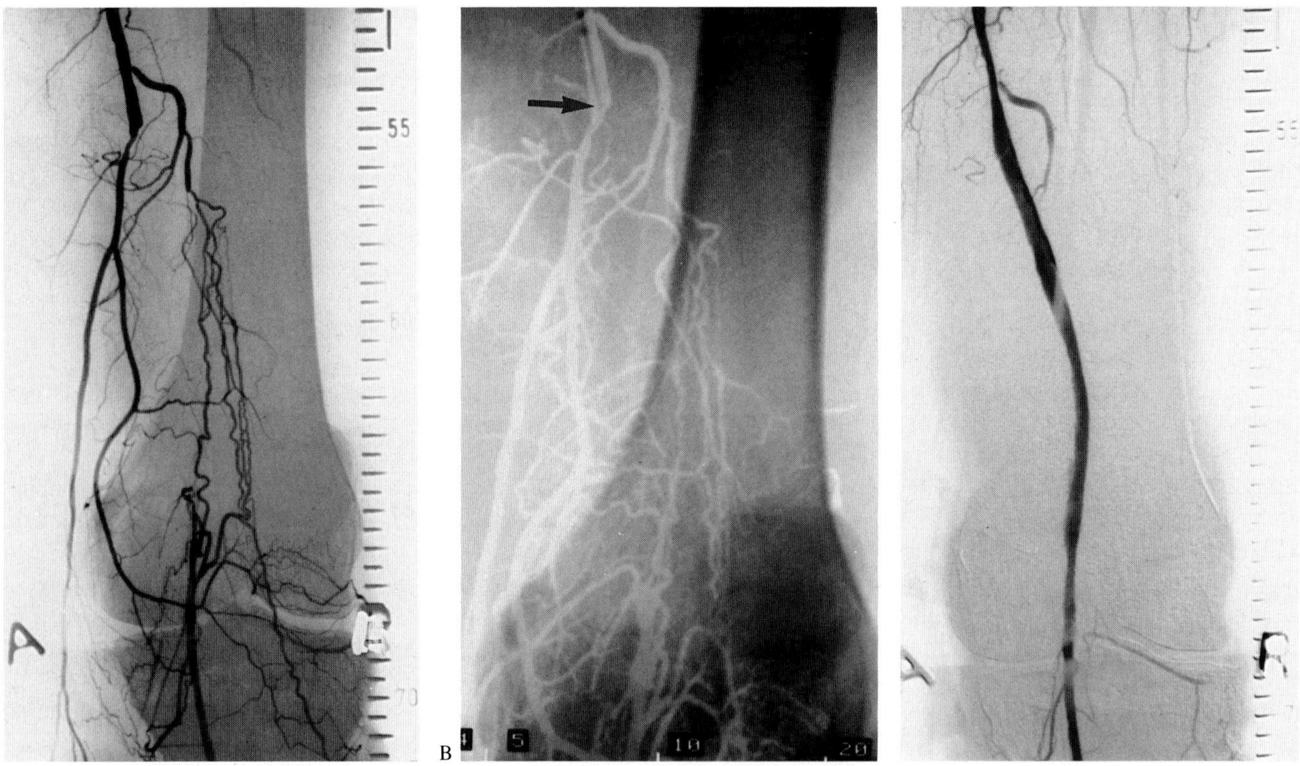

A B C

Figure 38–3. Fluorescence-guided laser angioplasty in a 60-year-old man with an 11 cm femoropopliteal occlusion. **A:** A preangioplasty arteriogram demonstrates the lesion. Attempts to recanalize the occlusion with a standard guide wire were unsuccessful. **B:** A roadmapped image of the lesion demonstrates the optical guide wire tip (arrow) positioned just proximal to the lesion. The position of the guide wire was adjusted using real-time fluorescence guidance until the fiber tip was in contact with the occlusion. Note that this device does not require the use of a centering balloon or saline irrigation or intermittent incremental repositioning of a guiding device. The tip of the optical fiber is placed in contact with the tissue to be ablated and is not damaged by this process. In actual clinical practice, roadmapping is rarely used for guidance, since fluorescence guidance is more accurate and not sensitive to patient movement. **C:** Following recanalization of the occluded segment with the laser, angioplasty was performed with a conventional balloon catheter.

2. Litvack F, Grundfest WS, Lee ME, et al. Angioscopic visualization of blood vessel interior in animals and humans. Clin Cardiol 1985;8:65–70.
3. Underhill DJ, Smith PD, Leon MB, et al. High resolution angioscopy: feasibility, limitations, and design considerations for laser coronary angioplasty. Surg Forum 1985;36:299–301.
4. Yock PG, Linker DT, Thapliyal HV, et al. Real-time, two-dimensional catheter ultrasound: a new technique for high-resolution intravascular imaging. (Abstr.) J Am Coll Cardiol 1988;11:130A.
5. Meyer, CR, Chiang EH, Fechner KP, et al. Feasibility of high-resolution, intravascular ultrasonic imaging catheters. Radiology 1988;168:113–6.
6. Leon MB, Lu DY, Prevosti LG, et al. Human arterial surface fluorescence: atherosclerotic plaque identification and effects of laser atheroma ablation. J Am Coll Cardiol 1988;12:94–102.
7. O'Brien KM, Gmitro AF, Gindi GR, et al. Development and evaluation of spectral classification algorithms for fluorescence guided laser angioplasty. IEEE Trans Biomed Eng 1989;36:424–31.
8. Lu DY, Leon MB, Smith PD, Balaban RS. Atherosclerotic plaque identification using surface fluorescence. (Abstr.) Clin Res 1986;34:630A.
9. Leon MB, Prevosti LG, Smith PD, et al. In-vivo laser-induced fluorescence plaque detection: preliminary results in patients. (Abstr.) Circulation 1987;76(4 part 2):IV–408.
10. Deckelbaum LI, Lam JK, Cabin HS, et al. Discrimination of normal and atherosclerotic aorta by laser-induced fluorescence. Lasers Surg Med 1987;7:330–5.
11. Sartori M, Henry PD, Roberts R. Estimation of arterial wall thickness and detection of atherosclerosis by laser induced argon fluorescence. (Abstr.) J Am Coll Cardiol 1986;7:207A.
12. Bartorelli AL, Almagor Y, Prevosti LG, et al. In vivo coronary plaque recognition by laser-induced fluorescence spectroscopy. Circulation 1988;78(4 Part 2):II–294.
13. Andersson PS, Gustafson A, Stenram U, et al. Diagnosis of arterial atherosclerosis using laser-induced fluorescence. Laser Med Sci 1987;2:261–6.
14. Bowker TJ. Laser-tissue interaction and arterial perforation thresholds in laser angioplasty. Semin Intervent Radiol 1986;3:39–46.
15. Prince MR, Deutsch TF, Shapiro AH, et al. Selective ablation of atheromas using a flashlamp-excited dye laser at 465 nm. Proc Natl Acad Sci USA 1986;83:7064–8.
16. LaMuraglia GM, Murray S, Anderson RR, Prince MR. Effect of pulse duration on selective ablation of atherosclerotic plaque by 480- to 490-nanometer laser radiation. Lasers Surg Med 1988;8:18–21.
17. Leon MB, Lu DY, Smith PD, et al. Arterial surface fluorescence becomes normal after laser atheroma ablation. (Abstr.) Am Heart Assoc Monogr 1986; 0(124):II–334 [Circulation 1986;74(4 Suppl II):II–334].
18. Leon MB, Prevosti LG, Smith PD, et al. Probe and fire laser angioplasty: fluorescence atheroma detection and selective laser atheroma ablation. (Abstr.) Circulation 1987;76(4 part 2):IV–409.
19. Deckelbaum LI, Stetz ML, O'Brian KM, et al. Fluorescence spectroscopy guidance of laser ablation of atherosclerotic plaque. (Abstr.) J Am Coll Cardiol 1988;11(2 suppl A):107A.
20. Geschwind HJ, Dubois-Rande JL, Bonner RF, et al. Percutaneous pulsed laser angioplasty with atheroma detection in humans. (Abstr.) J Am Coll Cardiol 1988;11(2 suppl A):107A.
21. Leon MB, Almagor Y, Bartorelli AL, et al. Fluorescence-guided laser angioplasty in patients with femoropopliteal occlusions. Circulation 1988;78(4 part 2):II–294.
22. Leon MB, Almagor Y, Bartorelli AL, et al. Fluorescence-guided laser-assisted balloon angioplasty in patients with femoropopliteal occlusions. Circulation 1990; 81:143–55.
23. Douek PC, Leon MB, Geschwind H, et al. Occlusive peripheral vascular disease: a multicenter trial of fluorescence-guided, pulsed dye laser-assisted balloon angioplasty. Radiology 1991;180:127–33.

39 Intravascular Stents: Experimental Observations and Anatomopathologic Correlates

Julio C. Palmaz, M.D.

INTRALUMINAL STENTING AS THE MECHANICAL SOLUTION TO BALLOON-ANGIOPLASTY FAILURE

Elastic recoil and subintimal or medial dissection often limit the success of transluminal balloon angioplasty. They cause a decrease of the diameter achieved by the inflated balloon and leave irregularities on the surface of the dilated vessel causing a hemodynamic disturbance and decreased flow. Balloon overdilatation of the stenotic segment has been advocated as a means of antagonizing elastic recoil by maximizing the stretching of the musculoelastic media. This is very often effective but definitely increases the risk of hemorrhage by transmural rupture. An intraluminal stent placed simultaneously or immediately after balloon angioplasty prevents elastic recoil by holding the vessel open to a predetermined diameter, corrects the effects of dissection by displacing the dissected layers against the arterial wall, and provides a cylindrical lumen by forcing asymmetrical plaques eccentrically.[1] This can be accomplished by a variety of stents, some of which are already undergoing clinical evaluation.[2–6] In general, stents are metallic coils or tubular mesh that are introduced into the body via a delivery catheter in a small or constrained diameter. After reaching a desired location the stent expands to a larger diameter by a variety of mechanisms previously described.[2] All intravascular stents currently in use are metallic. This is dictated by the need to have relatively high radial strength with the lowest possible bulk. In addition, metals in general are radiopaque, a feature needed for precise manipulation and positioning under fluoroscopy.

THE MAIN GOAL: ENDOTHELIALIZATION OF THE STENTED SURFACE

An important feature of an intravascular stent is to have an open design, which means having the lowest possible ratio of metal to open surface without compromising its mechanical properties. An open stent wall configuration is desirable because of the need to keep thrombogenicity of the metal surface at a minimum and to preserve as much endothelium as possible. This promotes multicentric endothelialization by allowing confluent growth of surviving endothelium between metal members.[7] Complete coverage of the treated surface by endothelium is the ultimate goal of vascular prosthetic implants because endothelium protects against low-flow thrombosis, a serious limitation of all currently used synthetic vascular bypass materials.

The endothelium covering stents is stable, as suggested by the mature appearance of the cells several months following implantation in dog, rabbit, and pig arteries. This is evident from the spindle shape of the endothelial cells with their long axis oriented in the direction of the flow, by their flat nuclei, and by the rare blood cell elements attached to the surface when examined by scanning electron microscopy.[8] In addition, positive immunospecific stains for arterial endothelium supports this assumption.[9]

Fascinating albeit unclear is the fact that rapid stent endothelization is also observed when these devices are placed in tracks of liver parenchyma serving as portocaval shunts.[10] The origin of the endothelial cells covering shunt tracks is unclear. It may originate from hepatic capillary sinusoids, from adjacent hepatic or portal veins, or from blood-borne precursors. Despite the uncertainty about its origin, this endothelium was found to have histologic and histochemical features similar to those of arterial stents.

STENT THROMBOGENICITY PRIOR TO ENDOTHELIALIZATION: THE ACHILLES HEEL

Since all metal surfaces are thrombogenic, the risk exists for a recently implanted stent to accumulate an excessive amount of thrombus to the point of occlusion. In prosthetic bypass tubular conduits, shear of the limiting flow layer with the prosthetic surface determines the amount of thrombus deposited.[11] This is a self-limiting phenomenon, since a low-flow situation increases thrombus deposition, narrowing the lumen and increasing flow velocity and shear. However, with critically low flow thrombus deposition continues until complete occlusion occurs. Stents in small vessels are also at increased risk of thrombosis because of the lower shear rates and unfavorable diameter to volume relationship. The same thickness of thrombus causing significant reduction of lumen area in a small diameter vessel may not be as obstructive in a comparatively larger vessel.

The amount of laminar thrombus initially deposited on a stented surface determines the thickness of the intimal tissue that will be present later. This was demonstrated in dogs with stents placed in femoral arteries with artificially induced distal stenosis, compared with stents placed in the opposite unobstructed femoral arteries.[12] Groups of animals with stents placed in this fashion were sacrificed at regular intervals for histologic examination of the stents. As expected, the amount of thrombus on the surface of the stents subjected to low flow was significantly larger than in arteries with normal flow. This thrombus was noted to be progressively replaced by fibromuscular tissue, which in turn was significantly thicker in low-flow stents compared with controls. It is obvious that, when a stent is exposed to low flow or it is placed in a small vessel, increased anticoagulation and antiplatelet medication is needed to assure patency.

The effect of a few anticoagulation-antiplatelet regimens on thrombus deposition on freshly implanted stents was studied in animals by using labeled platelets.[13,14] Particularly effective was a combination of heparin, aspirin, dipyridamole, and low molecular weight dextran. This regimen, adopted for coronary stent implantation in clinical trials, is followed by coumarin administration for a few months by most investigators in this field.[15,16] In contrast, stent implantation in large vessels with high flow, such as the iliac arteries, does not require any more anticoagulation than balloon angioplasty.[17] A similar experience was observed after caval and pulmonary artery stent placements.[18,19]

Ongoing research is underway to optimize the level and duration of anticoagulation to control thrombus deposition before endothelialization occurs. This is possible by the use of markers of focal platelet activity such as the technetium-99m-S12 antibody, which selectively attaches to the inner membrane of alpha granules of activated platelets[20] (Centocor, Malvern, PA). In addition, heparin-coated stents are currently being compared with noncoated stents regarding thrombus formation and long-term patency.

DOES STENTING INHIBIT RECURRENT ATHEROMATOUS PLAQUE FORMATION?

Stents placed in the abdominal aorta of rabbits subjected to balloon denudation and high cholesterol diet were incorporated in similar fashion to stents placed in normal rabbit aortas. The tissue covering the stent and the underlying plaque, 24 weeks following stenting, did not contain foamy macrophages and was essentially fibrous in nature, despite the maintenance of high serum cholesterol levels.[8] A possible explanation for this occurrence is the preservation of endothelium at the site of stent placement, followed by multicentric spread of endothelial cells. After this experimental observation, we had the opportunity to examine the autopsy specimen of a patient with an iliac stent placed 26 months prior to his death from a myocardial infarction. The tissue covering the stent was fibromuscular in nature and showed no evidence of cholesterol, calcium, or necrosis. Rousseau et al[21] had a similar experience using a self-expandable stent.

It is conceivable that stents provide a framework for fibrous tissue growth while maintaining favorable rheologic conditions. This tissue would cover faltering and ulcerated atheromatous tissue, avoiding thrombus formation and possible embolization. However, if biochemical or hemodynamic conditions that created the atherosclerotic plaque prior to stenting remain present, they should eventually lead to recurrence of such plaque. Failure of stenting by recurrence of the lesion within the stented lumen is therefore to be expected a few years following implantation of the device if atherogenic conditions such as cigarette smoking, high serum lipids, and hypertension persist.

FLEXIBLE VERSUS RIGID STENTS: A SUBJECT OF DEBATE

Several investigators working with intravascular stents have stressed the need for stent flexibility for ease of deployment and to accompany vessel movement when placed in segments subjected to bending, such as the femoral, axillary, or popliteal arteries.[6,22] Flexibility is certainly needed to negotiate curves in delivery catheters and tortuous vessels leading to the target area. This led to a change in our stent design in which one or more smaller stent segments are joined by a short bridge for certain applications, such as coronary and renal artery stenting. However, we still believe that stents should be rigid after placement to provide a stable, nonshifting surface for endothelial growth.

The assumption that dimensional change in a prosthetic surface causes increased endothelial slough, platelet and mononuclear cell attachment and ensuing muscle cell proliferation is supported by previous work. Barra et al[23] significantly decreased intimal hyperplasia in vein grafts by placing a perivenous mesh to render the grafts noncompliant. These authors demonstrated that the endothelium of meshed grafts was more mature and free of attached blood cells compared with nonmeshed grafts. Thubrikar et al[24] also emphasized the beneficial effect of relieving intramural stress by experimentally placing periarterial acrylic casts around branching points and bifurcations of large vessels of rabbits, where intramural stress was assumed to be maximal. After exposing the animal to a high cholesterol diet, the arterial segments with surrounding rigid casts were compared with segments covered with flexible silicone casts and to uncovered arterial segments. Areas relieved of stress by the rigid casts developed less intimal thickening and fat accumulation compared with arteries with flexible casts or to arteries not covered at all.

The importance of matching radial compliance between an artery and an interposed prosthetic conduit has been repeatedly stressed in the literature.[25] Compliance mismatch has been identified as one of the potential causes of anastomotic intimal hyperplasia in small caliber synthetic grafts. Therefore synthetic grafts are designed in such a way that their radial compliance matches that of the human arteries. Radial compliance mismatch could be present between rigid stents and adjacent artery, causing intimal hyperplasia at the transition point. However, in practice this was not observed.

Angiographic and gross examination of healed stents in arteries of animals and patients did not reveal a tendency of the intima to be thicker at the transition points between artery and stent. Whenever stent stenosis developed, the tissue causing it was generally distributed throughout the length of the stented lumen. It is possible that compliance mismatch is not relevant when rigid stents are placed in diseased vessels that are usually rendered rigid by wall thickening and calcification.

THE RESORBABLE STENT: A UTOPIAN DREAM?

In theory, resorbable suture materials should be mechanically sound before wound healing occurs. After healing, it should be phagocytosed without inducing chronic cellular reaction. It is conceivable that a stent of resorbable material could be constructed to keep intravascular atheromatous lesions open until the tissue replacing the stent would reorganize the vessel into a cylindrical conduit. This new tissue could then be considered a biologic stent. Unfortunately, all polymeric plastic materials, including the few available resorbable materials, are far from having the strength characteristics needed to perform as mechanical stents with reasonable bulk. This is particularly true in small vessels where a small decrease in diameter could produce a large flow restriction.

An additional concern regarding the concept of resorbable stents is the possibility of developing weakness at the level of the treated area, resulting in vessel rupture or aneurysm. After months to years following stent placement, the musculoelastic elements of the stented arterial wall atrophy for lack of use.[8] After stent placement the stress of the pulsatile blood pressure normally borne by the arterial wall is transferred to the stent, eventually causing atrophy of the wall. It is therefore conceivable that if the stent support is removed after atrophy has occurred, an aneurysm or rupture could develop. This would be of particular concern in large arteries subjected to large wall stress. Evidence to support this concept exists in previous experimental efforts at creating resorbable grafts. Aortobifemoral grafts of knitted polyglycolic acid filament were placed in pigs. Following reabsorption of the prosthetic material, aneurysms consistently developed.[26]

The idea of a resorbable stent is therefore not supported by currently available materials or experimental evidence.

THE FUTURE OF STENTING

In conjunction with emerging new diagnostic and therapeutic tools, intravascular stenting offers exiting new possibilities. Stents could expand the role of other revascularization techniques, such as thrombolytic therapy, atherectomy, or lasers, and its placement could be made more accurate by intravascular ultrasound and angioscopy. However, stent safety and efficacy are not completely proven. Randomized studies and 5-year patency rates are not available yet. Until then, areas where stents represent an alternative to proven, conventional therapy, such as iliac balloon angioplasty, should be undertaken with caution. In contrast, the use of stents in areas where no viable alternative is available is received with enthusiasm. This is true in percutaneous portocaval shunting in patients with bleeding esophageal varices and poor metabolic status,[27] caval,[18] portal, and hepatic vein obstruction,[28] and pulmonary branch stenosis.[29]

REFERENCES

1. Palmaz JC. Balloon-expandable intravascular stent. AJR 1988;150:1263–9.
2. Wright KC, Wallace S, Charnsangavej C, et al. Percutaneous endovascular stents: an experimental evaluation. Radiology 1985;156:69–72.
3. Sigwart V, Puel J, Mirkovitch V, et al. Intravascular stents to prevent occlusion and restenosis after transluminal angioplasty. N Engl J Med 1987;316:701–6.
4. Robinson KA, Roubin GS, Siegel RJ, et al. Intra-arterial stenting in the atherosclerotic rabbit. Circulation 1988; 78:646–53.
5. Rabkin J, Matevosov AL, Gotman LN. Radiological endovascular prosthesis. In Rabkin J (ed): Radiological Endovascular Surgery. Moscow: Moscow Medicine Publisher, 1987.
6. Strecker EP, Berg G, Weber H, et al. Experimentelle Untersuchungen mit einer neuen perkutan einfuhr baren und aufdehnbaren Gefabendoprosthese. Fortschr Rontgenstr 1987;147: 669–72.
7. Palmaz JC, Tio FO, Schatz RA, et al. Early endothelisation of balloon-expandable stents: experimental observations. J Intervent Radiol 1988;3:119–24.
8. Palmaz JC, Windeler SA, Garcia F, et al. Atherosclerotic rabbit aortas: expandable intraluminal grafting. Radiology 1986;160:723–6.
9. Palmaz JC, Kopp DT, Hayashi H, et al. Normal and stenotic renal arteries: experimental balloon-expandable intraluminal stenting. Radiology 1987;164:705–8.
10. Palmaz JC, Sibbitt RR, Reuter SR, et al. Expandable intrahepatic portocaval shunt stents: early experience in the dog. AJR 1985;145:821–5.
11. Sauvage LR. Externally supported, noncrimped external Velour, weft-knitted Dacron prostheses for axillofemoral, femoropopliteal, and femorotibial bypass. In Wright CB, Hosson RW, Hiratzka LF, Lynch TB (eds): Vascular Grafting: Clinical Applications and Techniques, Boston:Wright, 1983:168–86.
12. Noeldge G, Siegestetter V, Richter GM, et al. Palmaz stent: process of neointima formation in conditions of highly impaired flow. Radiological Society of North America meeting, Chicago, 1989.
13. Palmaz JC, Garcia O, Kopp DT, et al. Balloon-expandable intraarterial stents: effect of anticoagulation on thrombus formation. (Abstr.) Circulation 1987;76(suppl IV):45.
14. Palmaz JC, Garcia O, Kopp DT, et al. Balloon-expandable intraarterial stents: effect of antithrombotic medication on thrombus formation. In Zeitler E (ed): Pros and Cons in PTA and Auxiliary Methods. Berlin: Springer-Verlag, 1989.
15. Schatz RA, Leon BL, Baim DS, et al. Balloon-expandable intracoronary stents: initial results of a multicenter study. American Heart Association meeting, New Orleans, 1989.
16. Serruys PW, Beatt KJ, Bertrand M, et al. Restenosis rate after coronary stent implantation: angiographic assessment of the

initial series. American Heart Association meeting, New Orleans, 1989.
17. Palmaz JC, Garcia O, Schatz RA, et al. Balloon-expandable intraluminal stenting of the iliac arteries: The first 171 procedures. Radiology 1990;174:969–75.
18. Charnsangavej C, Carrasco CH, Wallace S, et al. Stenosis of the vena cava: preliminary assessment of treatment with expandable metallic stents. Radiology 1986;161:295–8.
19. Mullins CE, O'Laughlin M, Vick W, et al. Implantation of balloon-expandable intravascular grafts by catheterization in pulmonary arteries and systemic veins. Circulation 1988; 77:188–99.
20. Miller DD, Boulet A, Garcia O, et al. Monoclonal S-12 antibody imaging of in-vivo platelet activation after interventional procedures in atherosclerotic rabbit arteries. American Heart Association meeting, New Orleans, 1989.
21. Rousseau H, Joffre F, Raillat, et al. Iliac artery endoprosthesis: radiologic and histologic findings after 2 years. AJR 1989;153:1075–6.
22. Zollikofer CL, Largiader I, Bruhlmann WF, et al. Endovascular stenting of veins and grafts. Preliminary clinical experience. Radiology 1988;167:707–12.
23. Barra JA, Volant A, Leroy JP, et al. Constrictive perivenous mesh prosthesis for preservation of vein integrity. J Thorac Cardiovasc Surg 1986;92:330–6.
24. Thubrikar MJ, Baker JW, Nolan SP. Inhibition of atherosclerosis associated with reduction of arterial intramural stress in rabbits. Arteriosclerosis 1988;8:410–20.
25. Abbott WM, Megerman J, Hasson JE, et al. Effect of compliance mismatch on vascular graft patency. J Vasc Surg 1987;5:376–82.
26. Bowald S, Busch C, Erikson I. Absorbable material in vascular prostheses: a new device. Acta Chir Scand 1980;146:391–5.
27. Richter GM, Palmaz JC, Noeldge G, et al. Der transjugulare intrahepatische portosystemische stent-shunt (TIPSS). Radiologe 1989;29:406–11.
28. Palmaz JC. Development of a non-compliant balloon-expandable stent. Miami Vascular Institute meeting, Miami, 1989.
29. Mullins C. Personal communication.

40 Palmaz Balloon Expandable Stent

Wilfrido R. Castañeda-Zúñiga, M.D., S. Murthy Tadavarthy, M.D.

To overcome the problem of recurrence of stenosis following transluminal angioplasty, Palmaz developed a balloon expandable, intravascular stent. The device was intended to allow dilation and simultaneous placement of an intraluminal stent to support the wall, preventing elastic arterial recoil.[1] The initial design of the stent was a continuous, woven, stainless steel 150 μm diameter wire. The cross points of the wire mesh were soldered to give the stent high resistance to radial collapse.[1] Because of the 80% open design of the stent, rapid endothelialization occurred by 3 weeks, together with patency preservation of side branches.[2] In contrast to animal results, the inner surface of synthetic grafts in humans does not get covered by endothelium, but by a fibrin layer.[1]

The main disadvantage of the stent is its lack of longitudinal flexibility, which limits its application to straight vascular segments. The stent design was changed by replacing the woven mesh with a lath design obtained by electromechanical etching of thin-walled stainless steel tubing (Fig. 40-1). The etching produces a stent with parallel rows of staggered rectangular slots, allowing for a smaller diameter (3.1 F), thinner-walled stent (0.015 mm), with a length of 30 mm and an expansion range of 8 to 12 mm.[2] When the balloon is inflated, the rectangular slots open to form diamond-shaped spaces. Initially, the stents needed to be mounted and crimped out over an 8 mm to 3 cm long balloon with a crimping tool. A newer low profile version of the stent is available premounted on an 8 mm angioplasty balloon. Because of the stent tendency to slip back on the balloon, the stent-balloon assembly needs to be protected during introduction through the hemostatic valve by a stainless steel introducer. Furthermore, a 30 cm long introducer sheath needs to be used to advance the stent-balloon assembly through the artery to the level of the obstruction. Once the stent is located at the desired level, the sheath is withdrawn and the stent is expanded to the full 8 mm diameter. The balloon is deflated and carefully rotated within the stent to refold the balloon, which is then gently withdrawn over the guide wire. An angiogram and pressure measurements are obtained to assess the results. If needed, a 10 mm balloon can be introduced over the guide wire to further dilate the stent in larger diameter iliac arteries.

When long segments need to be stented, multiple stents can be placed, making sure their ends overlap. Although a guide wire or catheter can be manipulated across a freshly placed stent, it is better to keep the guide wire across the stent until it is decided that additional stents or balloon dilation are not needed. For each additional stent placement the 30 mm introducer sheath needs to be repositioned by advancing it over the guide wire across the previously placed stent. When multiple stents are needed, they should be placed from cephalad to caudad, with sequential stents overlapping by at least one third of the stent length.

CLINICAL RESULTS

Initial clinical trials with the Palmaz balloon expandable stent were undertaken as part of a multicenter study, including institutions from the United States and Europe, and were restricted to the iliac arteries. Some of the best reported results of transluminal angioplasty have been in the management of short, concentric stenosis of the iliac arteries (50 to 87%).[3] The results, however, are not so good when dealing with a long stenosis, complete occlusions, and in patients with diabetes mellitus or poor runoff vessels, with a reported patency rate at 5 years of only 55%.[4–7] Initial data included 154 patients: 28 women and 126 men, with an average age of 62 years. Risk factors included diabetes mellitus in 20%, smoking in 96%, hypertension in 52%, and obesity in 17.22%. Seventy patients were classified in stage II, 36 in stage III, and 48 in stage IV. Thirty-four patients had iliac artery stenosis and 20 had complete iliac artery occlusion. Average stenosis was 79% ± 15%; the average length of the iliac artery occlusion was 6.1 ± 2.8 cm. The average Dop-

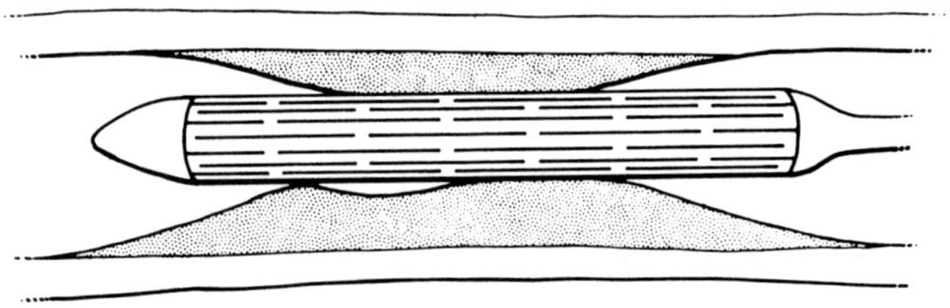

A

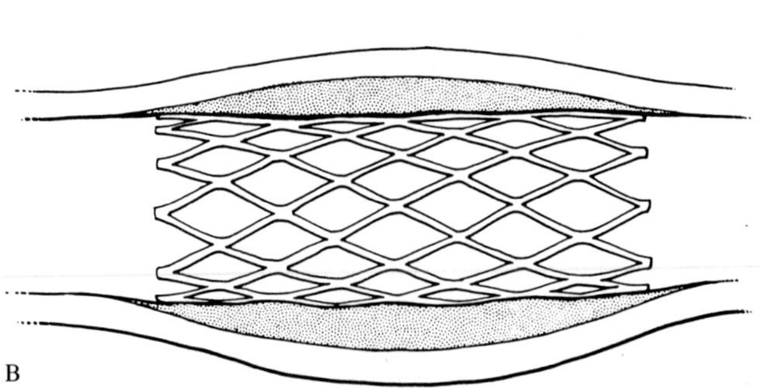

B

Figure 40–1. **A:** Diagram of Palmaz stent mounted on angioplasty balloon, placed at the level of the stenosis. **B:** Fully expanded stent holding lumen widely open. Balloon has been removed.

pler ankle to arm index (AAI) was 0.63 ± 0.2 in stage II patients, 0.54 ± 0.17 in stage III patients, and 0.49 ± 0.25 in stage IV patients.

The initial protocol included the placement of stents only to treat iliac artery stenosis or occlusion that failed to respond to conventional balloon angioplasty. Therefore, following percutaneous transluminal angioplasty (PTA), angiographic and hemodynamic studies were obtained to assess the results of PTA. Inadequate results were defined as the presence of intimal dissection (Fig. 40-2) or elastic recoil producing a residual gradient of 5 mmHg or more after the injection of vasodilators (Fig. 40-3). Other indications for stent placement included restenosis after previous PTA (Fig. 40-4) and total iliac artery occlusion (Fig. 40-5). Contraindications included extravasation after PTA, tortuous iliac arteries, and dense, extensive calcifications of the iliac arteries. Relative contraindications included iliac artery aneurysm, severe hypertension, impaired pain sensation, stenosis of the common femoral artery, and poor distal runoff.

One hundred eighty-one stents were placed in the common iliac arteries and 80 in the external iliac arteries. Seventeen patients had bilateral stent placement and 21 patients had stents placed in the ipsilateral external and common iliac arteries. The mean pressure gradient after vasodilation measured before stent placement was 36.4 ± 22 mmHg. The gradient fell to 1.6 ± 2.7 mmHg poststent placement. At the latest follow-up at an average of 6 months, with a range of 1 to 24 months, 113 patients were asymptomatic, 25 had moderate claudication, five had severe claudication, two had rest pain, and one had undergone a below-knee amputation. When correlating these data with the clinical stage of the disease apparent at the time of presentation, 71 patients had improved by one stage, 32 patients by two stages, and 31 patients by three stages. Eleven patients showed no initial improvement and six patients showed initial improvement with prompt recurrence of symptoms. On the early follow-up, an increase in the AAI to 0.91 ± 0.22 was found on the stage II patients, to 0.83 ± 0.22 in stage III patients, and to 0.75 ± 0.21 in stage IV patients. At the latest follow-up the reported indices were 0.90 ± 0.20, 0.85 ± 0.23, and 0.84 ± 0.28, respectively.[8,9] All stents have remained patent to the latest follow-up examination without evidence of migration or aneurysm formation. Complication related to the stent itself occurred in three patients (2%). Two of the patients had thrombosis of the stent that was successfully managed by thrombolytic infusion. The third patient had a small perforation secondary to balloon rupture during expansion. The patient had an uneventful recovery. Procedure-related complications occurred in 9.7% of patients, including groin hematoma in 3.9%, distal embolization in 2.6%, extravasation in 1.3%, pseudoaneurysm at the puncture site in 0.64%, and subintimal dissection in 0.64%.[9]

In close examination of the results, Palmaz et al[9] described a greater benefit of iliac artery stenting in patients with limbs at risk at the time of presentation, who underwent a combined iliac artery stenting and a femoropopliteal bypass procedure. The absence of initial response or the early recurrence of symptoms was directly correlated to either the presence of untreated distal disease or to the development of new lesions.[9] Patients were placed on an aspirin/dipyridamole regimen for 2 days before the procedure and continued for 3 months thereafter.[8,9] Similar results were reported by Bonn et al[10] in 19 patients. They stated that the angiographic results of stenting were uniform, independently of whether the lesion was focal or diffuse, eccentric or concentric, calcified or noncalcified, localized to the common or external iliac arteries. In addition, the results of stenting were not affected by whether stent placement was used to treat simple or complex complications of PTA (such as long intimal dissection).[10] They emphasized, however, that a precise localization of the lesion by anatomic landmarks and angiography is essential, not only for planning the procedure, but to prevent misplacement of stents.[10] They remarked on one of the main disadvantages of the stent, that is, the large diameter of the introducer system, which excludes patients with small diameter common femoral or external iliac arteries (less than 5 mm), since this predisposes to thrombosis at the puncture site level.[10] Improvements in the introducer system might decrease the occurrence of this problem.

Successful recanalization and stenting of completely occluded iliac arteries in 12 patients was reported by Rees et al.[11] Indications were limb salvage in seven patients and claudication in five. The AAI after stenting rose from a mean of 0.54 ± 15 to 0.94 ± 24. Transtenotic pressure gradients dropped from a mean of 42.1 ± 16.7 to 0.58 ± 1.4 mmHg. In follow-up ranging from 1 to 14 months, with a mean of 7.4 months, the mean AAI did not change significantly. Clinically all patients improved by one or more levels after stenting. Clinical status has remained unchanged in all, but one patient developed claudication of the contralateral leg at 6 months. Distal embolization occurred in two patients. Surgical embolectomy was used to manage these complications. Surgical exposure at the common femoral artery prior to PTA and stenting of completely occluded iliac arteries is suggested as a way to prevent these complications.[11]

Acute vascular occlusion following PTA has been reported in 3.8% of the cases in a series of 224 angioplasties. In 1.3% (three patients) there were complications of iliac PTA, but only one of these three patients (0.4%) had significant luminal compromise.[12] In the series reported by Becker et al[13] the incidence of severe PTA-induced dissection was 4.8%.[13] A correlation of severe intimal dissection with extensive calcification was reported by Maynar et al[14] based on postmortem studies of PTA and confirmed in the Becker et al[13] study on angiographic findings alone. In the past vascular occlusion after PTA was managed either by trying to tack the intima against the wall by a repeat balloon inflation, leaving the balloon inflated for several minutes, by a surgical bypass procedure, or by surgical endarterectomy. Currently, other therapeutic alternatives include stenting,[13] percutaneous atherectomy,[14] and intimal flap welding.[15–17] Of these options, only atherectomy is currently approved by the Food

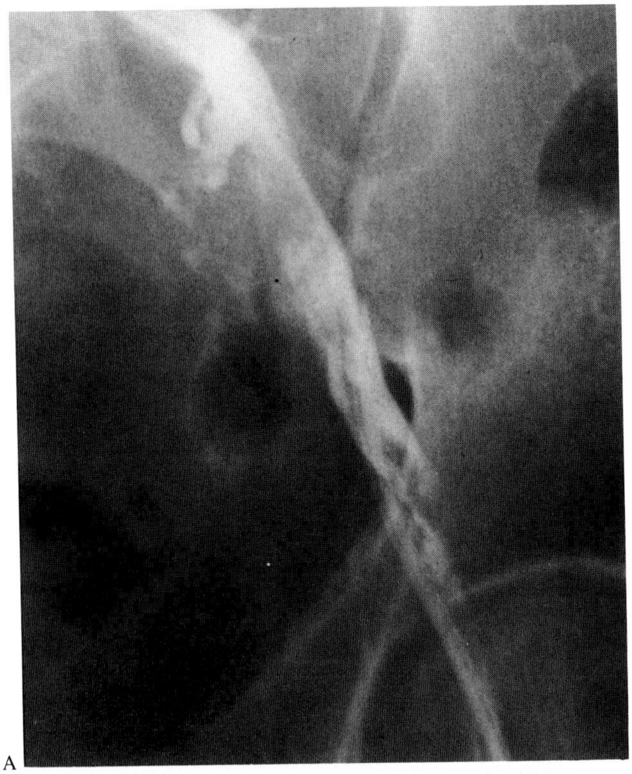

A

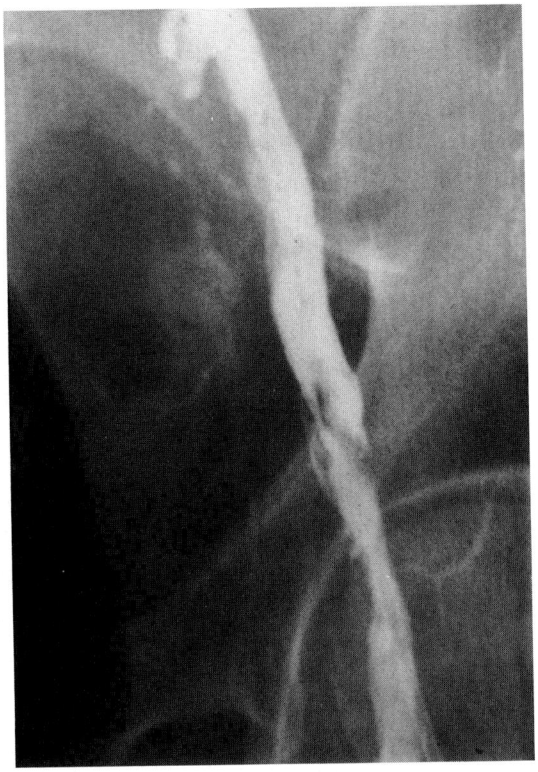

B

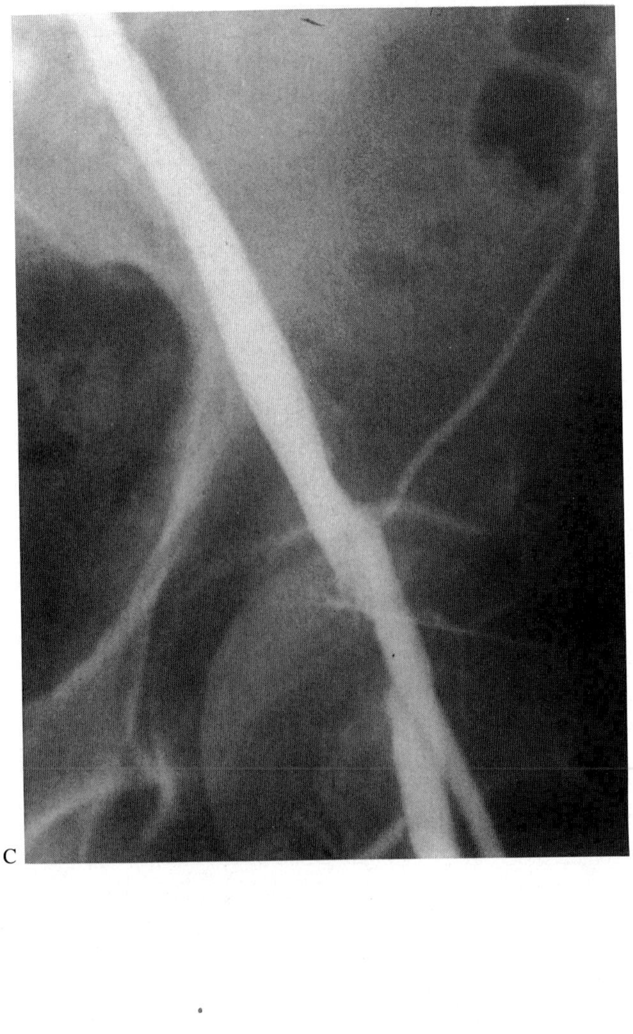

C

Figure 40–2. **A:** Postangioplasty thrombosis of left external iliac and common femoral artery. **B:** After thrombolysis, most thrombus has lysed and a large intimal flap can now be seen. **C:** Postplacement of two Palmaz stents; note a widely open lumen.

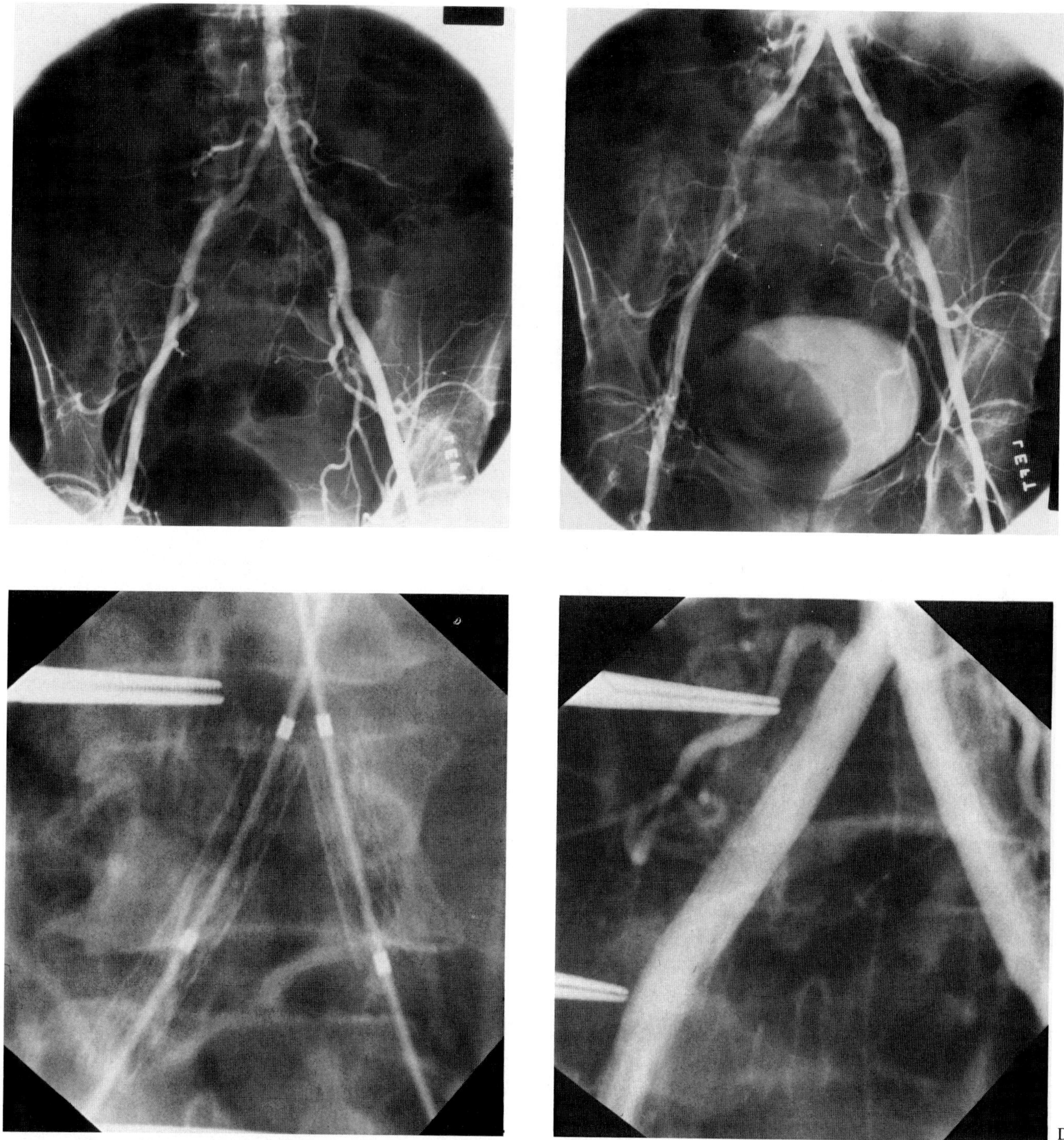

A B C D

Figure 40–3. A 48-year-old diabetic with bilateral claudication. **A:** Pelvic arteriogram long segment stenosis of both common iliac; 20 to 30 mmHg gradients were present bilaterally. **B:** Postangioplasty pelvic arteriogram shows extensive intimal flaps. Bilateral residual resting gradients were over 20 mm. **C:** Two stents on the right common iliac artery. Note the overlapping of the stents. One stent on the left common iliac artery. **D:** Pelvic arteriogram after placement of two Palmaz stents in both common iliac arteries shows widely patent lumens. No residual gradients.

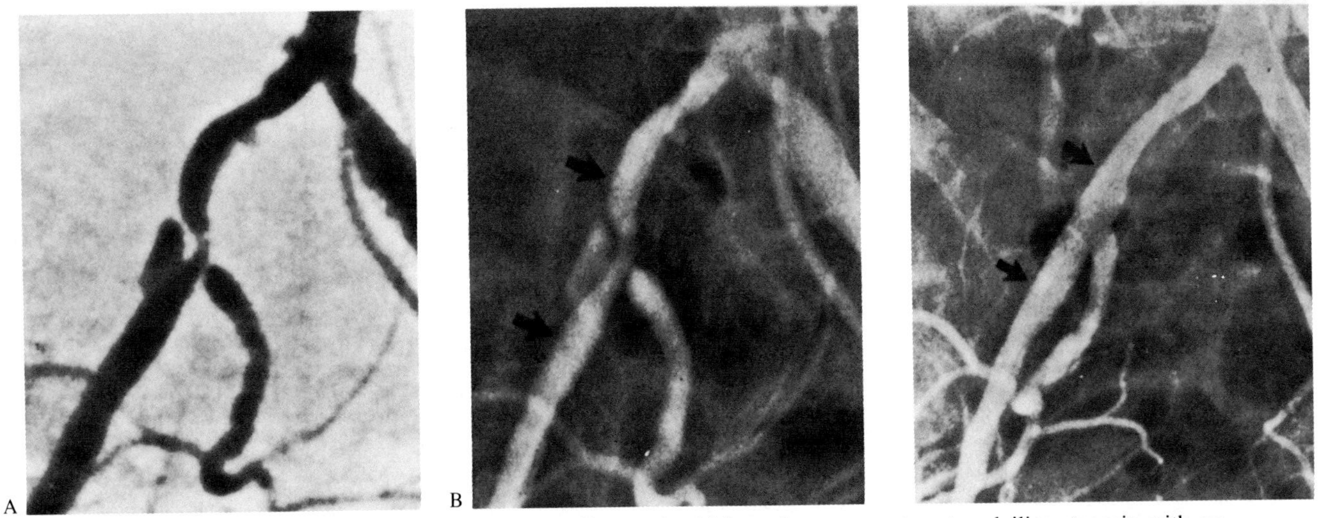

Figure 40–4. **A:** Pelvic arteriogram depicts an eccentric, high-grade common-to-external iliac stenosis with an associated dissection created during a previously performed external iliac artery angioplasty. **B:** After conventional angioplasty (performed between the arrows), there is little improvement in lumen diameter and no change in the dissection. **C:** After percutaneous transluminal angioplasty and stent placement (between the arrows), there is marked improvement in lumen size and wall contours, with elimination of the dissection and maintenance of patency at the internal iliac artery origin (Reprinted with permission from Bonn et al.[10])

and Drug Administration. The other devices are under investigational protocols. Because of the diameter of the iliac arteries, atherectomy has only a limited role in the management of these complications.[14]

Stenting is without doubt the best therapeutic option (Fig. 40-3). The management of angioplasty-induced dissection by intraluminal stenting was reported by Becker et al[12] in 12 iliac arteries. Stents were placed at the time of angioplasty procedure in six vessels and as a separate procedure in the other six. An average of three stents per vessel was used. On angiographic follow-up at a mean of 12.9 months on seven patients, only one stent showed evidence of intraluminal narrowing and in another patient clinical deterioration occurred despite a patent stent lumen.[13] Similar successful results with stenting after percutaneous transluminal coronary angioplasty (PTCA)-induced intimal flaps were reported by Haude et al.[18]

Polymer coating of the Palmaz-Schatz stent has been reported to decrease the occurrence of vascular spasm following stent implantation. The coating also decreases local

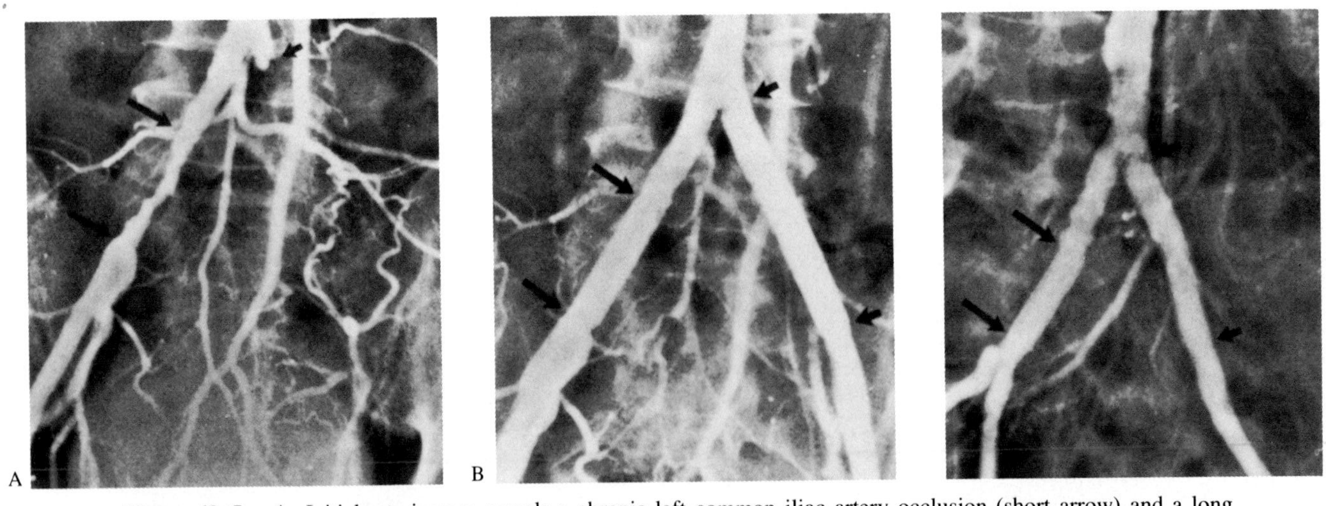

Figure 40–5. **A:** Initial arteriogram reveals a chronic left common iliac artery occlusion (short arrow) and a long segment right common iliac artery stenosis (between the long arrows). **B:** Subsequent arteriogram shows the result after recanalization and placement of two stents in tandem in the left common iliac artery (between the short arrows) and a single stent in the right common iliac artery (between the long arrows). **C:** Arteriogram 1 year after the initial procedure demonstrates only minimal formation of neointima in the distal aspect of the left common iliac artery. (Reprinted with permission from Bonn et al.[10])

platelet deposition. These two effects of polymer coating can therefore decrease the risk of stent thrombosis.[19] The purported decrease of the restenosis rate with the use of the Palmaz/Schatz stent in the coronary arteries is reportedly related to the improved initial results, rather than to a decrease in myointimal regrowth.[20] Delayed restenosis beyond 6 months is uncommon after intracoronary stenting. Stent implantation does not appear to delay, however, the temporal course of the restenosis process.[21] In a study of 50 of 186 patients with restenosis following stent implantation, Levine et al[22] reported that due to the firm incorporation of the stent into the arterial wall 4 to 6 months after placement, the artery tends to exhibit a plastic rather than an elastic behavior. This finding might contribute to a safe and effective redilation, since the neointima might be able to stretch rather than fracture. Twenty-two patients were redilated, with reduction of luminal stenosis from 81 ± 12% to 9 ± 13%. Only one patient had a minor dissection following PTCA.[22]

Recently, the Palmaz stent has been used to manage patients with hypertension due to osteal renal artery stenosis. Rees et al[23] reported on 24 patients with a mean age of 64 ± 9 years, with a mean duration of hypertension of 9.7 ± 10.7 years. Initial technical success (residual stenosis less than 30%) was obtained in 23 patients. Mean stenosis before PTA was 75% and 44% before stenting. In 17 patients with follow-up, up to 1 month with a mean of 6.8 months, cure or improvement of hypertension occurred in 14 patients (82%); four of seven patients showed a decrease in creatinine by 15% or more. Restenosis was angiographically demonstrated in 3 of 13 patients at a mean of 7.3 months.[23] Application of the stent in other areas, including the creation of portocaval shunts,[24] and in congenital heart disease have been recently described.[25,26]

Stenting with the Palmaz stent has proven its safety and efficacy in the iliac arteries, but disadvantages, such as its lack of flexibility and the large size of the introducer system, limit its application at this time. These problems may be overcome by improved designs in the future.

REFERENCES

1. Palmaz JC, Sibbitt RR, Reuter SR, et al. Expandable intraluminal graft: a preliminary study. Radiology 1985;156:73–7.
2. Palmaz JC, Sibbitt RR, Tio FO, et al. Expandable intraluminal vascular graft: a feasibility study. Surgery 1986;99:199–205.
3. Palmaz JC, Ritcher GM, Noeldge G, et al. Intraluminal stents in atherosclerotic iliac artery stenosis: a preliminary report of a multicenter study. Radiology 1988;168:727–31.
4. Doubilet P, Abrams HL. The cost of underutilization: percutaneous transluminal angioplasty for peripheral vascular disease. N Engl J Med 1984;310:95–102.
5. Johnston KW, Rae M, Hogg-Johnston SA, et al. Five-year results of a prospective study of percutaneous transluminal angioplasty. Ann Surg 1987;206:403–13.
6. Zeitler E, Richter EI, Roth FJ, Schopp W. Results of percutaneous transluminal angioplasty. Radiology 1983;146:57–60.
7. Kalman PG, Johnston KW. Outcome of a failed percutaneous transluminal dilation. Surg Gynecol Obstet 1985;161:43–6.
8. Palmaz JC, Garcia O. Cardiovascular radiology: newer percutaneous interventional techniques. Circulation (suppl III) 1990;82:III–102.
9. Palmaz JC, Garcia OJ, Schatz RA, et al. Placement of balloon-expandable intraluminal stents in iliac arteries: first 171 procedures. Radiology 1990;174:969–75.
10. Bonn J, Gardiner GA, Shapiro MJ, et al. Palmaz vascular stent: initial clinical experience. Radiology 1990;174:741–5.
11. Rees CR, Palmaz JC, Garcia O, et al. Angioplasty and stenting of completely occluded iliac arteries. Radiology 1989;172: 953–9.
12. Gardiner GA Jr, Meyerovitz MF, Stokers KR, et al. Complications of transluminal angioplasty. Radiology 1986;159: 201–8.
13. Becker GJ, Palmaz JC, Rees CR, et al. Angioplasty-induced dissections in human iliac arteries: management with Palmaz balloon-expandable intraluminal stents. Radiology 1990; 176:31–8.
14. Maynar M, Reyes R, Cabrera V, et al. Percutaneous atherectomy as an alternative treatment for postangioplasty obstructive intimal flaps. Radiology 1989;170:1029–31.
15. Lee BI, Becker GJ, Waller BF, et al. Thermal compression and molding of atherosclerotic vascular tissue using radiofrequency energy: implications for radiofrequency balloon angioplasty. J Am Coll Cardiol 1989;13:1167–75.
16. Spear JR. Percutaneous transluminal coronary angioplasty restenosis: potential prevention with laser balloon angioplasty. Am J Cardiol 1987;60:61B–4.
17. Spears JR, Reyes VP, James LM, Sinofsky EL. Laser balloon angioplasty: initial clinical experience. (Abstr.) Circulation (suppl II) 1988;78:II–296.
18. Haude M, Erbel R, Straub U, Dietz U. Intracoronary stent implantation in patients with symptomatic dissections after balloon angioplasty—short- and long-term results. Circulation (suppl III) 1990;82:III–658.
19. Bailey SR, Guy DM, Garcia OJ, et al. Polymer coating of Palmaz-Schatz stent attenuates vascular spasm after stent placement. Circulation (suppl III) 1990;82:III–541.
20. Ellis S, Fischman D, Hirshfeld J, et al. Mechanism of stent benefit to limit restenosis following coronary angioplasty: regrowth vs. larger initial lumen? Circulation (suppl III) 1990;82:III–540.
21. Savage M, Fischman D, Ellis S, et al. Does late progression of restenosis occur beyond six months following coronary artery stenting? Circulation (suppl III) 1990;82:III–540.
22. Levine MJ, Clemen MW, Schatz RA, et al. Management of restenosis following Palmaz-Schatz intracoronary stenting: multicenter results. Circulation (suppl III) 1990;82:III–560.
23. Rees CR, Palmaz JC, Becker GJ, et al. Palmaz stenting of atheromatous lesions involving the ostium of the renal artery. Circulation (suppl III) 1990;82:III–404.
24. Palmaz JC, Sibbitt RR, Reuter SR, et al. Expandable intrahepatic portacaval shunt stents: early experience in the dog. AJR 1985;145:821–5.
25. Mullins CE, O'Laughlin MP, Vick GW III, et al. Implantation of balloon-expandable intravascular grafts by catheterization in pulmonary arteries and systemic veins. Circulation 1988; 77:188–199.
26. O'Laughlin MP, Perry SB, Lock JE, Mullins CE. Implantation of balloon-expandable intravascular stents in patients with congenital heart disease. Circulation (suppl III) 1990;82:III–658.

41 Percutaneous Endovascular Stenting: Pathophysiologic Correlates

C. L. Zollikofer, M.D., F. Antonucci, M.D., F. Redha, M.D., T. Vollrath, M.D., G. Stuckmann, M.D., E. Salomonowitz, M.D.

Intravascular stenting is one of the most fascinating and challenging new subjects in research and treatment of vascular disease. The idea was conceived by Charles Dotter[1] only shortly after he had introduced percutaneous transluminal angioplasty (PTA).[2] It had a slow start, mainly because of technical limitations in delivering percutaneously large enough stents at that time. In 1980, Maass et al[3,4] began to investigate the applicability of an expandable endoluminal spiral coil system based on Dotter's early work.[2] About 2 years later, the first vascular endoprosthesis was inserted intraoperatively in a patient with a dissecting aortic aneurysm by Maass and Senning at the University of Zürich. Since then, numerous studies followed using a wide variety of stent designs, but all based on three main principles: thermal memory, spring load, and plastic deformation[1–10] (Figs. 41-1 through 41-5).

Common to all stents are the requirements for successful interluminal stenting: stable biomechanics, biocompatibility, low thrombogenicity, and easy and safe mode of stent implantation.

BIOMECHANICS

The design and material of intravascular stents must be such as to guarantee self-fixation and resistance to mechanical recoil of a stenotic vessel. Furthermore, metal fatigue from millions of cycles of stress caused by arterial pulsations must be excluded.

The ability to oppose the circumferential elasticity of a vessel to balloon-expanded stents and/or self-expanding stents may be varied by the elastic limit and modulus of the metal and the number and thickness of the wire filaments[8–10] (Figs. 41-3 through 41-5), wire bands[3,4] (Fig. 41-1), or the dimensions of struts and slots[7] (Fig. 41-2). The expansile force of a stent, however, should not be such as to cause serious damage or even perforation of the vessel wall. Studies by Maass et al[3] showed that expansion pressures of 1000 mmHg in the aorta and 300 mmHg in the vena cava in dogs were tolerated. An experimental study on mechanical stress of stents by Palmaz[11] showed that the fatigue limit of the stent during a forseeable life span of an average patient will not be approached.

Another important factor for percutaneous stent implantation is the expansibility ratio. The larger this ratio, the smaller the introducer catheter. Most stents currently used have an expansibility ratio between 1:4 and 1:5. The large Gianturco stents of 25 and 30 mm have a higher ratio of about 1:8.

BIOCOMPATIBILITY

Biocompatibility of endovascular stents is governed by a number of factors, such as the stent material, the stent design, and the pressure exerted on the arterial wall, which influences thrombogenicity and cellular reaction of the arterial wall. The various stent designs all have been extensively tested in animal experiments with follow-up of up to 3 years.[8,12–14] All stents showed the unique feature of early endothelial spread across the metal stents. However, fila-

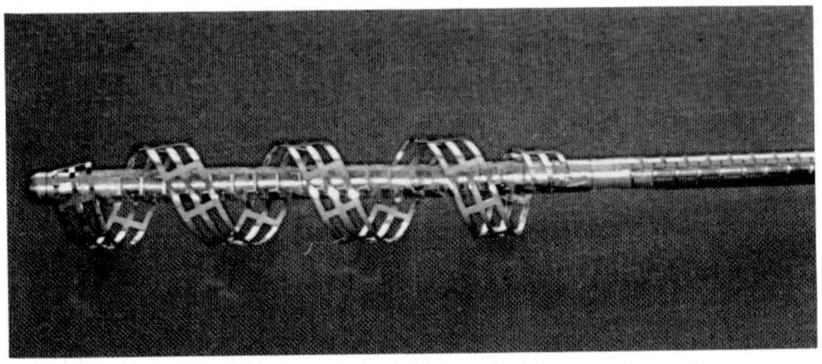

Figure 41–1. Maass double-helix spiral prosthesis partially released from the introducing instrument.

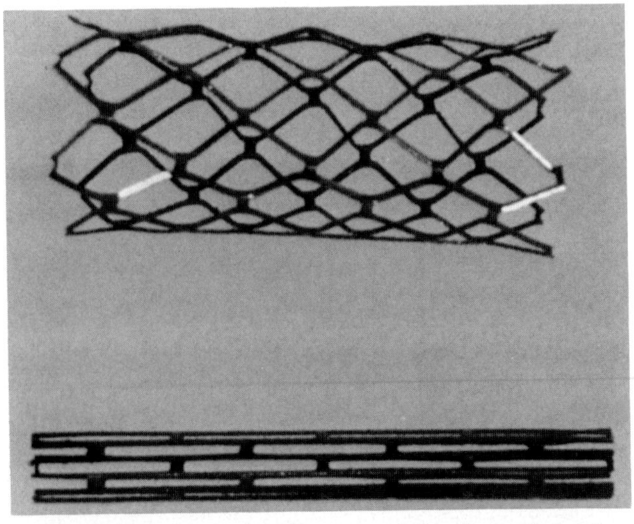

Figure 41–2. Palmaz stent in unexpanded and expanded state.

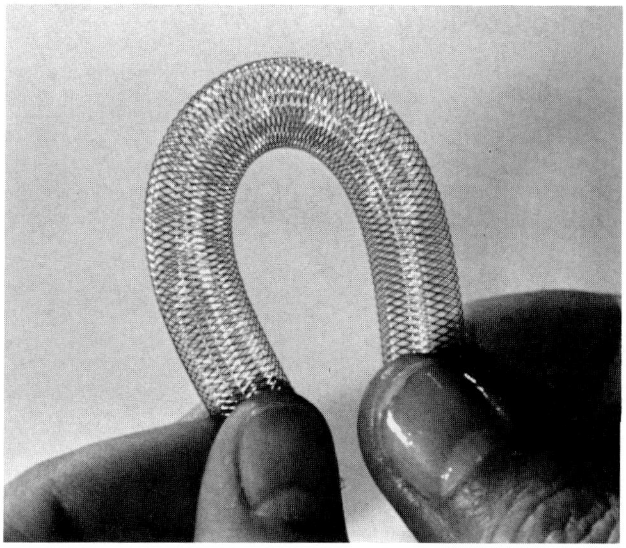

Figure 41–3. Wallstent.

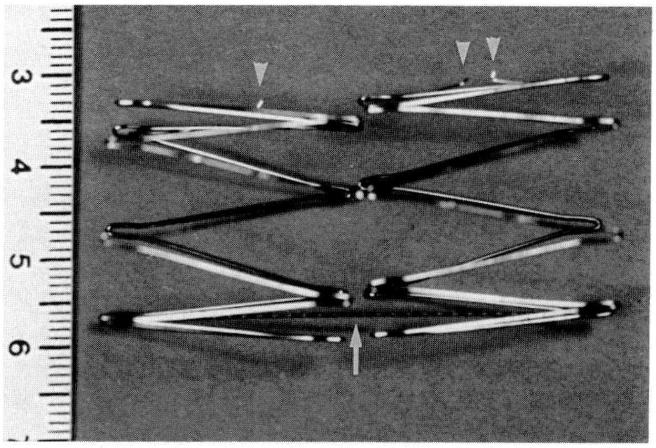

Figure 41–5. Gianturco double stent. Two stents are connected by a single wire (arrow). Small barbs (arrowheads) prevent migration of the stent.

ments of smaller diameter (less than 0.15 mm) were covered more rapidly.[8,13,15] In a study with Wallstents made from filaments of 0.08 mm diameter, a primitive endothelial layer was already found at 10 days and a multilayer neointima covering the stents at 3 to 4 weeks[15] (Fig. 41-6). Similar results were found by Maass et al,[14] Rousseau et al,[13] and Palmaz et al.[16] On the other hand, Wright et al[8] found only partial endothelialization of 30 to 80% at 4 months using stents made from 0.45 mm wire.

In most studies successive intimal hyperplasia in the order of 50 to 400 μm was found, which stabilized after 4 to 8 weeks.[4,13,16,17] However, restriction of flow or mismatch of stent and artery (more than 20%) resulted in increased intimal reaction that led to obstruction or thrombosis.[13,18,19] In a study on internal iliac artery stents in dogs (3.5 mm diameter stents) intimal hyperplasia was at the maximum at 4 weeks (average, 132 μm) decreasing to 46 μm at 6 months[19] (Fig. 41-7). We could also show that intimal hyperplasia was dependent on the stiffness or the expansile force of the stents using different filament thickness of 0.05 and 0.08 mm. At 4 weeks, the degree of intimal hyperplasia was 74 versus 102 μm. This means that increased expansile force leads to a more pronounced intimal reaction. On the other hand, there seemed to be no difference whether the arteries were pretreated with balloon dilatation before stenting.[19] Furthermore, most studies showed that side branches crossed by the stent filaments or struts usually remain patent[4,8,10,12,13] (Fig. 41-8).

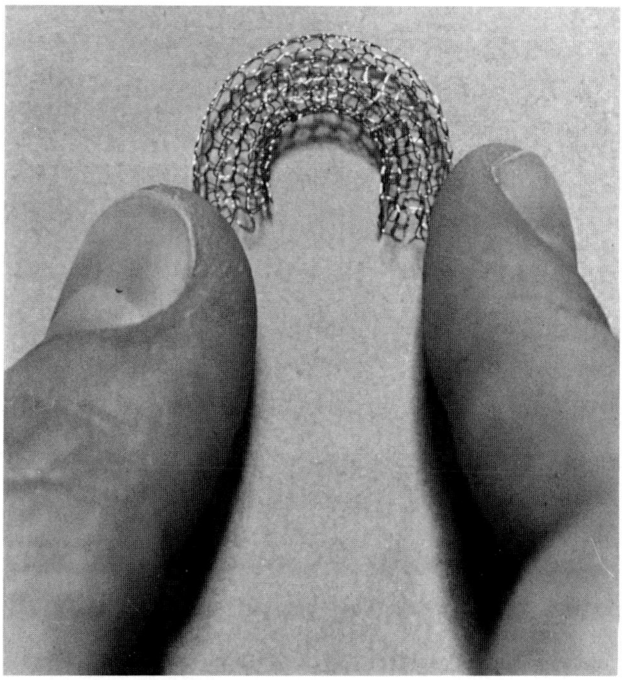

Figure 41–4. Strecker stent.

THROMBOGENICITY

Another critical element for stenting is thromboresistance. This depends on hematologic factors, such as thrombogenesis and thrombolysis; rheologic factors, such as blood flow patterns; and, finally, metallurgic properties, such as surface electric charge, critical surface energy, and texture.

Thrombogenicity is not altogether a negative feature, since a fibrin thrombus deposited over the metal surface allows for endothelialization of the stent. Therefore the rate of thrombus formation should be controlled by anticoagulation and turbulence or reduction of flow must be avoided. Several animal experiments studied the effectiveness of different anticoagulation regimens,[20,21] the effect of the metal surface, and reduction of flow.[8,21] In clinical experience of iliac artery stenting, however, various anticoagulation regimens using initial heparinization followed by oral anticoagulation with antivitamin K or aspirin with or without dipyridamole for various periods of time showed no signifi-

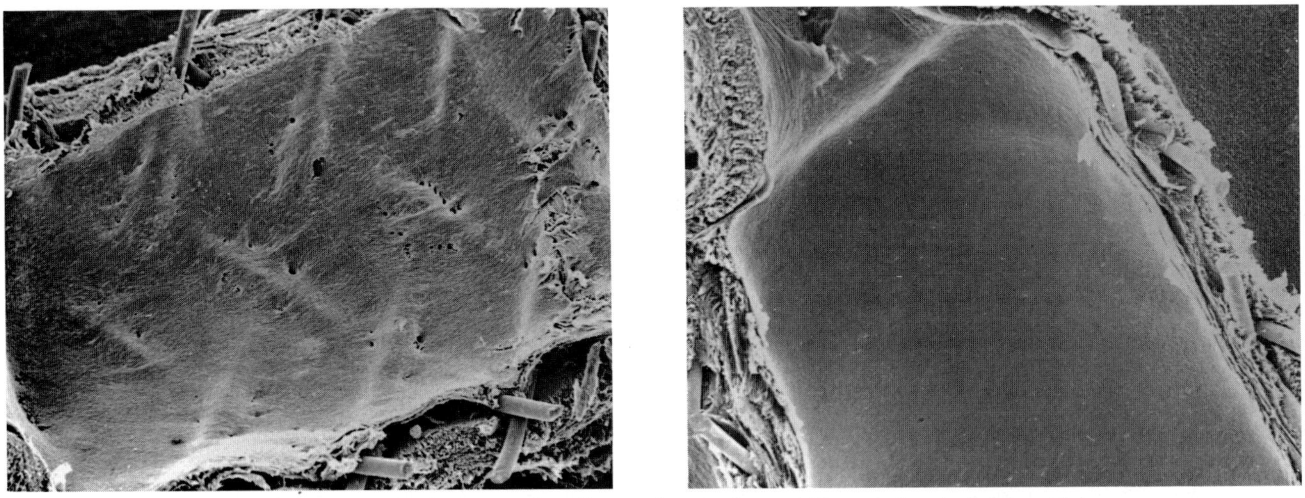

A B

Figure 41–6. Scanning electron microscope view of stented canine internal iliac arteries. **A:** A thin yet inhomogeneous layer covers the stent filaments at 10 days. **B:** At 4 weeks, the neointima is fairly smooth and regular.

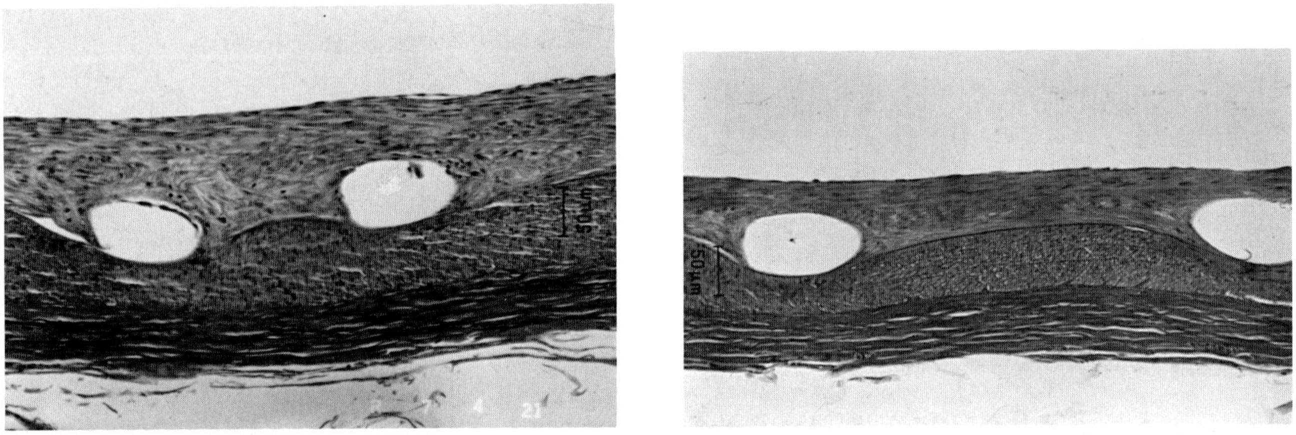

A B

Figure 41–7. Histologic section of stented canine internal iliac arteries at 4 weeks **(A)** and 6 months **(B).** Note the decreasing thickness of the neointima. At the area of the filaments, there is slight compression of the media.

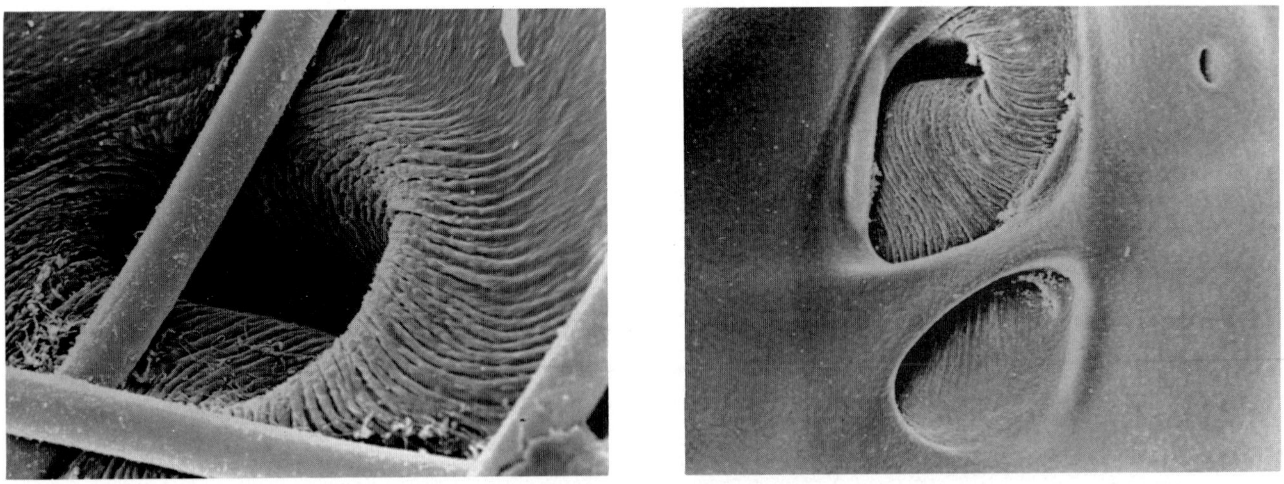

A B

Figure 41–8. A, B: Scanning electron microscope view of stented canine internal iliac arteries at 4 weeks and at 6 months. Note how the side branches crossed by stent filaments remain unobstructed and also the stent filaments are entirely covered by a neoendothelium after 6 months.

cant differences.[22–26] Whether oral antivitamin K improves the problem of severe intimal hyperplasia in femoropopliteal stenting is a matter of speculation, since the various experiences are difficult to compare.[22,24,26,27] However, animal studies performed by Palmaz et al[20] and Nöldge et al[21] also suggest that small diameter stents require aggressive anticoagulation.

For smaller arteries the stent design should be such that the metal surface is kept as small as possible by optimizing the mesh design, since the amount of fibrin-platelet thrombus deposited seems proportional to the total metal surface.[20]

CLINICAL EXPERIENCE AND CORRELATION

The largest group of vascular endoprostheses to date has been patients with iliac artery stenosis and occlusions. More than 500 iliac artery implants have been performed, mainly with the Palmaz stent, the Wallstent, and the Strecker stent.[23–26,28–32] The results have been excellent in view of the usually complex lesions with inadequate response to PTA that have been treated with stents. Patency rates of 90 to 100% after 6 to 12 months in iliac occlusions or iatrogenic-induced dissections or obstructions following PTA or surgery cannot be obtained by simple PTA alone. There have been few occlusions or problems with recurrent stenosis secondary to intimal hyperplasia after stenting of iliac arteries. As long as in- and outflow are not obstructed, the rate of acute thrombosis will be low. Furthermore, thrombosis and restenosis may be treated percutaneously with thrombolysis, percutaneous atherectomy, or repeated PTA.

The second largest group of patients treated are patients with coronary artery disease.[33,34] After initial enthusiasm, the hope that stent implantation may prevent or diminish restenosis has not been fulfilled. Uncontrollable intimal hyperplasia and acute thrombosis are the crux for all stents in small caliber vessels. The situation is worsened by low blood flow and poor runoff. The same problems apply to stenting of the femoropopliteal axis for long occlusions and poor results after PTA.[26,27] Even adequate runoff may not prevent intimal hyperplasia in femoropopliteal stents.

It has recently been suggested that active fibrocellular proliferation associated with restenosis after balloon angioplasty is further stimulated by stent implantation.[34] It has also been suggested that rigid stents may work better than the self-expanding stent because the limitation of vessel wall stress seems to be protective against atherogenesis.[7,12,35] The self-expanding stent through constant pressure on the wall or shear forces by the filaments of the mesh might be a source of stimulation for cellular migration into the intima or even damage of the neoendothelium. However, there is as yet no evidence for support of these speculations in clinical experience in spite of some support from experimental work.

Stenting of recurrent stenosis in hemodialysis arteriovenous fistula shunts is another indication in which it was hoped that the problem of recurrent stenosis would be solved. Again, intimal hyperplasia usually occurring after 5 to 9 months[36–38] calls for repeated interventions. In our experience, repeated PTA works astonishingly well in stented vessels, although atherectomy may give better long-term results.[39] Atherectomy specimens in a patient with recurrent stenosis from intimal hyperplasia after bilateral iliac artery stenting showed the excised intimal plaque to have a very low cellular content with most likely a high content of fluid. It is our belief that PTA in recurrent stenosis after stenting works by expression of the fluid by balloon compression. This may also explain the sometimes rapid recurrences after PTA of shunt restenosis,[39] although in our experience repeated PTA was never necessary at intervals of less than 3 months. Repeated PTA after stenting usually led to better function of the shunt compared with the situation before stenting.

Finally, stenting of large veins, such as femoral, iliac, subclavian, and the vena cava, have been performed very successfully. Long-term follow-up in benign disease is now available for more than 4 years.[38] In contrast to animal experiments, intimal hyperplasia seems to be less prominent in human veins compared with arteries[4] (Zollikofer CL: Unpublished data).

In conclusion, large vessels with rapid flow present the best conditions for successful stenting. Indications for iliac artery stenting and large veins may therefore be handled quite liberally. As stated before, the amount of fibrin-platelet thrombus deposited on the implanted stent is relatively constant for a given stent. Therefore the same amount of thrombus spread over a surface leads to decrease of lumen diameter and reduction of flow in a smaller artery but not in a large vessel. On the other hand, there is a limit as to how much the metal material of the stent can be reduced for small vessels in order not to cause collapse of the stent by the recoiling force of the vessel wall. Therefore stenting of the femoropopliteal axis should only be performed if other means, such as thrombolysis and atherectomy, fail to complete unsuccessful PTA. An exception to this rule may be made when stenting femoral arteries for smoothing of the lumen in patients with a dilative form of atherosclerosis and consequently a large diameter of the femoral arteries.

In addition to improving the thrombogenicity of the stent itself by modifying the metal surface, lowering the surface energy and a negative metal charge, a pharmacologic approach will be necessary to win the battle against restenosis.

REFERENCES

1. Dotter CT. Transluminally-placed coilspring endarterial tube grafts: long-term patency in canine popliteal artery. Invest Radiol 1969;4:327–32.
2. Dotter C, Judkins MP. Transluminal treatment of arteriosclerotic obstructions. Circulation 1964;30:654–63.
3. Maass D, Kropf L, Egloff L, et al. Transluminal implantation of intravascular "double helix" spiral prostheses: technical and

biological considerations. European Society for Artificial Organs Proceedings, 1982;9:252–6.
4. Maass D, Demierre D, Deaton D, et al. Transluminal implantation of self-adjusting expandable prostheses: principles, techniques and results. Prog Artif Organs 1983;2:979–87.
5. Cragg A, Lund G, Rysavy J, et al. Nonsurgical placement of arterial endoprostheses: a new technique using nitinol wire. Radiology 1983;147:261–3.
6. Palmaz JC, Sibbitt RR, Reuter STR, et al. Expandable intraluminal graft: a preliminary study. Radiology 1985;156:73–7.
7. Palmaz JC, Windeler SA, Garcia F, et al. Atherosclerotic rabbit aortas: expandable intraluminal grafting. Radiology 1986;160:723–6.
8. Wright KC, Wallace S, Charnsangavej C, et al. Percutaneous endovascular stents: an experimental evaluation. Radiology 1985;156:69–72.
9. Sigwart V, Puel J, Mirkovitch V, et al. Intravascular stents to prevent occlusion and restenosis after transluminal angioplasty. N Engl J Med 1987;316:701–6.
10. Strecker EP, Berg C, Weber H, et al. Experimentelle Untersuchungen mit einer neuen perkutan einführbaren und aufdehnbaren Gefässendoprothese. Fortschr Rontgenstr 1987;147: 669–72.
11. Palmaz JC. The current status of vascular prosthesis. Presented at the annual meeting of the Society of Cardiovascular and Interventional Radiology, San Diego, CA, March 1987.
12. Palmaz JC. Balloon-expandable intravascular stent. AJR 1988;150:1263–9.
13. Rousseau H, Puel J, Joffre F, et al. Self-expanding endovascular prosthesis: an experimental study. Radiology 1987; 164:709–14.
14. Maass D, Zollikofer CHL, Largiadèr F, Senning A. Radiological follow-up of transluminally inserted vascular endoprostheses: an experimental study using expanding spirals. Radiology 1984;152:659–63.
15. Redha F, Zollikofer CHL, Uhlschmid GK, et al. Combination of angioplasty and intraarterial stent: an experimental study. Presented at the 73rd Scientific Assembly and annual meeting of the Radiological Society of North America, Chicago, November 29–December 4, 1987.
16. Palmaz JC, Sibbitt RR, Tio FO, et al. Expandable intraluminal vascular graft: a feasibility study. Surgery 1986;99:199–205.
17. Schatz RA, Palmaz JC, Tio FO, et al. Balloon-expandable intracoronary stents in the adult dog. Circulation 1987; 76:450–7.
18. Duprat G Jr, Wright KC, Charnsangavej C, et al. Self-expanding metallic stents for small vessels: experimental evaluation. Radiology 1987;162:469–72.
19. Redha F, Zollikofer CL, Uhlschmid GK, Largiadèr F. Experimental combination of angioplasty and intraarterial stent. 23rd Congress of European Society for Surgical Research, Bologna, May 1988.
20. Palmaz JC, Garcia O, Kopp DT, et al. Balloon-expandable intraarterial stents: effect of anticoagulation on thrombus formation. (Abstr.) Circulation 1987;76(suppl IV):45.
21. Nöldge G, Richter GM, Siegerstetter V, et al. Tierexperimentelle Untersuchungen über den Einfluss der Flussrestriktion auf die Thrombogenität des Palmaz-Stentes mittels ^{111}Indium-markierter Thrombozyten. Fortschr Rontgenstr 1990; 152:264–70.
22. Rousseau HP, Raillat CR, Joffre FG, et al. Treatment of femoropopliteal stenoses by means of self-expandable endoprostheses: midterm results. Radiology 1989;172:961–4.
23. Becker GJ, Palmaz JC, Rees CR, et al. Angioplasty-induced dissections in human iliac arteries: management with Palmaz balloon-expandable intraluminal stents. Radiology 1990; 176:31–8.
24. Günther RW, Vorwerk D, Bohndorf K, et al. Iliac and femoral artery stenoses and occlusions: treatment with intravascular stents. Radiology 1989;172:725–30.
25. Palmaz JC, et al. Placement of balloon-expandable intraluminal stents in iliac arteries: first 171 procedures. Radiology 1990;174:969–75.
26. Zollikofer CHL, Antonucci F, Pfyffer M, Falah Redha, Salomonowitz E, Stuckmann G, Largiadèr J, Marty A. Arterial stent placement with use of the Wallstent: Midterm results of clinical experience. Radiology. 1991;179:449–456.
27. Triller J, Mahler F, Do D, et al. Die vaskuläre Endoprothese bei femoro-poplitealer Verschlusskrankheit. Fortschr Rontgenstr 1989;150,3:88–94.
28. Bonn J, Gardiner GA, Shapiro MJ, et al. Palmaz vascular stent: initial clinical experience. Radiology 1990;174:741–5.
29. Rees CR, Palmaz JC, Garcia O, et al. Angioplasty and stenting of completely occluded iliac arteries. Radiology 1989; 172:953–9.
30. Günther RW, Vorwerk D, Antonucci F, Beyssen B, Essinger A, Gaux JC, Joffre F, Raynaud A, Rousseau H. Zollikofer CHL. Iliac artery stenosis or obstruction after unsuccessful balloon angioplasty. AJR 156:389-393; February 1991.
31. Strecker EP, Liermann D, Wolf HR. Treatment of iliac and femoropopliteal artery occlusive disease with flexible tantalum stent. Presented at the Annual Meeting of the CIRSE. Brussels, May 1990.
32. Vorwerk D, Guenther RW. Mechanical revascularization of occluded iliac arteries with use of self-expandable endoprostheses. Radiology 1990;175:411–5.
33. Sigwart U, Puel J, Mirkovitch V, et al. Intravascular stents to prevent occlusion and restenosis after transluminal angioplasty. N Engl J Med 1987;316:701–6.
34. Serruys PW, Beatt KJ, Van der Giessen WJ. Stenting of coronary arteries. Are we the sorcerer's apprentice? Eur Heart J 1989;10:774–82.
35. Thubikar M, Baker J, Nolan S. Inhibition of atherosclerosis by reduction of arterial intramural stress in rabbits. Circulation 1987;76:314A.
36. Zollikofer CL, Largiadèr F, Bruhlmann WF, et al. Endovascular stenting of veins and grafts: preliminary clinical experience. Radiology 1988;167:707–12.
37. Günther RW, Vorwerk D, Bohndorf K, et al. Venous stenoses in dialysis shunts: treatment with self-expanding metallic stents. Radiology 1989;170:401–5.
38. Antonucci F, Salomonowitz E, Stuckmann G, Stiefel M, Largiadèr J, Zollikofer CHL. Placement of venous stents: Clinical experience with a self-expanding prosthesis. Radiology 1992;183:493-497.
39. Vorwerk D, Günther RW. Removal of intimal hyperplasia in vascular endoprostheses by atherectomy and balloon dilatation. AJR 1990;154:617–9.

42 Self-Expandable Intravascular Stent: Long-Term Results in the Iliac and Superficial Femoral Artery

F. Joffre, M.D., H. Rousseau, M.D., R. Chemali, M.D.

Since the pioneering work of Dotter and Judkins in 1964,[1] percutaneous transluminal angioplasty (PTA) has progressively become a preferred alternative to surgery for treatment of lower limb arterial lesions. However, this procedure has its limits, dominated by the immediate failure secondary to intimal dissection or recoil of the stenosis, and particularly by the restenosis at midterm, estimated to be 30% at the femoropopliteal level[2] and 10% at the iliac level.[3]

New methods seem to complete and to improve the results of the PTA and to widen the indications: atherectomy,[4] mechanical recanalization,[5] and laser angioplasty.[6] Among these methods, the use of percutaneous endoprostheses is very appealing.

Different kinds of endoprostheses have been proposed after Dotter.[7] They all maintain the vascular stenosis open after dilation and could play an important role in the prevention of both restenosis and early occlusion.

GENERALITIES ABOUT SELF-EXPANDABLE ENDOPROSTHESIS

In 1969, Dotter[7] reported the use of percutaneous endoprostheses to maintain an open artery after PTA, and since then different kinds of endoprostheses have been proposed and used during experimental works.[8–14]

The first clinical application appeared during the last few years using the Wallstent.[15] The Wallstent is the main self-expandable endoprosthesis used for arterial disease (Fig. 42-1). The endoprosthesis is composed of 20 spring steep filaments (surgical grade stainless steel alloy), each 75 μm in diameter, woven into a tubular braid configuration. The filament crossing points are not welded but are free to pivot over each other. The prosthesis can therefore be longitudinally reduced to a small diameter and will spontaneously recover its original diameter when released into the vascular lumen because of the spring characteristics of the individual filaments. When mounted in its reduced, small diameter format on the delivery catheter, the endoprosthesis is constrained by a rolling membrane that the operator can retract progressively via the control elements of the catheter. As the stent is deployed from the catheter, it expands radially, molding itself to the vessel wall, its longitudinal flexibility allowing perfect adaptation to vessel curvature.

The release of the stretched prosthesis leads to a spontaneous return to the initial shape, whose diameter and length are determined prior to insertion. The endoprosthesis is placed at the end of the catheter, the caliber of which varies according to the prosthesis caliber (5 F to 9 F). It can be used over guide wires of 0.014 to 0.035 inch. Different calibers and lengths of the prostheses are available (5 to 14 mm diameter). The delivery catheter is highly flexible, permitting tortuous access. The caliber tip is very flexible despite the presence of the mounted prosthesis.

The experimental results obtained with the Wallstent are similar, with some differences, to the results obtained with other types of prostheses.[12–14] These results can be summarized as follows: the implantation is very easy, the fitting of the stent to the arterial wall is excellent, no migration of the stent has been noted, and the microscopic studies have not shown host or inflammatory reactions. The essential phenomenon is the fast development of a neointima, which covers the filaments after 4 weeks.[5] The collaterals remained patent even when bridged by the stent.

TECHNIQUE

The implantation technique is analogous in many ways to that of PTA, since the devices can be delivered percutaneously over conventional guide wires, under local anesthesia, catheter introduction being performed through a sheath.

For iliac implantations, catheterization is achieved mainly via the ipsilateral femoral retrograde approach, but the contralateral access is possible. For the femoral lesions, the ipsilateral femoral antegrade approach is used except for proximal lesions, which need a contralateral access.

With self-expandable stents, PTA is always performed before stenting. The attempts at placement without dilation were mostly unsuccessful. The 7 F stent delivery catheter is introduced over a 0.035 inch (0.88 mm) guide wire. Implantation, performed under fluoroscopic guidance, does not exceed 5 minutes.

Stent diameters vary between 5 and 10 mm. The diameter is chosen to be slightly (15%) greater than the diameter of the native artery so that a residual pressure is generated against the vessel wall, preventing migration. The endoprosthesis is selected so that the length is sufficient to cover the entire diseased region, even if this requires several stents. Immediate radiologic and manometric controls are the rule.

Follow-up has to be based on clinical examination, Doppler determination of the systolic ankle-arm index, and

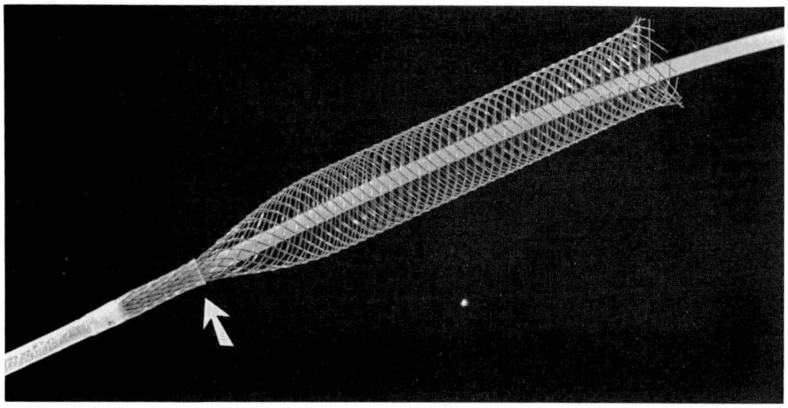

Figure 42–1. Photograph of Wallstent endoprosthesis: withdrawal of the sheath allows progressive release of the stent (arrow).

standard walking test, at 1, 6, and 12 months. Angiographic control is necessary if possible at 1, 6, and 12 months. Acetylsalicylic acid (300 mg/day) and dipyridamole (75 mg three times per day) are given 24 hours before implantation and for 6 months afterward. During implantation, an intra-arterial bolus of 5000 IU of heparin is given as well as dextran. Heparin is continued for 24 hours after placement, followed by oral anticoagulation for 2 months, mainly in cases of poor distal runoff femoral implants.

RESULTS

Immediate

The Toulouse group experience consists up to now of 27 patients with iliac lesions and 43 patients with femoropopliteal lesions, with a follow-up greater than 6 months.[16,17] The indications for iliac implants were mainly angioplasty failure or complex lesions: post-PTA restenosis (11 cases), occlusion (eight cases), iliac dissection (two cases), and post-PTA poor results (six cases). At the femoropopliteal level, the indications were similar: post-PTA poor results (seven cases), occlusions with 6 cm mean length (23 cases), miscellaneous (subadventitial cyst [one case]; bypass stenoses [two cases]). Ten patients have had implantation for simple femoropopliteal lesions without previous PTA.

Implantation was successful in all cases; a misplacement was very rare, related to the low radiopacity of the stent and concerned lesions located close to the origin of the iliac artery. In these cases it was necessary to place another stent in the appropriate site. No migration or traumatic dissection occurred. Angiographic studies showed a smooth vascular lumen, the stent eliminating the residual stenoses and subintimal dissection secondary to PTA (Figs. 42-2, 42-3). Pressure curves obtained with hemodynamic studies showed improvement compared with those obtained with PTA (Fig. 42-4). The main collateral vessels crossed by the stent remained patent in all cases.

Among the ten femoropopliteal lesions in which previous PTA was not performed, a residual stenosis between 20 and 30% was present in five patients. In all cases, results of clinical and Doppler evaluation showed improvement.

Early in our experience, some cases of acute thrombosis occurred. Iliac thrombosis occurred in two cases with poor distal runoff and in one case of previous iliac artery dissec-

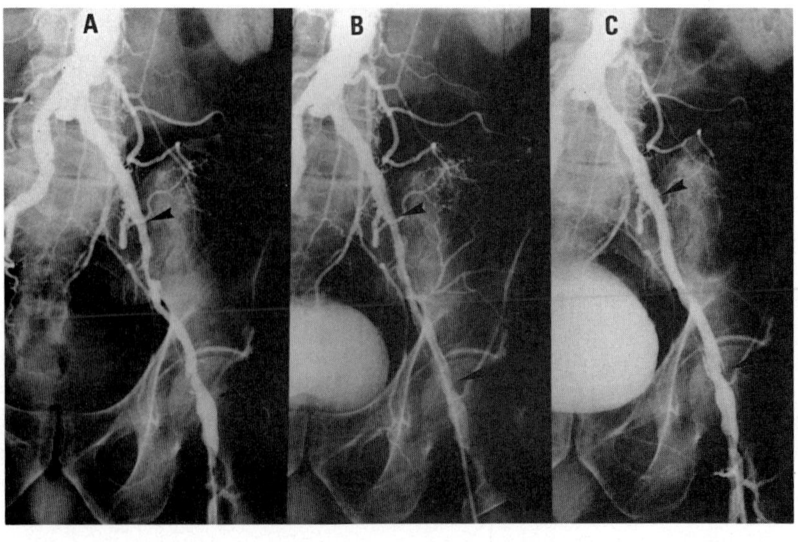

Figure 42–2. A: Angiogram shows severe, extensive and ulcerated lesions of the left iliac axis (arrowheads). **B:** Control after percutaneous transluminal angioplasty with important residual stenoses (arrowheads). **C:** Control after placement of two stents (arrowheads): excellent patency and clinical result.

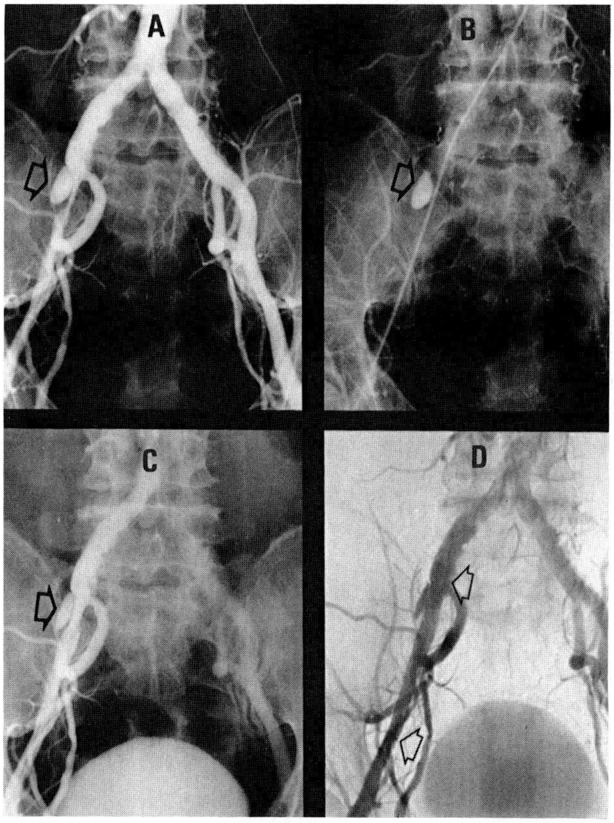

Figure 42–3. **A, B:** Angiograms with tight stenosis of external iliac artery, with important ulceration (arrows). **C:** Immediate control after dilation shows residual stenosis (arrow). **D:** Control 1 month after stenting: the ulceration is partially suppressed and the permeability is excellent (arrow).

tion. There were ten femoropopliteal thromboses, of which three were successfully treated with urokinase. Five of these ten thromboses occurred in patients who had not undergone PTA before stenting. Among these ten cases, only one case occurred in a patient treated with warfarin.

Late Results

The follow-up of these patients ranges from 6 to 46 months (Fig. 42-5). In the absence of early complications, late angiographic studies showed the presence of a thin, clear band on the inner surface of the stent corresponding to intimal proliferation. This hyperplasia remained stable with time and did not appear to progress after the third month. No case of iliac restenosis occurred in this group of patients, but a multicenter study concerning 100 patients and including our own patients showed three symptomatic restenoses between 30 and 50% of the stent diameter. Two patients showed a restenosis within the stent and at the extremities of the stent in one patient where the stent did not cover the whole lesion.

Among the 40 patients with implantation of femoropopliteal lesions treated with endoprostheses, five patients developed a symptomatic stenosis greater than 50%. The restenosis appeared at the extremities or inside the stent. Atherectomy was performed as a treatment of the stenosis in two of these cases using a Simpson catheter and showed that the material recovered was the result of intimal proliferation (Fig. 42-6). Three other patients showed stable (with a mean follow-up of 25 months) asymptomatic restenoses ranging from 30 to 50%. The anticoagulant therapy had no influence on the occurrence of restenosis. However, seven of eight cases occurred after the stenting of long lesions, longer than 5 cm.

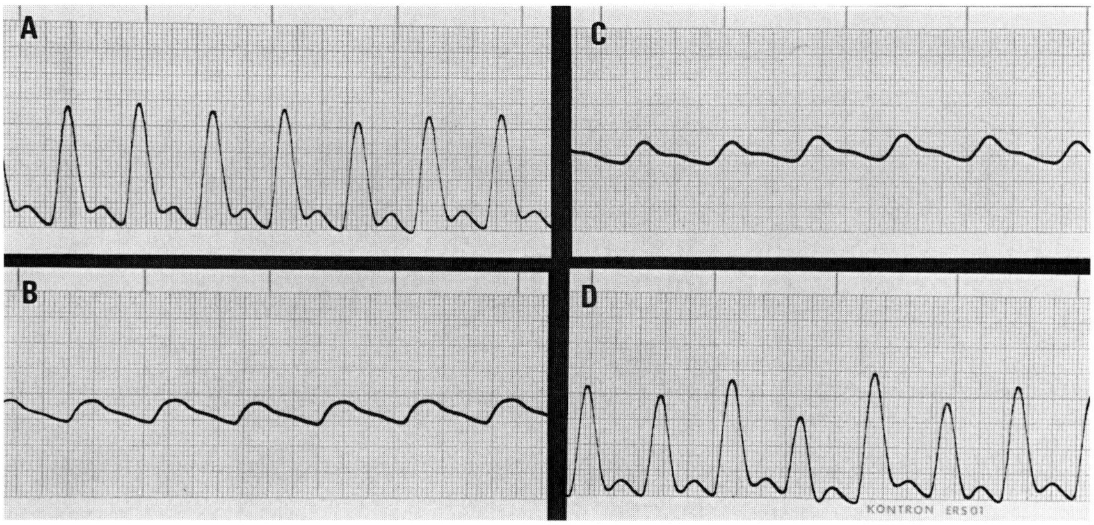

Figure 42–4. Hemodynamic studies reveal the improvement of the pressure below the stenosis after stenting. **A:** Aortic pressure. **B:** Femoral pressure before percutaneous transluminal angioplasty (PTA). **C:** Femoral pressure after PTA. **D:** Femoral pressure after stenting.

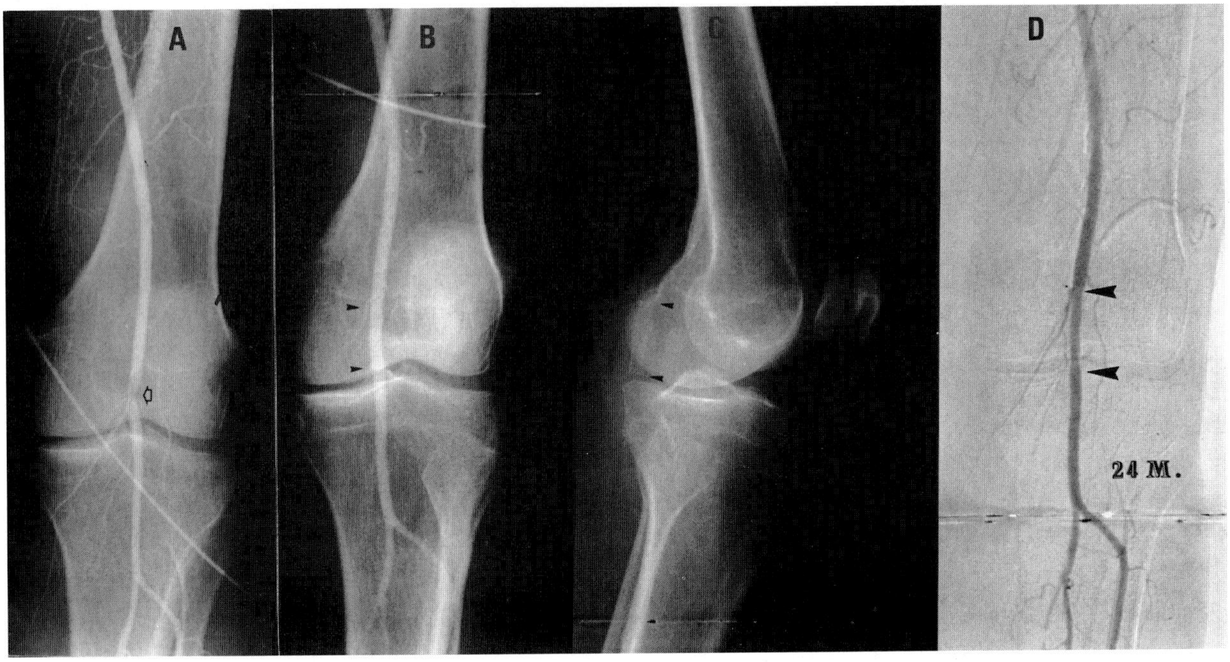

Figure 42–5. **A:** Simple atheromatous popliteal stenosis at the plicature level of the knee. **B:** Control after stenting without percutaneous transluminal angioplasty: excellent patency without residual stenosis. **C:** Profile view showing the stent in front of the plicature zone of the knee. **D:** Control 24 months after stenting: excellent clinical and angiographic result.

In four cases, stenotic lesions developed away from the stented area and were presumed to be associated with progression of atheromatous disease in patients who had made no attempt to reduce their risk factors.

Including the early thrombosis at the beginning of this experience, which declined strikingly with increasing experience, the overall long-term patency is about 90% for iliac artery lesions and 70% for femoropopliteal lesions.

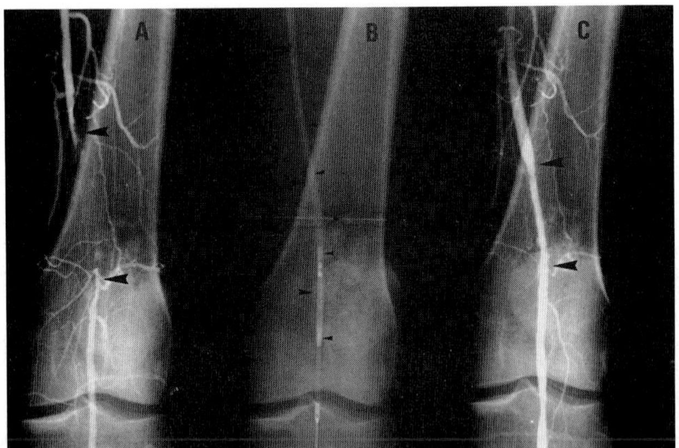

Figure 42–6. **A:** Angiography, 6 months after stenting, shows total occlusion of the stented area, by intimal hyperplasia and thrombosis. **B:** Recanalization and treatment with the Simpson catheter. **C:** Control after treatment.

COMMENT

PTA represents a considerable improvement in the treatment of vascular lesions. However, recurrences were still found at variable rates according to the territory. The presence of important longitudinal dissection secondary to PTA or persistent post-PTA stenoses seem to be the main factors of recurrence.

On the basis of the histologic appearance of arterial lesions treated by PTA and results of experimental animal studies, it appears that two essential phenomena play an important role in restenosis: the formation of a thrombus that progressively organizes to create a fibrous plaque, and intimal hyperplasia created by fibrocellular proliferation.[18,19] Both are related to the fissures and clefts of the initial parietal lesions caused by the PTA itself. In the same way, different retrospective clinical studies have shown that two factors play important roles in restenosis. The risk of restenosis is significantly higher when there persists a residual stenosis with a pressure gradient.[20] Van Andel et al[2,3] showed that the long-term patency rate was 75% when the intraluminal surface was smooth and 66% when irregular, 80% with short lesions, and 55% with long lesions. Until now, many authors considered the complex lesions (long, irregular, ulcerated) as poor indications for PTA.

The concept of a parietal "support" suppressing wall irregularities and dissection and so preventing recurrence after PTA seems to be particularly interesting. Multiple technical solutions can be suggested (metallic memory stent,[8] balloon expandable stent,[15] self-expandable stent[15]). All these different kinds of prostheses have the same goals: (1) to avoid immediate recoiling of the stenosis; (2) to reduce the pressure gradient; and (3) to achieve a smooth parietal surface, and so to decrease the frequency of restenosis. All articles dealing with clinical implantation show immediate good results with pressure gradient suppression and excellent patency with a regular lumen.[16,17,21,22]

Among the multiple stents available, the auto-expandable Wallstent prosthesis seems to have some advantages in comparison with other types. The thinness of its filaments gives it flexibility, which allows it to be introduced in the sinuous and low-caliber arteries guided by a thin catheter. Thus, the iliac or femoral contralateral access is permitted. It could be applied for arteries at a plication site (popliteal artery) without distortion and lumen deformation. The small caliber of the filament allows it fast intimalization, which depends on the thickness of the metallic elements. The absence of rigidity allows a progressive transition without angle between the healthy artery and the holding segment of the prosthesis. The fitness of the prosthesis to the lesion is excellent with multiple combinations of length (from 2 to 7 cm) and diameter (from 4 to 14 mm). On the other hand, this does not appear to be a problem for stenting a long segment by placing multiple stents side by side.

The main problem of the Wallstent is the low radiopacity, which could give some problems for exact positioning of the stent in obese patients, particularly for lesions near an ostium or a bifurcation.

The two-step placement (PTA and stenting) does not seem to be a disadvantage to balloon expandable stents. On the contrary, it allows avoidance of excessive stenting: we consider that prosthesis implantation is not necessary when we obtain good hemodynamic and radiologic post-PTA result. Besides, if a prosthesis is necessary the placement of a Wallstent is very easy.

The occurrence of early thrombosis or late restenosis does not seem to be related to the type of prosthesis. On the other hand, it is difficult to compare the different stents because the main problems occur at the femoropopliteal level and only the Wallstent has been used at this level in significant series of patients.

The experimental thrombogenicity of the Wallstent is comparable to the result reported by others.[13] Despite these results and the use of heparin, platelet antiagreggating agents, and dextran, the rate of early thrombosis is important compared with PTA alone. The main responsible factors seem to be poor distal runoff, the persisting lesions at the extremities of the stent when the length was insufficient, the residual stenoses when stenting was used alone without PTA, and insufficient anticoagulation. With good placement of the stent, good selection of the patients, and good anticoagulation, the thrombosis rate is very low and close to zero for the past 2 years. Nevertheless, it is important to check the patient very carefully for the first month after placement. An early thrombosis could be detected and successfully treated by thrombolysis.

Restenosis is a more worrisome problem, but its occurrence is rare and concerns mainly the femoropopliteal artery. The possibility of successfully treating these restenoses with Simpson atherectomy has to be evaluated in spite of satisfactory follow-up beyond 6 months in our two cases, as suggested by Vorwerk and Gunther.[23]

Because of the possibility of recurrence and although early clinical experience with self-expandable stents or stents in general are very promising,[16,17,21,22] the use of stenting has to be limited to selected cases. The unknown long-term results and the cost of the procedure are other arguments for careful selection of patients. The systematic implantation after every PTA seems to be abusive. On the other hand, implantation only for recurrence after PTA is a wrong choice. We suggest an intermediate attitude, which consists of performing an implantation for unsatisfactory results after PTA with residual stenoses greater than 30% or important intimal dissection with great risk of early thrombosis. This kind of result is sometimes obtained with simple stenoses, but more often with complex lesions, which are considered until now as poor indications for PTA: total obstruction or long and irregular ulcerated stenoses. It is clear now that stenting dramatically improves the immediate and late results of treatment of these kinds of lesions of the iliac arteries. It is not totally true for femoropopliteal lesions, where at present we only use stenting after the immediate failure of PTA.

External arterial compression, such as popliteal adventitial cysts, popliteal artery entrapment, or scalene syndrome, which are poor indications for PTA, may find a nonsurgical solution with stenting, but additional data are still required for this kind of patient.

After more than 3 years of clinical use and even though supplementary studies are necessary, it seems that arterial stenting is a very promising method. The main advantage is the treatment of, with reasonable success, iliac complex lesions, which were considered until now as a contraindication for PTA.

REFERENCES

1. Dotter CT, Judkins MP. Transluminal angioplasty of atherosclerotic obstructions: description of a new technic and preliminary report of its application. Circulation 1964;30:654–70.
2. Krepel VM, Van Andel GJ, Van Erp WFM, Breslau PJ. Percutaneous dilatation of femoral artery: initial and long term results. Radiology 1985;156:325–8.
3. Van Andel GJ, Van Erp WFM, Krepel VM, Breslau PJ. Percutaneous transluminal dilatation of the iliac artery: long term results. Radiology 1985;156:321–3.
4. Simpson JB, Zimmerman JJ, Selmon MR, et al. Transluminal atherectomy: initial clinical results in 27 patients. Circulation 1986;74(suppl 2):457.
5. Kensey KR, Nash JF, Abrahams C, Zarins C. Recanalization of obstructed arteries with a flexible rotating tip catheter. Radiology 1987;165:387–9.
6. Abela GS, Norman SJ, Cohen DM, et al. Laser recanalization

of occluded atherosclerotic arteries in vivo and in vitro. Circulation 1985;71:403–11.

7. Dotter C. Transluminally placed coil springs and arterial tube grafts: long term patency in the canine popliteal artery. Invest Radiol 1969;4:329–32.
8. Dotter C, Buschmann RW, McKinney MK, Rosch J. Transluminal expandable nitinol coil stent grafting: preliminary report. Radiology 1983;147:259–60.
9. Cragg A, Lund G, Raysavy J, et al. Nonsurgical placement of arterial endoprosthesis: a new technique using nitinol wire. Radiology 1983;147:261–3.
10. Maass D, Demiere D, Deaton D, Largiadèr F. Transluminal implantation of self-adjusting expandable prosthesis: principles, techniques, and results. Prog Artif Organs 1983;2:979–87.
11. Wright KC, Wallace S, Charnsangavej C, et al. Percutaneous endovascular stents: an experimental evaluation. Radiology 1985;156:69–72.
12. Rousseau H, Puel J, Joffre F, et al. Self expanding endovascular prosthesis: an experimental study. Radiology 1987; 164:709–14.
13. Palmaz JC, Sibbitt RR, Reuter SR, et al. Expandable intraluminal graft: a preliminary study. Radiology 1985;156:73–7.
14. Rousseau H, Joffre F, Raillat C, et al. Self-expanding endovascular stent in experimental atherosclerosis: work in progress. Radiology 1989;170:773–8.
15. Sigwart V, Puel J, Mirkovitch V, et al. Intra-vascular stents to prevent occlusion and restenosis after transluminal angioplasty. N Engl J Med 1987;316:701–6.
16. Raillat C, Rousseau H, Joffre F, Roux D. Treatment of iliac artery lesions by using the wallstent endoprosthesis: mid-term results. AJR 1990;154:613–6.
17. Rousseau H, Raillat CH, Joffre F, et al. Treatment of femoropopliteal stenoses by means of self-expandable endoprostheses: midterm results. Radiology 1989;172:961–4.
18. Essed CE, Van den Brand M, Becker AE. Transluminal coronary angioplasty and early restenosis: fibrocellular occlusion after wall laceration. Br Heart J 1983;49:393–6.
19. Faxon DP, Sanborn TA, Weber VJ. Restenosis following transluminal angioplasty in experimental atherosclerosis. Arteriosclerosis 1984;4:189–95.
20. Colapinto RF. Long-term results of iliac and femoropopliteal angioplasty. In Dotter CT, Grüntzig A, School W, Zeitler E, (eds). Percutaneous Transluminal Angioplasty. Berlin: Springer-Verlag 1983;202–6.
21. Palmaz JC, Richter GM, Noeldge G, et al. Intraluminal stent in atherosclerotic iliac artery stenosis: preliminary report of a multicenter study. Radiology 1988;168:727–31.
22. Gunther RW, Vorwerk D, Bohndorf K, et al. Iliac and femoral artery stenoses and occlusion: treatment with intravascular stents. Radiology 1989;172:725–30.
23. Vorwerk D, Gunther RW. Removal of intimal hyperplasia in vascular endoprostheses managed by combined use of atherectomy and balloon dilatation. AJR 1990;154:617–9.

43 Gianturco Self-Expanding Stents in the Management of Caval Obstructions

C. Humberto Carrasco, M.D., Chusilp Charnsangavej, M.D., Kenneth C. Wright, M.D., Sidney Wallace, M.D., William R. Richli, M.D., David Lawrence, M.D.

The caval veins are low-pressure, thin-walled vessels that can be easily compressed by adjacent disorders. Although caval obstruction may remain asymptomatic, it can result in the superior or the inferior vena cava syndromes, characterized by peripheral venous distension and edema, among others. Collateral circulation provides alternate pathways for venous blood return, moderating an otherwise life-threatening condition.

SUPERIOR VENA CAVA SYNDROME

Definition

In addition to venous distention and edema, the superior vena cava syndrome may comprise plethora, dyspnea, headache, and cyanosis.[1–3] In most patients, this syndrome improves within 2 weeks, regardless of the type of treatment instituted: irradiation, chemotherapy, or both.[1,4–9] The uniform outcome of different therapies suggests that other factors besides treatment may be responsible for the symptomatic improvement. A thorough review of the literature[10] showed that, in most treated patients, symptomatic improvement was not associated with reestablishment of luminal patency; instead, it depended primarily on the development of collateral circulation. In one publication ligation of the superior vena cava in seven dogs demonstrated the evolution of this syndrome, which spontaneously abated within 1 week in six of the seven animals, one of which died of infection.[11]

Etiology

Obstruction of the superior vena cava is most frequently caused by venous compression or invasion by malignant neoplasms. Approximately 3 to 15% of patients with bronchogenic carcinoma[12] and 3 to 8% of patients with lymphoma[13,14] develop the syndrome. Bronchogenic carcinoma is the cause of the syndrome in approximately 80% of the cases, with most of the remainder being produced by other malignancies, including lymphomas, germ cell tumors, and metastatic breast carcinoma.[3,10,15–17] At least 40% of the cases of bronchogenic carcinoma producing the superior vena cava syndrome are of the small cell type.[3,10] Caval thrombosis may also occur in patients with central venous catheters and in those with systemic diseases, such as Behçet's syndrome and systemic lupus erythematosus.[18]

Collateral Circulation

The syndrome's intensity depends on the level of the obstruction and the adequacy of the collateral venous circulation. The azygos vein provides the most important collateral pathway. Caval obstruction above the azygos orifice, occurring in 9% of one series,[19] results in collateral blood flow mainly into the azygos vein, the superior vena cava below the obstruction, and the right atrium. Obstruction below the azygos orifice, which occurred in 19% of the same series, reverses the flow in the azygos vein, causing blood to return to the heart via the vertebral plexus and the inferior vena cava. In most patients, however, the obstruction affects the azygos orifice, resulting in complex collateral pathways and a more severe syndrome, which may be further aggravated by secondary thrombosis.

Treatment

Purely symptomatic treatment of the superior vena cava syndrome has been attempted using diuretics, corticosteroids, anticoagulants, and even surgical bypass grafts and shunts.[20,21] Thrombolysis[22,23] and angioplasty,[24,25] alone or in combination,[26,27] have been successfully used to palliate obstruction secondary to thrombosis or fibrosis. Since most patients with this syndrome suffer from a malignancy, antineoplastic therapy is also indicated. The treatment of patients with non-small cell carcinoma of the lung includes irradiation, whereas those with the small cell type and the lymphomas[14] are treated primarily with various chemotherapeutic regimens. In addition, treatment is radically different for the few patients with benign diseases. For these reasons and because the superior vena cava syndrome rarely constitutes a medical emergency,[10,12,15] a thorough diagnostic workup prior to initiation of therapy is imperative.

INFERIOR VENA CAVA SYNDROME

Definition

In addition to peripheral venous dilation and edema, obstruction of the inferior vena cava about its hepatic segment may result in the Budd-Chiari syndrome.[28,29] Renal vein thrombosis and renal infarction may occur when the middle segment becomes occluded.[30] Lower extremity edema is usually bilateral, but it can be unilateral.[31] However, as in the case of superior vena cava obstruction, patients with occlusion of the inferior vena cava may remain asymptomatic, depending on the competence of their collateral circulation. Ligation of the inferior vena cava results in mild symptoms with morbidity being principally associated with lower extremity deep vein thrombosis.[32]

Etiology

The inferior vena cava may be obstructed by primary or metastatic neoplasms of the liver,[28] the right adrenal, the right kidney, lymph nodes, and other retroperitoneal structures as well as primary caval neoplasms.[33] Contrary to its incidence in Asia and Africa,[34] inferior vena cava obstruction in the United States is rarely caused by caval webs, membranes, or coarctation.[35] Obstruction of the inferior vena cava is also caused by retroperitoneal fibrosis,[36] compression by a cirrhotic liver,[37] liver transplantation,[38] and thrombosis that can be associated with the same systemic diseases that induce thrombosis in the superior vena cava.[18]

Collateral Circulation

Collateral venous return following obstruction of the inferior vena cava occurs principally through the vertebral venous plexus.[39] Blood flows through the azygos and hemiazygos systems to the superior vena cava territory and then into the right atrium. Additional collateral pathways include the hepatic veins,[40] the portal system (usually through the hemorrhoidal veins), and the veins of the abdominal wall.

TREATMENT

Membranous obstruction of the inferior vena cava has been treated with membranotomy and vascular bypass grafts and shunts.[29,34,41,42] Alternatively, transluminal membranotomy[43] and balloon angioplasty[44–46] in conjunction with laser recanalization[47] have been performed. Obstruction of the inferior vena cava by hepatic malignancies has been treated with a combination of strip radiotherapy with or without hepatic artery infusion chemotherapy, which palliates the syndrome in 83% of the patients.[48]

VASCULAR STENTS

The need to reestablish luminal patency by devices that could be inserted through relatively small caliber delivery systems has led to the development of endoprostheses that expand once they are deployed. Since 1969, when Charles Dotter[49] first reported on the experimental arterial placement of stainless steel coiled spring stents, endoprostheses of various designs have been used experimentally and clinically.[50–58] Some of the stents undergoing clinical trials include a malleable stent—the Palmaz stent—which expands by inflation of the balloon catheter on which it is crimped;[53,59–65] a self-expanding stent—the Wallstent—made of braided wire;[54] and another self-expanding stent—the Gianturco stent—constructed of wire bent in a zig-zag design.[55–57,66–69]

The Gianturco Stent

Although the experience with the Gianturco stent is still limited, it has been the most frequently used stent in the management of caval obstructions. This device is constructed of stainless steel wire varying in caliber from 0.018 to 0.022 inches. The wire is bent in a zig-zag pattern and its ends are soldered to form a cylinder; currently, most stents have six or seven bends. The expansile force of the stent is in direct relationship to the caliber of the wire, the diameter of the stent, the number and the angle of the bends, and in indirect relationship to the length of the stent. The stents are manufactured in various lengths and diameters to fit the structure in need of stenting.

Our initial experience in animals[55] demonstrated that, as with other metallic stents, intimal proliferation resulted in incorporation of the Gianturco stent into the vascular wall. In the venous system, this process was 80% complete by the fourth week after insertion. Orifices of tributaries remained patent even when bridged by the stent wires. There was no stent-associated thrombosis, luminal narrowing, or vascular erosion up to 6 months following insertion. The ability of the stent to distend experimental vascular stenoses was studied in canine inferior vena cavas that had been strictured with retroperitoneal injections of ethanol.[66] Dilation of the stenotic segment occurred in four of the seven dogs stented. Complications occurred in three animals: caval perforation in one and stent migration in two animals.

From its inception, the Gianturco stent has undergone several modifications. It is difficult to deploy a single stent precisely because it tends to suddenly spring open when released from the introducer catheter, thus becoming dislodged beyond its intended location. However, a tandem stent (two stents interconnected) allows controlled deployment. As the first stent is released, the second stent, which is still in the introducer system, prevents it from becoming dislodged. The endoprosthesis was further modified by the addition of barbs that prevent stent migration by anchoring the stent to the vessel wall. Initially, our stents were manufactured of 0.018 inch stainless steel wire, but we have tended to use larger caliber wire to achieve greater expansile force. In 1988, Uchida et al[70] reported on the use of a 4-0 nylon suture to connect two single Gianturco stents. This modification allows the stent to expand evenly to a predetermined diameter and prevents its hyperexpansion. Wire skirts may also prevent migration of the stent. Currently, the caval stent most commonly used at The University of Texas M. D. Anderson Cancer Center is a tandem made of 0.020 inch wire measuring 2.5 cm in diameter and 5 cm in length.

GIANTURCO STENT INSERTION

The length of the stenosis must be carefully identified by venography; radiopaque markers on the patient's skin may help identify the stenosis during stenting. Initially, using a right femoral venous approach, the stenosis is crossed using an angiographic catheter with a short tip such as a Headhunter or a Judkins right coronary catheter and a floppy straight guide wire such as a Bentson wire. Leaving the wire in place, the angiographer then exchanges the catheter for the stent introducer sheath and dilator measuring 80 to 100 cm in length. A 12 F sheath is sufficient for stents made of 0.018 inch wire, whereas those made of 0.022 inch wire require a 15 F sheath.

Once the sheath has crossed the stenosis, the inner dilator is removed and the stent, previously compressed in a loader, is advanced with a pusher cable into the introducer sheath. We are currently evaluating a delivery system that allows insertion of the stent already loaded on the tip of a catheter, thus eliminating the need to push the stent through the length of the introducer. Once the stent, still in the introducer sheath, has been centered on the stenosis, the sheath is pulled back while the stent is maintained stationary with a pusher. As the sheath is retracted, the stent expands to hug and distend the wall of the stenotic cava. Short stenoses require that one of the tandem stents be centered on the stenosis to prevent the stent from acquiring a cone shape with its apex in the stenosis and its base beyond it. The shape of the stenotic segment determines which of the tandem stents should be centered on the stenosis and which should be positioned proximally or distally. (Fig. 43-1A). Long stenoses may require more than one tandem stent.

THE GIANTURCO STENT IN CAVAL OBSTRUCTION

Stenting is performed as soon as malignant caval obstruction is suspected. As the occlusion becomes complete, the risk of secondary thrombosis increases, complicating the management of these patients. An occluding thrombus not only conceals the site and length of the stenosis, but also precludes reestablishment of flow by an endovascular stent. In the presence of thrombus, if no major contraindications exist, thrombolysis is begun prior to stenting. We use urokinase 2000 to 4000 U/kg/hr with the catheter embedded in the thrombus[69] until thrombolysis occurs, which usually results in significant initial symptomatic improvement. Caval stents are deployed once the site of the stenosis is clearly identified and the potential for reestablishment of flow is not hindered by clot. Following stent insertion, venography in two perpendicular views is performed because residual stenosis that might require additional stenting may be apparent in only one view. Pressure gradient measurement also helps to determine whether additional stents are required. Caval stenting does not preclude radiation therapy or chemotherapy, which can be started concurrently.

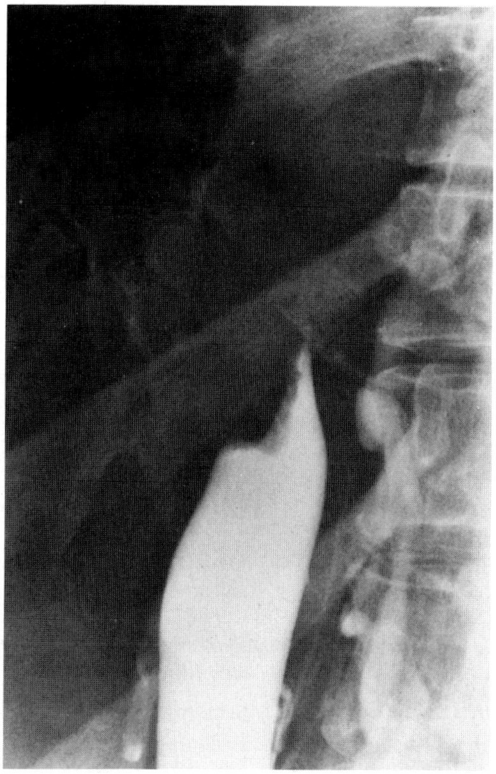
A

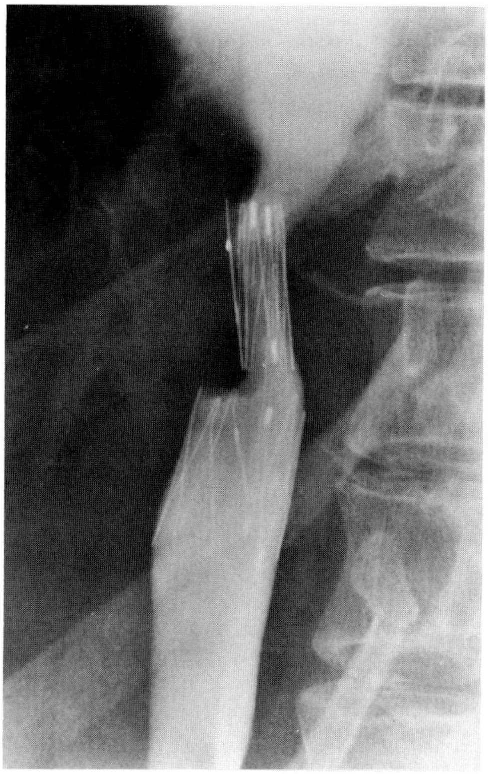
B

Figure 43–1. **A:** Complete obstruction of the inferior vena cava at its hepatic segment by a hepatic metastasis. Also note collateral veins overlying the spine. **B:** Reestablishment of flow through the inferior vena cava following insertion of a Gianturco stent.

We have used Gianturco stents in 15 patients with superior (13 patients) and inferior (2 patients) vena cava syndrome caused by neoplasms. Local thrombolytic agents were necessary in five patients to dissolve the clot above the stenosis prior to stenting. Three patients did not experience any improvement in their symptoms because of failure in clot lysis or stent expansion. The remaining 12 patients had complete (10 patients) or partial (2 patients) resolution of their syndrome for a median follow-up of 4 months (range, 6 days to 9 months).

The caval syndrome recurred in both patients with inferior vena cava obstruction at 4 months. In one of these patients, one stent migrated to the right ventricle within 24 hours of placement and another stent had to be anchored with a bird's nest filter in the inferior vena cava to prevent its migration. The patient did not suffer any untoward effects from the intraventricular stent and she died of progressive disease 4 months later. At autopsy, the stent was partially endothelialized. Since then, the use of tandem stents with barbs has prevented this complication.

CONCLUSION

Caval obstruction, in most patients caused by an incurable malignancy, leads to an extremely disabling syndrome. Although the majority of patients with the syndrome of caval obstruction improve within a week or two of presentation regardless of the treatment instituted, they usually require hospital care in the interim. The Gianturco stent allows reestablishment of caval patency leading to prompt symptomatic relief. Prompt resolution of the syndrome shortens hospital stay, which is a strong consideration in these patients whose life expectancy is very short.

REFERENCES

1. Perez CA, Presant CA, Van Amburg ALL III. Management of superior vena cava syndrome. Semin Oncol 1978;5:123–34.
2. Ehrlich W, Ballon HC, Graham EA. Superior vena caval obstruction with a consideration of the possible relief of symptoms by mediastinal decompression. J Thorac Surgery 1934;3:352–64.
3. Bell DR, Woods RL, Levi JA. Superior vena caval obstruction: a 10 year experience. Med J Aust 1986;145:566–8.
4. Davenport D, Ferree C, Blake D, Raben M. Radiation therapy in the treatment of superior vena caval obstruction. Cancer 1978;42:2600–3.
5. Levitt SH, Jones TK, Kilpatrick SJ, Bogardus CR. Treatment of malignant superior vena cava obstruction. Cancer 1969;24:447–51.
6. Rubin P, Green J, Holzwasser G, Gerl R. Superior vena caval syndrome. Radiology 1963;81:388–401.
7. Spiro SG, Shah S, Harper PG, et al. Treatment of obstruction of the superior vena cava by combination chemotherapy with and without irradiation in small cell carcinoma of the bronchus. Thorax 1983;38:501–5.
8. Citron ML, Fossieck BE, Krasnow SH, et al. Superior vena cava syndrome due to non-small-cell lung cancer. JAMA 1983;250:71–2.
9. Maddox AM, Valdivieso M, Lukeman J, et al. Superior vena cava obstruction in small cell bronchogenic carcinoma. Clinical parameters and survival. Cancer 1983;52:2165–72.
10. Ahmann FR. A reassessment of the clinical implications of the superior vena caval syndrome. J Clin Oncol 1984;2:961–9.
11. Carlson HA. Obstruction of the superior vena cava: an experimental study. Arch Surg 1934;29:669–77.
12. Nieto AF, Doty DB. Superior vena cava obstruction: clinical syndrome, etiology, and treatment. Curr Probl Cancer 1986;10:441–84.
13. Shimm DS, Logue GL, Rigsby LC. Evaluating the superior vena cava syndrome. JAMA 1981;245:951.
14. Perez-Soler R, McLaughlin P, Velasquez WS, et al. Clinical features and results of management of superior vena cava syndrome secondary to lymphoma. J Clin Oncol 1984; 2:260–6.
15. Schraufnagel DE, Hill R, Leech JA, Pare JAP. Superior vena caval obstruction: is it a medical emergency? Am J Med 1981;70:1169–74.
16. Lokich JJ, Goodman R. Superior vena cava syndrome. JAMA 1975;231:58–61.
17. Holbert BL, Libshitz HI. Superior vena caval syndrome in primary mediastinal germ cell tumors. J Can Assoc Radiol 1986;37:182–3.
18. Fassin D, Wechsler B, Herson S, Godeau P. Thromboses caves et maladies de système. Ann Med Intern (Paris) 1986;137:456–60.
19. Dyet JF, Moghissi K. Role of venography in assessing patients with superior cava obstruction caused by bronchial carcinoma for bypass operations. Thorax 1980;35:628–30.
20. Taylor GA, Miller HA, Standen JR Jr, et al. Bypassing the obstructed superior vena cava with a subcutaneous long saphenous vein graft. J Thorac Cardiovasc Surg 1974;68:237–40.
21. Doty DB. Bypass of superior vena cava: six years experience with spiral vein graft for obstruction of superior vena cava due to benign and malignant disease. J Thorac Cardiovasc Surg 1982;83:326–38.
22. Katz PO, Hackshaw BT, Barish CF, Powell BL. Venous thrombosis as a cause of superior vena cava syndrome. Rapid response to streptokinase. Arch Intern Med 1983;143:1050–2.
23. Meister FL, McLaughlin TF, Tenney RD, Sholkoff SD. Urokinase. A cost-effective alternative treatment of superior vena cava thrombosis and obstruction. Arch Intern Med 1989;149:1209–10.
24. Sherry CS, Diamond NG, Meyers TP, Martin RL. Successful treatment of superior vena cava syndrome by venous angioplasty. AJR 1986;147:834–5.
25. Rocchini AP, Cho KJ, Byrum C, Heidelberger K. Transluminal angioplasty by superior vena cava obstruction in a 15 month old child. Chest 1982;82:506–8.
26. Montgomery JH, D'Souza VJ, Dyer RB, et al. Nonsurgical treatment of the superior vena cava syndrome. Am J Cardiol 1985;56:829–30.
27. Capek P, Cope C. Percutaneous treatment of superior vena cava syndrome. AJR 1989;152:183–4.
28. Hartley JW, Awrich AE, Wong J, et al. Diagnosis and treatment of the inferior vena cava syndrome in advanced malignant disease. Am J Surg 1986;152:70–4.
29. Wang ZG, Zhu Y, Wang SH, et al. Recognition and management of Budd-Chiari syndrome: report of one hundred cases. J Vasc Surg 1989;10:149–56.
30. Stevens R, Tomyskoski A. Thrombosis of the inferior vena cava and renal veins with hemorrhagic renal infarction. J Urol 1984;72:120–8.
31. Ranniger K. Obstruction of the inferior vena cava with edema of thrombophlebitis of the lower extremities. AJR 1970;109:563–7.

32. Perhoniemi V, Salmenkivi K, Vorne M. Venous haemodynamics in the legs after ligation of the inferior vena cava. Acta Chir Scand 1986;152:23–7.
33. Pollanen M, Butany J, Chiasson D. Leiomyosarcoma of the inferior vena cava. Arch Pathol Lab Med 1987;111:1085–7.
34. Victor S, Jayanthi V, Kandasamy I, et al. Retrohepatic cavoatrial bypass for coarctation of inferior vena cava with polytetrafluoroethylene graft. J Thorac Cardiovasc Surg 1986;91:99–105.
35. Rector WG Jr, Xu YH, Goldstein L, et al. Membranous obstruction of the inferior vena cava in the United States. Medicine (Baltimore) 1985;64:134–43.
36. Mathew CV, Shanabo A, Zyka I, Eklof B. Retroperitoneal fibrosis with large-vessel obstruction. An uncommon vascular disorder. Acta Chir Scand 1985;151:475–80.
37. Rector WG. Pseudo-Budd-Chiari syndrome: extrinsic deformity of the intrahepatic inferior vena cava mimicking membranous obstruction. J Clin Gastroenterol 1989;11:88–91.
38. Barton P, Jantsch H, Pichler W, et al. Ultrasonic diagnosis following liver transplantation. Ultraschalldiagnostik nach Lebertransplantation. Rofo 1989;151:145–53.
39. Bellelli A, Teramo M, Gaudino G, et al. The vertebral venous plexus: its physiopathological aspects. A CT study in 2 patients with obstruction of the inferior vena cava. Radiol Med (Torino) 1989;77:564–7.
40. Takayasu K, Moriyama N, Muramatsu Y, et al. Intrahepatic venous collaterals forming via the inferior right hepatic vein in 3 patients with obstruction of the inferior vena cava. Radiology 1985;154:323–8.
41. Jennings RH, Henderson JM, Millikan WJ, Warren WD. Two-stage surgical management of Budd-Chiari syndrome with obstruction of the inferior vena cava. Surg Gynecol Obstet 1989;169:501–5.
42. Rao KS, Gupta BK, Banerjee A, Srivastava KK. Chronic Budd-Chiari syndrome due to congenital membranous obstruction of the inferior vena cava: clinical experience. Aust N Z J Surg 1989;59:335–8.
43. Yamasaki Y, Eguchi S, Terashima M, et al. Inferior vena caval obstruction: transvenous instrumental membranotomy. Cardiovasc Intervent Radiol 1988;11:18–20.
44. Loya YS, Sharma S, Amrapurkar DN, Desai HG. Complete membranous obstruction of inferior vena cava: case treated by balloon dilatation. Cathet Cardiovasc Diagn 1989;17:164–7.
45. Sparano J, Chang J, Trasi S, Bonanno C. Treatment of the Budd-Chiari syndrome with percutaneous transluminal angioplasty. Case report and review of the literature. Am J Med 1987;82:821–8.
46. Sawada S, Oshima T, Kato T, et al. Budd-Chiari syndrome treated by percutaneous transluminal angioplasty. Report of a case. Acta Radiol Diagn (Stockh) 1985;26:25–7.
47. Furui S, Yamauchi T, Ohtomo K, et al. Hepatic inferior vena cava obstructions: clinical results of treatment with percutaneous transluminal laser-assisted angioplasty. Radiology 1988;166:673–7.
48. Hartley JW, Awrich AE, Wong J, et al. Diagnosis and treatment of the inferior vena cava syndrome in advanced malignant disease. Am J Surg 1986;152:70–4.
49. Dotter CT. Transluminally placed coil-spring endarterial tube grafts: long term patency in canine popliteal artery. Invest Radiol 1969;4:329–32.
50. Dotter CT, Buschmann RW, McKinney MK, Rosch J. Transluminal expandable nitinol coil stent grafting: preliminary report. Radiology 1983;147:259–60.
51. Cragg A, Lund G, Rysavy J, et al. Nonsurgical placement of arterial endoprostheses: a new technique using nitinol wire. Radiology 1983;147:261–3.
52. Maass D, Zollikofer CL, Largiadèr F, Senning A. Radiological follow-up of transluminally inserted vascular endoprostheses: an experimental study using expanding spirals. Radiology 1984;152:659–63.
53. Palmaz JC, Sibbitt RR, Reuter SR, et al. Expandable intraluminal graft: a preliminary study. Radiology 1985;156:73–7.
54. Sigwart V, Puel J, Mirkovitch V, et al. Intravascular stents to prevent occlusion and restenosis after transluminal angioplasty. N Engl J Med 1987;316:701–6.
55. Wright KC, Wallace S, Charnsangavej C, et al. Percutaneous endovascular stents: an experimental evaluation. Radiology 1985;156:69–72.
56. Charnsangavej C, Wallace S, Wright KC, et al. Endovascular stent for use in aortic dissection: an in vitro experiment. Radiology 1985;157:323–4.
57. Carrasco CH, Wallace S, Charnsangavej C, et al. Expandable biliary endoprosthesis: an experimental study. AJR 1985;145:1279–81.
58. Jacob H, Maass D, Schmiedt W, et al. Treatment of major venous obstruction with an expandable endoluminal spiral prosthesis. J Cardiovasc Surg 1989;30:112–7.
59. Palmaz JC, Richter GM, Noeldge G, et al. Intraluminal stents in atherosclerotic iliac artery stenosis: Preliminary report of a multicenter study. Radiology 1988;168:727–31.
60. Alvarado R, Palmaz JC, Garcia OJ, et al. Evaluation of polymer-coated balloon-expandable stents in bile ducts. Radiology 1989;170:975–8.
61. Erbel R, Schatz R, Dietz U, et al. Balloon dilatation and coronary vascular stent implantation. Z Kardiol 1989;78:71–7.
62. Becker GJ, Cikrit DF, Lalka SG, et al. Early experience with the Palmaz stent in human iliac angioplasty. Ind Med 1989;82:286–92.
63. Erbel R, Schatz R, Dietz U, et al. Balloon dilatation and coronary vascular stent implantation. Versicherungsmedizin 1989;41:82–4.
64. Richter GM, Noeldge G, Fradrich G, et al. Treatment of acute iliac artery occlusion by catheter lysis, catheter dilatation and implantation of a new kind of metallic vascular endoprosthesis. Chirurg 1989;60:346–51.
65. Rees CR, Palmaz JC, Garcia O, et al. Angioplasty and stenting of completely occluded iliac arteries. Radiology 1989;172:953–9.
66. Charnsangavej C, Carrasco CH, Wallace S, et al. Stenosis of the vena cava: preliminary assessment of treatment with expandable metallic stents. Radiology 1986;161:295–8.
67. Wallace MJ, Charnsangavej C, Ogawa K, et al. Tracheobronchial tree: expandable metallic stents used in experimental and clinical applications. Radiology 1986;158:309–12.
68. Rösch J, Bedell JE, Putnam J, et al. Gianturco expandable wire stents in the treatment of superior vena cava syndrome recurring after maximum-tolerance radiation. Cancer 1987;60:1243–6.
69. Putnam JS, Uchida BT, Antonovic R, Rösch J. Superior vena cava syndrome associated with massive thrombosis: treatment with expandable wire stents. Radiology 1988;167:727–8.
70. Uchida BT, Putnam JS, Rösch J. Modifications of Gianturco expandable wire stents. AJR 1988;150:1185–7.

44 Intravascular Prosthesis: Experimental Results with the Strecker Flexible Stent

Klemens H. Barth, M.D., Renu Virmani, M.D., Ernst P. Strecker, M.D.

Intravascular endoprostheses or stents are devices designed to retain patency of a vascular lumen following failed or complicated balloon angioplasty. Indications include recurrent arterial stenosis, elastic recoil of atherosclerotic plaque, or arterial wall dissection complicating balloon angioplasty. Several types of stents are presently under laboratory or clinical investigation.[1–9] So far, all are made of a corrosion-resistant biocompatible metal mesh and allow intravascular expansion. All designs are attempting to keep the metal to open surface area ratio to a minimum. The main differences among the stent designs are both the type of metal, which determines the radiopacity and flexibility, and the expansion mechanism, self-expanding or passively expanded over an angioplasty balloon.[1–10]

The Strecker stent is made of a knitted tantalum wire and is balloon expandable.[10–12] Tantalum is considerably more radiopaque than stainless steel of equal caliber. In comparison to the Palmaz stent, the Strecker stent is much more flexible.

EXPERIMENTAL OBSERVATIONS

The reaction of the normal arterial wall to the Strecker stent was tested in healthy dogs. Detailed results of this study between 1 week and 6 months have been reported elsewhere.[12] The study period has been extended up to 1 year in a limited number of experimental animals (Fig. 44-1).

Pertinent observations can be summarized as follows. The Strecker stent, which is held on to the angioplasty balloon by proximal and distal silicone sleeves, is readily deployed by balloon expansion with pressures up to 6 atm (Fig. 44-2A,B). In some cases, a spasm-related minimal luminal narrowing has occurred immediately following stent placement. To test flexibility and resistance of the stent to extrinsic compression, a stent was placed in the femoral artery segment crossing the hip joint. The joint was then moved in all possible directions, and extrinsic manual compression was applied. No change in the luminal diameter or the contrast runoff was noted after these maneuvers (Fig. 44-2C–E).

The reaction of the arterial wall to the stent over 1-, 3-, 8-, 26-, and 52-week intervals showed initial endothelial denudation of the stented arterial segment followed by coverage of the stent struts by fibrin and platelet thrombus evident at 1 week (Fig. 44-3A). Within 3 weeks, endothelium had covered the stent almost completely (Fig. 44-3B). Neointima was forming rapidly inside the stent, chiefly by proliferation of smooth muscle cells from the media. The internal elastic lamella remained intact throughout the observation period up to 1 year. The neointima matured within 6 months (Fig. 44-3C). The highest buildup was seen at 2 months, with substantial decrease in thickness at 6 months (Table 44-1) and no further change at 1 year. The decrease in the intimal thickness is considered a result of decreased cellularity along with collagen formation. During maturation of the neointima, atrophy of the media outside the stent occurred with replacement of smooth muscle by collagen. At 6 months, it was about 50%, and at 1 year, close to 75%. A foreign body reaction was never observed. Some stent loops raised above the intimal surface and some of those crossing side branches never became covered with endothelium and occasionally showed fibrin thrombi.

COMMENTS

Intraluminal stents are to provide structural reinforcement of the arterial lumen in patients with atherosclerotic stenoses. When placed into normal arteries of experimental animals, the subject of interest is the reaction of the vessel wall to the stent implant. Experience with endartherectomy and surgical grafting has shown formation of a neointima and sometimes intimal hyperplasia as reaction to grafting and endartherectomy.[13,14] This reaction can compromise the vascular lumen by excessive tissue buildup similar in its effect to an atherosclerotic plaque. Neointima also forms inside all stents, as is evident from experimental studies (Table 44-1). We observed the peak in the neointimal thickness at 2 months. Schatz et al,[8] using the Palmaz stent, found a similar peak thickness at 2 months in the canine coronary arteries and a more pronounced decrease at 9 months than that observed in our studies at 6 months and 1 year. The decrease in neointimal thickness appears related to cell replacement by collagen fibers as the neointima matures. Important is the experimental evidence of limited neointimal growth insufficient to cause vascular lumen compromise. This is in contrast to some of the reactions observed during clinical stent placements in patients with atherosclerotic disease.[5,6]

The factors involved in excessive reparative wall reaction, often called myointimal hyperplasia, are presently subject to intense experimental investigations. Several peptides excreted by platelets and endothelium stimulate smooth muscle proliferation.[15,16] The question remains how to regulate this proliferative response, which, in part, is necessary to cover a thrombogenic surface. As demonstrated in our study and by others, nonendothelialized vascular stents remain thrombo-

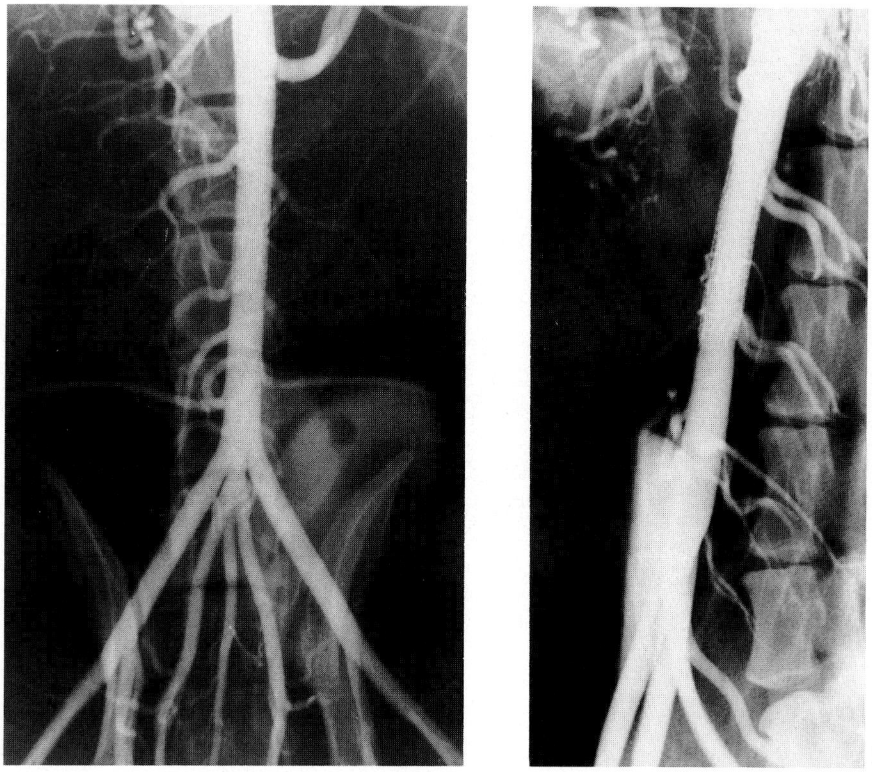

A B

Figure 44–1. **A:** Abdominal aortogram (posteroanterior view) 1 year after stent placement distal to renal arteries (arrows). Note minimal caliber change at proximal stent margin. **B:** Abdominal aortogram (lateral view) showing stent slightly outside the opacified lumen due to neointimal buildup inside the stent (arrows). Note that stent is still visible through angiographic contrast.

Table 44–1. Stent-Induced Neointimal Thickness in Canine Arteries (in microns)

	WEEKS				MONTHS		YEARS	
ARTERY/STENT NAME	*1*	*2*	*3*	*8*	*6*	*9*	*1*	*2*
Coronary/Palmaz,[8]	75		80	275		50		
Gianturco-Roubin[7]		300		270				
Femoral/Wallstent[3]			450					
Iliac/Nitinol[4]							229	223
Renal/Palmaz[5]				63				
Multiple/Wallstent[3]			250			50		
						45		
Aorta, Iliac/Strecker[12]			240	313	223			

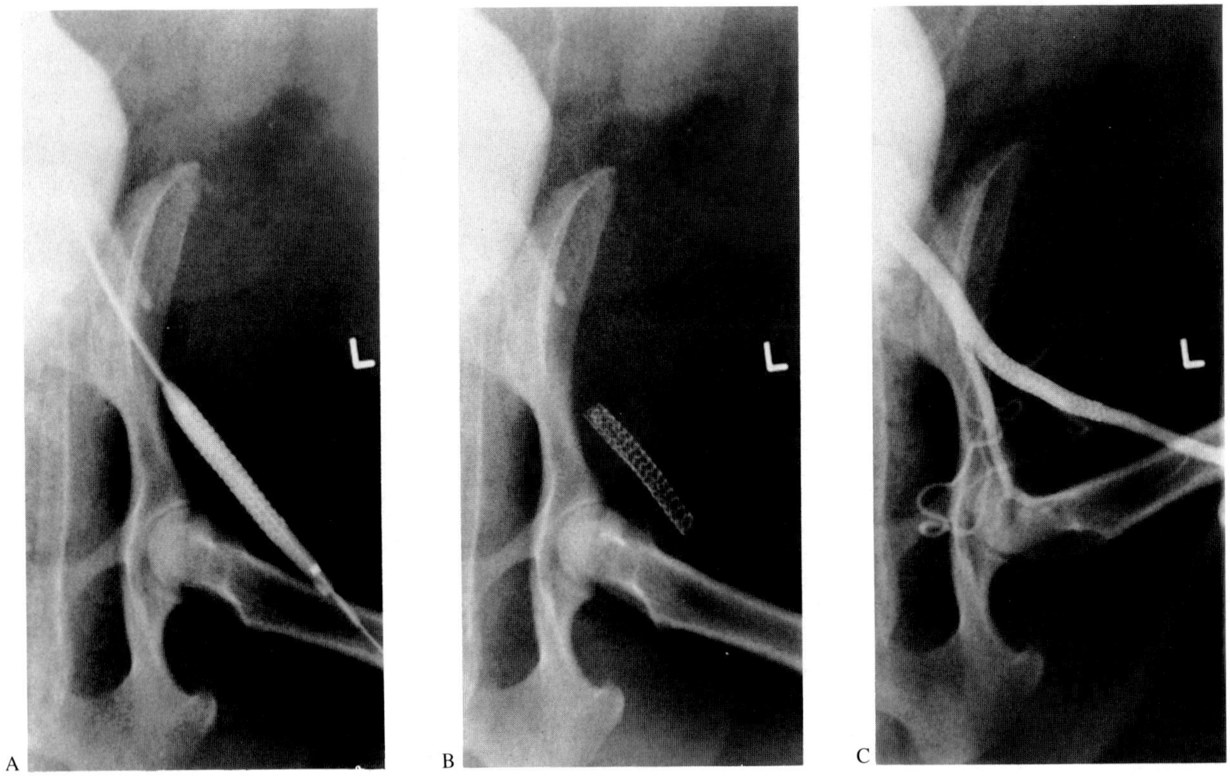

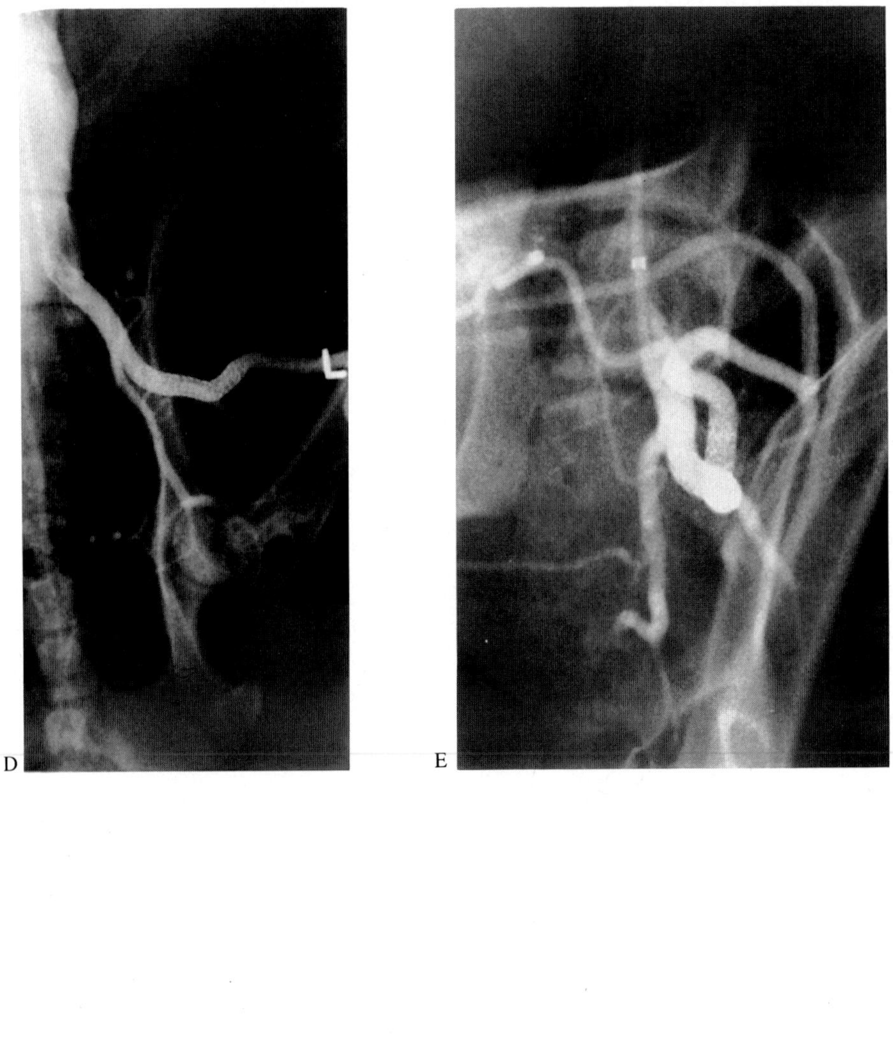

Figure 44–2. **A:** Stent expansion by balloon catheter in left common femoral artery. **B:** Deployed stent in left common femoral artery. **C:** Well patent arterial lumen inside stent and distal to stent during 90° flexion of left hip joint. **D:** Well patent lumen during maximal flexion (140°) and abduction. **E:** Well patent lumen during maximal flexion and adduction.

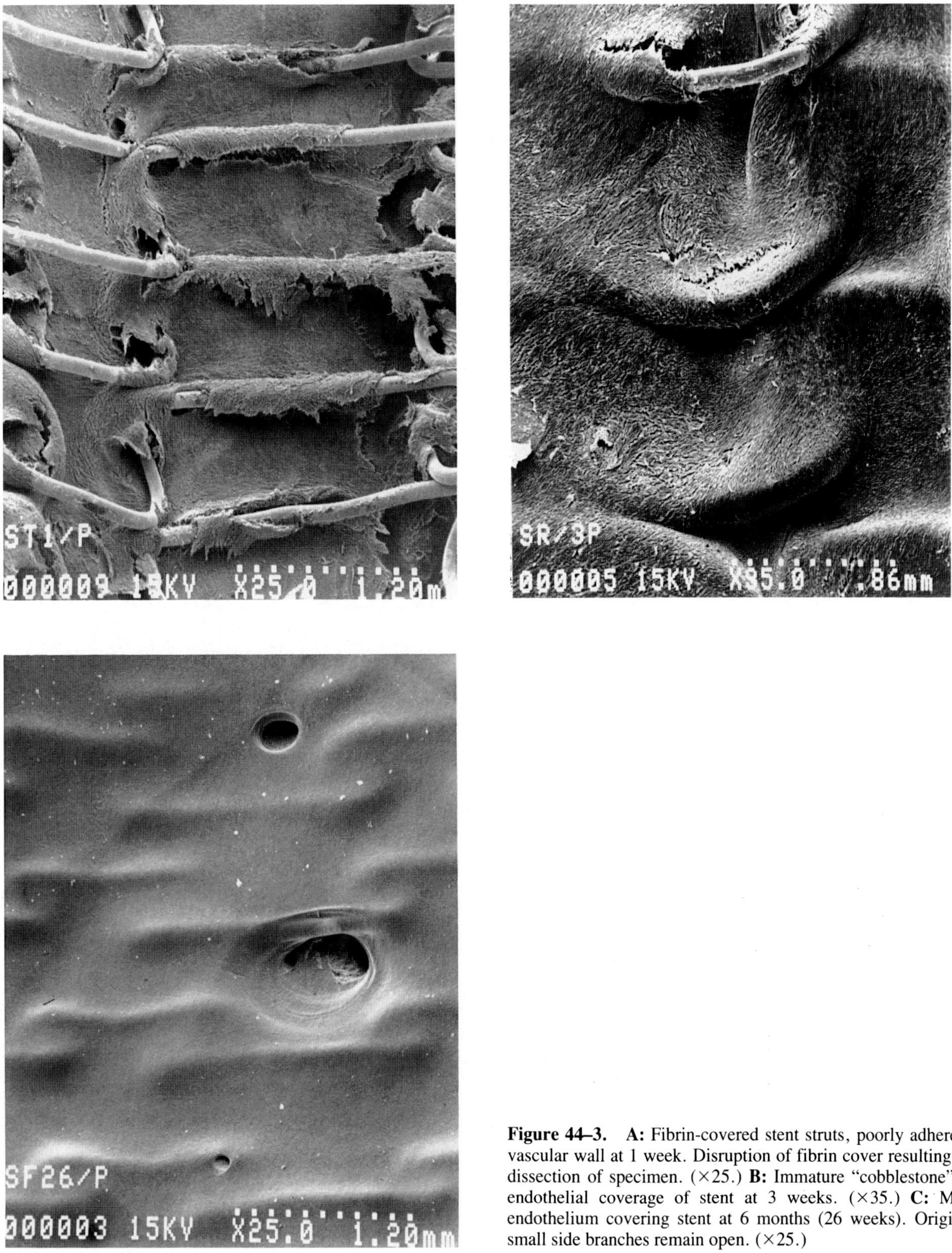

A B C

Figure 44–3. **A:** Fibrin-covered stent struts, poorly adherent to vascular wall at 1 week. Disruption of fibrin cover resulting from dissection of specimen. (×25.) **B:** Immature "cobblestone" type endothelial coverage of stent at 3 weeks. (×35.) **C:** Mature endothelium covering stent at 6 months (26 weeks). Origins of small side branches remain open. (×25.)

genic with the potential of lumen occlusion and distal emboli.

Anticoagulation and antiplatelet medication, with warfarin or aspirin, has not been demonstrated to reduce the incidence of neointimal hyperplasia after balloon angioplasty; even corticosteroids have been tried without success.[17] Unless appropriate pharmacotherapy can be established that controls the neointimal growth with little if any untoward effects, recurrent stenosis due to neointimal hyperplasia will remain a most frequent long-term complication of all transluminal recanalization techniques, including endovascular stents. The type of stent may modify the response slightly; however, conclusive comparison studies between the different stent designs have not been performed.

Passively expanded stents carry the theoretical risk of compressibility and lumen occlusion, particularly in areas exposed to external pressure, such as extremities; however, experimental studies are required to prove or refute such considerations. Stent flexibility may also play an important role in patency of rapidly moving arteries, such as the coronary arteries, and in arteries subjected to rhythmic respiratory motion, such as the renal arteries. Finally the long-term significance of the transformation of the muscular arterial wall into a fibrous wall outside the stent is also undetermined.

REFERENCES

1. Palmaz JC, Windeler SA, Garcia F, et al. Atherosclerotic rabbit aortas: expandable intraluminal grafting. Radiology 1986;160:723–6.
2. Duprat G Jr, Wright KC, Charnsangavej C, et al. Self-expanding metallic stents for small vessels: an experimental evaluation. Radiology 1987;162:469–72.
3. Rousseau H, Puel J, Joffre F, et al. Self-expanding endovascular prosthesis: an experimental study. Radiology 1987; 164:709–14.
4. Sutton CS, Oku T, Harasaki H, et al. Titanium-nickel intravascular endoprosthesis: a 2-year study in dogs. AJR 1988; 151:597–601.
5. Sigwart U, Puel J, Mirkovitch V, et al. Intravascular stents to prevent occlusion and restenosis after transluminal angioplasty. N Engl J Med 1987;316:701–6.
6. Palmaz JC, Richter GM, Noeldge G, et al. Intraluminal stents in atherosclerotic iliac artery stenosis: preliminary report of a multicenter study. Radiology 1988;168:727–31.
7. Roubin GS, Robinson KA, King SP, et al. Early and late results of intracoronary arterial stenting after coronary angioplasty in dogs. Circulation 1987;76:891–7.
8. Schatz RA, Palmaz JC, Tio FO, et al. Balloon-expandable intracoronary stents in the adult dog. Circulation 1987; 76:450–7.
9. Palmaz JC, Tio FO, Schatz RA, et al. Early endothelisation of balloon-expandable stents: experimental observations. J Intervent Radiol 1988;3:119–24.
10. Strecker EP, Berg G, Schneider B, et al. A new vascular balloon-expandable prosthesis: experimental studies and first clinical results. J Intervent Radiol 1988;3:59–62.
11. Strecker EP, Romaniuk P, Schneider B, et al. Perkutan implantierbare, durch Ballon aufdehnbare Gefassprothese. Erste klinische Ergebnisse. Dtsch Med Wochenschr 1988; 113:538–42.
12. Barth KH, Virmani R, Strecker EP, et al. Effects of flexible tantalum stents implanted in normal canine aortas and iliac arteries. Radiology 1990; 175:91–6.
13. De Weese JA. Anastomotic intimal hyperplasia. In Sawyer PN, Kaplitt MJ (eds): Vascular Grafts. New York: Appleton Century-Crofts, 1978;147–52.
14. Clagett GP, Robinowitz M, Youkey JR, et al. Morphogenesis and clinicopathologic characteristics of recurrent carotid disease. J Vasc Surg 1986;3:10–23.
15. Ross R. Platelet-derived growth factor. Annu Rev Med 1987;38:71–9.
16. Greisler HP, Dennis IW, Endean ED, Kim DU. Derivation of neointima of vascular grafts. Circulation 1988;78:16–21.
17. McBride W, Lange RA, Hillis LD. Restenosis after successful coronary angioplasty. N Engl J Med 1988;318:1734–7.

45 Intravascular Prosthesis: Flexible Tantalum Stent (Strecker), Technical Considerations

Ernst-Peter Strecker, M.D., Beate Schneider, Michael Savin, M.D., Alan H. Matsumoto, M.D.

Percutaneous transluminal angioplasty (PTA) is a definite advance in the therapy of atherosclerotic vascular disease. However, the patency rate of the angioplasty site is limited by a number of factors. Acute thrombosis, intimal and medial dissection, arterial recoil due to the elasticity of arterial walls, and intimal hyperplasia with smooth muscle cell proliferation may form acutely or chronically new stenoses and occlusions diminishing the advantage of PTA.[1,2]

In an attempt to improve on the apparent failures of conventional balloon angioplasty, balloon-expandable, flexible, intraluminal prostheses were tested in animal experiments and permanently implanted in patients with atherosclerotic, stenotic, or occluded iliac or femoropopliteal arteries. A prospective multiple center study in Germany was performed to evaluate the safety and clinical efficacy of the developed percutaneously implantable, flexible balloon-expandable tantalum stent. In this chapter, design and function of this arterial prosthesis, the preceding animal experiments and clinical results, including short- and long-term follow-up, are described.

DESCRIPTION OF THE VASCULAR PROSTHESIS

The developed vascular prosthesis, expandable by the balloon of an angioplasty catheter and percutaneously implantable, consists of a knitted tubular flexible metal wire mesh tube. Because of its structure of loosely connected wire loops, the prosthesis is within certain limits longitudinally and radially elastic and flexible (Fig. 45-1). The dimensions are determined by the number and size of loops (1.5 to 2.5 mm) and the inside diameter (depending on the core). All parameters regarding the dimensions of the vascular prosthesis can be changed at will. The vascular prosthesis (stent) is mounted on the nondilated balloon of a PTA catheter with radial force. In order to prevent any displacement of the stent on the balloon by friction with the inner arterial wall or during implantation through the introducer sheath, the prosthesis is additionally attached by silicone sleeves on the balloon section facing both tip and shaft of the catheter. After balloon expansion, the silicone sleeves will, while being shortened, roll back from the expanding balloon to the catheter shaft and will thus release the prosthesis (Fig. 45-2).

The metal filament consists of tantalum (99% purity) in order to obtain a good compatibility with the wire mesh and to avoid any thrombus formation. The implants are chemically electropolished. By this process the oxide film of the metal surface is reduced or fully removed and any microscopic irregularities of the surface are eliminated by dissolving existing projections and by the smoothing of rough areas. Those measures guarantee that the metal oxidation—as will occur in the bloodstream—will lead to a "uniform" oxide film.[3] Without such surface treatment, any contamination of the metal by traces of fat, oil, dirt particles, or the formation of a "nonuniform" oxide film inside a blood vessel located at the metal surface may induce thrombosis. The thin layer of inert tantalum pentoxide, which creates an electrically negative surface charge, will prevent the adhesion of platelets, which are negatively charged as well.[3]

Tantalum is superior to stainless steel or similar alloys because it is very radiodense and well visualized under fluoroscopy due to its high density and proton number. Tantalum can be regarded as an optimal, biologically inert material. Long-term studies of orthopedic implants and surgical clips did not show any corrosion caused by surrounding tissue fluids.[4–6]

Animal tests with intravenously implanted tantalum and medical grade stainless steel alloy wire segments reveal that both metals can be regarded as thromboresistant. It is of advantage that implanted tantalum stents are not disturbed by magnetic fields nor do they disturb magnetic resonance imaging. Magnetic resonance angiography techniques can be used to evaluate vascular patency in the presence of tantalum stents, whereas, in contrast, stainless steel implants will create signal loss appearing as black holes within the image.[7]

It is important to know to what extent stent shortening depends on the grade of expansion so as to be able to judge size and location of the implant within the artery to be treated. Measuring tests with gradual dilation show that stent shortening depends proportionally on the extent of radial expansion and that with the enlargement of the diameter from 2 to 7 mm, the stent is shortened by 50%.

In order to prevent such prosthesis shortening, the implant is, before dilation, longitudinally pressed or pushed together as far as possible from both ends, with the loops of the wire mesh almost completely overlapping.

When comparing the shortening of the tantalum stent, previously longitudinally stretched, with the stent longitudinally pressed together, it becomes evident that the latter type will also shorten to a certain extent with expansion, although the degree of shortening is, after previous longitudinal compression, reduced by half. This will also happen when

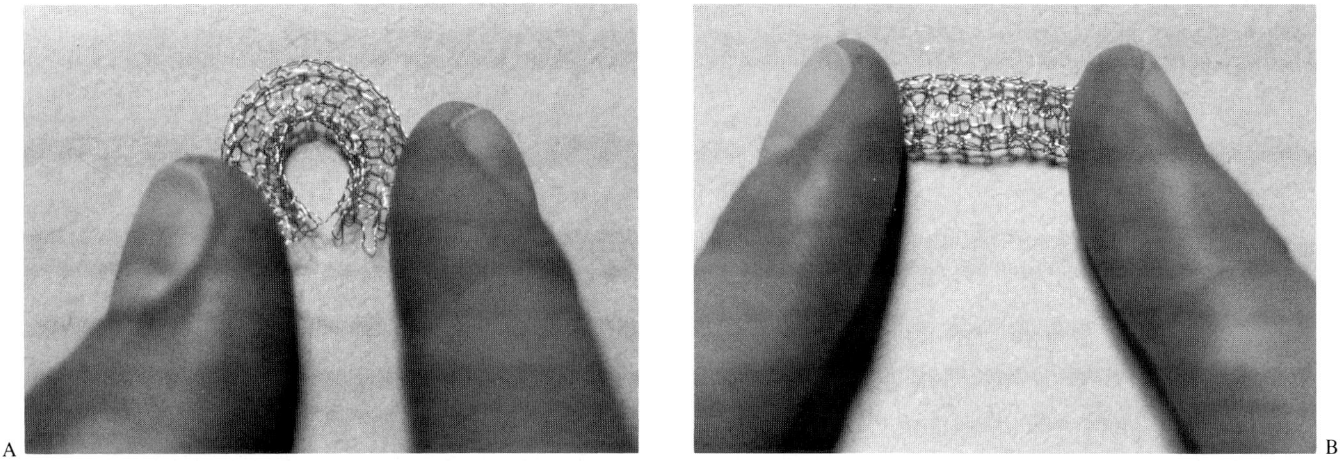

Figure 45–1. Expanded knitted tantalum stent. **A:** The balloon expanded vascular prosthesis consists of loosely connected metallic loops (0.1 mm filament) and is therefore flexible and pliable. **B:** The vascular prosthesis is elastic and within certain limits, it is compressible in the longitudinal and radial fashion.

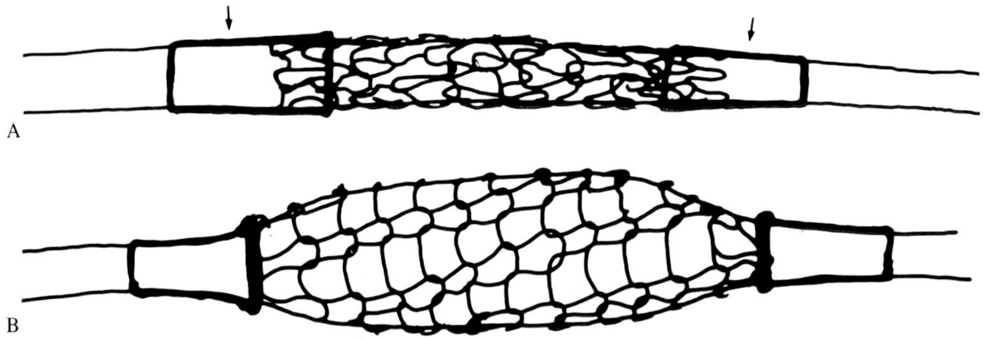

Figure 45–2. Diagram of the balloon stent assembly. **A:** Nonexpanded state: The knitted stent is compressed longitudinally with primarily loosely connected loops to prevent longitudinal shortening after expansion. It is held on the balloon by radial tension. In addition, the prosthesis is fixed by silicone sleeves at the catheter shaft proximal and distal to the balloon overlapping the ends of the prosthesis, preventing any stent dislocation during introduction. **B:** Half-expanded balloon. The wire loops have been widened by deformation and are almost firmly intersecting. The silicone sleeves are shortened and rolled backward, leaving the prosthesis free for implantation.

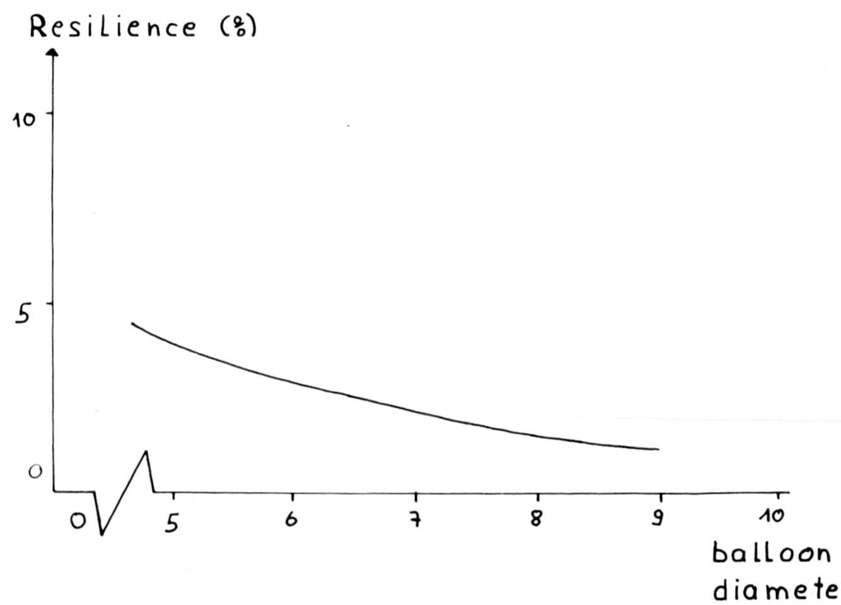

Figure 45–3. Resilience (elastic spring-back, in percent) of a knitted tantalum prosthesis after radial balloon dilation versus increasing balloon diameter. The elastic spring-back decreases with radial expansion and amounts to only 1% at a diameter of 9 mm.

the maximum diameter achievable is reduced. This will greatly help when the implant is placed in the patient.

Before accurate planning of arterial stent therapy, knowledge of the width of the dilated implant into the artery is essential. At the same time the mechanically induced spring-back of the stent after removal of the dilation balloon should be taken into consideration. To obtain this information, the outer diameter of the vascular prosthesis is measured with a sliding caliper at maximum expansion after evacuation of the balloon. The percentage of the decrease of the stent diameter after complete balloon dilation is demonstrated in a graph (Fig. 45-3). The percentage of decrease of the stent diameter, caused by elastic spring-back (resilience), is reduced after dilation, with the balloon diameters increasing. The effect of resilience is actually negligible. At maximum balloon expansion to 9 mm, the amount of radial resilience is extremely low (1%).

The favorable results obtained by preclinical examinations allowed us to perform various series of long-term animal experiments and consequently the implantation into diseased patient arteries.

REFERENCES

1. Sigwart U, Puel J, Mirkovitch V, et al. Intravascular stents to prevent occlusion and restenosis after transluminal angioplasty. N Engl J Med 1987;316:701–6.
2. Strecker EP, Romaniuk P, Schneider B, et al. Perkutan implantierbare, durch Ballon aufdehnbare Gefäßprothese: Erste klinische Ergebnisse. Dtsch Med Wochenshr 1988;113:538–43.
3. Sawyer PN, Stanczewski B, Srinivasan S, et al. Electronmicroscopy and physical chemistry of healing in prosthetic heart valves, skirts and struts. J Thorac Cardiovasc Surg 1974;67:25.
4. Kylberg F. The use of tantalum clips in general surgery. Acta Chir Scand 1975;141:242–4.
5. von Holst H, Collins P, Steiner L. Titanium, silver, and tantalum clips in brain tissue. Acta Neurochir 1981;56:239–42.
6. Rabenseifner I, Küsswetter W, Wünsch PH, Schwab M: Ist die Knochenbruchheilung bei den gewebeverträglichen Implantatwerkstoffen Tantal und Niob gegenüber Stahlimplantaten verändert? Z Orthop 1984;122:349–55.
7. Matsumoto AH, Teitelbaum GP, Barth KH, et al. Tantalum vascular stents: in vivo evaluation with MR imaging. Radiology 1989;170:753–5.

46 Flexible Tantalum Stent (Strecker): Clinical Long-Term Results

Ernst-Peter Strecker, M.D., Klemens H. Barth, M.D., Dieter Liermann, M.D., Hellmut R.D. Wolf, M.D., Nikolaus L. Freudenberg, M.D., Michael Westphal, M.D., Panagiotis Tsikuras, M.D.

PROSTHESIS IMPLANTATION TECHNIQUE

The procedure was performed percutaneously in all patients. The stenosis or occlusion is first dilated with a balloon to make sure it is balloon distensible. The balloon-mounted prosthesis is then introduced. During introduction through the hemostatic valve of a previously inserted introducer sheath (first cases, 10 F lumen; subsequent cases, 8 F), the stent-balloon assembly is protected by a 5 cm piece of thin-walled Teflon tubing. The tubing is pulled back to allow hemostasis after the stent is advanced within the sheath lumen. Positioning of the stent before expansion is accomplished with reference points: external metallic markers or contrast injection images either freeze-frame or road mapping. Balloon inflation expands the stent and the lesion simultaneously, leaving the stent mesh as a support within the lumen. Any residual irregularity or stenosis cranially or caudally to the stent is corrected by dilating the portion of the vessel without a stent with the same balloon after expansion of the stent or by placing a second stent. In some patients additional stents were installed overlapping the first by several millimeters. Inflation pressure values of at least 5 atm were required to ensure proper stent expansion and release. After stent expansion the balloon is deflated and carefully withdrawn to prevent a stent dislocation.

Before the first percutaneous transluminal angioplasty (PTA), 5000 U of heparin are injected intra-arterially, and an additional 5000 U are given immediately before introduction of the stent. After percutaneous placement of the stent, the puncture site was controlled with manual compression. All patients received heparin intravenously titrated to partial thromboplastin time (PTT) two to three times normally for 3 days.

In 23 of 24 patients, aspirin (325 mg/day) and in ten of these patients, dipyridamole (75 mg/day) were given for 2 days before the procedure and continued indefinitely thereafter. Two patients required warfarin due to the clinical history of gastric ulcers, contraindicating aspirin postprocedure.

FOLLOW-UP IN PATIENTS TREATED WITH ARTERIAL PROSTHESES

A total of 46 men and ten women (median age, 61 years; range, 38 to 81) were treated with the previously described balloon-expandable flexible tantalum stent. Of these, 39 received one stent, 14 received two stents, one received three stents, and three received four stents. Twenty femoropopliteal and 35 iliac lesions were treated with a total of 75 stents. The lesions had a median length of 5 cm (range, 0.5 to 50 cm).

Atherosclerotic cardiovascular disease risk factors included diabetes mellitus (11%), high blood pressure (30%), and a history of prolonged cigarette smoking (91%).

If necessary, PTA of additional ipsilateral lesions was performed. Five patients had rotation angioplasty and thrombolysis performed prior to stent placement, one patient had percutaneous aspiration embolectomy and fibronolysis, and one patient had an occluded iliopopliteal bypass graft, which was stented.

The four indications for stent placement were: restenosis after previous PTA (23 patients); poor initial PTA result with residual stenosis (33 patients); initial occlusion (18 patients); and intimal flaps (17 patients). Several patients had multiple indications.

RESULTS

Primary Results

ANGIOGRAPHIC SUCCESS

The median stenosis preprocedure (evaluated by angiography) was 84%, which improved to 49% postballoon angioplasty, then to 0% (range, 20 to 0%) immediately poststent placement (Fig. 46-1). The preprocedure to post-PTA improvement and the post-PTA to poststent improvement were both statistically significant ($p < 0.0001$, according to the Wilcoxon signed rank test). There was no thrombosis due to stent implantation during the first 3 months after implantation.

HEMODYNAMIC SUCCESS

Hemodynamic results were measured by the determination of the Doppler ankle to arm index (AAI), pre- and postprocedure in 26 lesions. The median AAI improved from 54% preprocedure to 89% poststent placement. The pre- to post-Doppler AAI improvement was significant ($p < 0.0001$, according to the Wilcoxon signed rank test). Of the lesions 55 were successfully treated by hemodynamic criteria (Fig. 46-2).

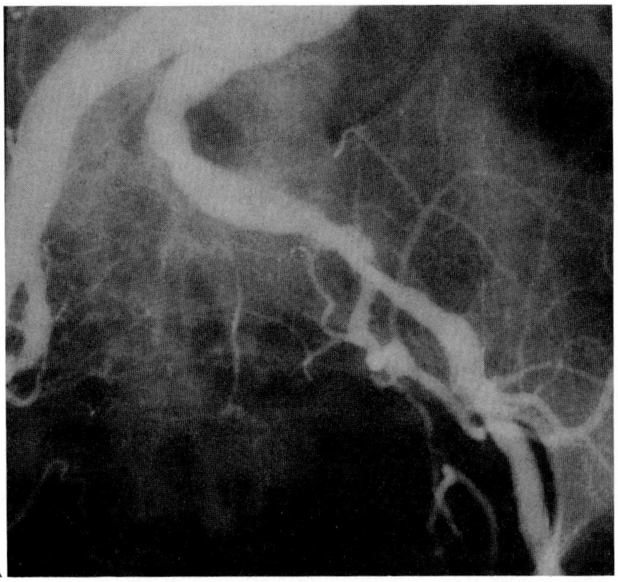

A

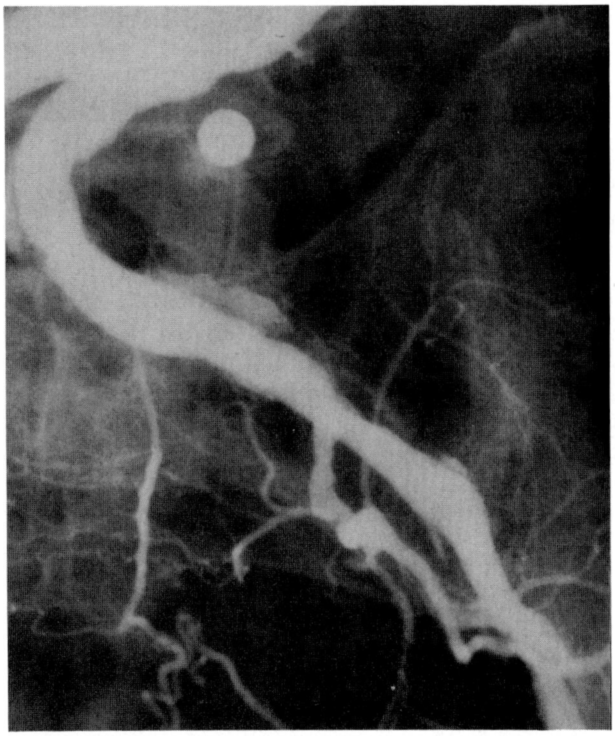

B

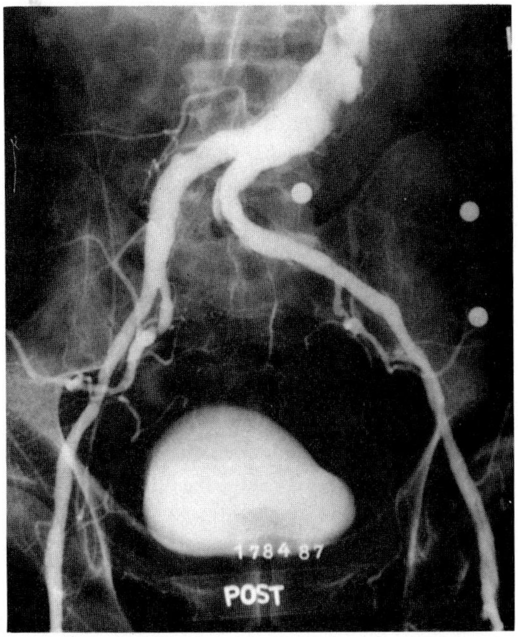

C

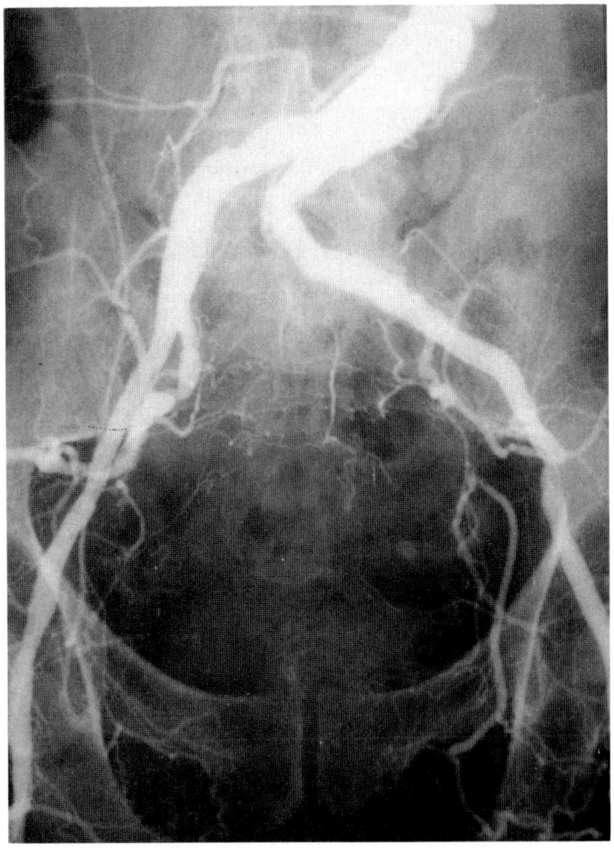

D

Figure 46–1. **A:** Severe atherosclerotic stenosis with life-style limiting claudication of the left external iliac artery. **B:** There is a considerable amount of residual stenosis after percutaneous transluminal angioplasty due to elastic arterial wall recoil, although overdilation was performed. **C:** The result is optimized by the implantation of a flexible tantalum stent. **D:** At 45 weeks after stent implantation, the internal surface of the treated arterial segment is covered with a thin tissue layer corresponding to a neointima.

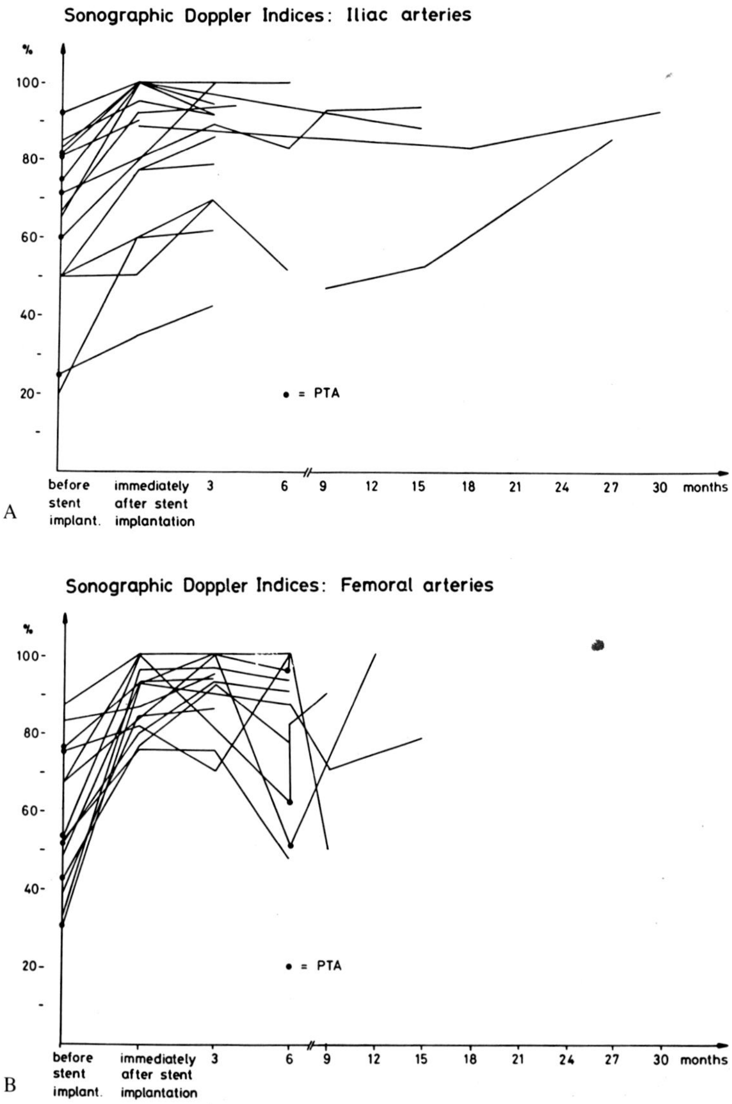

Figure 46–2. Long-term follow-up of Doppler ankle to arm indices. **A:** The follow-up curves of patients with iliac artery stents reveal any decline of the indices (maximum observation time, 30 months). **B:** The follow-up of patients with stented femoral arteries showed in four patients a decline of their indexes that corresponded to restenoses within the stent, demanding a repeat angioplasty.

One lesion improved by less than 0.15 Doppler AAI and was considered a hemodynamic failure. However, this case was successful by angiographic criteria. Also, this patient had a clinical follow-up and had improved by one level according to the classification of Fontaine.

CLINICAL SUCCESS

The clinical improvement was monitored by the Fontaine classification:

I. No symptoms
IIA. Claudication at more than 250 m
IIB. Claudication at less than 250 m
III. Rest pain
IV. Tissue loss

In all patients initially successfully treated, clinical function improved by a mean of 1.9 levels (range, 1 to 3 stages according to the Fontaine classification).

Long-Term Follow-up

The 6 months' (range, 5 to 9 months) control angiograms, mostly performed by intravenous digital subtraction angiography, revealed in patients treated with iliac artery stents very favorable results. There was no restenosis or reocclusion within, proximally, or distally to the implanted vascular prosthesis. The internal surface of the stent was covered by a thin smooth layer corresponding probably to a neointima (Fig. 46-1).

Four patients with a stent in the distal half, especially distal third, of the femoral artery showed restenosis occurring 4 to 7 months after implantation. Mainly, funnel-shaped filling defects could be detected within the midportion of the implants; the entrance and exit of the tubular stents remained uninvolved. Some filling defects narrowing the arterial lumen proximally or distally to the stent were observed as well. These stenoses were treatable by repeat balloon angioplasty, the Simpson artherectomy procedure, or laser angioplasty. Tissue specimens obtained by artherectomy and examined microscopically revealed intimal hyperplasia combined with thrombosis.

Doppler sonographic AAI determinations were performed until 36 months after iliac artery stent treatment. The follow-up curves reveal in all patients good results without any decline of the indices (Fig. 46-2). In contrast, four patients with distal superficial femoral artery prostheses showed recurrent disease, which correlates to the angiographic criteria described before (Fig. 46-2).

Long-term clinical success occurred in all patients with iliac artery stents with a maximum observation time of 36 months. In this group the primary improvement was obtained immediately after this new therapy and remained unchanged in all patients during the observation period.

As already mentioned, the prognosis was not as favorable in patients treated with stent placed into the distal part of the superficial femoral artery. The four patients with restenosis had a clinical deterioration of their early improved symptoms, with a clinical stage IIB according to Fontaine.

DISCUSSION

Intraluminal placement of flexible balloon expandable tantalum stents optimizes the geometric alterations following balloon dilation.[1–3] Because the expandable stent opposes elastic recoil, there is no need for overdilation. The smooth and regular lumen obtained with the stent decreases or prevents the development of luminal irregularity after angioplasty. These irregularities disturb normal blood flow patterns, creating turbulences and pressure gradients at arterial blood flow.

In six patients in our series the successful hemodynamic and clinical results of stent placement were not possible to obtain with conventional balloon angioplasty and made in three cases consecutive vascular surgery on an emergency basis unnecessary. There were totally occluding arterial flaps (one iliac, two femoral), which could not be permanently forced against the arterial wall by PTA, but by the placement of stents acute complicating problems could be resolved. One patient had rest pain and a 50 cm long thrombotic occlusion of the iliopopliteal bypass graft. The occlusion was lysed, but the graft had an occlusive kink at the distal anastomosis. This kink would have led to immediate rethrombosis; therefore a stent was placed that successfully opened the kink. An emergent redo bypass operation was avoided and the patient is asymptomatic at 6 months follow-up.

The incidence of acute occlusion during PTA is generally reported as 4 to 6%.[4–6] Many of these occlusions are due to intimal flaps. It is possible to reopen acute occlusions due to intimal flaps through the use of stents. It is also possible to improve the geometry of bypass graft anastomoses in cases in which the graft is kinked. In the other two cases the PTA result was diminished by serious intimal flaps creating 80 to 90% stenoses (renal and popliteal arteries). These complicating lesions could be treated by stents as well.

Other than the six cases of lesions unresponsive to balloon dilation just discussed, the promising hemodynamic and clinical results in our series have been obtained with conventional balloon angioplasty in some patients. However, stent placement improved the luminal diameter from a mean residual reduction of 31% post-PTA to 3% poststent placement. Residual stenoses of 30% or greater are known to result in higher restenosis rates.[5] Therefore it is possible that stents can improve the long-term patency rate for PTA when there is a residual lumen reduction after balloon dilation. To test this hypothesis, a comparison between the stent cohort and a control angioplasty group will be made when long-term follow-up is achieved in a sufficiently large series. There is a risk of restenosis secondary to intimal hyperplasia combined with thrombosis until the formation of a functionally mature neointima of the inner stent surface occurs; therefore all patients should be treated with aspirin postprocedure.[1,7]

The knitted prosthesis offers a high degree of mechanical flexibility. Therefore this implant can be introduced through curved arteries and over the aortic bifurcation. The prosthesis can maintain its configuration after expansion, since the loosely connected loops, made of tantalum wire filaments, are elastic within certain limits. Percutaneously implanted expandable stents will improve PTA results and may extend the indications for PTA. More experience is necessary to determine the indications for this new therapy for occlusive atherosclerotic disease in the iliac and femoral arteries.

REFERENCES

1. Strecker EP, Romaniuk P, Schneider B, et al. Perkutan implantierbare, durch Ballon aufdehnbare Gefäßprothese: Erste klinische Ergebnisse. Dtsch Med Wochenschr 1988;113:538–76.
2. Palmaz CJ, Richter GM, Noeldge G, et al. Intraluminal stents in atherosclerotic iliac artery stenoses: preliminary report of a multicenter study. Radiology 1988;168:727–31.
3. Triller J, Mahler F, Thälmann, R: Die vasculäre Endoprothese bei femoro-poplitealer Verschlußkrankheit. Fortschr Rontgenstr 1989;150:328–34.
4. Crowley MJ, Dorros G, Ralsey SF, et al. Acute coronary events associated with percutaneous transluminal coronary angioplasty. Am J Cardiol 1989;53:12c.
5. Holmes DR, Holubkov R, Vlietstra RE, et al. Comparison of complications during percutaneous transluminal angioplasty from 1977 to 1981 and from 1985 to 1986. The National Heart, Lung, and Blood Institute Percutaneous Transluminal Coronary Angioplasty Registry. J Am Coll Cardiol 1988;12:1149–55.
6. Mayorovitz MF, Friedmann PL, Ganz P, et al. Acute occlusion developing during or immediately after percutaneous transluminal coronary angioplasty: nonsurgical treatment. Radiology 1988;169:491–4.
7. Austin GE, Ratliff NB, Hollman J, et al. Intimal proliferation of smooth muscle cells as an explanation for recurrent coronary artery stenosis after percutaneous transluminal angioplasty. J Am Coll Cardiol 1985;6:369–75.

47 The Rabkin Nitinol Coil Stent: A Five-Year Experience

J.K. Rabkin, M.D., V.G. Germashev, M.D.

It took only 2 years to introduce the method of stent endoprosthesis placement into clinical use. Roentgenoendovascular dilation (RED) has been advocated as an effective method of restoration of vascular status of organs and tissues by treatment of occlusions and stenoses of the vessels. Among the advantages of the method are its nontraumatic, preserving, and painless character. The procedure is relatively easy to perform and it results in quick restoration of blood flow. However, a more cautious attitude and a more selective choice of patients for RED are necessary. According to different authors, the rate of restenosed and reoccluded zones after RED for various arteries reaches 41.1% in a 2-year period, and, for smaller vessels, even up to 68.6%.[1–16] The results of thousands of RED suggested a possible means of preventing restenoses and having a positive effect on the procedure, making it irreversible. The choice of methods could go in two directions:

1. Medicamentous influence on blood rheology and arterial endothelium.
2. Insertion of the supporting stent device into the vessel's wall, arterial lumen.

The first way has demonstrated no independent effect. The implantation of a steel device in the form of spiral, made in the United States by Charles Dotter,[17] showed no positive results either. Later, in 1983 Dotter[18] performed experimental implantations of nitinol stents into the vascular lumen.[19,20] However, technical imperfection of the prostheses, in particular, 60°C heating of the alloy in order to restore its form, did not allow introduction of the method into clinical use.

Endovascular stent devices, made of special medical shape-memory nitinol (37°C) have been developed at the National Research Center of Surgery under the guidance of Academician B.V. Petrovsky (J. Rabkin, D. Rabkin) in cooperation with engineers and metallurgists under the guidance of P.I. Polukhin. (They obtained authorship of invention N 1237201 with the priority dated April 4, 1985.) Thus, for the first time, we used endovascular stent in our clinic in March 1984.[8,21,22] A special department for cardiovascular roentgenosurgery of 25 beds was organized, and special outpatient selection of patients was conducted.

At present, we have gained experience that allows long-term (6 months to 5 years) evaluation of the effectiveness of the new technique.

Nitinol spiral stent made of nickel and titanium alloy, according to special technology, possesses a shape-memory effect, meets all specially developed medical and technical requirements: biologic compatibility, corrosion resistance, athrombogenic, apyrogenic, self-adhesive to the vascular wall. It can be easily guided through the angiographic catheter of 7 to 9 F when it is cooled and straightened. Similar to porous shunts, ion exchange occurs as do endothelialization and neointima formation.[23–26] Histologic studies demonstrated fine, nonadhesive, nonthrombogenic intima coating without any signs of hyperplasia; that is, a kind of implantation process took place during the first 14 postimplantation days. It is interesting that during the first postimplantation hours, the albumin filament deposition on the stent devices were revealed, not of fibrin, as usually occurs in case of insertion of a foreign body into the arterial vessel's lumen.

For the 5-year period, 295 endoprostheses were placed in 268 patients into different anatomic areas.[21] Localization and extent of the procedure are shown in Table 47-1.

Bifurcational prosthetics were implanted in both common iliac arteries for stenotic or occlusive processes in the proximal sites of iliac arteries. Multiple prosthetics indicate implantation of two or more stents into one or different arteries.

All implantations were performed transcutaneously, by femoral artery approach; in the case of brachiocephalic branches of the aortic arch, we used transaxillary approach in three of five cases.

Endovascular stent implantation was performed using a specially developed technique of stent placement into the area of damage through an angiographic catheter following dilation (sometimes endovascular dilation was preceded by recanalization). The choice of the endovascular stent is based on the angiographic data, taking into account the diameter of the arterial lumen. The endovascular stent diameter must be wider than the lumen diameter by 0.15 to 0.20 mm.

The length of the stent depends on the length of the lesion and varies from 0.5 to 3.5 cm. In two cases the implanted stents were 100 mm in length with 20 mm diameter.

The whole procedure, including dilation and postimplantation angiographic control generally took 45 minutes. The interventions were performed under topical anesthesia. Patients who had no complications in the early postimplantation period (95.4%) could walk independently in 15 minutes.

Among the etiologic factors that led to occluding and stenotic lesions were: atherosclerosis, 232 cases (87%); nonspecific aorto-arteritis, 28 cases (10%); fibromuscular dysplasia, 8 cases (3%). The period from the onset of the disease to the stent endoprosthesis placement ranged from 6

Table 47–1. Localization and Type of Stent Implantation

	NO. PATIENTS	BIFURCATION PROSTHESIS	SINGLE PROSTHESIS *After Dilation (Recanalization)*	SINGLE PROSTHESIS *After Laser Recanalization*	SINGLE PROSTHESIS *After Rotor Recanalization*	MULTIPLE PROSTHESES	NO. STENTS
Common iliac	69	4	55	8	—	2	75
External iliac	53	—	45	5	—	3	56
Common femoral	3	—	3	—	—	—	3
External femoral	90	—	60	20	10	8	106
Popliteal	24	—	19	5	—	1	26
Subclavian	13	—	9	4	—	—	13
Brachiocephalic branch	2	2	—	—	—	—	2
Renal	14	—	11	3	—	—	14
Total	268	6	202	45	10	14	295

months to 12 years; the age of the patients varied from 21 to 72 years. Of the patients, 76.6% had severe associated pathologic conditions, limiting possible direct interventions or absolutely excluding them. Among them were postinfarction cardiac failure, 90 patients; angina pectoris, 35 patients; severe diabetes, accompanied by angiopathy and retinopathy, 65 patients; following cerebral circulation disturbances, 14 patients, four of whom demonstrated hemiparesis and one with sensory and motor aphasia; visual acuity in one patient was 0.01 for both eyes. Combinations of these diagnoses occurred in 20.0% of cases.

Following conservative therapy 3 to 5 days prior to endovascular stent implantation, repeated blood platelet aggregation and adenosine diphosphate studies are usually performed, coagulation profile and platelets are checked and necessary corrections in the antiaggregant therapy are made (aspirin, ticlopidine, rheopolyglukine). Dextran 400 and vasodilators are infused daily. Indirect anticoagulants are given 2 days before the procedure. The dosage of aspirin varies from 125 to 250 mg/day, ticlopidine 0.5 to 3 tablets per day, depending on blood platelet aggregation. During the procedure, intravenous infusion of dextran with 5000 to 10,000 U of heparin (intravenous or intra-arterially) is performed. After RED, 2500–5000 U of heparin and vasodilators are administered through the angiographic catheter; the same treatment is repeated after the endoprosthesis has been placed. Postimplantation therapy is usually identical to that given preoperatively. Aspirin and phenindione are indicated for 4 to 6 months postoperatively.

One case, during the first 4 hours after the endoprosthesis placement, demonstrated signs of acute occlusion, requiring fibrinolytic therapy with avelyzin and heparin in the total dosage of 4,000,000 U and 1,000,000 U for a period of 3 days. The acute thrombosis in the iliac artery endoprosthesis was eliminated successfully immediately following treatment, 3 days later, and 6, 12, and 18 months after the procedure.

Pre- and postimplantation blood circulation was evaluated by means of rheovasography (RVG), Doppler technique, radioisotope scintigraphy, angiography, and digital subtraction angiography. General state of patients, local manifestations of ischemia, and subjective sensations were studied. The immediate, annual, and, if indicated, early results were also evaluated angiographically and by noninvasive methods. According to the data obtained, the following results of the stent endoprosthesis placement have been established: 1, good; 2, satisfactory; 3, without effect; 4, deterioration. Thus, a good result means definite pulse in the distal part of the diseased artery, complete restoration of blood flow, normal perfusion in the crus and foot according to radioisotope studies, the lack of difference in temperature between sides, and angiographic evidence of patency of the vessel at the site of former stenosis or occlusion. Also, lack of clinical manifestations of the disease: intermittent claudication, rest pain, or trophic lesions.

Satisfactory results of the procedure mean higher physical load tolerance, intermittent claudication every 750 to 1000 m, absence of trophic lesions of the lower extermites, lack of marked difference in skin temperature of foot and crus, compensated circulation of the lower extremities at all levels according to RVG, scintigraphy, no more than 15% deviation in the pulse blood flow rate compared with the healthy extremity.

A case of a 60-year-old patient is an example of satisfactory result of the procedure. In 1985 the patient was admitted to the hospital with clinical evidence of occlusion of the middle third of the left superficial femoral artery, circulatory decompensation of the left crus, trophic ulcer of the dorsal part of the left foot, insulin-dependent diabetes (96 U/day), postinfarction cardiac failure, angina pectoris, intermittent claudication (left) every 30 m. Recanalization and dilation of the damaged segment of the femoral artery were done (Figs. 47-1, 47-2, 47-3). Early noninvasive blood flow studies demonstrated compensated circulation in the left crus and

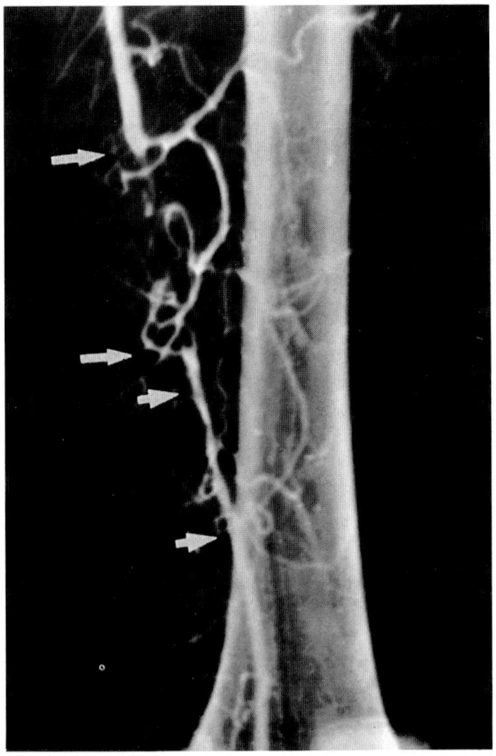

Figure 47–1. Complete occlusion of left superficial femoral artery (arrows).

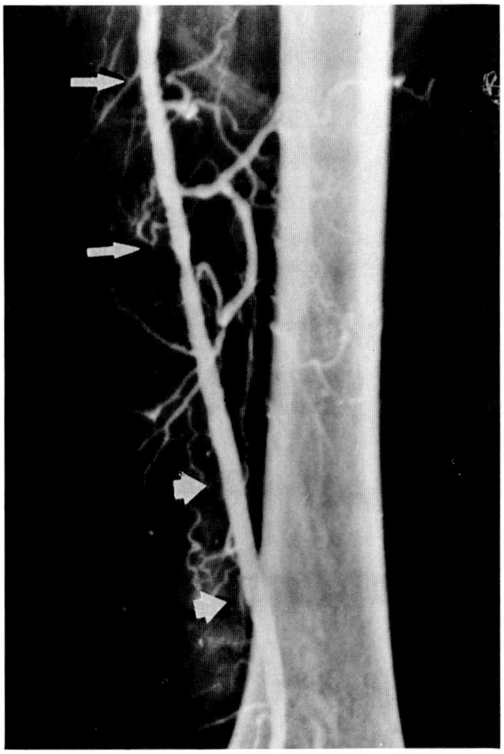

Figure 47–3. Follow-up arteriogram post PTA and stenting of occluded segment. Stents were placed (arrows).

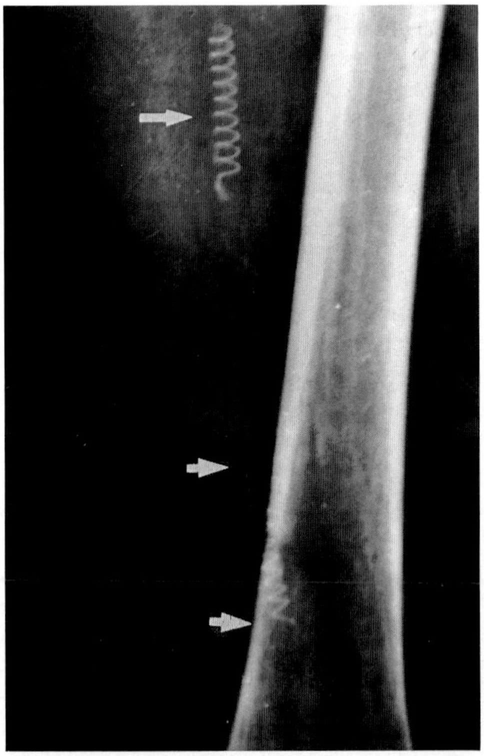

Figure 47–2. Plain film showing location of stents (arrows).

foot, with absence of intermittent claudication. There appeared to be a tendency toward epithelialization of the foot trophic ulcer. Intermittent claudication occurred during climbing every 800 to 1200 m. Deterioration of the patient's state manifested itself in clinical signs of the main disease, which resulted in an emergent operation.

Successful dilatation of brachiocephalic branches of the aortic arch can result in disappearance of vertebrobasilary insufficiency scintigraphically and RVG proved normal circulation in the brain vessels and symmetrical pulse in the radial arteries.

A case of endovascular stent placement in the subclavian artery in a 48-year-old patient is an example of the abovementioned effect. The patient was admitted to hospital in March 1987. There was no pulse in the right hand. The patient had headaches, unstable gait, sudden stagger. Angiographic study revealed right subclavian artery occlusion (Fig. 47-4). Scintigraphy demonstrated sharp decrease in the pulse of the right hemisphere; RVG showed decompensated circulation in the right parieto-occipital region. Recanalization, dilation, and endoprostheses of the right subclavian artery were performed through the femoral approach. As a result of the treatment, we could detect pulse in the radial artery, and the symmetrical AD in both hands was 145/70 mmHg.

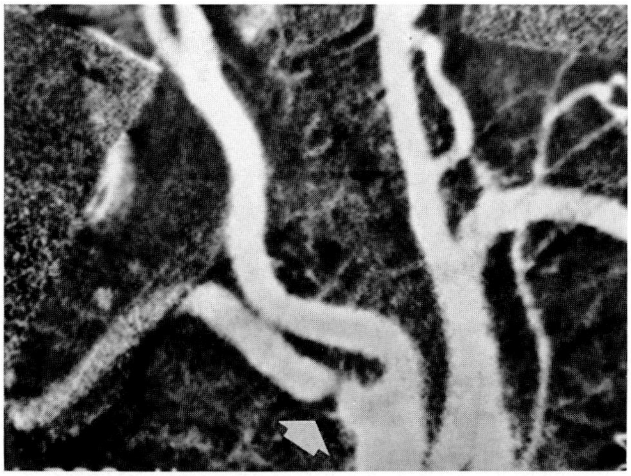

Figure 47–4. High-grade stenosis of the right subclavian artery (arrow).

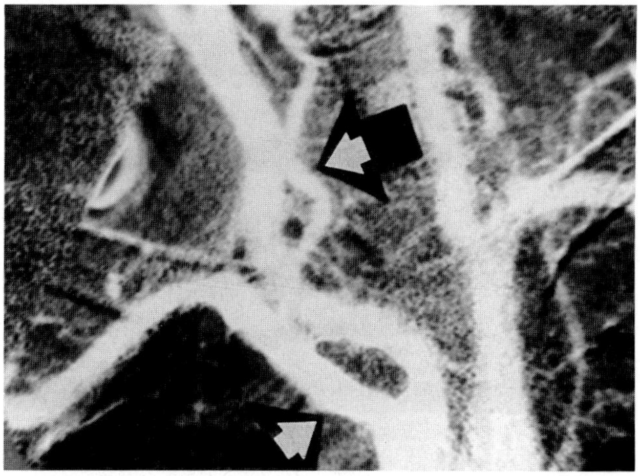

Figure 47–6. Follow-up angiogram following PTA and stent placement (arrow). Shows normal lumen.

Angiograms showed good patency of the subclavian artery, and vertebral and axillary arteries became visible. No signs of vertebrobasilary insufficiency were observed. In 2 years, good patency of the endoprosthesis area (Figs. 47-5, 47-6), compensated circulation in the hemispheres, restored muscle strength, and no headaches were noted.

Satisfactory results of the stent placement into the brachiocephalic branch of the aortic arch can be characterized by the improved brain circulation, according to scintigraphy and RVG, but 25 mmHg AD gradient in the brachial arteries persists, as well as 10 to 15 kg difference in the muscular strength.

As far as good effect of the treatment of renal arteries is concerned, we regard it as such, if no hypotensive drugs are used and normal AD 155/85 mmHg and normal radioactive drug perfusion in the kidneys, according to scintigraphy, are observed. Long-term results of 6 months to 5 years were studied in 209 of 295 patients who received endovascular prostheses of various major arteries (70.8%). The results are presented in Table 47-2, which shows that the success of the procedure (in percent) depends on localization of the stenotic or occlusive processes. The best results have been obtained for iliac, brachiocephalic, and renal arteries. If the distal arteries were diseased (superficial femoral or popliteal), the procedure was less effective, depending on linear and volume blood flow. Majority of thromboses occurred in the first 6 months following stent placement.

The detailed analysis of the results revealed distal crus circulation disturbances due to diabetic angiopathy in patients with postimplantation thrombosis of the superficial femoral and popliteal arteries. Acute thrombosis occurred as the result of incorrect manipulations during stent implantation into the superficial femoral artery in five cases and popliteal artery in 2 cases. Deterioration was registered in 30 cases, nine of them required urgent reconstructive operation, and 17 patients were operated on 6 to 18 months following implantation. There were no complications resulting in amputation of the extremity or patient deaths.

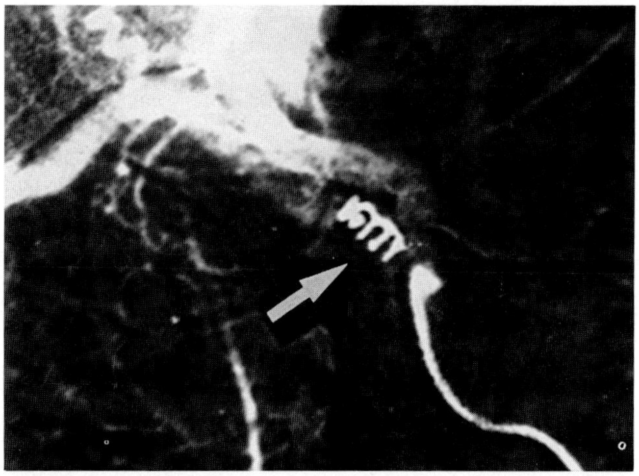

Figure 47–5. Position of stent is better shown in late film (arrow).

CONCLUSIONS

1. Stent endoprostheses implantation is a new, atraumatic, painless method of revascularization of organs and tissues.
2. Nitinol prostheses do not produce toxic effect on the organism and tissue and do not lead to any changes in the blood rheology.
3. Total positive results reaches 82.7% for arteries of all localization.
4. Unsatisfactory results of 17.3% occur in the treatment of superficial femoral and popliteal arteries.
5. In case of thrombosis of the artery involved in stent implantation, urgent or delayed operations are performed. The effect of the operation is normally good. No fatal outcome or amputation followed stent implantation.

Table 47–2. Results of Nitinol Stent Endoprosthesis Placement

	IMMEDIATE RESULTS				LONG-TERM RESULTS							
	1–7 days				*1–3 years*				*3–5 years*			
ARTERY	*No. stents*	*Good*	*Satisfactory*	*Deterioration*	*No. stents*	*Good*	*Satisfactory*	*Deterioration*	*No. stents*	*Good*	*Satisfactory*	*Deterioration*
Common iliac	75 25.4%	75 100%	—	—	50	48 96.0%	2 4.0%	—	30	29 96.6%	—	1 3.4%
External iliac	56 100%	56 100%	—	—	38	35 92.1%	3 7.9%	—	20	19 95.0%	1 5%	—
Common femoral	3 1.01%	3 100%	—	—	2	2 100%	—	—	1	1 100%	—	—
External femoral	106 35.9%	78 73.6%	—	28 26.4%	80	52 65.0%	8 10%	20 25%	45	25 55.5%	10 22.2%	10 22.2%
Popliteal	26 8.59%	17 65.3%	—	9 24.7%	18	9 50%	—	9 50%	10	5 50%	—	5 50%
Subclavian	13 4.32%	13 100%	—	—	9	9 100%	—	—	6	6 100%	—	—
Brachiocephalic branch	2 0.67%	2 100%	—	—	2	2 100%	—	—	1	1 100%	—	—
Renal	14 4.62%	14 100%	—	—	10	9 90.0%	1 10.0%	—	7	6 85.7%	1 14.3%	—
Total	295 100%	258 88.8%	—	37	209	166 79.4%	14 6.6%	29 14%	120	92 76.6%	12 10%	16 13.4%

6. Indications for stent endoprosthesis implantation are: restenosis or reocclusion after angioplasty for atherosclerotic artery disease; stenosis and small occlusions in case of fibromuscular dysplasia or arteritis, to prevent restenosis and create hemodynamically patent vessel; pathologically tortuous arterial vessel in cases of clinically manifested ischemia; stenoses of the anastomoses of the vascular shunts, to restore their patency; and stenotic or occlusions in patients with a severe accompanying disease process, preventing direct surgical intervention.

REFERENCES

1. Dzhoraev IG. Application of RED for treatment of arterial stenoses and occlusions of extracranial brain vessels and arteries of the upper extremities. Proceedings of the All-Union Conference of young scientists and specialists "Urgent Problems of Profylaxis and Treatment of Cardio-Vascular Diseases," Moscow, 1987:57.
2. Litvinov AP. Effect of RED in stenosed renal arteries in patients with arterial hypertensia. In: Urgent Problems of Cardio-Vascular Surgery. Proceedings of the All-Union Conference of Cardio-Vascular Surgeons, Vilnus, 1986:57–8.
3. Matevosov AL, Natzvlishvili ZG. Long-term results of RED of the renal arteries stenoses in patients with vasorenal hypertensia. In Urgent Problems of Cardio-Vascular Surgery. Proceedings of the All-Union Conference of Cardio-Vascular Surgeons, Vilnus, 1986:73–4.
4. Procubovsky VI, Koshkin VM, Farber AJ. Immediate and long-term results of RED in obliterating lesions of the arteries of the extremities. In Roentgenoendovascular Surgery. Abstracts of the VII All-Union Symposium, Moscow, 1985: 49–51.
5. Rabkin JK, Matevosov AL, Shechter Yu I. RED of subclavian artery. Thorac Surg 1988:76–8.
6. Rabkin JK, Matevosov AL, Dzhoraev IG. RED of the stenoses of the subclavian and vertebral arteries. In Urgent Problems of Cardio-Vascular Surgery. Proceedings of the All-Union Conference of Cardio-Vascular Surgeons, Vilnus, 1986:76–8.
7. Rabkin JK. Roentgenoendovascular surgery. In Roentgenoendovascular Surgery. Abstracts of VII All-Union Symposium for Angiography, Moscow, 1987:5–11.
8. Tarakanov YP, Zvirin GE, Kuleshov VI, et al. Immediate and long-term results of endovascular balloon dilatation. In Urgent Problems in Cardio-Vascular Surgery. Proceedings of the All-Union Conference of Cardio-Vascular Surgeons, Vilnus, 1986:78–80.
9. Connoly JE, Rwaan JH, McCart PM. Complications after percutaneous transluminal angioplasty. Am J Surg 1981; 142:60–6.
10. Cumberland DC. Percutaneous transluminal angioplasty. A review. Clin Radiol 1983;34:25–30.
11. Galichia JP, Bajaj AR, Vine DL, et al. Subclavian artery stenoses treated by transluminal angioplasty: six cases. Cardiovasc Intervent Radiol 1983;6:78–81.
12. Grüntzig A, Hopff H. Percutane Rekanalisation chronischer arterieller Verschlüsse mit einem neuen Dilatacionskatheter Modification der Dotter-Technik. Dtsch Med Wochenschr 1974;99:2502–5.
13. Greenfield AJ. Femoral, popliteal and tibial arteries: percutaneous transluminal angioplasty. AJR 1980;135:927–34.
14. Motarjeme A, Koifer J, Zurka A. Percutaneous transluminal angioplasty of the brachiocephalic arteries. AJR 1982; 138:457–62.
15. Samson RH, Sprayregen S, Veith FG, et al. Management of angioplasty complications, unsuccessful procedures and early and late failures. Ann Surg 1984;199:234–40.
16. Zeitler W, Richter EJ, Roth FJ, et al. Results of percutaneous transluminal angioplasty. Radiology 1983;145:57–60.
17. Dotter CT. Transluminally placed coil springs and arterial tube grafts: Long-term patency in the canine popliteal artery. Invest Radiol 1969; 329–32.
18. Dotter CT, Krippaehne WW, Judkins MP. Transluminal an-

grafts: Long-term patency in the canine popliteal artery. Invest Radiol 1969:329–32.
18. Dotter CT, Krippaehne WW, Judkins MP. Transluminal angioplasty in atherosclerotic obstruction of femoral popliteal system. Am Surg 1969;35:453–9.
19. Cragg A, Lund G, Rysavy J, et al. Nonsurgical placement of arterial endoprostheses: a new technique using nitinol wire. Radiology 1983;147:261–3.
20. Cragg A, Lund G, Rysavy J, et al. Percutaneous arterial grafting. Radiology 1984;150:45–9.
21. Rabkin JK, Zajmovsky VA, Khmelevskaja YI, et al. Experimentally based first clinical experience in endovascular prosthetics. Radiology Herald, 1984;4:59–64.
22. Rabkin JK. Revascularisation par implantation d'une prothese radioendovasculare. Toulousi, Radiologie interventionelle en pathologie cardiovasquaire. (Abstr.) 1988.
23. Vitjugov IA, Kotenko VV, Ghünter VV, et al. Tissue response to implantation of the devices from nickel titanium for osteosynthesis. In Superelasticity, shape-memory effect and its application in new technologies. Tomsk: All-Union Scientific Conference, 1985:143.
24. Zajmovsky VA, Kolupajeva TL. Uncommon properties of ordinary metals. Moscow; Scoence: Nauka, 1984:192.
25. Kurdjumov VA, Khandros LG. Thermoresistant balance of the phases in martensite conversion. Reports of the USSR Academy of Science 1949;66:211–5.
26. Kotenko VV, Zakluchajeva VN, Günter VE, et al. Nickel content in the organs and muscles of dogs in experimental implantations of nickel-titanium alloy TN-10. In: Superelasticity, shape-memory effect and its application in new technologies. Tomsk: All-Union Scientific Conference, 1985:147.

48 The Maass Double-Helix Spiral Stent

C.L. Zollikofer, M.D., D. Maass, M.D., F. Antonucci, M.D.

In 1980 Maass and coworkers[1,2] at the University of Zürich took up Charles Dotter's idea[3] of transluminal insertion of a vascular endoprosthesis. They first started experimenting with spiral surgical steel alloy coils made from wire (0.3 to 0.5 mm diameter). Because of problems with insufficient mechanical control of the spirals made from wire or narrow metal bands (mainly tilting), which resulted in migration or thrombosis,[2] a double-helix spiral prosthesis made from metal bands with diameters from 12 to 35 mm was developed.[2,4] This prosthesis consists of heat-treated steel alloy metal bands (0.10 to 0.15 mm thick and 1.5 mm wide) (Figs. 48-1, 48-2). Under torsion these spirals had a smaller tilting momentum and therefore allowed high expansion ratios (relationship between relaxed and minimal diameter). A special implantation instrument allowed transluminal insertion under fluoroscopy via arteriotomy or venotomy (Figs. 48-1, 48-2). With this instrument of 7 mm diameter, stents of 12 to 35 mm diameter could be placed. For smaller vessels, stents of 12 to 15 mm diameter mounted on a 4 mm instrument were available. The pressure exerted by the expanding spirals on the vascular wall could be planned in advance or calculated in retrospect.[4] The insertion was carried out by means of the flexible instrument with the stent tightened, then expanded, and released to spirals.

Macroscopic, microscopic, and scanning electron microscopic (SEM) samples of aorta and vena cava of dogs and calves showed that intimal proliferation started within the first postoperative days. After 2 to 3 weeks, the metal was largely overgrown by a neointima. This process was completed after approximately 6 weeks and no further changes were visible (Fig. 48-3). A combination of intimal proliferation and microthrombi was found more frequently in the veins. These thrombi became organized and smooth. Further experiments showed that expansion pressures of 1000 mmHg in the aorta and 300 mmHg in the vena cava were tolerated without any damage to the vessel wall. Side branches of the aorta or the vena cava remained patent even when they were crossed by several spiral coils (Fig. 48-4).

CLINICAL APPLICATIONS

Since this prosthesis had been designed for larger vessels, such as the aorta or the vena cava, the new technique was first used intraoperatively via a surgical cutdown. As early as 1982, double-helix Maass spirals have been used clinically. In two patients with dissecting aneurysms of the aorta type B, such stents were implanted into the abdominal aorta intraoperatively to prevent further dissection (Fig. 48-5). With further improvements of instrumentation, this technique may offer the unique feature of treating dissecting aneurysms nonsurgically, as these two preliminary intraoperative experiences have shown.

More than 20 patients received the Maass spiral for compression of the vena cava at the time of surgical treatment for Budd-Chiari syndrome with the so-called Senning operation.[5,6] In spite of operative thrombosis obliteration and recanalization of the hepatic veins, the massively hypertrophied caudate lobe of the liver frequently compresses the vena cava also postoperatively, causing inferior vena caval obstruction. Using the Maass spiral, this problem can be solved[6,9] (Fig. 48-6).

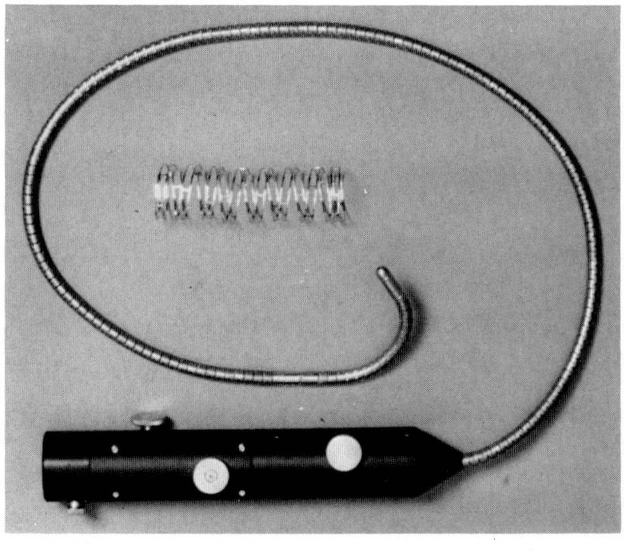

Figure 48–1. Introducing instrument with released double-helix spiral. The instrument is highly flexible with a bidirectional steering tip. Controls located at the handle release the spiral at its target site by retortion.

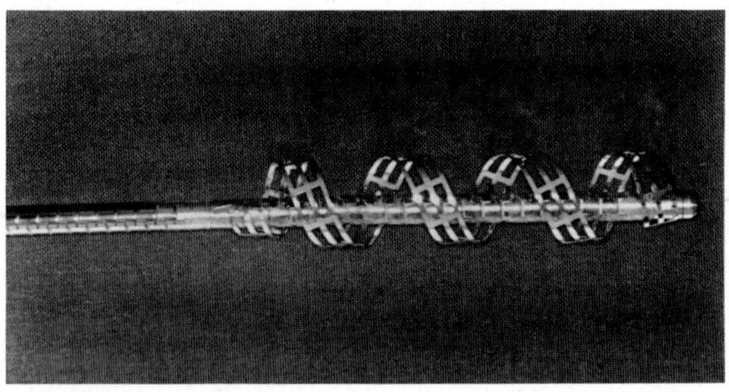

Figure 48–2. Tip of instrument with partially released endoprosthesis.

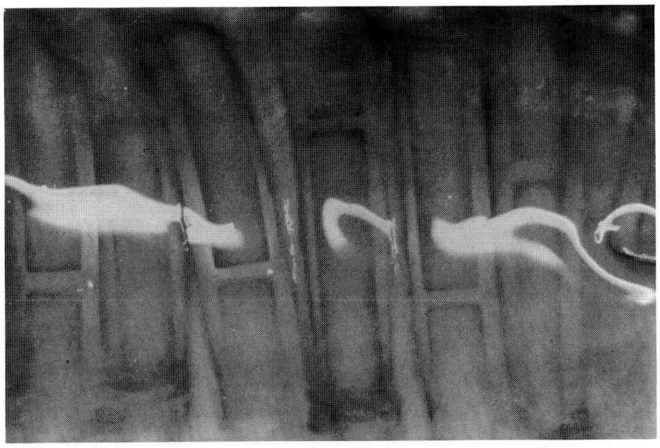

Figure 48–3. Specimen of dog aorta 6 weeks following stent implantation. The entire endoprosthesis is covered by a smooth, regular neointima.

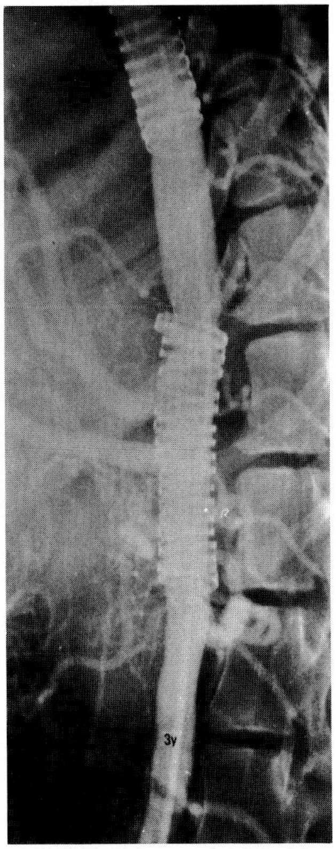

Figure 48–4. Two double-helix spirals in a canine aorta 3 years after implantation. There are no signs of obstruction of the celiac trunk and superior mesenteric artery despite the stent in the abdominal aorta.

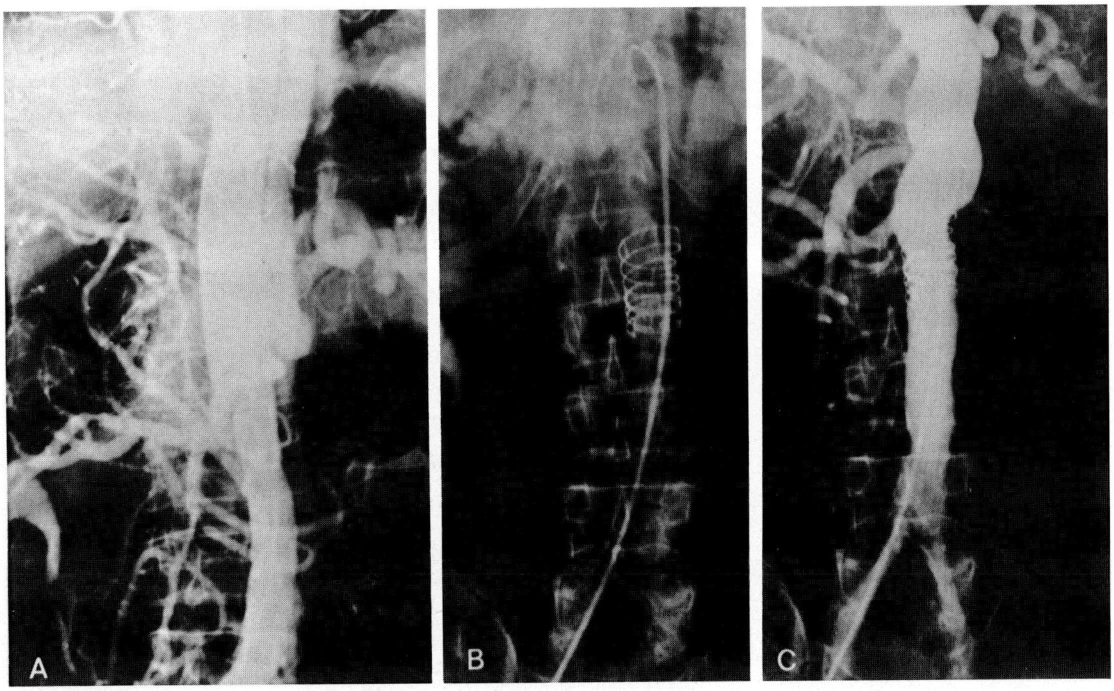

Figure 48–5. A 63-year-old patient with dissecting aneurysm type B. **A:** Dissection extends to the abdominal aorta with occlusion of the left renal artery. **B:** The patient was operated on with Dacron graft of the lower thoracic and upper abdominal aorta. To prevent further dissection, a double-helix endoprosthesis was implanted with additional external banding. **C:** Control angiogram 18 months later shows open lumen of the aorta with mild intimal hyperplasia.

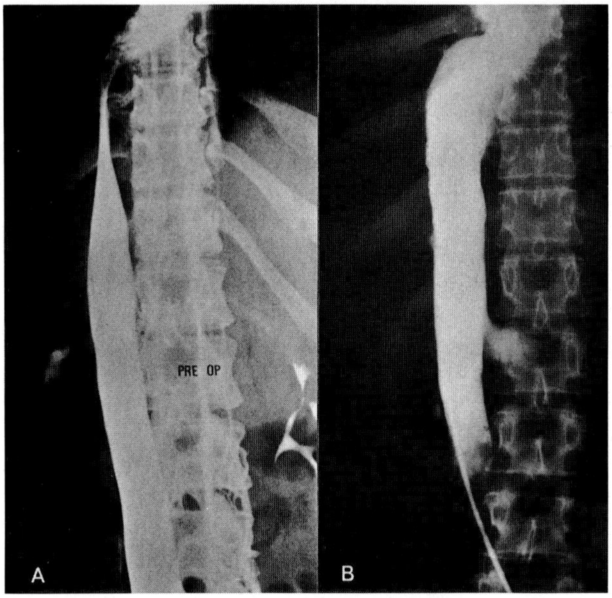

Figure 48–6. Patient with Budd-Chiari syndrome. **A:** Preoperative cavogram demonstrates compression of intrahepatic portion of vena cava. **B:** Cavogram of inferior vena cava 7 days after implantation of double-helix spiral shows widely patent lumen.

Several cases of Maass implants in patients with obstruction of the inferior vena cava and pelvic veins secondary to venous thrombosis have been performed successfully with follow-up of up to 34 months.[7,8] Mechanical obstacles that cause inferior vena cava or ileofemoral thrombosis present problems that cannot be solved by thrombectomy and balloon angioplasty or other conventional means. Percutaneous transluminal angioplasty (PTA) alone often fails because of the elastic recoil of the stenotic lesion. Even after surgery, success is only 50 to 80%[10–12] and thrombolytic treatment may not solve the problem either.[13–14] Treatment of an underlying lesion, such as a venous spur, scar traction, congenital stenosis, or external tumor compression is essential but may involve major surgery or may be contraindicated in malignant disease. Therefore endoluminal stents such as the Maass stent are a promising alternative to treat these patients, avoiding major surgery (Figs. 48-7, 48-8). However, further improvements are necessary, particularly miniaturization of the introducing instrument for easy and safe percutaneous use. Finally the Maass endoprosthesis has also shown its usefulness in tracheobronchial compression secondary to tumor or vascular compression[15] (Fig. 48-9).

In conclusion, the Maass double-helix spiral endoprosthesis has shown its usefulness particularly in stenting of large lumina, such as the aorta, vena cava, and tracheobronchial tree.

REFERENCES

1. Maass D, Kropf L, Egloff L, et al. Transluminal implantation of intravascular "double helix" spiral prostheses: technical and biological considerations. European Society for Artificial Organs Proceedings 1982;9:252–6.
2. Maass D, Demierre D, Deaton D, et al. Transluminal implantation of selfadjusting expandable prostheses: principles, techniques and results. Progr Artif Org 1983;2:979–87.
3. Dotter CT. Transluminally-placed coilspring endarterial tube grafts: long-term patency in canine popliteal artery. Invest Radiol 1969;4:327–32.
4. Maass D, Zollikofer CHL, Largiadèr F, Senning A. Radiological follow-up of transluminally inserted vascular endoprostheses: an experimental study using expanding spirals. Radiology 1984;152:659–63.
5. Senning A. The cardiovascular surgeon and the liver. J Thorac Cardiovasc Surg 1987;93:1–10.
6. Zollikofer CH. Interventionelle Behandlungsmöglichkeiten beim Budd-Chiari-Syndrom. In: Friedmann G, Steinbrich W,

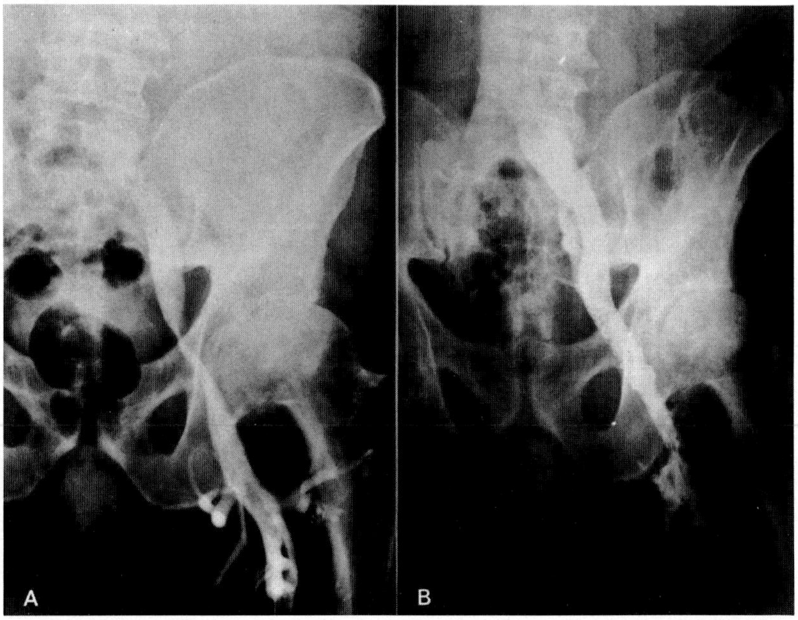

Figure 48–7. Patient with post-thrombotic stenosis of the external iliac vein. **A:** Venogram shows tight stenosis. **B:** Poststenting there is a widely patent lumen.

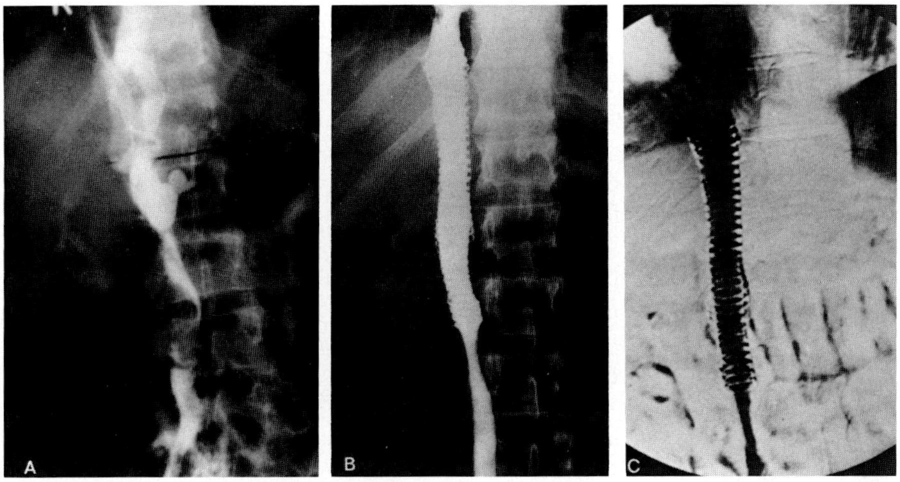

Figure 48–8. Patient with thrombosis of pelvic vein and the inferior vena cava. **A:** Phlebography shows clots in the infrarenal vena cava, stenosis of the suprarenal cava, and drainage via collaterals. **B:** There is free flow after surgical thrombectomy and two Maass spirals. **C:** Follow-up after 3 months shows continued patency.

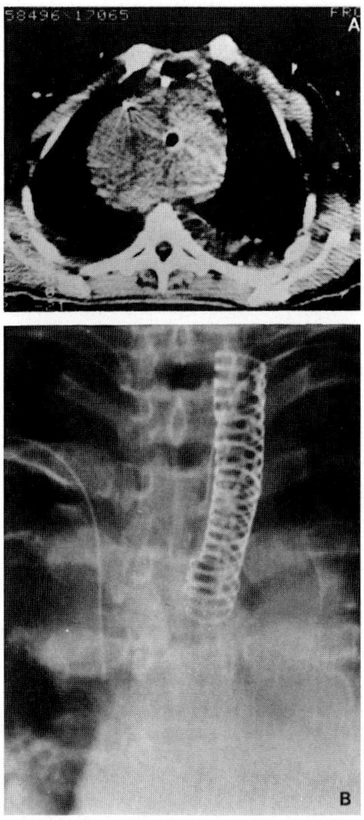

Figure 48–9. A 40-year-old patient with massive compression of the trachea secondary to carcinoma of the thyroid. **A:** Computed tomography scan shows mediastinal tumor mass causing circular compression of the trachea. **B:** Maass spiral is seen in trachea with normal tracheal lumen.

Gross-Fengels W (eds): Angioplastie, Embolisation, Punktion, Drainagen. Konstanz: Schnetztor Verlag, 1989:129–37.

7. Jakob H, Maass D, Schmiedt W, et al. Treatment of major venous obstruction with expandable endoluminal spiral prosthesis. J Cardiovasc Surg 1989;30:112–7.
8. Jakob H, Oelert H, Schmiedt W, et al. Initial clinical experience with an endoluminal spiral prosthesis. Texas Heart Inst Jo 1989;16:87–94.
9. Bansky G, Ernest C, Jenni R, et al. Treatment of Budd-Chiari-syndrome by dorsocranial liver resection and direct hepatoatrial anastomosis. J Hepatol 1986;2:101–12.
10. Hutschenreiter S, Vollmar J, Loeprecht H, et al. Rekonstruktive Eingriffe am Venensystem: Spätergebnisse unter kritischer Bewertung funktioneller und gefässmorphologischer Kriterien. Chirurg 1979;50:555–63.
11. Stiegler H, Sunder-Plassmann J, Becker HM. Indications and technics in pelvic and leg vein thromboses. Chirurg 1985;56:73–80.
12. Lindhagen J, Hagland M, Harland U, et al. Iliofemoral venous thrombectomy. J Cardiovasc Surg 1978;19:319–27.
13. Theiss W, Schlund J, Kriesmann A, et al. Die Behandlung tiefer Venenthrombosen mit Urokinase, Klin Wochenschr 1980;58:521–6.
14. Van de Loo JCW, Kriesmann A, Trübestein G, et al. Controlled multicenter pilot study of urokinase-heparin and streptokinase in deep vein thrombosis. Thromb Haemost 1983;50:660–7.
15. Buchmann P, Maass D, Geroulanos S. Die Doppelhelixspirale zur Überbrückung von hochgradigen Tracheastenosen. Schweiz Rundschau Med 1988;42:1142–3.

INDEX

(*Numbers in italics indicate references to tables and figures.*)